KU-733-397

WHAT WORKS FOR WHOM?

HS 616.891 ROTH

WHAT WORKS FOR WHOM?

SECOND EDITION

A CRITICAL REVIEW OF PSYCHOTHERAPY RESEARCH

Anthony Roth and Peter Fonagy

with contributions from
Glenys Parry, Mary Target, and Robert Woods

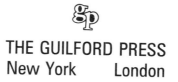

THE GUILFORD PRESS
New York   London

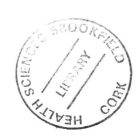

i16616674

© 2005 The Guilford Press
A Division of Guilford Publications, Inc.
72 Spring Street, New York, NY 10012
www.guilford.com

All rights reserved

No part of this book may be reproduced, translated, stored in a retrieval system, or
transmitted, in any form or by any means, electronic, mechanical, photocopying,
microfilming, recording, or otherwise, without written permission from the Publisher.

Printed in the United States of America

This book is printed on acid-free paper.

Last digit is print number: 9   8   7   6   5   4   3   2   1

Library of Congress Cataloging-in-Publication Data

Roth, Anthony.
   What works for whom?: a critical review of psychotherapy research / Anthony
Roth and Peter Fonagy; with contributions from Glenys Parry, Mary Target, and
Robert Woods.—2nd ed.
      p.   cm.
   Includes bibliographical references and index.
   ISBN 1-57230-650-5 (hardcover: alk. paper)
   1. Psychiatry—Differential therapeutics.   2. Psychotherapy—
Evaluation.   3. Psychotherapy—Research.   I. Fonagy, Peter, 1952–   II. Title.
   RC480.52.R669 2005
   616.89′14—dc22

                                                          2004015791

ABOUT THE AUTHORS

Anthony Roth, PhD, is Joint Course Director of the Doctoral Course in Clinical Psychology at University College London (UCL). He joined the UCL program in 1990 and has contributed to the development of clinical training both in London and at a national level. He has worked in hospital and community settings within the National Health Service for over 20 years. Reflecting a research interest in the development of a clearer evidence base for training, Dr. Roth was commissioned by the English Department of Health (along with Peter Fonagy) to identify evidence for the impact of the psychological therapies, a review that emerged as the first edition of *What Works for Whom?* He has written widely about the application of evidence in standard clinical settings, and has contributed to the development of national treatment guidelines, most recently *Guideline on Treatment Choice in Psychological Therapies and Counselling* and *Policy Guidance for the Development of Services for People with Personality Disorder.* His clinical interests focus on interventions for adult mental health problems. His research interests include links between psychotherapy process and outcome and the challenges of implementing evidence-based therapies into clinical settings. Dr. Roth's recent research has focused on the relationship between patient and therapist attachment patterns and the therapeutic alliance, the impact of therapist attachment patterns on therapist behavior, and the application of family interventions for people with schizophrenia within clinical settings.

Peter Fonagy, PhD, FBA, is Freud Memorial Professor of Psychoanalysis and Director of the Sub-Department of Clinical Health Psychology at University College London; Chief Executive of the Anna Freud Centre, London; and Consultant to the Child and Family Program at the Menninger Department of Psychiatry at Baylor College of Medicine, Houston, Texas. Dr. Fonagy is also a clinical psychologist and a training and supervising analyst in child and adult analysis in the British Psycho-Analytical Society, as well as cochair of the Research Committee of the International Psychoanalytic Association and a Fellow of the British Academy. His work attempts to integrate empirical research with psychoanalytic theory, and his clinical interests center on issues of borderline psychopathology, violence, and early attachment relationships. Dr. Fonagy's most recent books include *Attachment Theory and Psychoanalysis, What Works for Whom?: A Critical Review of Treatments for Children and Adolescents* (with Mary Target, David Cottrell, Jeannette Phillips, and Zarrina Kurtz), *Psychoanalytic Theories: Perspectives from Developmental Psychopathology* (with Mary Target), and *Psychotherapy for Borderline Personality Disorder: Mentalization-Based Treatment* (with Anthony Bateman).

CONTRIBUTING AUTHORS

Glenys Parry, PhD, FBPsS, is Professor of Applied Psychological Therapies at the University of Sheffield School of Health and Related Research and Visiting Professor at University College London and the University of Leeds. She is also a Consultant Clinical Psychologist in the Sheffield Care Trust, and a cognitive analytic psychotherapist, trainer, and supervisor. President of the Society for Psychotherapy Research, United Kingdom, and chair of the research committee of the British Association for Counselling and Psychotherapy, Dr. Parry is lead author of the Department of Health reports *NHS Psychotherapy Services in England: A Strategic Review* and *Guideline on Treatment Choice in Psychological Therapies and Counselling.* Her interests include the application of research to policy and practice, process and outcomes of psychotherapy in health service settings, and psychotherapeutic competence. Dr. Parry has conducted research in the fields of mental health, life event stress, social support, health inequalities, and psychotherapy. Her recent research includes studies of the prevalence of panic-fear in asthma, the efficacy of cognitive-behavioral therapy in asthma-related anxiety, the mental and physical health of Gypsies and Travellers in England, and psychological therapy for severe and complex mental health problems.

Mary Target, PhD, is a clinical psychologist with experience in adult mental health, child and family psychiatry, and pediatric liaison. She is also an Associate Member of the British Psycho-Analytical Society, a Reader in Psychoanalysis at University College London (UCL), and Professional Director of the Anna Freud Centre. A member of the Scientific Committee and Chair of the Research Committee of the British Psychoanalytic Society and founding Chair of the Working Party on Psychoanalytic Education of the European Psychoanalytic Federation, Dr. Target is also a member of the Research Committee of the International Psychoanalytic Association, Course Organiser of the UCL MSc in Psychoanalytic Theory, and Academic Course Organiser of the UCL/Anna Freud Centre Doctorate in Child and Adolescent Psychotherapy. She is Consultant to the Child and Family Program at the Menninger Department of Psychiatry at Baylor College of Medicine, Houston, Texas, and has active research collaborations in many countries in the areas of developmental psychopathology, attachment, and psychotherapy outcome. Dr. Target serves as joint series editor for psychoanalytic books for Whurr Publishers, and her most recent publications include *What Works for Whom?: A Critical Review of Treatments for Children and Adolescents* (with Peter Fonagy, David Cottrell, Jeannette Phillips, and Zarrina Kurtz), *Psychoanalytic Theories: Perspectives from Developmental Psychopathology* (with Peter Fonagy), and *Affect Regulation, Mentalization, and the Development of the Self* (with Peter Fonagy, György Gergely, and Elliot L. Jurist), which received the Gradiva Prize of the American Psychology and Psychotherapy Institute for Best Theoretical and Clinical Contribution of 2003.

Robert Woods, MA, MSc, is Professor of Clinical Psychology of Older People at the University of Wales, Bangor. He serves as Codirector of the Dementia Services Development Centre Wales and is a member of the Medical and Scientific Advisory Panels of the Alzheimer's Society, Alzheimer's Europe, and Alzheimer's Disease International. He has been a clinical psychologist working with older people for nearly 30 years, working initially in Newcastle-upon-Tyne and subsequently at the Institute of Psychiatry, London, and University College London. Professor Woods has been greatly involved in training clinical psychologists in work with older people as well as in service developments, and he continues to work clinically in a memory clinic in Bangor. His research interests in dementia care include family caregiving, psychosocial interventions, and quality of care. He has published numerous research papers on dementia care and depression in older people, as well as caregiver guides and training packages, and is coauthor of three Cochrane reviews. His books include the edited volumes *Cognitive Rehabilitation in Dementia* (with Linda Clare), *Psychological Problems of Ageing, Handbook of the Clinical Psychology of Ageing,* and *Positive Approaches to Dementia Care* (with Una Holden).

ACKNOWLEDGMENTS

The first edition of this book was based on a report commissioned by Glenys Parry on behalf of the National Health Service Executive of the English Department of Health, which formed a part of the Department's Strategic Policy Review of Psychotherapy Services. A draft was peer-reviewed by experts in the field: Mark Aveline, David Barlow, Ivy Blackburn, Paul Crits-Christoph, Ellen Frank, Chris Freeman, Ray Hodgson, Michael King, Marsha Linehan, John C. Markowitz, Isaac Marks, Jane Milton, Paul A. Pilkonis, Jan Scott, Eugene Paykel, and Digby Tantum, coordinated by David Shapiro. A number of colleagues also contributed observations and comments on earlier drafts of chapters: Chris Barker, John Clarkin, Keith Hawton, Rose Kent, Deborah Lee, Emanuelle Peters, and Anne Richardson.

The second edition of this work represents a substantial revision. Though it retains the tone of the original, much of its content is new. A number of individuals were kind enough to review drafts of chapters, and we would like to thank David Barlow, Paul Davis, Jan Scott, Dominic Lam, Katherine Pike, Anne Richardson, and Kerry Young for their help and advice. Particular thanks go to Amanda Williams for her close reading of, and commentary on, several chapters, and to Liz Allison for her calm and capable editorial assistance.

Finally, special thanks are due to Seymour Weingarten of The Guilford Press, who has patiently awaited the arrival of this second edition with only gentle reminders of the original schedule for submission, and with little indication of anxiety about its lengthy gestation.

CONTENTS

INTRODUCTION

The first edition of this book, published in 1996, was based on a report commissioned in 1994 by the U.K. Department of Health as part of its review of the planning and provision of psychological therapy services. At that time, there was a growing expectation that psychotherapy—along with any other form of publicly funded treatment—should be demonstrably effective and cost-effective. Since then, this expectation has become normative, and there are few countries where the demand for "evidence-based practice" does not apply.

This book attempts to identify and review evidence that can help answer the challenging question "What works for whom?"—in other words, which psychotherapeutic interventions are of demonstrated benefit to which patient groups? This question—originally posed by clinical researchers—is now seen as being of direct relevance to both service users and service providers, clinicians and researchers.

With the growth in the number of interested parties, there is a critical need to understand the nature of the evidence on which important decisions can rely. The questions posed by researchers (and the techniques used to answer them) rarely produce data that are directly applicable to funders or to individual consumers of health care (Parry, 1992). Just as we cautioned in 1996, readers need to understand that there is no direct relationship between research and clinical practice: The one needs translation into the other. While we believe that research evidence can be used to improve the structure and planning of psychotherapy services, we also recognize that, without careful interpretation, this evidence can be misconstrued, to the detriment of all parties (Roth & Parry, 1997).

There is, of course, no single entity called "psychotherapy," and in order to help the reader distinguish between therapies, we begin this book with a description of the theory and practice of the major schools of psychological therapy. Since Freud's pioneering work in the 19th century, psychotherapy has undergone a process of evolution, and it has long been more accurate to talk of a range of psychological interventions, each employing more or less distinctive techniques. Whereas some have retained the models of unconscious motivation of psychoanalysis, others have eschewed it; some focus on the remoter aspects of the patient's past, whereas others are interested only in present experience and functioning. To a great extent, the tensions created by the emergence of new models and ideas have been helpful and creative, forcing an examination of practice, and leading to the development of further methods of intervention. Equally they have the potential to overemphasize what is distinctive about therapies at the cost of neglecting their commonalities.

In Chapter 2, we outline the methodologies used by psychotherapy researchers and the way in which these limit the application of research findings to clinical practice. In the final introductory chapter, Chapter 3, we try to place research in the context of health care delivery systems and present a model relating research findings to clinical practice. In many ways, the model is a guide to interpretation of all that follows.

The body of the book contains research evidence relating to the treatment of each of a wide range of psychological problems. Our strategy has been to examine available reviews of treatments, together with individual studies, where these are relevant. On methodological grounds, we have had to be selective, making judgments about the form of study that we consider contributes best to our task. For this reason, the majority of trials in this book represents controlled studies of psychotherapy outcome; less frequently, open trials; and only rarely, case reports. After reviewing this evidence, we present a number of conclusions and consider their implications for research, practice, and service delivery.

Although we have for the most part retained the structure of the first edition, there are two substantive changes. First, the chapter on substance abuse now considers treatments for cocaine and opiate abuse, as well as alcohol. Second, we have removed the chapter on "counseling and primary care interventions," largely on the grounds that considering outcomes from treatments in relation to the context in which they are practiced fits uneasily with the structure of the book. However, most chapters include reports of studies conducted in primary care, and there has been little loss of coverage as a result of this decision.

As is usual for any systematic review, some indication of our search strategy will be helpful. Our aim was to be as comprehensive as possible, and to build on and extend the coverage of the first edition. The first and most obvious procedure was to search the MEDLINE, EMBASE and PsychINFO databases from 1995 through 2003, covering the period from our last review to the present. Within each topic area, we sought both reviews and individual studies, and used the former to identify further relevant trials, with citation indices providing a further check when we were uncertain that coverage was comprehensive. We also hand-searched the content pages of major journals over this period (including *Acta Psychiatrica Scandinavica, American Journal of Psychiatry, Archives of General Psychiatry, Behavioural and Cognitive Psychotherapy, Behaviour Research and Therapy, British Journal of Psychiatry, British Journal of Clinical Psychology, Clinical Psychology Review, Clinical Psychology: Science and Practice, European Eating Disorders Review, International Journal of Eating Disorders, Journal of Consulting and Clinical Psychology,* and *Psychotherapy Research*). It is probably helpful to add that—unlike many systematic reviews—this process was undertaken by the authors both before and during the process of review. This allowed a more evolutionary (and to our minds clinically relevant) approach to identifying studies than when junior researchers undertake this task on the basis of search criteria supplied by senior authors. Nonetheless, it is inevitable that we have omitted some relevant studies, and we acknowledge that our work is weakest in relation to reports in dissertations and in non-English-language journals. While we feel our search strategy has been systematic and hope it has achieved its aims, we welcome comments from readers who note important gaps in our coverage.

CHAPTER 1

DEFINING THE PSYCHOTHERAPIES

Psychosocial treatments are common in the mental health field—indeed, almost any intervention can be seen as assisting patients to cope with impairments in their psychological functioning. Psychotherapies are inevitably psychosocial treatments but usually share a set of distinguishing characteristics. Strupp's (1978, p. 3) well-known definition describes psychotherapy as "an interpersonal process designed to bring about modifications of feelings, cognitions, attitudes and behavior which have proved troublesome to the person seeking help from a trained professional." This definition draws attention to three characteristics of psychotherapy: the presence of a therapist–patient relationship; the interpersonal context of the psychotherapies; and, implied by the notion of training and professionalism, the sense that therapies are conducted according to a model that guides the therapist's actions. Psychotherapies are defined in part by their setting and in part by the presence of an explicit model of psychopathology, which in turn generates procedures for relieving distress.

Within this broad definition, it is worth noting that a large number of interventions can be described as psychotherapeutic; Kazdin (1986) identified over 400 different therapies, a number that has certainly grown since that time. The diversity of interventions is hard to encompass in any single review, though the task is made easier by the fact that many of these therapies represent subclasses of a smaller number of major orientations. In this book, we differentiate therapies primarily in terms of the following major classes:

- Psychodynamic psychotherapy
- Behavioral and cognitive-behavioral psychotherapy
- Interpersonal psychotherapy
- Strategic or systemic psychotherapies
- Supportive and experiential psychotherapies
- Group therapies
- Counseling

Each of these orientations provides a model of human behavior, as well as a heuristic focus for the level to which an intervention is ideally addressed. Whether this is the best way of clustering interventions could be debated. We recognize that in clinical practice, few practitioners make use of orientations in their pure form, and in recent years, there have been developments that render classification based on "grand theories" less pertinent. There are several reasons for this. One has been the pressure to implement empirically based treatments, which has led to a focus on treatment packages addressing particular problems and a shift of interest from general principles to particular therapeutic skills. A further trend has been the development of therapies whose rationales place them outside traditional psychological theory and render them difficult to classify (e.g., eye movement desensitization and reprocessing, studies of which are detailed in Chapter 8). While not wishing to anticipate our review, evidence of a close relationships between the theoretical justifications for a technique and empirical outcome is often difficult to find, and it is possible that, in the future, therapies will be more influenced by organizing principles based on novel perspectives (such as cognitive neuroscience). While this implies that change may be afoot, most outcome investigations concern themselves with treatment approaches clearly nested within the theoretical framework of one of these orientations, and this pragmatic consideration seems to justify our approach.

A further parameter distinguishing treatment approaches is the context or format within which treatment is offered. Psychotherapeutic treatment may be offered to individuals, to families, or to groups. It may be offered for relatively short periods or be open-ended. The format of treatment also differs in terms of the intensity (e.g., five times a week compared to once a week or once a month), the setting (inpatient or community-based), and the extent to which nonpsychosocial treatments (such as medication) are offered adjunctively.

Whereas it is clear that a comprehensive psychotherapy service would cover a range of orientations, it is less evident that significant benefit may accrue from a single individual's mastery of a range of approaches. Nonetheless, it seems reasonable to argue that a therapist's capacity to intervene flexibly with a range of problems requires at least rudimentary knowledge of a number of the orientations listed earlier.

PSYCHODYNAMIC THERAPY

The origin of the psychodynamic approach is a relatively brief, focused therapy (Breuer & Freud, 1893–1895/1955). Classical psychoanalysis developed into a long-term, intensive treatment aimed not at removing single symptoms or troublesome problem behaviors, but at attempting to restructure the entire personality. More pertinent to providing managed care services are the focal therapies designed by pioneers such as Alexander and French (1946), Sifneos (1972), Mann (1973), Malan (1976), Davanloo (1978), Luborsky (1984), and Strupp and Binder (1984). Such focal approaches no longer aim at pervasive transformations of the personality, but assume that cognitive understanding of personal problems may initiate symptomatic change, which continues after termination of the formal treatment. Long-term exploratory psychodynamic psychotherapy may span 1 year or more. Its focal implementation is more likely to comprise 4–6 months of once- or twice-weekly sessions. Whereas long-term exploratory therapy aims to consider a wide variety of transference distortions, focal therapy tends to be aimed at circumscribed character change. Both exploratory and focused treatment have the resolution of unconscious conflict as their goal; unlike cognitive and behavioral psychotherapies, these are not primarily or only concerned with achieving symptomatic change.

The technique of psychodynamic therapy is a focus on the provision of conscious understanding, primarily through the use of interpretation of the patient's verbalizations and behavior during the session. Modern psychoanalysis also highlights the experience of problematic internal states of feelings, desires, and beliefs in conflict, encoded into relationship patterns that are exposed to scrutiny within the therapeutic situation and in relation to the therapist. Conscious insight may not be as important a component of the treatment as previously thought; the emotional experience associated with the therapist tolerating thoughts and feeling previously considered intolerable by the patient may be equally or even more important. Other potentially therapeutic aspects of the treatment include promoting the assimilation of emotionally painful and previously warded-off experiences (catharsis), suggestions, and support. The more structured approach of the focal therapist calls for a more active therapist, who identifies for the patient recurring patterns of behavior consistent with the presence of a hypothesized unconscious conflict.

BEHAVIORAL AND COGNITIVE-BEHAVIORAL THERAPIES

The roots of behavioral and cognitive-behavioral interventions are in classical learning theory (conditioning and operant learning) and in social learning theory. Wolpe's systematic desensitization method was probably the first rig-

orous attempt to adapt Pavlovian conditioning to a clinical situation. At the
same time, Skinner and colleagues used operant conditioning techniques to
modify the behavior of psychotic inpatients. Largely for epistemological reasons, behavioral approaches ignore the importance of cognitive processes.
Under the influence of Bandura, Ellis, Meichenbaum, and Beck, the balance
has been redressed, and cognitions (both conscious and unconscious) have
come to occupy an increasingly prominent role in models of psychopathology (as indeed is the case in the academic discipline of psychology as a whole).
Cognitive therapies share with dynamic therapies the assumption of irrational
cognitive processes. However, within cognitive therapy, cognitions are seen
as having been learned and maintained through reinforcement; challenges to
these assumptions may therefore be made directly rather than via unconscious
determinants, as implied by dynamic theory. In addition, the proposed links
between symptomatology and specific cognitions are somewhat less complex
in cognitive than in dynamic approaches. Nevertheless, there is considerable
overlap between modern cognitive therapy and traditional psychoanalytic
ideas, and indeed, many cognitive propositions derive from analytic formulations. Examples of overlap between these two traditions include the notion of
helplessness; the discrepancy between the perceived self and the ideal self; the
self-destructiveness of negative cognitions implied in the negative view of the
self, the world, and the future; and the tendency defensively to avoid the
scrutiny of painful cognitions.

   At least traditionally within this orientation, the clinician is less concerned than his/her dynamic counterpart with how maladaptive ideas and
behaviors have emerged. Behavioral and cognitive-behavioral clinicians focus
on how these maladaptive aspects of functioning are maintained by the individual's environment and through properties inherent to his/her belief systems. In the early days of cognitive therapy, considerable emphasis was placed
on the primacy of cognitions over emotional responses—in other words, the
proposition that emotional reactions could be predicted on the basis of belief
and expectations. More recently, there has been a general recognition by
both dynamic and cognitive theorists that the separation of these two modes
of functioning is an oversimplification of little heuristic value, and one that
has no credibility either within philosophical tradition or in modern cognitive science.

   Because of the intellectual roots of this orientation in positivist episte-
mology, the focus of behavioral interventions is on definable behaviors
that can be readily monitored and addressed in therapeutic interventions.
Cognitive-behavioral treatments represent an integration of this level of analysis, with consideration of thoughts and beliefs that may lead to dysfunctional
behavior. The goal of such interventions is to change maladaptive beliefs,
using a wide range of techniques at the clinician's disposal. These commonly
include elements of self-monitoring, identifying, and challenging negative

thoughts and assumptions that maintain problematic behavior and experiences; decatastrophization; and scheduling activities that in turn aid further self-monitoring and challenge to dysfunctional beliefs. Although interpretation may at times be a part of the cognitive therapist's armamentarium, finding reasons for particular beliefs is not regarded as an essential or necessarily very effective component of the intervention. The goals of intervention tend to be clear, and the patient's motivation is strongly reinforced by suggestion and support from the therapist.

The distinction between cognitive and behavioral interventions is a controversial one. Clinicians from a primarily behavioral tradition consider that interventions such as cognitive restructuring may be effective only through their impact on patients' behavior, which in turn modifies their subjective states. By contrast, "pure cognitivists" consider directly induced behavioral changes (e.g., through selective reinforcement, or *in vivo* exposure) to have a long-term impact only in that they force a change in the patient's expectations. In this review, we do not concern ourselves with this distinction, which is of limited relevance to technique, although it may have implications for training.

Dialectical behavior therapy (DBT) is an adaptation of cognitive therapy, originally developed for parasuicidal patients. It uses a mix of individual and group psychotherapy to address problems of impulse control and affect regulation, using specific techniques such as social skills training, psychoeducation, contingency management, and problem solving. The therapy has a declared stance to "validate" patients' perceptions of their actions and beliefs, while negotiating more appropriate (or more "mindful") strategies for management of their mental states. The cognitive roots of DBT are apparent in its focus on the patient's cognitive style (e.g., in assisting the patient to alter all-or-none thinking). However, it also makes use of the patient–therapist relationship, especially at points of crisis, helping the patient replace maladaptive actions (such as self-destructive acts) with more adaptive responses. In this respect, it mirrors the psychodynamic emphasis on resistance and transference.

INTERPERSONAL PSYCHOTHERAPY

Interpersonal psychotherapy (IPT) is based on the ideas of the interpersonal school (Sullivan, 1953), and was initially formulated as a time-limited weekly therapy for depressed patients. It makes no assumptions about etiology but uses the connection between the onset of depressive symptoms and current interpersonal problems as a focus for treatment. It therefore focuses on current relationships rather than enduring aspects of the personality, and therapists take an active and supportive stance.

IPT is normally a brief treatment, usually administered in the acute phase of depression. Therapy starts with a diagnostic phase, in which the patient's disorder is identified and explained. The therapist highlights the ways in which the patient's current functioning, social relationships, and expectations within these relationships may have been causal in the depression. There is an educational aspect to this process, whereby the therapist links depressive symptoms to one of four interpersonal areas: grief, interpersonal role disputes, role transitions, or interpersonal deficits. In the second phase of treatment, the therapist pursues strategies specific to one of these problem areas—for example, he/she may facilitate mourning and help the patient to find new relationships and activities to compensate for the loss. Role disputes may be tackled by helping the patient explore problem relationships and consider options available to resolve them. In the final phase of the treatment, the patient is helped to focus on therapeutic gains and to develop ways of identifying and countering depressive symptoms, should they arise in the future. Though originally intended for application only to depression, IPT has more recently been adapted for use with a wider range of populations (e.g., Agras et al., 2000b; Weissman & Markowitz, 1994).

SYSTEMIC ORIENTATIONS

Whereas the roots of both dynamic and cognitive approaches date back to the turn of the last century, the systemic approach is a relatively new model of psychological disturbance. The intellectual roots of the approach lie in anthropology, as well as cybernetics. Early workers in this field (e.g., Bateson, Haley, and Erickson) identified some general properties of human systems that ran across a number of domains. A basic assumption of the model is that neither symptoms nor insight can be an appropriate focus for treatment interventions. Rather, the system that generates the problem behavior is the appropriate target for intervention. The approach is most usefully applied to the system of the family, where each family member is seen as a unit within the system and the client's problem behavior is generated by its malfunctioning. The therapist's task is to identify the strategic role that the client's problem has in maintaining the family system and to address this aspect of its functioning. Although symptomatic change is not seen as an appropriate goal, a change in symptomatic behavior may help toward identifying dysfunctional aspects of the system. Thus, systemic therapists also use a number of techniques for directly tackling symptomatic behavior as a preliminary to bringing about systemic modification. Although the setting of systemic therapy often includes the entire family, this is neither a necessary nor a sufficient condition for systemic change.

Systemic therapists use advice, suggestion, paradoxical injunctions, symptom prescription, marking of boundaries, and an emphasis on the positive value of symptoms for the whole family as ways of bringing about change to the family system.

SUPPORTIVE AND EXPERIENTIAL THERAPIES

The philosophical tradition behind supportive and experiential therapies has roots in the humanistic, existential, and phenomenological ideas proposed by Nietzsche, Sartre, and Husserl. In different ways, all these authors reject the mechanistic philosophies underpinning psychodynamic, behavioral, and systemic therapies. The roots of disturbance are seen to lie in the dehumanizing and disintegrative effect of social conditions. In their view, any therapy that imposes directive and mechanistic methods compounds rather than solves this problem. Supportive and experiential therapists eschew intellectual solutions and prescribe interventions aimed at reinforcing and validating spontaneous and immediate experience, which is seen as facilitating the integrity of the self and a sense of personal authenticity. Emotional problems arise when circumstances prevent an individual from actualizing his/her potential and force the individual to inhibit essential aspects of his/her personality. Supportive and experiential approaches do encourage self-awareness, but not awareness of unconscious forces (rather, awareness of experience itself, including emotional reactions and the experience of interactions with others). The therapist's role is one of a facilitating observer, who aids clients in extending their awareness of their subjective world. Again, insight and symptomatic improvement are not seen as appropriate goals for therapy. Instead, clients are offered support in their natural striving toward self-determination, personal meaning, and self-awareness.

Because of its nonmechanistic philosophy, technique plays a less important part in experiential treatments than it does in many therapies. Experiential therapists place emphasis on intuitiveness, openness, receptiveness, empathy, and unconditional regard for the patient as key elements that facilitate change. However, the very insistence that psychotherapy is not a "treatment" but rather a growth experience represents a technical stance, as is the focus on therapist attitudes rather than on specific maneuvers. Specific exemplars of this orientation, such as psychodrama, Gestalt therapy, or the client-centered approach, do make use of specific techniques such as role play and strategies for encouraging various forms of abreaction.

GROUP THERAPIES

Group psychotherapy has been used to address the needs of children, adolescents, adults, and the elderly. It was developed particularly during World War

II, when understaffed military hospitals were forced to use group treatment to attend to the overwhelming number of psychiatric casualties.

The growth of group therapy to some degree transcends theoretical orientations. While it has common roots with psychoanalysis, even in its early days, it was associated with clinicians who became disillusioned with Freud's ideas. Yalom's (1975) influential contribution came from a Sullivanian perspective and focused on correcting here-and-now interpersonal problems. Group sessions were seen as enabling the expression and understanding of problems such as mistrust, anger, and dependency.

The mechanisms of change were seen as hope, corrective emotional experience, modeling, and the promotion of self-awareness. Alongside this interpersonal tradition, the psychoanalytic influence continued, with an emphasis on eliciting the interpersonal derivatives of unconscious conflicts through the manifestations of transferences both to the group leader and to other group members (Slavson, 1964). Foulkes (1975) originated group analysis based on the concept of the "group matrix," a hypothetical web of communication in which the group serves to represent the feelings of individuals. Other therapists developed innovative, action-based group methods. For example, Moreno's (1953) emphasis on spontaneity and action led him to develop the technique of psychodrama. This and other methods were adopted by Gestalt and experiential therapies, and the encounter group movement, including role playing, doubling, role reversal, and vicarious therapy.

Group therapies encompass clinical outpatient groups and their derivatives, such as psychoeducational, human development, and self-help groups. The community mental health movement in the United States in the early 1960s led to a further rapid growth in the application of group techniques and the development of short-term group therapies with a limited focus on the enhancement of ego functioning and social competence. In addition, modified group approaches that were developed do not require specialist training in psychotherapeutic techniques and are frequently found in mental health settings, such as drama, art, and dance therapies.

The many theoretical positions listed here represent a small sample of those that exist in contemporary group psychotherapy. Furthermore, many group therapists practice in a pluralist fashion, using theories drawn from a wide range of orientations (Scheidlinger, 1994). Consequently, it is not surprising that group therapy research is hard to examine as an entity in and of itself.

Many treatments originally described for use with individuals are also administered in group formats. This review includes a number of group-based interventions, though within the context of the patient groups for which treatments were delivered and the theoretical orientation guiding the therapy.

COUNSELING

Unlike the models described earlier, counseling is a term used to denote a varied set of techniques used to address a wide range of problems. While some of these are pertinent to this book, a number (such as genetic or HIV counseling) lie outside it, even though they incorporate psychotherapeutic techniques.

Counseling is not a unitary theoretical framework, but tends to be defined by the setting in which it takes place. Regardless of the theoretical model employed by the counselor (and in contrast to some psychotherapies), the relationship between the client and the counselor is often intended to be one of equals. The focus is usually on current problems facing the individual, and the approach taken is frequently pragmatic. Classically, it is very strongly influenced by client-centered ideas of empathy, warmth, and genuineness. Though these remain important, more recently, counseling has developed as an integrative approach that combines a range of therapeutic orientations. It has also specialized to focus on particular clinical settings (such as primary care) or problems (such as bereavement).

DIFFERENTIATION AND INTEGRATION OF TREATMENT APPROACHES

The previous discussion represents prototypes of therapeutic orientations that rarely exist in pure form. Psychodynamic intervention is probably impossible to carry out without a substantial supportive, experiential component. Similarly, cognitive and strategic interventions overlap. Some approaches (e.g., Kohutian psychoanalytic psychotherapy; Kohut, 1977) deliberately combine supportive and dynamic components. Other therapies (e.g., Ryle, 1990) aim deliberately to integrate orientations. In a clinical setting, the orientation adopted by a clinician will depend to a large measure as much on the characteristics of the client as on the therapist's own training and orientation. A psychologically minded individual may well demand expanded self-understanding, whereas a less psychologically minded person may insist on practical help and advice. The degree to which problems are "encapsulated" may also influence the specificity of treatment approach. For example, whereas a monosymptomatic phobia might be managed solely by behavioral techniques, dysthymic disorder may require a wider repertoire of approaches to tackle the interpersonal problems associated with this presentation. Although there have been attempts at providing a theoretically coherent integration of techniques derived from these orientations, there are as yet few satisfactory theories to provide the clinician with a rationale for integrating these approaches. In the United Kingdom, Ryle's (1990, 1995) cognitive analytic therapy (CAT) has gained increasing acceptance. This integrates psychodynamic therapy with a more structured approach reflecting personal construct therapy and cognitive-behavioral therapy (CBT). At its core is the "procedural sequence object relations" model (PSOR), which describes the procedures an individual evolves to cope with his/her difficulties. These are conceptualized as habitual patterns of "reciprocal role relations"—the differing but often reciprocating positions the individual can occupy in relation to the dilemmas he/she confronts. As an example, the expectation of abandonment may generate an oscillation between involvement (which risks loss) and avoidance of intimacy; critically, the individual is potentially able to occupy both positions, being both the person who rejects and is him/herself rejected. By describing the way in which the person is positioned within a pattern of reciprocal roles, CAT attempts to clarify how the person becomes locked into his/her problem, and also the way in which it could be resolved. Crucially—and in contrast to many therapies—this formulation is shared explicitly with the client and used to shape the therapy (which is not restricted to any one technical procedure). In the United States, cognitive therapists working with individuals with personality disorders are in the process of expanding cognitive therapy using schema theory. A particularly significant contribution has been made with borderline patients by Young and Lindeman (1992), whose approach extends the traditional cognitive framework in terms of both theory and technique. Theoretically, the additional focus is on the origins of maladaptive and preverbal cognitive structures; in terms of technique, these workers recommend long-term structured interventions, which sometimes come close to psychodynamic therapies. However, in clinical practice, considerations for integration tend to be pragmatic.

Of course, therapists and the theories that guide them do not exist in isolation from each other. To some degree, the techniques applied determine the kind of data to which therapists of particular orientation are exposed and, indeed, to which they are responsive. Nonetheless, there is considerable cross-fertilization between treatment approaches in terms of both theory and technique. Currently, for example, there is a degree of convergence among clinicians rooted in psychoanalytic practice and those whose interests lie primarily in cognitive-behavioral techniques. Whereas the latter are increasingly interested in nonconscious processes and the impact of the therapeutic relationship, the former have shown more concern about the nature of knowledge representation and the significance of cognitive factors that may account for slow progress within psychotherapy. Ultimately, theoretical orientations will have to be integrated, since they are all approximate models of the same phenomenon: the human mind in distress. For the moment, however, integration may well be counterproductive, because theoretical coherence is the primary criterion for distinguishing false and true assertions in many psychotherapeutic domains. To the extent that it removes the applicability of this criterion, integration would create confusion rather than clarify controversies. There may be notable exceptions to this objection among emerging integrative psychotherapy approaches—for example, Ryle's (1990) CAT. In any case, this objection does not apply to the desirability of integration at the level of technique. In everyday clinical practice, there is much that is "borrowed" from different orientations by all practitioners. From the point of view of evaluation, what remains crucial is that all such borrowed techniques should make sense in the context of the theory into which they are borrowed.

CHAPTER 2

RESEARCH AND PRACTICE

Methodological Considerations
and Their Influence on This Review

Research into psychotherapy necessarily and inevitably changes the nature of the therapy it investigates: Quantification requires a compromise between the usual procedures of the clinic and the demands of scientific inference. Clear thinking about the applicability of research findings rests on an understanding of these compromises.

CLINICAL EFFICACY AND CLINICAL EFFECTIVENESS

At the outset, a clear distinction needs to be drawn between the *efficacy* of a therapy (the results it achieves in the setting of a research trial) and its *clinical effectiveness* (the outcome of the therapy in routine practice). In order to demonstrate reliability and validity, clinical trials are required to conform to a number of criteria (Cook & Campbell, 1979). In particular, they usually aim to achieve a high degree of *internal validity*. This can be defined as the extent to which a causal relationship can be inferred among variables, or where the absence of a relationship implies the absence of a cause. If internal validity is low, *statistical conclusional validity* is compromised, and the results of a study would be hard to interpret. However, achieving internal validity requires the use of techniques rarely seen in everyday practice, examples of which would be studying highly selected, diagnostically homogenous patient populations; randomizing the entry of these patients into treatments; and employing extensive monitoring of both patients' progress and the types of therapy used by therapists. All of this poses a threat to *external validity*—the extent to which we can infer that the causal relationship can be generalized. In the present case, this translates into the problem of inferring clinical effectiveness from any demonstrations of efficacy.

The apparently contrary demands of internal and external validity pose a considerable problem to clinical researchers, because they create an inevitable dialectic: At the one pole is ambiguity; at the other, lack of relevance. This tension is not resolved simply by relocating research into clinical contexts, since the advantages of such a move are counterbalanced by threats to internal validity. For example, participants would be more representative of clinical populations but would also be more heterogenous, and this would make it difficult to draw conclusions about the impact of treatment on specific groups. Treatments offered in a clinical setting are more likely to reflect the common clinical practice of combining approaches; while this could yield information about their likely impact, the dose and appropriateness of adjunctive treatments would be uncontrolled, treatments might be suboptimal and outcomes misleading, and interventions would probably be responsive to patient variables. In this sense, increasing the representativeness of research diminishes its explanatory power.

The tension between naturalistic assessment of outcome and experimental measures of efficacy is a real one, and it should be recognized that the bridge between research trials and routine treatment is difficult to span. It is reasonably clear that, in general, "research therapy" appears to be more effective than everyday clinical practice (Shadish et al., 2000; Weisz et al., 1995a). There are many reasons why this could be. Some of the more obvious reasons relate to methodological issues—among them the use of focused and structured treatments, regular access to supervision, participants recruited by advertisement rather than through clinical services, and greater exclusion rates. However, the vicissitudes of biology and individual psychological differences in treatment response may also be relevant. Psychotherapy is a highly complex interchange in which a large number of factors interact, any one of which could significantly influence outcome. Patients differ along many dimensions, including their socioeconomic circumstances, the stage of their disorder at the time of presentation, and in their premorbid psychological functioning. Similarly, therapists vary in their personality, their skills, their motivation, their ability to comprehend their patients' problems, and their adherence to treatment modalities. Service provision also varies in important ways, including the length of treatment offered, the quality of liaison with other services, the support and supervision offered to practitioners, and the physical resources available.

All these factors are known to interact in a highly complex manner and are subjected to systematic scrutiny in research on psychotherapy process. In principle, much of this work is beyond the scope of this review. Orlinsky et al. (1994) provide a comprehensive overview of progress in this field. However, they note that the distinction between process and outcome research can become blurred. Indices of therapeutic process can often be informative of outcomes in the course of therapy, which in turn contribute to measures of end-state functioning employed in outcome research. The conclusions that can be drawn from trials of therapeutic efficacy will be influenced and modified by these considerations. Thus, where possible, we have attempted to identify some critical process factors in our review of treatment outcome.

METHODOLOGIES AND STRATEGIES
IN PSYCHOTHERAPY RESEARCH
The Hierarchy of Evidence

A hierarchy of evidence has been developed (Sheldon et al., 1993) that usefully distinguishes studies according to their susceptibility to bias. Quite deliberately, this privileges internal over external validity, and research priorities over clinical considerations. This hierarchy should not be misunderstood as indicating the clinical utility of different research designs; depending on the research question being asked, methodologies lower in the hierarchy may be completely appropriate. There is no "ideal" research design, since researchers need to match their aims to their methods, and the design of trials often represents a compromise reflecting the intents, interests, and resources of investigators.

The first category in the hierarchy is randomized controlled trials and their aggregation in systematic reviews and meta-analyses. Next come controlled trials without randomization, or quasi-experiments and experimental single-case designs. At the third level are cohort studies (in which groups of patients are allocated to treatments) preferably from more than one center. Fourth are case–control studies (in which patients with similar outcomes are grouped and an attempt is made retrospectively to account for differences in outcomes), again, preferably from several centers. At the lower levels of the hierarchy come large differences reported in comparisons between times and/or places, with or without interventions, professional opinion based on clinical experience, descriptive studies, uncontrolled studies, and reports of expert committees.

Principal design strategies are considered in turn, together with their strengths and weaknesses. A full account of methodological issues in psychotherapy research is given in Kazdin (1994b).

Randomized Controlled Trials

Randomized controlled trials (RCTs) explicitly ask questions about the comparative benefits of two or more treatments. Patients are randomly allocated to different treatment conditions, usually with some attempt to control for (or at least examine) factors such as demographic variables, symptom severity, and level of functioning. Attempts are made to implement therapies under conditions that reduce the influence of variables likely to influence outcome—for example, by standardizing factors such as therapist experience and ability, and the length of treatments. The design permits active treatments to be compared, or their effect to be contrasted with no treatment, a waiting list, a "placebo" intervention, or a treatment of known efficacy. Increasingly, studies also ensure that treatments are carried out in conformity with their theoretical description—for example, ensuring that cognitive-behavioral treatments do not include psychodynamic elements, and vice versa. To this end, many treatments have been "manualized" (a process that specifies the techniques of the therapy programmatically), with adherence to this manual carefully monitored.

This design has the potential to distinguish the impact of treatments and to provide a control for changes in patient status that reflect the natural history of the disorder rather than the impact of treatment. However, in practice, there are inherent limitations of this approach.

Problems of Randomization

In a perfectly conducted trial, random assignment of participants to treatments allows investigators to assume that any differences that emerge in outcome are attributable to the intervention they received. Unfortunately, this assumption is true only when trials are large. Since many psychotherapy trials have less than 20–30 participants in each treatment condition, it is probable that groups will differ in critical ways, despite the fact that investigators can attempt to balance entrants to each arm on a small number of critical variables. Smaller trials are also especially vulnerable to the consequences of patient attrition, which threatens randomization simply because loss of participants is unlikely to be a random process.

Problems of Control Groups

The notion that a contrast intervention acts as a "control" for an experimental therapy is probably misleading, since all forms of control have their strengths and weaknesses, and trial designs often reflect pragmatic as much as theoretical considerations. At least in some respects, the ideal design of a trial would be to contrast treatment to no treatment, but it is rarely the case that this is either ethically or practically possible. Though comparison with a wait list is a reasonable (and indeed a common) contrast, it is not unproblematic. For example, it could be argued that motivation for change in this group in at least some individuals will be deferred until they receive treatment and, strictly speaking, any form of control in which treatment is absent or deferred acts only to contrast doing something with doing nothing, yielding little information about specific aspects of the intervention that might be helpful (Kazdin, 1997). The alternative of offering a placebo treatment—one that is considered inactive, at least from the point of view of the active treatments offered—is beset by the difficulty of finding an activity that could be guaranteed to have no therapeutic element, that controls for the effect of attention, and that is also viewed by patients as being as credible as the active interventions. Problems of interpretation will arise if the control condition is not specified clearly. For example, though "treatment as usual" (TAU) can be a sensible control in many settings, it is (by definition) a heterogeneous intervention. This makes it harder to attribute differences in outcome, since a number of confounds are possible, such as differences in the frequency of treatment sessions, the size of clinicians' caseloads, their commitment to the treatments they are offering, and their level of expertise (Borkovec & Castonguay, 1998). There is also the practical and ethical issue of restricting control patients to the control treatment; for example, if allocated to a minimal treatment arm, it is likely that at least some patients would seek their own treatment. Many recent studies restrict themselves to the comparison of active treatments; as evidence has accumulated for the general efficacy of therapy, ethical committees have become unwilling to sanction trials that could be seen to deprive patients of help (e.g., Elkin, 1994).

Clearly the effect size of a treatment depends as much on outcomes in the control group as it does on impacts in the group whose treatment was under scrutiny. Contrast to an ineffective or weak control will enhance apparent efficacy—for example, a manualized therapy delivered as part of a well-organized treatment program may perform better than a wait list, but since this could reflect the influence of many processes over and above the therapy itself, such an outcome would need to be interpreted with caution.

For many researchers, the application of a rigorous control (e.g., contrast to a treatment with best-established efficacy) represents a powerful test of a treatment's efficacy. While there is much to be said for this approach, this would substantially reduce the likelihood of observing a between-group difference. Although there are statistical techniques for showing the null hypothesis to be true (i.e., that there is genuinely no true difference between groups), in these cases, the power requirements that imply the need for a large sample are too big for most trials to muster. The import of this point is that nonsignificant results are not the same as showing no difference between treatments.

Manualization and Monitoring of Treatment

If results are to be replicated, it is critical to define the treatment offered in a trial. Treatment manuals are used to describe and to specify the procedures carried out by therapists, and sessions are monitored to ensure that therapies are delivered as intended (checking for "treatment integrity" or adherence). Although highly desirable from a research perspective, the use of manuals is not uncontroversial. For example, there are claims that some treatments are more readily manualized than others, and objections that manuals distort the usual conditions of therapy by restricting the therapeutic strategies open to clinicians. In order to ensure treatment fidelity, many trials are careful to see that regular supervision is available to therapists, a feature of manualization and monitoring that often passes unremarked. Given that the impact of supervision is rarely monitored, it is difficult to know whether its presence or absence will impact on outcomes in routine settings. Despite these concerns regarding generalizability, the use of manuals in therapy trials now seems to be accepted.

One strength of manualization is that it helps reviewers to identify when a treatment has been delivered in a manner congruent with that advocated by its proponents. This establishes the issue of adherence, independent of outcome, making it harder for null or negative findings to be attributed to poorly conducted therapy, and minimizing the opportunity for postpublication controversy based on claims that results relate to issues of implementation.

Length of Therapy

Setting up an RCT is a major undertaking and consequently a great expense. Although there are exceptions, most trials limit the amount of intervention offered (frequently to around 16 weeks). While this may be appropriate for some therapies (principally behavioral or cognitive-behavioral approaches), psychodynamic therapists (e.g., Fonagy & Higgitt, 1989) could and do argue that the techniques they employ were never designed for delivery over such a short time frame.

Diagnostic Homogeneity

In order to protect internal validity, many trials screen out patients with significant comorbid diagnoses, despite the fact that these presentations are usual in clinical settings. Although some regard this as a definite barrier to generalization, this is an assumption rather than being empirically based. For example, in a preliminary report, DeRubeis and Stirman (2001) determined that of 126 outpatient cases, only two could not be assigned to treatment on the basis of current outcome literature, even though in 31 cases there was significant comorbidity.

Patient Preference and Random Allocation to Treatment

Patients are not passive recipients of treatment, and their preferences for different forms of treatment may be critical to their participation in clinical trials (Brewin & Bradley, 1989). The bias introduced by consequent attrition from treatment is invisible within studies but may be particularly relevant to clinical practice.

Although random allocation is often seen as the "gold standard" in medical research, its application to psychological therapy is often seen as controversial. Clearly, RCTs are a powerful tool, helping researchers to draw relatively clear clinical implications from trials. Equally, however, their methodological power should not blind reviewers to their limitations, especially when examining the effectiveness of treatments for conditions that have high levels of comorbidity with Axis I or Axis II conditions, or that tend to be complicated by their presentation in the context of major adverse life events (all factors that tend to be underrepresented in research trials). There is also the risk that RCTs are inappropriately privileged over other research strategies, without the recognition that each design is best applied to answer different research questions, and that in this sense, all have both strengths and weaknesses.

Finally, it is common for data from RCTs to be aggregated into meta-analyses in order to make better sense of general patterns of outcome. However, it is important to remember that within these, the control and logic of their experimental designs (focused on increasing the capacity to make causal inferences) are often substituted for a quasi-experimental correlational approach (Cook & Campbell, 1979), constraining the conclusions that can legitimately be drawn (e.g., when post hoc analyses are performed in order to pinpoint groups for whom a treatment might be particularly effective).

Meta-Analysis

Meta-analysis is a procedure that enables data from separate studies to be considered collectively through the calculation of an effect size from each investigation. Effect sizes refer to group differences in standard deviation units on the normal distribution. Following Cohen (1988), an effect size of 0.2 is considered small, one of 0.5 is medium, and 0.8 is large. Their intuitive meaning is made clearer by translating them into percentiles, indicating the degree to which the average treated client is better off than control patients. A table giving this information and an explanatory guide to interpretation is included in Appendix I at the end of the book.

Effect sizes can be calculated in different ways. Most commonly, they are calculated from the difference between the treatment and control group means divided by the standard deviation of the control group (see Appendix I). Within-treatment, rather than between-treatment, effect sizes can also be calculated (by taking the difference between the pre- and posttreatment means on an outcome variable and dividing by the standard deviation). However, these can be hard to interpret, since (as is always the case when there is no contrast treatment) effect sizes could be influenced by many factors beyond the treatment itself.

More recently, meta-analysts have elaborated their techniques. For example, correlations, recovery rates or time to relapse, and other indices can be used to estimate treatment effects. Increasingly binary measures are used that distinguish between patients who have improved or not improved using a variety of criteria (e.g., no longer meeting diagnostic criteria, or having a posttreatment score below a clinically defined cutoff point). In addition, methods have been developed that enable results to be displayed more clearly (usually graphically), and that also indicate "confidence limits"—the likelihood that the same results would be found were the study replicated.[1]

Meta-analysis is a powerful and relatively straightforward statistical tool. Its capacity to integrate research literature on a specific topic overcomes the problem of inconclusive results from individual trials; aggregating studies enables researchers to make more accurate estimates of the likelihood that a particular treatment will be effective. It can also cast light on process factors by overcoming the problem that patient samples and settings in individual studies can be homogenous, making it harder to detect differential responses to treatment among subgroups of participants. Aggregation of data across studies can also reveal treatment effects previously hidden because of the low statistical power of individual studies.

Despite its utility, there are problems with the meta-analytic approach. Aggregating data across different types of treatment may make inappropriate assumptions concerning the homogeneity of any data set of studies. For a meta-analysis to yield meaningful aggregated effect sizes, the homogeneity assumption must be met. When there is variability between studies along spe-

---

[1] Increasingly means, mean differences, estimates of numbers needed to treat, or odds ratios are given with "confidence intervals." This is done because a single study provides only one estimate of the "true" result. If the study were repeated 100 times, 95 of the 100 resultant estimates of the "true" result would lie within the 95% confidence interval. This confidence interval can be considered to describe the range of values in which we can be 95% confident that the "true" value lies. The 95% confidence interval is calculated as a ratio of the observed variability in the samples and the size of the sample. It follows that the larger the sample, the more confident we are that the observed value is the "true" one, and the narrower the confidence interval is around the observed value.

cific dimensions, such as treatment standardization, average treatment length, or the severity of disorders treated, these may be used to help account for the variability in the outcomes observed. However, when the differences along these dimensions are very large, it is possible that the studies are no longer sensibly considered as addressing the same research question, in which case the analysis is inappropriate. Such instances would be referred to as a violation of the homogeneity assumption, and most recent meta-analyses apply statistical tests to examine whether this assumption applies to the studies under review. Meta-analyses could be restricted to studies that directly compare different treatments within the same study, using the same measures, and controlling for treatment duration and other methodological features (e.g., Robinson et al., 1990; Shapiro & Shapiro, 1982a), but even here, there are likely to be further differences between the conditions (e.g., in terms of therapist expertise and researcher allegiance; Luborsky et al., 1999).

A second issue is the need to ensure that studies included in reviews as exemplars of a particular approach are appropriately classified, since unreliability at this first stage of analysis will lead to misleading conclusions. For example, in a reexamination of the Weisz et al. (1995b) meta-analysis of child psychotherapy, Shirk (1998; Shirk & Russell, 1992) demonstrated that few of the studies categorized by the original meta-analysis as psychodynamic could be seriously considered to be so. Less than one-fourth of the studies met basic criteria, such as an established psychodynamic theoretical frame of reference or trained therapists.

Third, meta-analytic studies are vulnerable to "publication bias" (a bias against publishing small trials, or those with negative findings) that can have the effect of causing the support for a proposition in the published literature seem stronger than it really is (Sutton et al., 2000). Lipsey and Wilson (1993), in a meta-analysis of 92 meta-analyses of outcome research, found that average effect size for published studies was 0.53, while in unpublished research it was only 0.39. Over 95% of published studies yield significant findings, yet it seems implausible that such a high percentage of research conducted actually confirms the hypotheses with statistical significance. Some have suggested that publication bias may be large enough to account for the generally positive findings of meta-analyses of treatment outcomes (Sohn, 1996).

Fourth, not all meta-analyses meet appropriate standards of statistical analysis and as a consequence draw inappropriate conclusions. For example, analyses could multiply sample measures taken from the same patient and from the same study, leading to effect sizes computed on the basis of dependent data, or they could fail to weight the means for sample size. A particular issue is the averaging of effect sizes, which is legitimate only if these are homogenous; otherwise, significant negative and positive effect sizes will cancel each other out. In at least some cases, a lack of statistical sophistication in the way treatment effects are computed has led to claims of exaggerated differences between treatments, which evaporate when these methodological considerations are taken on board (Wampold et al., 1997).

Finally, it should be remembered that effect sizes can only speak to treatment effects for the average client, and though this is informative of general treatment effects, further elaboration of therapeutic impacts is usually required to detail the more specific effects of treatment.

In this book, reviews of treatment conditions lead with conclusions from meta-analyses, in line with the hierarchy of evidence cited here. However, it should be clear that meta-analyses, just like the primary studies on which they are based, need to be carefully reviewed; the current state of methodology means that their findings cannot be uncritically accepted as accurate summaries of the literature. Quantification of the review process brings with it the risk that findings are reified, and that even sophisticated reviewers make inadequate use of their clinical judgments in drawing conclusions from the literature.

Single-Case Studies

In these designs, the focus is on the individual patient rather than a group average, even when a group of patients is studied. Single-case studies may be descriptive or quantitative. Within this latter group, some are naturalistic reports of outcome or quasi-experiments (Cook & Campbell, 1979); others are reports of the experimental manipulation of interventions. In cases where appropriate baseline measures are taken, or where treatments are applied and withdrawn in a controlled manner, the patient acts as his/her own control. This methodology has been widely used by behavioral and cognitive-behavioral researchers (Morley, 1987, 1989) but is equally applicable to psychodynamic investigators (e.g., Fonagy & Moran, 1993) and to the investigation of process factors (e.g., Parry, 1986).

Single-case studies have a number of attractive features. They can be carried out in routine clinical practice, do not (necessarily) require the facilities associated with more complex research, and can be conducted fairly quickly. Although of great importance in the demonstration or refinement of clinical technique and especially in treatment innovation, their results can be difficult to generalize to the broader clinical population (indeed, the design is not intended for such a purpose); therefore, they do not play a major part in this and other reviews of psychotherapy. Patients are often highly selected (necessarily so when studies are aiming to show the effectiveness of a technique for particular clients). More fundamentally, however, interpretation of results is limited by the fact that (as will become evident in the body of this book) therapeutic interventions have both general and specific impacts on the welfare of patients. A contrast intervention is required in order to be clear that any demonstrated benefits are attributable to specific therapeutic techniques—a strategy adopted in the RCT.

Open Trials

Although entry to treatment may be governed by strict criteria and trials can include a control group, results from open trials are generally regarded as less conclusive than RCTs. The absence of randomization means that differences between groups could be accounted for by whatever factors determined assignment to treatment. To some degree, this difficulty is managed by more rigorous open trials—for example, when there is careful matching of patients, or when quasi-random processes determine allocation to treatment (as would be the case when allocation is based on catchment area). At the other end of the scale, cohort studies may risk administering treatments to groups that differ from each other in important ways, making it difficult to interpret outcomes.

Open trials have the potential to examine therapies under more naturalistic conditions—for example, the impact of two or more treatments for the same disorder, as practiced in different settings. In reality, differences in case mix and the failure to control specific components of treatment usually place drastic limitations on the implications that may be drawn from such studies. Given a sufficiently large data set, it may be possible to derive conclusions about the relative value of treatments even in the absence of random assignment. However, even where this has been done, the conclusions have often been ambiguous, because post hoc analysis reveals systematic case mix by treatment interactions. While RCTs are not immune from this problem, they can attempt to reduce this risk through methodologies such as stratification or minimization, which help balance groups on factors known to influence treatment outcome (though this is true only to the extent that researchers know which factors to control for, and that randomization itself controls those variances of which they are unaware).

RESOLVING CONFLICTS BETWEEN INTERNAL AND EXTERNAL VALIDITY IN RESEARCH DESIGNS

We have already noted that a major problem for psychotherapy researchers is the tension between satisfying the demands of internal and external validity when developing research strategies. Current designs have to reach a compromise between these factors; bridging the gap between them requires innovative attempts at integrating an apparent incompatibility between scientific rigor on the one hand and generalizability on the other. Single-case designs may come to play a more important role in this respect, since external validity is not an inherent problem in designs of this type (Kazdin, 1994a). When replicated across randomly sampled cases, they have considerable generalizability. They can be employed to answer most of the questions that concern researchers, such as the appropriateness of a particular form of treatment, the length of treatment required to achieve a good outcome, the relative impact of treatment on particular aspects of the problem, or the relevance of particular components of treatment. However, there is one critical exception: Within this research strategy, client and therapist factors are difficult to study. If there is no replication across subjects (clients and therapists), the design will not yield information about their influence on outcome. Thus, methodology that is truly adequate to the task of simultaneously ensuring internal and external validity in psychotherapy research has probably yet to be developed. In the meantime, the best—though possibly inadequate—answer lies in reviews (such as the present one), which include critical appraisal of likely threats to external validity posed by current research.

MEASUREMENT TECHNIQUES

There is some consensus (e.g., Kazdin, 1994a) that single measures of outcome are unsatisfactory, that measures should be unreactive to experimenter demand, and that they should be drawn from the following:

- Differing perspectives (such as those of the patient, close relatives, or friends of the patient, and those of the therapist or independent observers)
- Differing symptom domains (such as affect, cognition, and behavior)
- Differing domains of functioning (such as work, social, and marital functioning)

Although this position is reasonable, there is a risk that studies using multiple measures of outcome selectively report only on those measures for which statistical or clinically significant change is evident. On this basis, there is an argument for employing (or at least basing reports on) a single but robust measure chosen for its pertinence to the problem under examination. Unfortunately, and more generally, there is rarely consensus on which specific measures should be used, and this leads to some difficulty in comparisons among studies and on occasion to problems of interpretation within trials when measures assumed to converge on similar target areas give discrepant results.

Establishing the reliability and validity of measures used within a trial may also be complex. For example, a measure based on a patient diary may be subject to fatigue effects and be reactive to the treatment offered (accurately completing a diary may have a different meaning in patients for whom it is integral to their treatment, as opposed to those for whom it is experienced as a burdensome form of record keeping). Similarly, direct observation of behavior can suffer from deceasing sensitivity with time ("instrument fatigue") that may bias results. Often studies report the reliability of instruments as found in other investigations, but the reliability of their use in the particular trial is untested, which may be particularly relevant (e.g., in the use of interviews to establish symptomatic status or post-termination service use for individual patients).

There are several levels or domains of outcome measurement, and distinguishing between them may be helpful (Fonagy et al., 2002). Most studies monitor outcomes at the symptomatic or diagnostic level, using both categorical and dimensional assessments. Although these are used with great reliability, there can be differences between informants, such as therapists, patients, or carers; not infrequently, these are obscured by aggregation in quantitative reviews. Symptom severity does not always predict outcome or follow-up very closely, perhaps because whereas symptoms are an indicator of pathological processes, they are not necessarily directly linked to the underlying problem (e.g., in a person with chronically poor relationships, depressive symptoms are an indicator of the person's difficulties but are not isomorphic with them).

The second level concerns adaptation to the psychosocial environment. A number of meta-analyses have demonstrated that evaluating treatments solely in terms of their impact on core symptoms leads to an overestimation of the effects of treatment (Weisz et al., 1995b). The most likely reason for this is the high reactivity of many symptom measures. Some measurement techniques may tap domains of change close to those targeted by the therapies employed, and may therefore indicate greater degrees of success than would be found using broader assessments. For example, the Beck Depression Inventory (BDI) assesses the level of depression largely through more cognitive representations of this disorder. In contrast, the Hamilton Rating Scale for Depression (HRSD) focuses more on biological symptoms. It may be that trials of cognitive therapy could achieve better outcomes using the BDI, and trials of medication better outcomes using the HRSD, reflecting less the "true" outcome than the bias of scoring instruments.

A third level of outcome measurement concerns mechanisms, the cognitive and emotional processes that probably underlie both symptomatology and problems of adaptation. As discussed below, Kazdin and Kendall (1998) argue that specifying the processes and mechanisms through which treatments achieve their effects may be a productive strategy for developing innovative treatments and assessing their outcomes (e.g., by testing for the operation of implicit psychological processes, such as attentional bias or dysfunctional schemas). At the next level come "transactional" issues, reflecting the fact that many interventions take place in the context of an index patient's wider social environment. On this basis, it is often relevant to determine the impact of treatments on the quality of these relationships and to include not only the perspective of carers but also the impact treatment has on them. A final area of measurement is the level of service utilization. Often (and appropriately), it is assumed that intervention leads to a reduction in service use (e.g., posttermination treatment seeking could be seen as one measure of effectiveness). However, in some areas, increased contact may be a goal (e.g., in substance abuse, or in the management of individuals previously nonadherent to medication for psychosis). The acceptability of a treatment can also be important in evaluating its value, since, no matter what its efficacy, if it is experienced as aversive by users, attrition from treatment will ensure that it has minimal effectiveness.

PATIENT SAMPLING

At every level of patient recruitment, a filtering process operates; quite apart from the selection criteria applied by researchers, only participants who agree to be randomized are available for trial entry, already an unrepresentative group. A traditional criticism of research trials is that they tend to focus on patients with relatively mild and simple presentations. Though this is less true than it was (for example, many trials utilize exclusion criteria to screen out subthreshold cases), the severity, complexity, and diversity often seen in clinical settings is not well represented in research. This is a cause for worry, because meta-analyses have demonstrated an association between the number of cases excluded from a trial and effect size (Westen & Morrison, 2001).

With some exceptions (notably in the field of substance abuse), patients are sampled from a fairly a restricted ethnic group, largely Caucasian, and usually drawn from North American or European cultural backgrounds. Although this reflects the predominance of research reports from these areas, many researchers fail to capture the diversity of their resident populations. Though they are increasingly attentive to this problem, and demographic characteristics are now regularly reported, the impact of ethnicity is rarely examined as a potential moderator of the effect size. The implicit assumption is that what we know of treatment effectiveness generalizes across groups with widely varying cultural beliefs and treatment expectancies, a proposition that is largely untested.

FOLLOW-UP

For many conditions, the success of therapy may be indicated not only by its ability to improve patient functioning but also by its capacity to maintain that improvement after therapy ends. The length of follow-up required to demonstrate a clinical effect is governed by the natural history of a disorder, which will suggest both the probability of relapse and the usual length of time between episodes. Therapeutic efficacy can only be demonstrated in the context of both factors; for example, a 3-month follow-up for a condition known to show greatest relapse over a period of 1 year would clearly be inadequate. Although this is a reasonable position, rather few trials report follow-up data, and interpreting long-term follow-up is not a straightforward matter.

When follow-up is carried out, it can vary markedly in length. Sometimes it is a matter of weeks, more usually months; rarely is it more than 1 year. Reasons for this variability are hard to account for, though it is relevant to note that researchers face practical problems maintaining contact with patients over time, and the cost of repeated measurement and assessment is substantial. Even studies with well-conducted follow-up procedures suffer significant attrition, and this increases with length of follow-up, creating biased samples. Life events beyond the researchers' control are inevitable, and patients often seek further treatment (e.g., Shea et al., 1992a), particularly if they are more severely distressed. All this means that the longer a patient is followed up, the more difficult it is to ascribe change to original treatment: The original randomization will have been lost, making it harder to attribute any group differences to treatment allocation.

Since, over time, RCTs degenerate into a naturalistic study, they are better suited to answering questions about proximal rather than distal outcomes. This is a particular problem when treatments aim not only to manage symptoms but also to foster adaptations that protect the individual against later relapse. On this basis, results may not be apparent until the individual is exposed to further challenges, but by this point, attribution to experimental manipulation is often clouded by a range of intercurrent processes, most importantly, additional treatments and life events.

Finally, the stability of symptomatic change over the follow-up period may be an issue of concern in its own right. The monitoring of individual patients suggests that a proportion will change their symptom status more than once (e.g., Brown & Barlow, 1995; Shapiro et al., 1995). Reporting of group averages tends to obscure this variability, leading to an overestimation of longer term outcomes in clinical practice.

ATTRITION

All clinical trials will lose patients at various points in treatment; the point at which they are lost will have differing impacts on validity. Early loss from an RCT may disrupt the randomization of treatment, threatening internal validity. Even when there is no differential attrition from treatments, it may be the case that significant attrition could lead to results applicable only to a subgroup of persistent patients, threatening external validity. Alternatively, attrition rates across treatment conditions may not be random and may reflect the acceptability of therapies, suggesting that attrition may be an important variable in its own right.

Significant levels of attrition restrict the conclusions that can be drawn from a study and complicate reporting of results. A number of statistical solutions to this problem are available to researchers that utilize the last available data point to overcome the likely bias introduced by loss of patients (e.g., Flick, 1988; Little & Rubin, 1987). However, this strategy can itself generate bias if an individual patient was present at the end of treatment but lost to followup, conflating these two sets of observations (e.g., Foa et al., 1999b). Alternatively, data can be reported on the basis of an "intention-to-treat" sample, including all subjects entered into the trial, as well as presenting separate data for those completing all or a specified length of therapy (e.g., Elkin et al., 1989).

Allegiance Effects

A number of meta-analytic reviews suggest that effect sizes can be predicted by knowledge of the declared theoretical allegiance of the primary authors of the investigation. Though there is some evidence that allegiance effects may be less apparent in more recent studies (e.g., Gaffan et al., 1995), the therapeutic equipoise posited by the design of the RCT appears vulnerable to researcher orientation. In one study, 69% of the variance in outcome across studies was predicted if three different ways of measuring theoretical allegiance were simultaneously introduced (Luborsky et al., 1999). Looked at another way, this suggests that if the allegiance of investigators is known, 92% of the time we can predict which of two treatments is likely to be more successful. There are different ways of interpreting this. In a more benign sense, it is reasonable to expect individuals committed to a treatment approach to have greater expertise in its delivery. However, it is unlikely that, by chance, the allegiance of the investigator would emerge favorably in over 90% of his/her investigations. It may be that a form of publication bias operates, in which investigators are unwilling to publish trials that do not support their position. It is also possible that allegiance effects reflect the relatively unsystematic way in which control groups have been constituted, with selection of comparison conditions that are biased in favor of the experimental treatment, or simply not implemented with the same level of competence or enthusiasm.

Identifying Process Elements

Therapies comprise a package of interventions, and when these are tested for efficacy, it remains unclear which of their many components were necessary or sufficient for ensuring change. Most commonly, investigators conduct post hoc analyses, seeking patterns of association in their data, an approach that is useful for exploring possible mechanisms but cannot establish causality. A more robust approach would be to conduct an RCT in which process elements are manipulated as part of the initial randomization, but examples of this are rare, presumably because funding for such studies is difficult to obtain. Such a trial also make the dual assumption that (1) we know what components are relevant, and (2) there is no interaction between the components that generate outcome (there is a risk that experimental disaggregation underestimates their true impact). Finally, investigators may not recognize the pertinence of relevant process factors, and may therefore fail to monitor them (e.g., when a treatment achieves its impact by increasing the likelihood of receiving social supportive experiences but failed to monitor these).

STATISTICAL ISSUES IN PSYCHOTHERAPY RESEARCH
Clinical and Statistical Significance of Change

Much of this report is based on journal articles examining the truth of the null hypothesis—in essence, the proposition that psychological therapies have no effect, or no effect greater than a placebo. It is conventional to report the statistical significance of differences between treatments in terms of a confidence level of $p < .05$ or $< .01$. However, researchers may be able to reject the null hypothesis at relatively high levels of statistical significance, without simultaneously demonstrating that this finding is worthy of clinical attention (Kukla, 1989). Demonstration of statistical effects may not be equivalent to a clinically significant—or clinically meaningful—therapeutic change, and a number of strategies have been used to detect this (discussed further in Kazdin, 1994b; a helpful synoptic overview is given in Evans et al., 1998).

1. One approach is to specify a return to functioning with a range of scores representative of normal functioning. Where the distribution of scores on a measure is available both for the normal and clinical populations, clinically significant change is indicated when a person who has previously scored within a dysfunctional range obtains posttreatment scores that are more likely to come from a normative population sample (Jacobson & Truax, 1991). In a similar way, some studies adopt a criterion of recovery that enables categorical rather than continuous scoring of outcomes—for example, using a BDI score ≤9 to indicate treatment response in depression (e.g., Elkin et al., 1989).

2. A second approach assesses the significance of change by setting a criterion measure of change, expressed in standard deviation units. This could be set at a level that exceeds chance fluctuations, adjusted for the reliability of the instrument (Jacobson & Revenstorf, 1988) (though this approach has the disadvantage that changes will depend not only on the effectiveness of the

treatment but also on the reliability of the measure). Another example would be to specify as a criterion that, at posttherapy, scores for treated clients should be at least 2 standard deviations from the mean of the untreated group (Jacobson & Truax, 1991).

3. A third strategy is applicable when individuals who previously met diagnostic criteria for a disorder no longer do so after treatment. Though this approach has obvious merit, the arbitrary nature of the diagnostic criteria sometimes makes this a misleading indicator. For example, Westen and Morrison's (2001) meta-analysis suggests that whereas individuals receiving treatment for panic disorder may no longer meet diagnostic criteria, the average treated patient continues to panic only slightly less than once per week and endorses a total of four of the seven panic symptoms required for a *Diagnostic and Statistical Manual of Mental Disorders* (DSM) diagnosis of panic disorder. By contrast, treatment for a disorder such as autism may make a substantial and meaningful impact, without any expectation of effecting a change in the diagnosis.

There have been attempts by epidemiologists and others to design ways of representing outcome data that make more intuitive sense to clinicians (McQuay & Moore, 1997; Sackett et al., 1996). These are outlined in Appendix II. It is increasingly common to see outcomes expressed as the "number needed to treat" (NNT). This figure is based on categorical criteria of successful or unsuccessful intervention and expresses the success rate of an intervention as the number of patients who would need to be treated in the experimental condition in order for one of them to receive a benefit that he/she would not have received had he/she been treated in the control group. A small NNT (between 2 and 3) would indicate that a treatment is quite effective.

A useful criterion for deciding when to adopt a categorical or a dimensional approach to clinical significance is whether clinically desirable outcomes are better captured by one or the other method. For example, the number of suicide attempts may be reduced by an intervention, but from a clinical standpoint, one attempt a week is just as much cause for concern as two; a more meaningful criterion is presence or absence. Equally, a categorical outcome, such as abstinence for individuals with substance abuse, may be inappropriate in some trials, or may represent an unacceptable goal for certain clients. Finally, there may be instances in which neither approach fully captures clinical impact, particularly when movement across a threshold produces stepwise rather than incremental change. For example, even small improvements in the capacity for self-care in a psychotic individual who is highly dependent on his/her family could have a major impact on his/her caretakers' functioning; in this instance, a quantitative approach may be difficult to map onto the social utility of an intervention.

One final approach to this issue is worthy of mention. Novel statistical models are increasingly helping to bridge the gap between research and clinical perspectives. For example, within conventional analyses, the subsample of patients meeting criteria for recovery at one time point may not be the same subsample as that so categorized at another time: Analysis based on group means obscures rather than clarifies each patient's trajectory of change. The application of growth curve analysis (such as hierarchical linear modeling or survival analysis) allows researchers to model the progress of individual patients through treatments and contrast groups in terms of the differences in the shape of these curves. Analysis determines whether knowing which treatment the person received improves our capacity to predict its shape. Clearly, this should be the case when a therapy is successful. The ability to track individual changes in clinical status across time is more sensitive than traditional methods of analysis, and likely to result in more realistic appraisal of outcomes.

Multiple Data Sampling and Type I Error

Researchers frequently report numerous results of statistical significance without being clear as to how each test relates to the prediction they are examining. Dar et al. (1994) illustrated this problem by suggesting a hypothetical study in which two treatments for flying phobias are contrasted, with levels of anxiety and coping skills being the dependent variables. In practice, there may be a number of procedures for measuring these variables, all of which are likely to be intercorrelated. Each of these variables could be examined separately, though, in reality, there are only two hypotheses under investigation—the impact of the treatment on anxiety and its effect on coping skills. More than two statistical analyses are therefore redundant and represent an overstatement of the data available to the researchers. A real-life example of this process is the much-cited National Institute of Mental Health study of treatments for depression (Elkin, 1994), which shows statistical significance on only some of a relatively large family of variables pertaining to dysfunctional emotional states.[2] A consequence of multiply sampling related data sets is to increase the risk of Type I errors—rejecting the null hypothesis when that hypothesis is true (e.g., in practice, claiming that one treatment works better than another, when, in reality, the two work equally well).

Because it is well recognized that a series of measures tapping similar domains may be interrelated, investigators often employ multivariate tests, which permit some understanding of relationships between dependent measures. Though this procedure overcomes some of the problems noted earlier,

---

[2] This study is discussed fully in Chapter 4; a caveat to this criticism (Ogles et al., 1995) should be noted.

problems can arise when multivariate tests that indicate overall significance are then followed by univariate tests. Not only does this increase the risk of Type I error but results can also be difficult to interpret, once again, because of possible relationships among variables under test.

Atheoretical Analysis

Dar et al. (1994), in a review of the use of statistical tests in psychotherapy research from the 1960s to the 1980s, noted a high level of inappropriate significance testing, which they attributed to the pragmatic concerns of psychotherapy researchers. The determination to find statistically significant associations is seen by them as motivated by "a flight from theory into pragmatics" (p. 79). Because psychotherapy research frequently has very little theoretical guidance leading to meaningful hypotheses and testable predictions, there has been an explosion of exploratory procedures, leading to a state of affairs in which even in the best journals, "much of the current use of statistical tests is flawed" (1994, p. 80).

Statistical Power

Statistical power is the extent to which an investigation is able to detect differences between samples when such differences exist in the population: in other words, when there is a true difference among the groups under test. Power is a function of the criterion for statistical significance, or alpha level; the sample size; and the effect size, or the magnitude of the difference that exists between the groups. Statistical power in perhaps the majority of psychotherapy trials may be relatively weak, primarily because of low sample sizes (Kazdin, 1994b). Cohen (1962) distinguished three levels of effect size (small, 0.25; medium, 0.50; and large, 1.0) and evaluated the ability of published studies to detect such differences at the conventional alpha level of $p <$ .05. Power within these studies was generally low; for example, studies had a one in five chance of detecting small effect sizes, and less than a one in two chance of detecting medium effect sizes. Despite the cautionary note struck by Cohen's paper and the date of its publication, Dar et al. (1994) found that a significant proportion of even recent research continues to neglect these issues. Most particularly, there continues to be a neglect of measures of effect size in favor of citing statistical significance. The problems inherent in this procedure can be readily illustrated by considering a study with a large sample but a small effect size; although statistical significance may well be achieved, this does not speak to the magnitude of the effect, nor to its likely reliability or validity.

It should be clear that all of these issues threaten the external validity of psychotherapy research; Dar et al. (1994) detailed a number of strategies for ensuring that such threats are minimized—for example, by employing theory-guided predictions, planned rather than post hoc statistical decisions, reduced use of omnibus multivariate techniques, stricter control of type I error rates by using single rather than multiple tests, "families" rather than a multiplicity of hypotheses, and the avoidance of stepwise statistical procedures and testing of hypotheses not against a difference of zero, but rather against a predetermined interval.

THE USE OF THE *DIAGNOSTIC AND STATISTICAL MANUAL OF MENTAL DISORDERS* IN ORGANIZING THIS REVIEW

This book is organized in relation to client presentation rather than treatment modality. To some degree, our findings justify this problem-oriented approach, since specific interventions appear to have particular applicability to certain disorders, and considerations of the relative efficacy of treatment techniques are nested within major groups of disorders. This strategy has its own limitations, particularly, that service provision is currently largely organized according to specific approaches rather than mental health problems. However, because the results of this review suggest advantages for a multimodal psychotherapeutic service, we feel that our appraisal is service-relevant. A further advantage of the approach we have taken is to be found in the obvious fact that the challenge a disorder presents to psychotherapy services greatly depends on its prevalence, comorbidity, and natural history, both in the clinic and in the community.

Our chapter headings largely reflect the classification of psychological disorders in the text revision of the fourth edition of the *Diagnostic and Statistical Manual of Mental Disorders* (DSM-IV-TR; American Psychiatric Association, 2000). The DSM system classifies patients on five axes (though this report focuses largely on only the first two). Axis I represents clinical syndromes; Axis II, developmental disorders and personality disorders; Axis III, physical disorders and conditions; Axis IV, severity of psychosocial stressors; and Axis V, a global assessment of functioning. In large part, the logic of this organization is pragmatic. Most treatment studies are conducted on the basis of samples selected according to DSM and less frequently ICD (World Health Organization, 1992) criteria. It is relatively rare to find studies focused on referral problems (e.g., individuals who are bereaved, or who have been victims of childhood sexual abuse).

There are many virtues in the DSM system, both for clinical and research purposes. Its reliability is high if appropriate instruments are used for data collection (although this is true only for major categories of disorders, and the reliability of Axis II diagnoses are more questionable [Shaffer et al., 1996]). In addition, knowledge of the natural history of these diagnoses, based increasingly on epidemiological surveys, creates a context against which the efficacy of treatments can be judged. However, data from this source indicate the first problem with diagnostic systems, which is that individuals with the same initial diagnosis can expect to have different patterns of outcome. For example, it is well known that whereas about one-third of individuals with depression remit rapidly, others' depression is enduring and recurring. Obviously, there are many reasons for this variability, but it is relevant to note that, viewed from the perspective of developmental psychopathology, diagnostic presentations represent the common end point of a range of interactions between constitutional vulnerabilities and environmental challenges. It is also the case that the same set of experiences can lead to quite different outcomes; for example, exposure to a traumatic event (such as child sexual abuse) may lead to a range of diagnostic presentations at a later date.

Recent longitudinal birth cohort studies have made it clear that adult psychopathology rarely arises de novo (Kim-Cohen et al., 2003). In approximately three-fourths of cases, adult presentations were anticipated by a diagnosable childhood disorder, and though adult disorders were generally preceded by their juvenile counterpart, this was not invariably the case, suggesting that childhood and adult diagnoses do not always correspond. For example, depression in women is frequently anticipated by conduct disorder in middle childhood and adolescence. From a treatment point of view, this raises questions about the apparent homogeneity of diagnostic categories, since it implies that they represent heterogenous pathways, with clear implications for variation in outcome.

Whatever its utility, diagnosis, in and of itself, is insufficient to describe a condition. The nature of the problem that the condition represents can only be understood if the context in which it occurs is explored. This suggests the relevance of the history of the condition and its current determinants (usually addressed in a psychological formulation), factors not addressed by diagnosis.

LIMITATIONS OF THIS REVIEW

Methodological Quality of Research Studies

In this chapter, we have detailed the many issues relating to the methodology underpinning research trials. In carrying out our review, we note that the quality of studies is improving as members of the research community recognize the standards to which they need to aspire. However, many of the trials we review do have methodological problems—some minor, some more serious. We have made a decision, largely on the grounds of limitations of space, not to identify or itemize the deficiencies of each study except where these seem especially relevant. Instead, we rely on the discussion contained in this and the next chapter to alert readers to the general problems likely to be contained in studies, and trust that they will examine individual studies and reviews when these seem particularly pertinent to their practice or interests.

The Range of Disorders and Problems

Readers of this review will note a number of omissions. Those of which we are aware relate to limitations of time and resources, and a concern that we would not be able to do justice to reviewing areas in which we had limited clinical experience. For this reason, we have not reviewed treatments within the health psychology setting, despite the fact that this is an increasingly important area of practice. The structure of our review makes it difficult to include information about interventions when problems rather than diagnoses are to the fore; for example, we have not considered studies that focus on improving relationships between and within couples or families, and in which neither partner has a psychiatric presentation, despite its relevance to mental health. Also, we have excluded trials such as interventions for adult survivors of childhood abuse, in which clients are recruited on the basis that they have experienced a common problem rather than presenting with the same diagnosis. For similar reasons, we have not been able to include treatments for people with mental retardation (or learning disorders). These are reviewed by Beail (2003) and Prout and Nowak-Drabik (2003), and their exclusion from this report is not intended to indicate that such treatments are ineffective (an issue considered further in Chapter 17). Finally, though we report on studies that employ counseling and counselors, we usually subsume these in relation to the technique adopted rather than the professional identify of the person delivering the intervention. We feel justified in this because, although counselors may approach their work with a potentially different frame of reference, their practice is often similar to that of psychotherapists. Furthermore, our review of outcomes in relation to therapist training and values in Chapter 16 indicates that the manner in which therapies are implemented is more pertinent than professional descriptors. There are attempts to establish an evidence base for counseling independent of psychotherapy, but quite apart from definitional problems (with these terms often used interchangeably depending on treatment context), few trials are currently available for review (Bower et al., 2003b).

Literature Covered

Our review is heavily dominated by English-language journals most frequently reporting trials carried out in the United States, Europe, and Australia. Although we had no resources for translating non-English-language papers, inevitable and extensive use of abstracting systems such as PsychINFO, MEDLINE and EMBASE, as well as citation indices, suggests to us that, in the main, our monolingualism has denied us access to reviews rather than to original articles. Nonetheless, we are aware of a substantial body of literature (from France and Germany in particular) relevant to this review but inaccessible to us, because it tends not to be republished in Anglocentric journals, with their orientation toward empiricist tradition. Just as (if not more) pertinent, very few trials are reported from Africa or Asia, raising questions about the degree to which our report is culturally representative. We have no definitive response to this question. Informal comparison between equivalent European and American studies suggests that findings from outcome studies are generalizable at least across these national boundaries, despite the apparent diversity of cultures covered by the research. Whether this is more broadly true is unclear.

Contrasts of Psychopharmacological and Psychological Treatments

Many of the conditions we discuss are commonly treated using both medication and psychological interventions. Many researchers have contrasted the relative benefits of these treatments, both alone and in combination, and we consider these studies at a number of points in this review. Our comments regarding medication are based on these contrasts; it is beyond the scope of this book to provide definitive statements regarding the benefits of psychopharmacology, nor are we qualified to do so. In chapters where we discuss conditions in which medication is particularly relevant to treatment, we have tried to indicate sources of further information for the interested reader.

The Problem of Comorbidity

Throughout this review, we find that comorbidity of Axis I and Axis II disorders is extensive. Both clinicians and researchers are increasingly recognizing the importance of comorbidity in the application of therapeutic technique and its impact on efficacy. As noted by Clarkin and Kendall (1992), there is irony in the fact that as awareness of this challenge to the efficacy of therapy grows (and is becoming the focus for research), the pressures of resource management dictate shorter treatments. It is clear from evidence we review that comorbidity impacts on treatment delivery, usually resulting in more challenging therapies with poorer outcomes (Coryell et al., 1988; Coryell & Noyes, 1988; Grunhaus, 1988). Comorbid conditions are also likely to lead to poorer end-state functioning, because at the end of treatment, patients may continue to exhibit symptomatology related to the untreated comorbid condition—an example of which would be panic disorder with comorbid generalized anxiety disorder (Brown & Barlow, 1992).

This fact makes the relationship between diagnosis and treatment planning more complex than might be indicated by research we have reviewed, and while not necessarily an insurmountable problem (e.g., DeRubeis & Feeley, 1991), it makes it more difficult to transfer data directly into the clinical context.

Patients with comorbid conditions are particularly likely to be seen in specialist mental health settings. They are also likely to constitute the majority of patients receiving long-term therapy or multiple episodes of short-term therapy. This creates a major problem in that recommendations regarding appropriate treatment (e.g., their modality and length) must be considered in the context of patients who present with multiple and possibly changing diagnoses. We are uncertain whether appropriate treatment length is best considered as an additive or multiplicative function of the number of diagnoses, or whether particular combinations of diagnoses may be better treated as separate disorders from the point of view of psychotherapeutic treatment.

Different therapeutic orientations take very different views of this problem, and it may be impossible to arrive at a formulation of comorbidity that is genuinely independent of the theoretical orientation of particular practitioners. Some Axis II diagnoses, such as borderline personality disorder, are so constructed as to inevitably include multiple Axis I disorders—such as depression and anxiety. No clinician would mistake problems of depression in such individuals with those presented by a patient without significant Axis II pathology. Thus, the applicability of findings from RCTs fails even at the level of face validity with such patients. Given the current state of research-based knowledge, caution should be shown in generalizing research results to those with comorbid Axis I disorders and severe deficits in personality functioning.

Biased Representation of Theoretical Orientations in the Research Literature

In the previous chapter, we identified the range of commonly practiced psychological therapies. However, there is a marked and continuing variation in the extent to which these differing orientations have been subjected to systematic evaluation. The consequence of this fact is that, relative to the frequency with which they are employed, certain orientations—most particularly psychodynamic therapy—are underrepresented in this review.

Treatment trials of psychodynamic treatments have been particularly constrained by the following:

- An absence of a quantitative research tradition within this orientation.
- The related fact that appropriately trained clinicians are rarely available to participate in research trials.
- The expense and difficulty of mounting trials of long-term treatment.
- The absence of appropriate measures to encompass the more ambitious aims of these treatments.

It would he inaccurate to claim that no research on the efficacy of psychodynamic therapy has been carried out (e.g., Crits-Christoph, 1992; Leichsenring, 2001; Svartberg & Stiles, 1991), but it should be acknowledged that this research is limited in volume.

There are a number of approaches taken by psychodynamic therapists to address the skew inherent in the research literature and its corollary, the lack of research representative of actual clinical practice. The first is to rely on clinical intuition and judgment. There is a feeling, prevalent among clinicians of all orientations, that their clinical experience, rather than research findings, guides their clinical practice (Morrow-Bradley & Elliot, 1986). This may be a realistic perception in terms of research on psychotherapeutic process, but it does not seem to us either pertinent or viable as a response to the absence of outcome research. No single clinician can accumulate experience sufficient in quantity to ensure generalizability. A second strategy commonly used to describe outcomes in psychodynamic journals is the use of case reports. Although of great clinical interest, these cannot be used as evidence for effectiveness, since they rely on a small group of clinicians and nonrandomly sampled patients, which necessarily limits the possibility of generalization to other settings and other therapists. Ultimately, and perhaps unfortunately, in the absence of data, clinicians tend to rely on their intuition, which, when put to empirical test, tends to lack both reliability and validity (Garb, 1989).

There have been objections to randomized controlled trials for long-term treatment because of the ethical implications of withholding treatment from needy individuals for a long period. In our view, there is no special ethical problem presented by RCTs for psychodynamic psychotherapy, particularly since the limited availability of these services implies that very few of the individuals who may need such treatments would ever receive them. Furthermore, maintenance therapy is an effective control for most long-term interventions (e.g., Frank et al., 1991). We do, however, see an ethical problem in administering a treatment to patients without firm evidence of the absence of negative effects. Open trials are not an appropriate alternative (for reasons considered earlier), since they fail to avoid many of the problems associated with RCTs, while adding the ambiguity inherent in nonrandom assignment to treatment groups.

Thus, although we can see that the absence of evidence of efficacy cannot and must not be equated with absence of evidence of effectiveness, this scientific review can only draw conclusions from the evidence available. It cannot use different evidential criteria for different orientations. In the absence of evidence, broader organizational and less formal considerations may be used to guide policy, but these are beyond the scope of this review.

Restricted Coverage of Analyses of Economic Impact

Although the costs of mental health problems to the community are demonstrable (e.g., Katon, 1991; Stroudemire et al., 1986), so are the direct costs of implementing psychosocial interventions. As in most areas of health care, there are demands for these to be justified in relation to their economic benefit. We have not systematically or separately considered this issue, though where evidence is available, we have included it. Illustrative reviews have been conducted by Healy and Knapp (1994), Gabbard et al. (1997), and Chiles et al. (1999); Kaplan and Groessl (2002) considered procedural issues.

The paucity of available data probably reflects the difficulty of conducting meaningful econometric analyses. Part of the challenge is the fact that many of the outcomes measured by psychotherapy researchers are not economically meaningful, and that the data for such analyses need to be drawn from a wider range of perspectives than are commonly considered. For example, the cost-effectiveness of an intervention is an indication of the amount of health benefit that is gained using the resources that are required to deliver it. However, assessment of cost-effectiveness depends on the perspective applied. Benefit to society may not be the same as benefit to the specific agencies charged with delivery of the service, and this may differ again from impacts for an individual patient and his/her associates. Although there is some consensus that a societal perspective should be adopted (e.g., Gold et al., 1996), this implies accounting for all possible impacts. Because comprehensively monitoring and costing these would challenge the resources of most researchers, in practice, many studies assess cost–offset in relation to services—for example, reductions in health care use as a result of the intervention (though this implies that observed reductions in utilization reflect actual health benefit, an assumption that is not usually directly assessed). Cost–offset is well-illustrated in Gabbard et al.'s (1997) review, which identified 18 trials published between 1984 and 1994 in which economic costs were evaluated with appropriate rigor. The majority of these suggested that there was a reduction in total costs consequent to therapy. The greatest potential for cost savings related to use of inpatient and emergency services, though these benefits were most evident when the target group included potentially intensive users of such facilities (e.g., individuals with psychotic disorders or borderline personality disorder).

Although it is appropriate for costs to be related to outcome, being cost-efficient is not equivalent to being cost-effective. Put simply, a brief but ineffective treatment is likely to be less cost-effective than one that has greater cumulative costs but better outcomes, and choice of treatment should therefore reflect the balance of costs against outcomes. This issue is considered more fully in Chapter 3.

CHAPTER 3

PSYCHOTHERAPY RESEARCH, HEALTH POLICY, AND SERVICE PROVISION

Glenys Parry, Anthony Roth, and Peter Fonagy

HEALTH SERVICE DELIVERY SYSTEMS

Research on psychotherapy effectiveness takes place, and its findings are exploited, within the context of a health service delivery system. Although there are major differences in how psychotherapy services are funded and provided internationally, concerns about the accountability of health care professionals and the costs and effectiveness of psychotherapy are universal (Miller & Magruder, 1996). A comparison of the American and British health systems illustrates this.

In both countries, there have been significant changes in how health services have been delivered over the past 20 years, and in both systems, mental health service usage and service costs have been accelerating. In the United States, between 1967 and 1980, the proportion of the population using mental health services increased from 1 to 10%, with outpatient services accounting for the bulk of this. The proportion of mental health reimbursements relating to outpatient services rose from less than 1 to 12% in the same time period (Klerman, 1983). Government and employers pay for 80% of health-related expenditure (Austad & Berman, 1991), and these parties, along with the health insurance industry, have been increasingly concerned about containing mental health costs. An early attempt to regulate which psychological therapies would be reimbursable under Federal insurance plans (Inouye, 1983) foundered, but the concerns have endured. Following the 1973 Health Maintenance Organizations Act, a variety of health maintenance organizations (HMOs) and other models of managed behavioral health care have proliferated in the United States. Mental health care is included by a Federal statute requiring an HMO to offer short-term outpatient mental health evaluation and crisis intervention services, as well as 60 days of inpatient psychiatric care (DeLeon et al., 1985). Professional responses have been to provide pragmatic, brief interventions and to seek more cost-efficient ways of treating chronically mentally and emotionally disabled patients in prepaid health care systems (Austad & Berman, 1991). Managed care has attempted to change clinician behavior through the greater use of clinical protocols for reimbursement decisions (Cummings, 1991). Concurrent reimbursement review caused clinicians deep concern about their ability to provide optimal treatment (Gabbard et al., 1991), and psychological therapy practices were felt to be particularly vulnerable (Cummings, 1987), although, in practice, this era has also brought significant new roles for some practitioners (Sanchez & Turner, 2003).

The National Health Service (NHS) in the United Kingdom provides health services to the public free of charge at the point of delivery, funded through government revenue. Health care, including mental health care, is provided by primary care trusts and the staff they employ, family physicians (known as general practitioners), and by NHS hospital and mental health trusts. There are also contributions from the charitable sector, particularly in relation to bereavement and couple counseling, and for other specific groups (such as abused women, children, and some ethnic minorities). Compared to the United States, there is still a very small proportion of psychological therapies for mental ill health provided by the private sector. Despite a different infrastructure for funding, the themes of containing costs and ensuring clinical effectiveness are just as salient within the NHS (Parry, 1996). Increased investment in mental health services is restricted to specific initiatives within a program of "modernization" linked to a National Service Framework for mental health, which sets performance standards for services. Psychological therapies were included in the 1999 National Service Framework, when access to safe and effective psychological therapies was set as a national standard. Public health specialists within primary care trusts and strategic health authorities assess the needs of the local population and allocate resources on behalf of the public to achieve the best services for the lowest cost. Managers of NHS services also strive to increase the volume of clinical activity to meet contractual targets.

Pressures to examine value for money and cost-effectiveness led to the debate that took place in the United States in the early 1980s being recapitulated in the United Kingdom in the 1990s. Concerns about efficacy and cost-effectiveness of psychotherapy and counseling led some U.K. health authorities to examine more closely the types and lengths of psychological treatments they purchase. A National Institute for Clinical Excellence (NICE) was established to produce nationally authoritative guidance to the NHS, with systematic and formal processes for health technology assessments, cost-effectiveness review, and guideline commissioning. There is a suite of NICE mental health guidelines on depression, schizophrenia, and anxiety disorders, each incorporating recommendations on psychological therapies (*www.nice.org.uk*). Thus, high-level generalizations from meta-analyses are being used to determine which psychological therapies are (or are not) provided in the United Kingdom health care system. There is an explicit commitment to drive policy, to make commissioning decisions, and to allocate resources on the basis of research evidence on what is clinically and cost-effective. This not only includes assessing evidence of need for a service or an intervention (basically defined in terms of people's capacity to benefit) but also the measurable health gain for a given investment of revenue, the latter being an important but complex issue.

ECONOMIC EVALUATION

Most trials in the field of health technology assessment include an economic evaluation, and this is increasingly common for psychological therapies. All use methods for comparing costs with outcomes, but there is a wide variation in the methods used and, hence, how the results can be applied.

Cost–benefit analysis (CBA) assigns a monetary value to both costs and outcomes, so that they can be directly compared. If costs are less than the monetary value of the outcome, there is a net benefit. Costs are assessed from a broad, societal perspective to capture the socially worthwhile use of resources—for example, by estimating the wider economic impact of an individual's unemployment due to ill health. In order to assign monetary value to a given outcome, empirical evidence of people's willingness to pay for that health care benefit can be gathered using survey methods with hypothetical scenarios. CBA is the least-used form of economic evaluation in psychological therapy research.

Cost-effectiveness analysis (CEA) aims to support policymakers and service managers in achieving the best outcomes for a given resource, or in choosing between alternative interventions for a specific client group. Costs estimates are often from a narrow perspective (e.g., the cost of the intervention itself), and the health outcome is often appraised on a single index and is usually measured in natural units (e.g., the costs of preventing relapse, readmission to the hospital, or a repetition of deliberate self-harm). For example, Scott et al. (2003) calculated the cost of preventing relapse using cognitive therapy in patients with partially remitted depression (i.e., residual symptoms after treatment). The incremental cost-effectiveness ratio ranged from £4,328 to £5,027 per additional relapse prevented.

This form of CEA is helpful for some purposes but has a number of drawbacks. For example, it is hard to relate any specific outcome (such as a repeated incident of self-harm) to the patient's overall experience of health. It is also impossible to compare cost-effectiveness across different patient groups with different interventions. Cost–utility analysis (CUA) is a specific development of cost-effectiveness research that addresses these limitations. CUA measures and then values the impact of an intervention on a patient's health-related quality of life. Ideally, cost estimation is based on a broad perspective and conforms to the economic principles of using opportunity costs rather than charges, marginal not average costs, resource use rather than transfer payments, and total resource use, not just the mental health resource use (Kamlet & Kleinman, 1999). It is common for costs in CUA to be limited to the budget that the analysis is seeking to inform. In the NHS, for example CUAs are limited only to those costs falling on health and social care. The usual denominator in the cost–utility ratio is the quality-adjusted life year (QALY; Torrance, 1986). To estimate the QALY, generic health utility measures that address the impact of the health state over broad domains such as mobility, pain or discomfort, and role function are required. Using survey techniques in large samples, values are derived for the resulting health states from 0 (death) to 1 (full health). The value of this method is that health outcomes from psychological therapy can be directly compared with those from other medical or surgical interventions, in terms of the cost–utility ratio. This offers policymakers and service commissioners the prospect of comparing the health outcomes of a psychological therapy with more familiar interventions, such as hip replacement in osteoarthritis or chemotherapy in cancer care. On the other hand, Chisholm et al. (1996) argue that current QALY measures have limited relevance to mental health outcomes, and this may be one reason why CUA has rarely been applied to psychological therapy.

Cost–offset is an aspect of cost estimation in economic evaluation that has attracted considerable attention in the field of mental health (Hunsley, 2003; Kocakulah & Valadares, 2003). There is the potential for expenditure on mental health interventions to result in cost savings on more general medical services, if overall health service usage is reduced. For example, Bateman and Fonagy (2003) found that the cost of partial hospitalization for patients with borderline personality disorder was more than offset by savings in inpatient and emergency room treatment in the 18 months following the termination of the therapy. Cost–offset studies therefore quantify costs and savings across a broader health care system, although methodological issues leave enough room for debate over whether the "cost–offset phenomenon" exists (Kashner & Rush, 1999).

Including health economic evaluation in randomized clinical trials creates practical difficulties, in addition to appropriately rigorous cost estimation and outcome measurement. The sample size needed for an adequate cost-effectiveness analysis is typically much greater than that for a simple clinical trial, usually with $n > 100$, and most psychotherapy trials are underpowered for economic analysis (Briggs, 2000; Knapp & Healey, 1999). There may be some scope for meta-analysis of smaller trials to be conducted by aggregating individual patient data, although this raises methodological problems, such as sensitivity to assumptions on costs (Bower et al., 2003a). Most trials have too short a follow-up period for good cost–utility analysis, which requires estimation of health effects that persist for a number of years. However, it is possible to extrapolate from trial results given various assumptions. For example, Kamlet et al. (1995) constructed a Monte Carlo simulation to estimate the lifetime impact of different maintenance treatments in depression. They found that for patients meeting the eligibility standards of the RCT, interpersonal therapy maintenance treatment of recurrent depression led to an estimated cost–utility ratio of $5,000/QALY, well below the typical threshold for judging an intervention to be cost-effective. Such a strong result gives some confidence to the conclusion, despite the methodological limitations.

Given the methodological and practical challenges in conducting trials with economic analysis, it is not surprising that few are undertaken. Byford et al. (2003b) reviewed 28 economic evaluations in the field of mental health, published over a 12-month period. Of these, 11 were RCTs. They found that cost–utility analyses in adequately powered RCTs are rare and concluded that the evidence base on cost-effectiveness is still too sparse to inform resource allocation decisions.

SERVICE MANAGEMENT AND USE OF RESEARCH

For many years, there was little trade between psychotherapy research, service delivery, and clinical practice. Clinicians rarely consulted research journals, researchers undertook psychotherapy studies in laboratory conditions outside routine service contexts, and no systematic systems existed for research to influence service planning and delivery (Parry, 1992). This picture has changed dramatically, although not beyond recognition, in the last two decades.

As described in Chapter 2, the priority of researchers undertaking "explanatory" clinical trials is to protect against threats to internal validity, to show underlying causal relationships between improvement and intervention. This requires tight controls on the way the treatment is structured and administered, the way the sample is selected, and how outcomes are assessed. By contrast, the clinician's priority is usually more pragmatic, concerned less with the demonstration of which component of a complex intervention is responsible for change than with achieving change itself. Clinicians and funders have different concerns, interests, and needs, and they view research from contrasting standpoints. Clinicians sometimes complain that research fails to capture the complexity of the clinical situation, where permutations of diagnosis, psychological characteristics, and social circumstance make the choice of treatment a complex decision-making process. Each patient can be seen as presenting a unique puzzle, rendering research evidence that suggests matching treatment to diagnosis is irrelevant, because it is seen as over-simplistic.

In contrast, those paying for psychological therapy would like to identify treatments and delivery methods that are both effective and cost-effective and, from this standpoint, it is unhelpful to be told that planning should be constructed on the basis of each individual case. Psychological therapy services are provided within a finite budget and, in principle, funders and service managers wish to ensure optimum outcomes for a given expenditure. As research evidence is collated, there is a temptation to turn to these findings as though they provide a definitive answer, without noting the cautions researchers almost universally attach to them. In any case, much research is designed to answer scientific questions rather than practical and applicable ones, and results are not straightforwardly applied to service provision. Tunis et al. (2003) argue that pragmatic trials on representative populations and clinically relevant interventions are vitally needed but will continue to be in short supply, because current research commissioning systems do not value trials designed to answer decision-makers' questions.

There are, therefore, many difficulties in applying scientifically sound research on treatment efficacy in a complex system where decisions on investing funds are governed by multiple drivers and constraints. In practice, it is often easier for funders and service managers to think and act in terms of cost reduction rather than cost-effectiveness, in part because the latter relies on more complex and subtle judgments than the former. It may be helpful to consider two illustrative examples—reducing treatment length, and getting better value for money from the investment in skilled professionals by supple-menting them with computerized delivery or facilitated self-help.

Advocates of "stepped care" (Haaga, 2000; Katon et al., 1999) suggest that briefer, simpler, and the most accessible therapies should be offered first, and that more complex, expensive, and effortful therapies be offered only if the patient has not responded to the simpler approach. Research here is informative but does not remove the need for service managers to make con-sidered choices. There is no general rule for determining the shortest treat-ment length commensurate with achieving appropriate and stable change, since this depends on many factors, including the type of problem and the patient's history. As is clear from evidence reviewed in this book, while shorter treatments can be offered with no loss of efficacy for some disorders, for others, longer therapies, though more costly, are more effective.

A second example is the application of computerized cognitive-behavioral therapy (CBT) and guided self-help, where packages have been developed for patients with anxiety and depression, with the aim of reducing therapist contact time and making CBT more accessible to the large numbers of individuals who may benefit from it. Internet delivery methods are being developed, both as Web-based versions of computer programs for behavioral interventions, with the goal of symptom reduction (Ritterband et al., 2003) and interactive support group methods using Internet "chat room" technology (Taylor & Luce, 2003). These methods have potential advantages in terms of accessibility, convenience, user empowerment, and cost-effectiveness, but with some potential for harm as yet unexplored, such as unmonitored deterioration. A systematic review of 16 studies of computerized CBT, of which 11 were randomized controlled trials, suggested that computerized CBT may be as effective as therapist-led CBT and better than standard care, although the evidence was by no means conclusive (Kaltenthaler et al., 2004). The amount of psychological therapy delivered via the Internet is certain to increase, although how much of this will emerge in the public health sector remains to be seen. However, the case for computerized delivery in terms of cost-effectiveness has not yet been made. In fact, this promising use of new technology may involve considerable clinician time and may itself be expensive to install and use. It has not yet demonstrated a benefit over and above the use of books and self-help manuals in clinician-assisted methods.

These examples demonstrate that research at any given time can only provide evidence to inform investment choices; it does not provide answers that obviate the need for such choices. Psychotherapy research (particularly outcome research) can only be expected unequivocally to answer a very narrow range of questions. Researchers, practitioners, and purchasers all have different and internally coherent requirements of research but sometimes act as if these were identical rather than overlapping. Research findings cannot be "all things to all people"; we need to recognize research as one part of a broader process. We believe that this broader process is capable of offering useful insights to all parties.

Where funders use research simplistically in the design of managed care programs and directives regarding first-line treatments, the reaction of many clinicians is to become suspicious of moves toward (or demands for) evidence-based practice. This adversarial process threatens to set those paying for care against those providing it, and indeed, providers against researchers. In this context, there are clear perils along the path of applying research findings to clinical practice. On the one side is the risk that practitioners reject

psychotherapy research out of hand; on the other is the possibility that purchasers might embrace it uncritically, leading to a cookbook approach to
planning.

EMPIRICALLY SUPPORTED TREATMENTS:
A SIMPLE APPROACH TO RESEARCH-BASED PRACTICE

Partly to protect psychological therapies in a mental health care system dominated by the combined might of biological psychiatry and pharmaceutical com-
panies, the Division of Clinical Psychology of the American Psychological
Association set up a "task force" on the Promotion and Dissemination of Psychological Procedures (American Psychiatric Association, 1993b; Chambless et
al., 1996). Different forms of therapy for different diagnostic categories of mental health problems were appraised to determine which therapies met an explicit
set of criteria for "specific" or "probable" efficacy, in this way generating published lists of "empirically supported therapies" (ESTs). The initiative was controversial (Elliott, 1998). Although many researchers supported it (Barlow,
1996; Crits-Christoph, 1996; Kendall, 1998), others have been highly critical
(Garfield, 1996; Henry, 1998; Shapiro, 1996; Slife, 2004) on scientific, philosophical, and pragmatic grounds.

The majority of therapies meeting efficacy criteria were cognitive-
behavioral. Opinions differ over whether this means that these therapies are
actually more efficacious than others, whether the method is intrinsically
biased in favor of CBT (Messer, 2001), or whether CBT simply had a "head
start" in terms of the quantity of research available (Parry, 2000). If the latter,
one way or another, evidence on the efficacy of other therapies will emerge
from new trials (although there is a risk that once CBT acquires the sobriquet
"empirically supported," research funders may prove reluctant to commission
research on other approaches). This argument has particular force in relation
to psychodynamic therapies that, while widely practiced, were harder to justify solely on the basis of outcome research. For example, in the early 1990s,
two meta-analyses (Crits-Christoph, 1992; Svartberg & Stiles, 1991) found
that psychodynamic therapies had at best equal, and at worst less efficacy than
cognitive-behavioral therapies, particularly in relation to some diagnostic categories, such as depression. More recently, as more RCTs on psychodynamic
and relational approaches are conducted, it becomes plausible to argue that
they also have efficacy, particularly for more complex conditions (e.g., Bateman & Fonagy, 1999; Guthrie et al., 1999).

This debate can easily overemphasize historical differences between therapies and fail to notice the fact that theoretical developments make these
demarcations less clear. For example, some forms of cognitive therapy incorporate some of the strengths of psychodynamic therapy by making links

between unconscious cognitive processes and emotion, and by drawing attention to the role of early life in developing maladaptive interpersonal schemas (Safran & Segal, 1990; Young et al., 2003). At the same time, methods that integrate cognitive and relational approaches have been developed (Ryle & Kerr, 2002; Safran & Muran, 2000). Equally, there are an increasing number of systems for producing replicable psychodynamic formulations (e.g., Horowitz, 1989; Horowitz et al., 1989; Luborsky & Crits-Christoph, 1990; Perry et al., 1989), with good evidence for their reliability and construct validity (Luborsky et al., 1994), and for a link between the capacity of a therapist to utilize these formulations accurately and better outcome (Piper et al., 1991a, 1993).

Whatever arguments there may be against the notion of ESTs alone, this does not justify the hostility of some psychodynamic therapists to evidence-based practice. Historically, psychodynamic therapists have tended to be antipathetic toward scientific investigation on the grounds that the product of such therapy was beyond measurement, or that the changes detected by empirical methods would be so inappropriately unsophisticated as to be not worth collecting. We view this position as demonstrably untenable; there is a large body of empirically sophisticated, high-quality outcome and process–outcome research conducted by a number of psychodynamic research teams (detailed in this book, most particularly in Chapter 16). Even without this research, it would be curious to suggest that *none* of the products of a successful psychodynamic therapy could be measured.

However, the EST approach to evidence-based psychotherapy requires that each separate psychotherapy type, with its theoretical base and set of specific techniques, be treated as if it were a drug. Like a pharmacological substance, each therapy would be tested against placebo or the standard treatment in an RCT, in order to have its safety and efficacy established. Apart from the practical difficulties of funding the hundreds of RCTs required, there are powerful arguments in principle against this approach.

The Department of Health in the United Kingdom in 1996 explicitly eschewed the EST model of evidence-based psychotherapy. This was partly on the grounds that such an approach is a wrong use of research evidence. It fails to take account of strong evidence that although therapy types and specific techniques have an influence on outcome, they do not account for much of the variance in outcome, and that all successful psychotherapies share many common factors (Wampold, 1997). This is well exemplified by the results of another American Psychological Association "task force," mounted by the Psychotherapy division, on the important role of therapy relationships in good psychotherapeutic outcomes, irrespective of therapeutic "brand names" (Norcross, 2001, 2002).

Though it is a truism to state that psychological therapy requires the active participation of the patient, this fact is overlooked in the EST

approach. It should not be surprising to discover that carrying out a therapy
"as planned" requires a coordination of effort between patient and therapist.
A number of patient characteristics are associated with better outcomes, such
as their capacity for thinking about problems, readiness for therapy, motivation, and general adjustment (Clarkin & Levy, 2004). Undoubtedly, some
patients are more responsive to treatment than others. However, the skill of
the good therapist may lie in his/her ability to detect obstacles that would
make it difficult to implement therapy—in other words, a capacity to monitor and maintain the therapeutic alliance. The alliance is a common factor
across therapies (Horvath & Symonds, 1991), but it is more than a reflection
of a bond between patient and therapist. Most models of the alliance (e.g.,
Gaston et al., 1991) note that it also involves a series of technical factors that
are related to the implementation of the particular therapy—not only how to
achieve this implementation but also in what areas. In this context, the therapist's ability to apply clinical judgment and to formulate becomes critical, and
the importance of these factors to successful outcome is recognized across the
spectrum of therapeutic orientations. For example, Persons (1989, 1991) criticized research into cognitive therapy because of its neglect of case formulation in favor of manualization, with the attendant risk that therapy become
formulaic (and by implication less effective). In Stiles and Shapiro's (1994)
comprehensive attack on the drug metaphor in psychotherapy research, a key
argument was the observation that therapists often adapt technique in the service of the therapy relationship and the needs of the patient. This means that
therapy is not a static entity, passively delivered or passively received. More
empirically (and illustrating some of the complexity that this position
implies), Strupp et al. (1988) monitored the progress of trainees in psychodynamic therapy, and found that though they showed increased technical
adherence, they also showed decreased efficacy. Though at first sight this
result is surprising, it appears that trainees focused on psychodynamic technique to the detriment of the therapeutic alliance. A similar phenomenon in
cognitive therapy was noted by Castonguay et al. (1996).

   Therapeutic effectiveness therefore rests on more than narrow technical
competence. There is a risk that the technical sophistication of research trials,
which demand clear causal inference, can overregulate therapy content and
underemphasize the freedom of action available to individual clinicians. This
could widen further the gap between clinical trials and clinical practice in
terms of a relative neglect of the role of clinical judgment. Paradoxically, the
task of applying research findings may call for precisely this capacity on the
part of the clinician—in other words, the ability to see the pertinence of specific discoveries to the individual case.

   This research review might be seen as providing backing for the claim
that there is no good efficacy evidence, one way or the other, for many clinical practices—for example, many psychoanalytic interventions and the eclec-

tic approach that characterizes much psychotherapeutic treatment in practice. Although outcomes of eclectic practice have been underresearched, there is good evidence for the importance of nonspecific, pantheoretical factors. It is possible to argue (e.g., Goldfried, 1995) that the difference in effectiveness of therapies may lie in the differential extent to which they allow common curative factors to come into operation rather than the extent to which specific factors are brought to bear. Where the appropriate research has not yet been done, the absence of evidence for efficacy is not evidence of ineffectiveness, and valuable approaches that offer appropriate and demonstrably clinically effective care should not perish for lack of funding.

Although the EST approach has an appealing simplicity, achieving evidence-based practice in the psychotherapies is not simple. Basing payment decisions on research evidence of efficacy is an apparently straightforward and justifiable process but one that needs to be undertaken with care if it is not to do more harm than good. In particular, there are dangers in funding, purchasing, or reimbursing for only a limited range of treatment "packages" that meet a stated efficacy criterion in relation to certain specified diagnostic groups. Four concerns can be briefly outlined: the issue of comorbidity, the impact of researcher allegiance, the need for effective second-line treatments, and the danger of stifling innovation.

One obvious concern with this funding pattern is that it overlooks the very high rates of comorbidity found in clinical settings (e.g., Kessler et al., 1994). Many presentations of mental ill health are complex, with dual diagnoses; in addition, mental and physical health are closely related in a number of different ways. As well as simple comorbidity, psychological issues are crucial in the prevention, treatment, and management of physical health problems such as cancer, asthma, and heart disease. Psychophysiological processes are directly implicated in many physical diseases (e.g., irritable bowel syndrome, functional dyspepsia, chronic fatigue syndrome, chronic pain, and pelvic inflammatory disorder). Some patients present their emotional and mental health difficulties through physical symptoms (e.g., in somatization disorders). This also has economic consequences. For example, Chisholm et al. (2003), in a study of the economic consequences of depression, found that the physical ill-health associated with depression was associated with increased costs, rather than the depression itself. The cost–offset of psychological therapies in reducing use of other health care services is an important consideration for service provision (Hunsley, 2003; Kocakulah & Valadares, 2003), but is not considered in single-diagnosis treatment guidelines.

As noted in Chapter 2, researcher allegiance effects have been well demonstrated (Luborsky et al., 1999) to the point that in some meta-analyses, the significance of many treatment effects disappears when allegiance is accounted for. Often, the people conducting research on a specific method are themselves enthusiasts for the method, and there is not enough "independent" research, or research led by a team with mixed allegiances. The impact of researcher allegiance may have many causes, such as unconscious bias, choice of measures, and the competence with which a therapy is conducted. For some, this is a major caution in the overreliance on outcome research alone.

A more pragmatic concern is the need for effective second-line treatments. Even an EST, competently delivered, will fail to help a substantial proportion of clients. Some clients may also have strong preferences in the way they wish to be treated. In many health care systems, this gives rise to an imperative to find effective therapies for those who fail to benefit from first-line treatments or reject them. Research rarely focuses on this specific issue.

There is the further danger that in a system in which public sector or insurance-based funding is the determining influence on psychotherapy service delivery and research, overprescriptive purchasing or reimbursement could stifle innovation and development. The history of clinical practice over the past 40 years suggests that this is not an empty, abstract point. Most psychotherapists recognize that clinical practice has seen major developments in this time. Perhaps few would have seen the light of day had overenthusiastic funders constrained treatments to those available and validated during the 1960s; clinicians would have been restricted to a narrow range of behavioral techniques, some effective but of limited application. In fact, cognitive therapy has greatly extended the potential scope and potency of behavior therapy, and even those diminishingly few practitioners who decry what is often referred to as the "cognitive revolution" recognize the enormous stimulus to practice, research, and innovation arising from these newer developments. For us, this represents both a powerful caution against premature foreclosure on therapy provision and a model of good practice; cognitive therapy has developed in the context of a strong commitment to research—a factor that contributes to its current status.

We also take seriously the possibility that those reimbursing for therapy or commissioning services preempt, through funding decisions, clinical judgments on, for example, treatment length and modality. Ironically, rather than encouraging clinical assessment and formulation to be based on research evidence and fostering a model of evidence-based practice, such a policy could actually delay its development.

A BROADER APPROACH TO EVIDENCE-BASED PRACTICE

We have argued that the relationship between research, policy, and practice is complex, and indeed, it can be demonstrated that simple interventions in complex systems are liable to produce unintended outcomes (Willems, 1973). It is therefore important to have a formulation of evidence-based practice that does justice to this complexity and addresses the interplay between different elements of the system.

In 1996, in the first edition of this book, we outlined a formulation of evidence-based practice in psychological therapies in which research, professional consensus, individual clinical practice, service delivery systems, evaluation, and training all play their part in improving patient care through the use of evidence. The same model was promulgated in the United Kingdom in a strategic review of policy on psychotherapy services published by the Department of Health in the same year. We saw this as a way of resolving the potential conflict between researchers, funders, and clinicians to the benefit of the patient. The end point of the model (see Figure 3.1) is the improvement of patient care, and it tries to locate and integrate the differing domains, interests, and concerns of all stakeholders in psychotherapy provision. This approach relates clinical innovation to research, and research to evidence-based practice. It also emphasizes the value of practice-based evidence from service audit, evaluation, and benchmarking, and locates the role of evidence-based practice in maintaining and improving the quality of a clinician's work.

The model can be briefly summarized as follows:

- Psychological therapists develop new approaches, building on existing theory, knowledge, and practice.
- Promising new therapies are not only formally researched to establish efficacy but also field-tested in large samples in natural service systems.
- Both research evidence and clinical consensus inform clinical practice guidelines, in order to clarify areas in which general statements can (or cannot) be made about best practice.
- Standards derived from research-based guidelines are set, and clinical audit is used to determine whether they are achieved.
- Skills deficits revealed by audit are addressed by training.

The model illustrated in Figure 3.1 is explored in more detail in the following sections.

GENERATING KNOWLEDGE: CLINICAL INNOVATION

The starting point for our model is the clinician's wish to improve patient care. Observations from clinical practice, sometimes in combination with theoretical development, result in the development of new techniques or innovation. This can take the form of new therapeutic approaches to traditional clinical problems, or the application of established methods to new areas. Two illustrative examples of the former include dialectical behavior

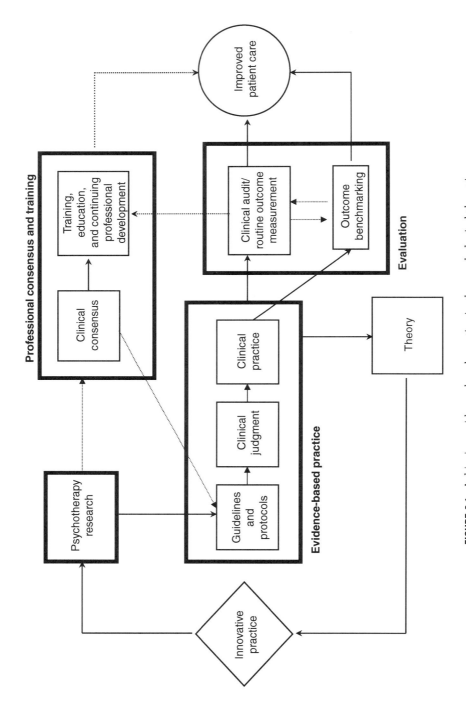

FIGURE 3.1. Achieving evidence-based practice in the psychological therapies.

therapy (DBT) and cognitive analytic therapy (CAT) in the treatment of borderline personality disorder. Examples of the latter (reviewed in this book) are the development of cognitive-behavioral techniques specifically oriented to the management of panic disorder, and the extension of ideas from cognitive therapy to the management of delusions and hallucinations in people with schizophrenia.

Recent years have seen rapid growth in the field of psychotherapy, during which we have learned a great deal about techniques that may be powerful in combating mental health problems. From some perspectives, the very richness of this development represents a major obstacle for rational health care: There are now well over 400 different named therapies, which can be seen as variations on the basic themes within a smaller number of families of theories and techniques. The vast majority of these "brand-name" therapies are totally unevaluated. Outcome research challenges the assumption that each of these approaches is uniquely beneficial, and, in any case, it would be an impossible (and prohibitively expensive task) to test each one in a definitive randomized trial. Process–outcome research, especially "dismantling" studies, has the potential to clarify the degree to which an innovative technique is truly distinctive, or best seen as part of an already established family of therapies.

Clinical creativity is essential both in adapting methods to the needs of the individual case and in ensuring genuine and generalizable innovation. The critical task is to establish systems that do not jeopardize innovation in the effort to standardize practice, systems that manage the tension between clinical creativity and the need for demonstrable effectiveness.

GENERATING KNOWLEDGE: THE RESEARCH CYCLE

Although the development of new therapeutic approaches ultimately calls for formal evaluation, in practice, this is often preceded by a phase of small-scale research aimed at developing the theory and practice of the technique. Salkovskis (1995) describes this process of clinical development in his "hourglass" model, within which initial ideas about technique are first tested through single-case studies. Sometimes relatively less stringent methodological criteria are used at this stage, reflecting both the exploratory nature of the work and likely constraints on time and resources. However, once initial development is complete, there is a requirement for research that conforms to the most rigorous standards of inquiry—equivalent to the pinch in the hourglass. Salkovskis (1995) notes that at this point, considerations of internal validity take priority, recognizing the fact that this raises questions about generalizability (or external validity) but that these can be answered in a subsequent phase of research that returns to an externally valid form of inquiry.

These phases of development are well illustrated in Salkovskis's (1995) account of the development of panic control therapy, along the lines of the hourglass model. A similar progression is recognized by the Medical Research Council in its framework for development and evaluation of randomized controlled trials for complex interventions to improve health (Medical Research Council, 2000).

Formal research evaluation is a process involving several well-recognized and distinct phases. For example, evaluation frequently starts by comparing a new treatment with an established treatment or a "treatment as usual" control group. This form of "pragmatic" trial selects clinically relevant alternative interventions to compare, includes a diverse population of study participants from heterogeneous practice settings, and collects data on a broad range of health outcomes (Tunis et al., 2003). Its aim is to test the efficacy of the new therapy against a relevant alternative or standard care.

Most pragmatic trials in the field of health technology assessment include an economic evaluation, and this is becoming increasingly common for psychological therapies. Costs can be calculated in terms of £/QALY, or specific health outcomes can be costed, for example, the costs of preventing a relapse in depression, or a repetition of deliberate self-harm. However, cost–utility analyses in adequately powered RCTs are rare, and the evidence base on cost-effectiveness is still too sparse to inform resource allocation decisions (Byford et al., 2003b).

This "pragmatic" trial method can be contrasted with the "exploratory" trial (Schwartz & Lellouch, 1967), which is usually undertaken only at a later stage. This addresses scientific questions in a more refined analysis—for example, varying the components of treatment to see which are necessary and sufficient, examining what new components may be added to enhance the likelihood of change, or exploring how much of any particular component (e.g., number of sessions or intensity) is optimally required.

Even later in the research cycle comes the question, Which of two reasonably well-optimized treatments is more effective for a particular population? And later still come questions about patient or therapist characteristics (or other individual-difference factors) that significantly moderate the effectiveness of an approach. Alongside all these lines of inquiry run questions of process: At each of the levels distinguished, we may legitimately ask, "What processes occurring within therapy contribute to treatment outcome?" Process–outcome research is excluded from the narrow "EST" approach but is a vital contribution to our understanding of what processes are effective, irrespective of the therapy "brand-name" and allegiance of the researcher (Luborsky et al., 1999).

Clearly, this body of outcome research takes considerable time to accumulate, and few, if any, psychotherapies have been taken programmatically through this full cycle. It would be impractical and indeed unnecessary to insist that research findings be integrated across all these levels before being applied to clinical guidelines and standards of practice.

SUMMARIZING KNOWLEDGE: CLINICAL PRACTICE GUIDELINES

"If only we knew what we know." This wistful phrase captures the difficulty all health care professionals (including psychological therapists) face in staying up to date with their field in the age of information overload. There is now a massive endeavor to search for, appraise, and summarize evidence in heath care: The field of "knowledge management" includes systematic reviews and meta-analyses, technology appraisal, and guidelines development.

Psychologists and psychotherapists have often used the term "guidelines" when describing recommendations for clinical practice based on clinical experience or unsystematic reviews (e.g., Horvath, 1993; King et al., 2001b; Leibenluft & Goldberg, 1987; Lipsius, 1991), but these rarely meet criteria for systematically developed clinical practice guidelines based on research evidence. Clinical practice guidelines differ from standard literature reviews, chapters, and textbooks in the way they are constructed. Their development is systematic and explicit, usually involving a guideline development group representative of professional and lay interests, and a systematic approach to identifying, evaluating, and incorporating evidence in the guideline. Research evidence is combined with clinical consensus in most guidelines: The research evidence taken from existing or specially commissioned systematic reviews and structured consensus methods is used in developing the guideline recommendations. Different guidelines vary in how research and clinical opinion are weighted and combined. A key factor of clinical guidelines is that whatever evidence base is used, it is clearly indicated for each recommendation, so users of the guideline can evaluate this. Many guidelines grade recommendations using a "hierarchy of evidence," with meta-analyses of RCTs having most weight and clinical opinion least.

Very few systematically developed research-based guidelines have been targeted at psychological therapists or deal with psychological treatments (Parry et al., 2003). One exception already noted is the "empirically supported treatments" guideline arising from the American Psychological Association task force (Chambless & Hollon, 1998). Another is the guideline *Treatment Choice in Psychological Therapies and Counselling* (Department of Health, 2001). This was developed over a 2-year period by a multidisciplinary group, under the auspices of the British Psychological Society. Its recommendations were based on three sources of evidence: a systematic review of existing reviews and meta-analyses, a supplementary review of research evidence appearing more recently than those reviews, and structured, expert consensus. The guideline incorporated service user feedback, was subject to independent peer review, and was formally appraised against criteria for guideline quality. About half the recommendations are general considerations, for example, on recommended length of therapy, the impact of patient and therapist characteristics, and the importance of the therapeutic alliance, irrespective of therapy type. The other recommendations are for first-line therapies for specific conditions, and some contraindications. Although closer to the concept of ESTs than the 1996 Department of Health policy statement (Department of Health, 1996), the guideline explicitly warns against assuming that absence of evidence implies evidence of ineffectiveness, particularly in a field where very few studies demonstrate relative rather than absolute efficacy.

Although there is a lack of research-based guidelines for psychological therapies, medically oriented guidelines increasingly include psychological treatments. Examples include eating disorders (American Psychiatric Association, 1993a), schizophrenia (American Psychiatric Association, 1997; Kendall et al., 2003), and bipolar disorder (Kahn et al., 1996).

Most clinical practice guidelines in medicine are disease or condition-based guidelines of the form "What are the most effective treatments/interventions for condition X?" Parry et al. (2003) argue that this form of guideline is more appropriate to the practice of medicine, where practice decisions are primarily about choice of intervention (e.g., the type of drug to prescribe). Unlike psychological therapists, the practitioner does not have responsibility for quality control of the intervention itself, because it is the pharmaceutical company that is liable for the quality of the drug prescribed. In this respect, psychological therapists are more akin to physical therapists and surgeons, who, as well as deciding on the type of intervention (type of operation or therapy), are responsible for the quality of the intervention delivered. Effectiveness depends as much or more on the skillful undertaking of the intervention by the practitioner, such as the choice of the most appropriate intervention/procedure.

Intervention guidelines define the steps required in the skillful practice of an intervention over time. Treatment manuals, although designed to ensure the integrity of therapy delivery in research trials, are in effect clinical practice guidelines for carrying out that intervention. Such manuals are now available for a wide variety of psychotherapies (Addis, 1997; Najavits et al., 2000; Wilson, 1998), and teaching programs based on these manuals are increasingly delivered (Calhoun et al., 1998). Formal measures of therapist competence (Chevron & Rounsaville, 1983) are another potential source of intervention guidance. The use of these rating scales in practice is not dissimilar to process guidance; therapeutic skills and tasks are derived from professional consensus (in some cases, using structured methods) and specified with clarity and precision in a way that can be rated reliably. Where these measures have been found to predict clinical outcome (Crits-Christoph et al., 1988; Shaw et al.,

1999) there is an evidence-base for their use. Evidence related to measures of the therapeutic alliance (Martin et al., 2000; Safran & Muran, 1996) can be similarly incorporated.

THE ROLE OF CLINICAL JUDGMENT

The challenge of protocol-driven practice is to ensure that clinicians combine clinical experience and sensitivity, together with their knowledge of the research base, recognizing the value and limitation of each resource. Guidelines are designed to assist practitioners and patients in making complex clinical judgments, not to replace the judgment process (Baker, 2001; Haynes et al., 2002). Clinicians retain clinical freedom to do something different but also responsibility for their judgments. Our view is that guidelines and protocols represent the default position for treatment, a statement about the treatment most likely to benefit the average patient presenting with a particular principal diagnosable condition. This statement is consonant with the research base, most of whose conclusions are derived from statistics, and, by definition, therefore rests on findings that are known to apply to perhaps a majority of, but certainly not all, patients in any trial. Against this background, clinicians should be making judgments about whether a particular presentation is normative, and if it is not, whether factors can be identified that militate against the recommended treatment. Practitioners and patients need to decide whether the circumstances of the patient and point of therapy are such that the guideline recommendations are appropriate. Slavish adherence to their recommendations (i.e., 100% adherence) would be equally as worrisome as clinical practice that is never in accordance with guidelines (Parry et al., 2003).

Clinical judgments can only be made in the context of a clear formulation of the patient's difficulties, which requires the integration of skills training, theoretical knowledge, and past clinical experience, as well as an acquaintance with the research literature. This, in combination with the protocol, allows for the fact that, as Kazdin (1991) has commented, no manual (or indeed protocol) of psychological therapy can ever reflect the complexity of treatment and scope of the exchanges between therapist and patient.

In our view, the critical step in this process is the derivation of a formulation of the patient's problems, which the clinician derives through the initial assessment and revises during the course of an intervention. Formulation is the process of constructing explanations of current and past behavior in terms of mental attributes, beliefs, emotions, goals, and intentions—arriving at a set of hypotheses that offers a psychologically coherent model for the patient's problems and suggests the most appropriate mode of intervention (Eells, 1997).

APPLYING KNOWLEDGE: GUIDELINE IMPLEMENTATION, SERVICE AUDIT, AND BENCHMARKING

We have discussed how psychological therapy knowledge is generated and summarized, but despite these activities, there is no evidence-based practice without the successful application of knowledge. This is an essential but highly problematic domain. For example, despite very strong evidence for CBT as a first-line treatment for phobic anxiety, a U.K. national survey showed that very few people with this problem received it (Office of National Statistics, 2000).

Passive dissemination of guidelines does not work: Clinicians do not adopt guideline recommendations without specific intervention, and those interventions that improve standards of care are typically complex, resource-intensive ones (Bauer, 2002; Gilbody et al., 2003). These include academic detailing (termed educational outreach in the United Kingdom), reminders, audits, and feedback.

Traditional clinical audit of therapy delivery derives locally agreed-upon, measurable standards and monitors these over a period of time. This involves choosing the criteria for judging service quality, defining the norms for good care, and setting specific standards of performance. Adherence to these standards is then monitored to determine whether acceptable-quality therapy has been delivered. This process should yield relatively quick feedback for the audit cycle to reveal useful information about what steps can be taken by psychotherapists to improve their practices. The audit of therapy delivery will reveal gaps in therapists' skills and knowledge, and this in turn should help to set the agenda for continuing professional development of the clinicians involved. Though an audit of therapy process might appear to be beyond the resources of many services, in practice, it can be achieved by drawing up a set of guidelines for the broad characteristics of a particular intervention, and establishing the degree to which these match the methods employed by therapists—for example, through a process of peer review or self-administered checklists. Reaudit checks that standards have improved. Clinical practice guidelines have the advantage of focusing and clarifying the audit effort, since the guideline states "the right thing to do," whereas the audit asks, "Has the right thing been done?" and "Has it been done right?" By targeting an audit on those processes derived from research- and consensus-based protocols, a clear link can be established between research and the audit (Firth-Cozens, 1993). The growth of quality-assurance methods in psychological therapies was marked by a special section in the *Journal of Consulting and Clinical Psychology* (Lambert, 2001).

An extension of the clinical audit in psychotherapy is patient-focused research, which aims to improve psychotherapy outcome by monitoring client progress and providing this information to clinicians to guide ongoing treatment, thus bridging the gap between efficacy and effectiveness research and clinical practice (Lambert, 2001, discussed further in Chapter 17). This uses the concept of "expected treatment response" (Lueger et al., 2001) to identify clients who are progressing poorly. Whipple et al. (2003) alerted practitioners to clients whose early progress was poor and helped them use a hierarchical problem-solving strategy derived from research evidence on factors important in psychotherapy outcome. They provided "clinical support tools"—resources intended to assist therapists in assessing the quality of the therapeutic alliance, client motivation to change and its match to treatment tactics, the client's social support network, accuracy of the diagnostic formulation, and appropriateness of a referral for medication. In a randomized controlled trial in a university counseling center, they found that providing feedback on client progress improved outcome, and that the use of clinical support tools significantly improved outcomes over the feedback condition alone.

Service-level outcomes are also an important part of this broader approach to evidence-based practice. It is now much more common for clinical outcomes to be monitored in routine clinical practice, often through the use of outcome measures designed for this purpose (Barkham et al., 2001; Lambert et al., 1996). Service profiling methods allow case mix and service-level outcomes to be summarized and benchmarked against other, similar services (Barkham et al., 2001).

COMPLETING THE FEEDBACK LOOP:
NEW RESEARCH QUESTIONS

A key feature of this approach to evidence-based practice is the ability of the system to reveal gaps in knowledge, which feed back into new theoretical and empirical questions. If all parts of the model are implemented, the system has the opportunity to become self-correcting over time, in a way that is hard to achieve with a simpler method.

For example, therapist competence is an important piece of the evidence-based psychotherapy jigsaw. Competence encompasses skills and knowledge, going beyond technical adherence to a treatment protocol, to describe how well an intervention is delivered. Practice-based evidence, both at the practitioner level and the service level, has great potential to identify gaps in skills where further training is required. Illustrating this, early client-focused research on expected treatment response led Whipple et al. (2003) to devise hierarchical problem-solving strategies and clinical support tools for clinicians, which can be seen as delivering a training intervention.

The ability of the individual practitioner to deliver a specific therapeutic intervention tailored to the needs of the individual client is as important, if not more important, as matching the type of therapy to the presenting mental health problem of the client. As such, it is a key link between evidence-based guidelines and good outcomes in practice, and deserves much more attention than it commonly receives both in research and research-based guidelines. A good example from the United Kingdom is the NICE guideline on the treatment of schizophrenia (Kendall et al., 2003). On the basis of a meta-analytic review of outcome research, NICE recommended that people with positive symptoms in schizophrenia should have access to CBT in the British NHS. However, there are insufficient practitioners with the skills required to implement the methods to the standards that were found effective in the original research, and without monitoring service-based outcomes to identify skills gaps, this could be a very wasteful recommendation. Indeed, putting such an apparently simple recommendation into practice would have implications for many parts of the complex mental health care system, since changes would be required in the practice and roles of psychologists, doctors, nurses, in how teams function, in commissioning of workforce training, in the use of resources, and in the organization of care delivery. There is as yet almost no research evidence on the wider systemic impact of implementing guideline recommendations through health services management, and this form of evidence has to derive from practice settings.

Where outcomes in clinical practice are poorer than those predicted by research, and this cannot be accounted for by failings in the quality of service delivery, attention is drawn to gaps in our knowledge concerning that treatment method. Considering ways of accounting for these discrepancies yields further research questions—for example, in terms of either client or therapist characteristics, or the necessary and sufficient components of a treatment strategy. Ideally, further clinical development and innovation follow, as does refinement of the clinical protocol.

The evaluation process as a whole should permit a more general evaluation and planning of a service on the part of management. Naturally, this should include lead clinicians, as well as purchasers of services. Given that all these groups have improvement of patient care as their collective priority, there is a priori little need for conflict in making appropriate changes to a service in line with data obtained. Even more important, a good-quality service becomes defined as the end result of a process of integration, linking research with clinical findings arising from clinical practice, and using this as a springboard to further innovation, in this way ensuring a fully recursive process and that improvements in patient care are continuous.

SUMMARY

Changes in the health care delivery system in the United States, the United Kingdom, and other Western European countries have inevitably led to increased concern about the cost-effectiveness of all medical interventions. Psychological therapies, along with other forms of mental health intervention, are increasingly subject to scrutiny from funders of these services. They, along with clinicians and service managers, raise questions about the likely efficacy of therapy for particular patient populations. At root, these are the same questions psychotherapy research has attempted to answer from a scientific stance. However, since the motives each has for asking its questions are quite distinct, it follows that the criteria used for judging whether the answers are helpful will also be different.

No single answer can meet the requirements of these stakeholders; each is addressing different issues within an ongoing process, which we describe in our model of evidence-based practice. A simple reliance on "ESTs" will not deliver improvements in services. For research to be put to effective use requires other components, such as the achievement of a professional consensus, the preparation and implementation of guidelines for good practice, service-based evaluation methods, and feedback loops to new research questions. It is our view that if all these components are in place, improvements in patient care will result.

CHAPTER 4

DEPRESSION

DEFINITIONS

DSM-IV-TR describes a number of subcategories of depression; those particularly relevant to research studies are defined as follows (adapted from Wells, 1985).

Major Depressive Disorder

Major depressive disorder (MDD) is characterized by one or more major depressive episodes and the absence of manic episodes. A major depressive episode is defined by depressive mood or loss of interest or pleasure in almost all usual activities, accompanied by other depressive symptoms. These include disturbances in appetite, weight, and sleep; psychomotor agitation or retardation; decreased energy; feelings of worthlessness or guilt; difficulty concentrating or thinking; and thoughts of death or suicide, or suicidal attempts. DSM-IV-TR specifies that at least five of nine specific depressive symptoms must be present nearly every day for at least 2 weeks to make a diagnosis of MDD, and that the symptoms cause clinically significant distress or impairment in social, occupational, or other important areas of functioning. Depressive episodes are distinguished from normal bereavement reactions.

Dysthymic Disorder

This disorder is characterized by depressed mood or loss of interest in nearly all usual activities, though symptom severity is not sufficient to meet the criteria for MDD. The disorder is, by definition, chronic. Symptoms should be present for at least 2 years, and a diagnosis cannot be made if patients are symptom-free for more than 2 months in any 2-year period. It is character-ized by depressed mood for most of the day, together with at least two of the following six symptoms: poor appetite, insomnia or hypersomnia, low energy, low self-esteem, poor concentration, and feelings of hopelessness. For diagnostic purposes, these symptoms should be severe enough to cause clini-cally significant distress or impairment in social, occupational, or other areas of functioning.

"Double Depression"

Patients with dysthymic disorder frequently present with a superimposed MDD; this is usually referred to as "double depression."

PREVALENCE AND NATURAL HISTORY
Prevalence

Only a portion of individuals with mental health problems present to family physicians or mental health professionals (e.g., Bebbington et al., 2000a; Goldberg & Huxley, 1980). Because of this, estimating treatment need is better done through community-based surveys rather than relying on data from clinical services. Two large-scale community surveys provide data on the prevalence of psychiatric disorders in the United States. The National Institute of Mental Health (NIMH) Epidemiologic Catchment Area (ECA) program was a five-site project sampling approximately 20,000 adults (Robins & Regier, 1991). The National Comorbidity Survey (NCS; Blazer et al., 1994) had a slightly more restricted age range, and interviewed approx-imately 8,000 adults between ages 15 and 54. The prevalence rates derived from these surveys need to be interpreted cautiously; for example, there is a risk that they are inflated by individuals whose distress is transient. Deriving a "correct" prevalence rate that accounts for the clinical significance of symp-toms is difficult and controversial. Narrow et al. (2002) have recomputed prevalence rates from the ECA and NCS surveys, taking into account the degree to which symptoms resulted in help-seeking behavior and led to sig-nificant levels of distress (see Table 4.1). In addition, they attempted to rec-oncile differences in prevalence rates between the surveys, some of which relate to methodological differences. Their approach has been criticized as inappropriately robust (Wakefield & Spitzer, 2002), and it is clear, that while presentation to services appears to be linked to the severity of symptoms (Bebbington et al., 2000b), lack of help seeking cannot be assumed to indi-cate that distress is unimportant. Nonetheless, the revised rates are cited here (and in Appendix III), since they probably yield a more accurate indicator of service need.

TABLE 4.1. One-Year Prevalence Rates for MDD and Dysthymic Disorder for Adults Ages 18–54

	ECA (corrected for clinical significance)	NCS (corrected for clinical significance)	Combined ECA + NCS estimate after correction for clinical significance
MDD	5.4 (4.6)	8.9 (5.4)	4.5
Dysthymia	5.7 (1.7)	2.5 (1.8)	1.6

Note. Data from Narrow et al. (2002).

The ECA and NCS estimate 1-year prevalence for MDD at 5.4% and 8.9%; corrected for clinical significance, these figures lower to 4.6% and 5.4%, respectively. Narrow et al.'s (2002) estimate, which combines data from both surveys, is 4.5%. For dysthymic disorder, the ECA and NCS estimates are 5.7% and 2.5%, respectively; with correction for clinical significance, these reduce to 1.7% and 1.8%, respectively; the combined estimate is 1.6%. Other reviews derive somewhat different (uncorrected) rates. Angst (1992), reviewing 17 studies, suggests that 1-year prevalence rates for MDD lie between 2.6 and 6.2%, and for dysthymic disorder, between 2.3 and 3.7%. Lifetime prevalence rates vary between 4.4 and 19.5%. Angst also reports data from a Swiss prospective community survey carried out (to date) over 10 years. This was based on multiple interviews and hence avoided problems of estimating prevalence based on recall. Lifetime prevalence to age 30 of MDD was 14.5%, with around half of affected individuals seeking treatment.

The prevalence of depression varies by gender and age; prevalence of MDD in the ECA and NCS was almost twice as high in women as men, and greater in younger adults. In part, this may reflect the greater willingness of younger adults to admit to mental health problems (Taube & Barrett, 1985; Weissman et al., 1988), or problems of recall when older respondents are interviewed in cross-sectional surveys (Fombonne, 1994). However, there is evidence that prevalence within younger age groups is increasing (Burke et al., 1991), though the degree to which this is associated with comorbid substance abuse is unclear. Furthermore, there is some agreement that overall rates of depression are increasing (Fombonne, 1998b; Klerman & Weissman, 1989).

Natural History

Most studies of "natural" history monitor longitudinal outcomes for patients offered "treatment as usual" (TAU). Over a 2-year period, Wells et al. (1992)

followed up 626 outpatients; the sample included patients diagnosed with MDD, dysthymic disorder, and double depression, and also contained clients with subthreshold depressive symptoms. Patients with MDD had a 42% probability of remission[1] in the first year, and a 60% probability of remission in the second year, if none had occurred in the first year. Clients with double depression had a rather different course, depending on the severity of their symptoms. Those with more severe symptoms had a 37% likelihood of remission in the first year; if no remission occurred by this point, there was only a 16% probability of remission in the second year. Both dysthymic patients and those with subthreshold symptoms of depression were at considerable risk of suffering an episode of MDD over the study period. Half the patients with an initial diagnosis of dysthymic disorder and 25% of patients with subthreshold symptoms of depression (with or without a prior history of depression) experienced an episode of MDD over the 2-year period. Data from patient samples in field trials for DSM-IV-TR confirm this pattern; 79% of patients with dysthymic disorder eventually developed MDD (McCullough et al., 1992). The poorest clinical outcomes were found in patients with double depression; there was a particularly low rate of remission in patients with both double depression and high initial symptom severity. Patients with dysthymic disorder (even in the absence of MDD) had higher levels of depressive symptoms over the 2-year period of the study than patients with MDD alone, despite the fact that dysthymic disorder is defined by the presence of less severe (if persistent) depressive symptoms. In addition, patients with dysthymic disorder were rated as having poorer social and emotional functioning than those with MDD.

Keller and Shapiro (1982) and Keller et al. (1983) suggest that patients with double depression tend to have a shorter episode of MDD but are also likely to relapse more quickly than those with MDD alone. Double depressives appear to have a faster "cycle time"; over a 2-year period, 62% of them had completed a cycle of recovery and relapse, compared to 33% of the MDD group.

---

[1] Recovery and relapse are problematic terms unless specified, and are used inconsistently in the literature (Prien et al., 1991). Frank et al. (1991) have proposed the adoption of the following definitions, many of which have been adopted by researchers but (where relevant) with somewhat differing time courses:

Partial remission: A period when improvement of a sufficient magnitude is observed, but during which the patient continues to show more than minimal symptoms.

Full remission: A relatively brief period during which the individual is asymptomatic.

Recovery: A remission of a longer period, usually indicating recovery from the index episode (though not from the illness per se).

Relapse: A return of symptoms satisfying criteria for the full syndrome that occurs during the period of remission, but before recovery.

Recurrence: The appearance of a new episode of MDD arising during a period of recovery.

Long-term monitoring confirms a pattern of vulnerability to relapse for people with MDD. Piccinelli and Wilkinson (1994) reviewed 50 naturalistic follow-up studies of in- and outpatients with unipolar depression, carried out between 1970 and 1993. Although recovery rates increase over time (on average, 53% of patients will recover at least briefly by 6 months), one-fourth of the patients will have suffered a recurrence of the index episode within 1 year. Seventy-five percent of patients followed up for 10 years suffered a further episode of depression, and 10% of patients suffered persistent depression. Mueller et al. (1999) followed up patients over 15 years; all were in receipt of TAU. Of 380 patients who had recovered from an index episode of MDD, a cumulative proportion of 85% relapsed over this period. Of a further 105 patients who had recovered and remained well over 5 years, a cumulative proportion of 58% relapsed. Though there were indications that TAU included suboptimal delivery of medication, there was little information available regarding the use of psychosocial interventions. Demographic or clinical characteristics did not predict relapse, though there were indications that individuals who had recovered but continued to experience subthreshold symptoms were particularly vulnerable, a pattern found in other studies (e.g., Judd et al., 1998b).

Summary

Studies of the prevalence and natural history of depression have a number of implications for research. Although precise estimation is complicated, it is clear that depression is a relatively common syndrome affecting at least 4.5% of the population, with prevalence among women about double that among men. The course of depression appears to differ according to subtype (MDD, dysthymic disorder, or double depression). It is likely that 80% of patients with dysthymic disorder will eventually develop an MDD, suggesting that dysthymic disorder and acute depression are variants of a similar condition. Relapse is a serious challenge: 85% of patients followed up over 15 years, and 75% of patients followed up over 10 years will have suffered a further episode of MDD, and 10% of these will have endured persistent depression. The probability of relapse is increased in patients with more than three previous episodes of MDD but is greatest in patients with a diagnosis of dysthymic disorder; these patients show a faster cycle of recovery and relapse than those with MDD alone. Even among those patients who have "recovered," subthreshold symptoms are common and are associated with an increased likelihood of relapse.

The risk—indeed, the probability—of relapse has obvious implications for treatment trials. The effectiveness of a treatment needs to be judged not only by its capacity to manage an index episode but also by its ability to maintain remission. This poses a challenge, in part, because on the basis of figures given above, long-term follow-up of at least 2 years would be necessary to provide a conclusive result that is not confounded with the natural history of this disorder. It is also likely that outcome in clinical trials will be influenced by case mix, and particularly by the presence of patients with double depression or a history of recurrent MDD. Because of the exclusion criteria applied in at least some research trials, it is possible that the clinical population will contain comparatively more patients with chronic depression and dysthymic disorder. This may lead to overestimation of treatment effects; poorer outcomes might be expected in clinical practice than in trials. However, as an increasing number of studies concern themselves with "treatment resistant" patients, this may be a less pertinent issue than before.

LANDMARK STUDIES OF EFFICACY

Subsequent chapters review individual studies in the context of meta-analyses and qualitative reviews. This chapter adopts a different strategy, describing in some detail a small number of high-quality individual studies that help to contextualize the broader body of evidence. These trials give indications of the acute and longer term efficacy of the major treatment approaches in this area (cognitive-behavioral therapy, interpersonal psychotherapy, short-term psychodynamic therapy, and medication), and of the challenge posed by relapse.

Cognitive-Behavioral Therapy and Interpersonal Psychotherapy: NIMH Treatment of Depression Collaborative Research Program

This major and widely cited research program (summarized in Elkin, 1994) set a standard against which other studies can be judged. Patients were randomized to receive one of four interventions: cognitive-behavioral therapy (CBT; Beck et al., 1979), interpersonal psychotherapy (IPT; Klerman et al., 1984), imipramine plus clinical management (IMI-CM), or placebo plus clinical management (PLA-CM). Clinical management consisted of a weekly meeting of 20–30 minutes to discuss medication, side effects, and the patient's clinical status. In addition, and where necessary, support, encouragement, and direct advice were also offered. On this basis, it is worth noting that both medication conditions contained psychotherapeutic elements. This research design has been misinterpreted as a test of therapy against medication (Elkin, 1994); more accurately, the intention was to use medication condition as a "benchmark" against which to compare the psychological therapies.

The study was carried out at three research sites in the United States. Five hundred sixty outpatients were initially screened, essentially ensuring that patients met criteria for a DSM-III-R diagnosis of unipolar depression.

Two hundred fifty patients, all moderately to severely depressed, were selected for the trial; 239 actually entered it. Of these, 60% had been depressed for more than 6 months; for only 36% was this a first episode of depression.

Treatments were carried out by experienced therapists (10 each in IPT and pharmacotherapy, eight in CBT) chosen for their expertise in applying their respective therapy and supervised regularly throughout the clinical trial. To ensure that therapies were conducted as intended, sessions were taped, and the process of therapy was checked against measures of therapy adherence. Though there were some differences in attrition from each condition, these were not statistically significant. Rates of dropout across treatment modalities were as follows: 23% ($n = 14$) for IPT, 32% ($n = 19$) for CBT, 33% ($n = 19$) for IMI–CM, and 40% ($n = 25$) for PLA–CM.

Patients were assessed before treatment and at 4, 8, 12, and 16 weeks, and followed up at 6, 12, and 18 months. During therapy, a number of standardized measures of symptomatic status were employed (including the Hamilton Rating Scale for Depression [HRSD] and the Beck Depression Inventory [BDI]). After discharge, progress was assessed using a semistructured interview designed to assess the longitudinal course of psychiatric disorders (the Longitudinal Interval Follow-Up Evaluation II [LIFE-II]; Keller et al., 1987).

Analyses were carried out on three overlapping sets of patient samples: a completer sample ($n = 155$) that had received at least 12 sessions or 15 weeks of therapy; the sample of patients that had entered treatment and received at least four sessions of therapy ($n = 204$); and the total (intent to treat) sample of patients that had entered the trials ($n = 239$).

Posttherapy, the general direction of results was similar on all measures and in all samples (Elkin et al., 1989), with patients who received IMI–CM having the lowest symptomatic scores, PLA–CM the most symptomatic, and the psychotherapies in between and usually closer to IMI–CM. The magnitude of these differences was not large, and pairwise comparison of treatment conditions revealed no differences between therapies or between therapies and IMI–CM.

In addition to comparisons of relative scores, a comparison of "recovery rates" was carried out—clearly a more stringent and clinically relevant analysis. Recovery was defined as an HRSD score ≤ 6 and a BDI score ≤ 9. No significant differences between treatment groups were found employing the BDI data, though, in part, this seems to reflect the degree of improvement in the PLA–CM condition. Using HRSD data, significant differences were apparent. Pairwise comparisons using the complete sample of patients indicated that those who received IMI–CM and IPT were significantly more likely to recover than those who had received PLA–CM; a trend toward significance was apparent in the other two patient samples. There were, however, no significant differences between therapies or between therapies and IMI–CM in any patient sample.

All treatment conditions resulted in a significant improvement pre- to posttreatment—perhaps surprisingly, this included PLA–CM. Outcome for patients in the therapy conditions was equivalent to that in other treatment trials (reviewed below). The lack of significant differences seems attributable to the good performance of PLA–CM. However, as already noted, PLA–CM does contain a number of nonspecific therapeutic elements; in a sense, comparisons between it and the psychotherapies may reflect differences between such elements and the technical interventions embodied in the therapies.

Ogles et al. (1995) reanalyzed data for the completer sample of patients, arguing that the Elkin et al. (1989) analysis did not consider the reliability of change from pre- to posttherapy, that there was no attempt to consider the clinical significance of multiple measures simultaneously, and that the possibility of reliable deterioration was not determined. Using Jacobson and Truax's (1991) method, it is apparent that the proportion of clients showing reliable change was statistically equivalent across treatments, with little evidence of deterioration—in fact, observed at a rate of between 2 and 5% dependent on the measure employed. If clinically significant change is determined by movement into the functional distribution of scores across instruments (within 2 standard deviations of the mean for the normal population), the immediate impact of therapy across all treatments was equivalent when using the BDI and the HRSD. This further emphasizes the substantial improvements achieved by clients within the PLA–CM group (e.g., 62% achieved clinically significant change using the BDI as a measure). However, there were significant differences across treatments on measures of general symptomatology (using the Hopkins Symptom Checklist [HSCL-90, Lipman et al., 1979], equivalent in most respects to the Symptom Checklist 90 [SCL-90; Derogatis, 1977]). Thus, on this instrument, 78%, 93%, and 87% of the CBT, IPT, and IMI–CM groups, respectively, were placed in the functional distribution, contrasted to 65% of the PLA–CM group.

Although (as noted earlier) Elkin et al.'s (1989) analysis found statistically significant differences between treatments only when the HRSD was employed as a measure, Ogles et al. (1995) noted that reanalysis for both clinical significance and concordance across measures showed a high level of agreement. Thus, for 118 (73%) of 162 clients, all three measures were in agreement regarding the clinical significance of the change pre- to posttreatment.

A secondary analysis (Elkin et al., 1989) considered the degree to which initial symptom status influenced outcome. Two definitions of severity were employed. In the first, severity was defined as an HRSD score of ≥ 20; in the second, a Global Assessment Scale (GAS) score of ≤ 50 was used (tapping both depressive symptomatology and functional impairment). The results suggested that for the less depressed group, there were no significant differences between treatments. However, for the more depressed group (and contrasting the three patient samples), pairwise comparisons using the HRSD revealed consistently lower scores for IMI-CM than for PLA-CM, and some significant differences for IPT compared to PLA-CM. Using the recovery criterion, there were no significant differences between treatment groups for less severely depressed patients, but, again, patients receiving both IMI-CM and IPT were significantly more likely to recover than those in PLA-CM. However, no significant differences were found between therapies.

Reanalysis of these data (Elkin et al., 1995) using more powerful statistical techniques (random regression models) confirms the equivalence of intervention methods for less depressed patients but indicates greater differentiation among the therapies for the more depressed sample. For these patients, using both HRSD and BDI scores as outcome measures, IMI-CM and IPT appeared equally effective. IMI-CM was significantly more effective than CBT or PLA-CM; IPT showed a trend ($p < .08$) toward greater efficacy. CBT was no more effective than PLA-CM. When the GAS was used as an outcome measure, a different pattern emerged, with IMI-CM being more effective than the other three interventions, all of which showed equal relative efficacy.

These analyses are exploratory, but they do suggest that initial patient severity may be an important factor in considering treatment allocation—particularly the finding that for patients with lower levels of depression, PLA-CM (which could be considered a "minimal support" intervention) was as effective as the active therapies. Although there is evidence that IMI-CM was particularly effective with more severely depressed and functionally impaired patients, it should be noted that it was no more effective than IPT when patients were symptomatically rather than functionally impaired. A number of researchers have interpreted these results to indicate that medication is necessarily the treatment of choice in more severe depression (Elkin, 1994). These results suggest that some caution should be taken in this regard.

Follow-up of patients continued over 18 months and is reported in Shea et al. (1992a). In this analysis, the question of interest was the fate of the patients who had met a stringent criteria for recovery—at least 8 weeks following completion of treatment with minimal or no symptoms. Relapse was defined as the presence of at least 2 weeks of MDD-level symptoms over the 18-month follow-up period.

Only 20% of the original sample and 24% of the patients with follow-up data met the criteria for recovery with no relapse. Of those entering therapies, 24% of those receiving CBT remained recovered without relapse at 18 months, compared with 23% for IPT, 16% for IMI-CM, and 16% for PLA-

CM. Of those with follow-up data at 6 months, 30% in CBT, 26% in IPT, 19% in IMI-CM, and 20% in PLA-CM were recovered without relapse at 18 months. Despite the presence of a trend for psychotherapy to be superior to IMI-CM, there are no statistical differences in these rates. However, it should be noted that, as is the case for any study that attempts a naturalistic long-term follow-up, there are problems in interpreting the data statistically: Because the groups no longer benefit from the original randomization, attributions about effects cannot be traced to the treatment modality employed (Shea et al., 1992a).

Overall, it is clear that rather few patients recover and remain well with 16 weeks of treatment, and a clear conclusion from this study is that interventions of this length are not sufficient to maintain functioning in the majority of patients. This result is not, perhaps, surprising in the light of evidence considered earlier regarding the natural course of depression.

Although the differences between CBT and IPT in this trial were not substantive, relative to other studies, CBT did perform less robustly than many of its practitioners would have expected, and this has led to debate about the competence of its delivery and supervision (e.g., Hollon & Beck, 1994). There are suggestions that CBT performed much better at one site, and IPT performed more poorly at another (Elkin, 1994). Though these data have not been confirmed in later analyses (Elkin et al., 1996), these results have continued to be contested (Jacobson & Hollon, 1996a, 1996b). Unfortunately, even in a trial as large as this, statistical power reduces markedly when investigators seek site differences for specific forms of therapy conducted with high-severity patients, because at this level of stratification, the number of available "data points" is very low.

Notwithstanding the need to accept the data as reported, there may be some indications that CBT and IPT were delivered at different levels of competence, though whether this reflects an actual or methodological difference is unclear. As before, sessions were taped and monitored, and therapists were alerted when their performance was felt to be problematic. On this basis, alerts were issued for 33% of monitored CBT tapes but only 3% of IPT tapes (Elkin, 1999). However, CBT and IPT supervisors had different procedures for scoring competence, and in some respects, the standards for CBT do seem to have been more stringent. While this may—or may not—be grounds for questioning the "adequacy" of treatment delivery, it may also raise questions about the impact of deviations from treatment fidelity in routine clinical settings, where expert therapists and intensive supervision are rarely available.

The data set from this trial is now publicly available, and a number of post hoc analyses have been undertaken, attempting to link therapy, therapist, and patient characteristics to outcome. These are considered later in this chapter and in Chapter 16, along with other process studies.

Cognitive-Behavioral Therapy Alone and in Combination with Medication: University of Minnesota and University of Pennsylvania–Vanderbilt University Studies

Perhaps because of its scale and rigor, findings from the NIMH trial have been highly influential, particularly in its conclusions regarding the relative efficacy of CBT and medication. This issue is addressed in two trials by Hollon, DeRubeis, and colleagues, who have examined the impact of these therapies in moderately to severely depressed individuals.

The first trial at the University of Minnesota (Evans et al., 1992; Hollon et al., 1992) aimed to examine both response to acute treatment and patterns of posttherapy relapse. On this basis, 107 patients (all with BDI scores ≥ 20) were randomized to one of four treatment arms. In the first, three patients received 12 weeks of acute treatment: CBT alone, IMI-CM, or CBT and imipramine combined. The fourth condition comprised 12 weeks of acute treatment with imipramine, followed by 12 months of maintenance medication. Clinical management was similar to that employed in the NIMH trial. Treatments were administered by experienced therapists and were somewhat more intensive than in the NIMH study, with 20 sessions planned for the 12-week period. Sixty-four patients completed all treatments; although attrition was high, there was no significant difference in the rate between conditions.

At the end of treatment (and, at this stage, considering both medication conditions together), all three treatments showed equal efficacy, though with a nonsignificant trend toward better results for the combined treatment group. In contrast to the NIMH study, there was no indication of a differential response with more severely depressed patients (although the sample size was perhaps too small to allow this comparison).

At 2-year follow-up, clear differences were found between treatment groups. Recovery was defined along the same lines as in the NIMH trial, though relapse was indicated by a consistently elevated BDI score. Although 44 patients (of the 64 completing treatment) were followed up, the low number of patients in each treatment cell necessitates some caution in interpreting the treatment results. Nonetheless, adjusting for patient attrition from the study, patients receiving medication without continuation showed the greatest rate of relapse (50%), all within the first 4 months of follow-up. In contrast, the relapse rate of patients receiving cognitive therapy (either alone or in combination with medication) was 18%. Most of these relapses occurred later than in the medication–no–continuation condition; mean survival times were 17.4 ± 1.2 months and 3.3 ± 0.4 months, respectively. Relapse rate in the medication continuation condition was intermediate, with a 32% relapse rate and a mean survival time of 17.3 ± 2.1 months. A secondary analysis indicated that relapse rates in the two cognitive therapy conditions were not different from one another.

More recent (and more substantive) research conducted at the University of Pennsylvania and at Vanderbilt University extends this work in a larger sample of moderately to severely depressed patients treated both with CBT and selective serotonin reuptake inhibitors (SSRIs) (DeRubeis & Amsterdam, 2002; Hollon & Shelton, 2002). Entry criteria included a current episode of MDD, with an HRSD score ≥ 20. Two hundred forty patients met these criteria, and selection for appropriate severity and refractoriness appears to have been successful: Approximately half met criteria for chronic depression, with a mean duration of the current episode of 46 months; about 75% met criteria for recurrent depression, with a mean of 2.4 prior episodes of MDD.

In order to carry out the study of relapse described below, treatment assignment was asymmetric: 120 patients received antidepressant medication, 60 received pill placebo, and 60 received CBT. Active treatments were delivered over 16 weeks; those in receipt of placebo were monitored over 8 weeks, at which point active treatment was offered (on the basis that withholding active intervention over a longer period would be unethical). Medication was delivered by pharmacotherapists expert in treating depression, who met with patients once weekly in the first 4 weeks, then biweekly for the remaining 12 weeks. All patients were initially treated with paroxetine; those who showed no evidence of a response at 8 weeks had their medication augmented with lithium, desipramine, or Wellbutrin.

A similar pattern of results was obtained using both a categorical analysis (which identified patients as responders if they had an HRSD score ≤ 12) and hierarchical linear modeling (a form of growth curve analysis that models the progress of each individual patient rather than aggregating patients' scores in the form of means). At 8 weeks, medication patients showed a faster rate of response than those receiving CBT or placebo; respective response rates were 50%, 43%, and 25%. At 16 weeks, both active treatments showed an equivalent response rate of 58%, though there was a significant treatment-by-site interaction; on one site, CBT was superior to medication, at the other, medication was superior to CBT. Response rates at each site for medication were 48% and 67%, and for CBT, 63% and 53%. Further post hoc analysis is required to determine any reasons for these differences, but initial observation suggests that on one site, therapists were less experienced in CBT, and their patients tended to be more comorbid (two factors that might be expected to reduce response rates). Cross-site differences in CBT were less striking than for medication. While differences in prescribing practice may be relevant, it is not clear why such a large difference should emerge, especially given the particular care taken in this study to ensure that pharmacotherapy was delivered according to the highest standards.

One hundred four patients (58% of the sample assigned to active treatment) were classified as treatment responders and entered the next 12-month follow-up phase of the study, which focused on relapse prevention. The 69 responders to medication were randomized either to continue their medication or to be switched to pill placebo; all continued to receive regular clinical management. Patients who had responded to CBT ($n = 34$) were permitted up to three maintenance sessions. Relapse was defined by an HRSD score ≥ 14 over 2 successive weeks, or if patients met criteria for MDD. Patients who had received CBT were significantly less likely to relapse than those switched to placebo (31% vs. 76%); patients maintained on medication showed statistically equivalent relapse rates to those who had received CBT (47%). Adjusting these figures for patients who were nonadherent to medication gave a relapse rate for continuation medication of 42%.

Taken together, these studies suggest that CBT may be a robust intervention in individuals with moderate to severe depression. The more recent trial was conducted to rigorous methodological standards, and indicates that the capacity of CBT both to achieve and to maintain recovery from acute episodes is equivalent to a regimen of carefully administered maintenance pharmacotherapy, This result stands in contrast to that from the acute-phase of the NIMH study, though the extent of cross-site differences—most particularly for medication—reinforces the need for caution in interpreting outcomes from individual studies, no matter how well conducted.

Cognitive-Behavioral Therapy
and Short-Term Psychodynamic–Interpersonal Psychotherapy:
Sheffield Psychotherapy Project

As well as contrasting CBT and short-term psychodynamic/interpersonal therapy (and representing a rare empirical test of the latter technique), this trial was designed to explore a number of methodological and clinical issues raised by prior research. Most pertinent to this review, the study design stratified patients in relation to symptom severity and allocated them to treatments of different length (either 8- or 16-session treatments). The first issue emerged as a concern in the NIMH trial, but on the basis of a secondary analysis of their data. The second reflects early work on dose–response relationships (Howard et al., 1986), which suggested that treatment gains are most rapid early in therapy, with improvements in subsequent sessions showing a negatively accelerating "dose–response relationship."

The study was therefore concerned with (1) the efficacy of the two different therapies, (2) the influence of initial symptom severity, and (3) the impact of offering differing lengths of treatment (and relatedly, any evidence for a differential speed of action between the therapies). A total of 257 patients was assessed; 169 met criteria for DSM-III-R and Present State Examination (PSE; Wing et al., 1974) definitions of major depressive disorder. Thirty-nine percent were referred by their family physicians or mental health services; the remainder were self-referred. Clients were stratified into those with low (BDI score 16–20), moderate (BDI score 21–26), or high (BDI score ≥ 27) levels of depression.

Following assessment, patients were randomly allocated to CBT or psychodynamic/interpersonal therapy, with treatment lasting either 8 or 16 weeks. Because randomization took place in the context of stratification by the severity of depression, the design had 12 "cells," and patient allocation continued until each cell had been occupied by 10 patients (see Table 4.2).

Overall, both therapies were found to be equally effective, to exert their effects with equal rapidity, and to have equivalent results for clients at all three levels of symptom severity. However, an interaction was found between initial symptom level and duration of therapy. Patients with mild or moderate depression did equally well with either 8 or 16 weeks of therapy. In contrast, those with severe depression showed significantly better outcomes when they received 16 weeks of therapy compared to those who received only 8 weeks.

One hundred three of the 117 completer patients were followed up at 1 year (Shapiro et al., 1995) and classified as recovered (asymptomatic at least 4 months, defined as a BDI score < 9), as having relapsed (a BDI score ≥ 15 during a period of remission from the previous episode but before meeting the criterion for recovery), or as having a recurrence (BDI score ≥ 15 after the criterion for recovery has been met). Of the 103 patients, 52% were treatment responders: 57% maintained their gains, 32% partially maintained gains, and 11% relapsed or had a recurrence. Thus, the proportion of all patients entering the trial and remaining asymptomatic from posttreatment to 1-year follow-up is 29% (a figure comparable to that found in the NIMH study).

No overall differences were found in outcome or maintenance of gains between CBT and psychodynamic/interpersonal therapy, nor was the interaction between initial symptom severity and duration of therapy maintained. However, there was an interaction between treatment type and duration, with those patients receiving eight sessions of psychodynamic/interpersonal therapy doing less well at 1 year on all measures. In addition, there was a nonsignificant trend toward better maintenance of gains with 16-session CBT, contrasted to the three other treatment combinations. Furthermore, there was some evidence that the patients who were more depressed initially

TABLE 4.2. Allocation of 120 Patients to Treatment Cells in Shapiro et al. (1994)

Level of depression	Treatment type	Length of treatment
High	CBT *or* psychodynamic/exploratory	8 *or* 16 sessions
Moderate	CBT *or* psychodynamic/exploratory	8 *or* 16 sessions
Low	CBT *or* psychodynamic/exploratory	8 *or* 16 sessions

tended not to maintain their gains, regardless of treatment modality or duration.

Shapiro et al. (1994) tentatively raise a number of questions about the degree to which their findings have direct implications for service delivery. Their posttherapy data suggest that patients with mild or moderate depression will gain no more from 16 sessions than they would from eight; only patients with severe depression would derive extra benefit from (and hence justify) longer therapy. However, follow-up data suggest a more cautious interpretation, since the pattern of maintenance of gains suggests that simple recovery is not an adequate measure of the efficacy of brief interventions. In particular, eight sessions of exploratory therapy appears to be too little, and there is some evidence favoring 16 sessions of CBT. Overall, poorer maintenance was evident in patients with greater levels of initial distress. This may caution against too marked a contraction of therapy contact time, particularly for more depressed patients.

A further concern regarding this study is the extent to which its results can be generalized from a research to a clinical sample. Although it is clear that patients met study criteria for depression, the majority (approximately 60%) were self-referred or referred through occupational sources, raising some questions about the comparability of these patients to the usual clinical population. This question was partially addressed by the Collaborative Psychotherapy Project (CPP; Barkham et al., 1996a), an explicit attempt to replicate the Sheffield project within a standard clinical context. This was carried out by colleagues of those involved in the Sheffield project, and, though (for practical reasons) smaller scale, used a similar methodology and research design. Thirty-six patients of low, medium, and high depression severity were allocated to CBT or psychodynamic IPT for 8 or 16 sessions (see Table 4.2).

Two main effects were found. First, CPP patients fared significantly better in therapies carried out over 16 sessions than in 8-session treatments. Second, while posttherapy gains made by patients in the CPP and the Sheffield project were similar, at 3-month follow-up, there was strong evidence that CPP patients were failing to maintain their gains. The severity × duration interaction found at posttherapy in Shapiro et al. (1994) was not replicated, though there is good reason to believe that the low statistical power of the CPP study may have contributed to this null finding (Barkham et al., 1996a).

Taken together, the Sheffield study and the CPP provide evidence that both therapy modalities under study are—broadly—equally effective and equally rapid in their initial response. However, some caution is necessary in considering "dose–response" relationships found in the Sheffield project, particularly where these appear to indicate that very brief periods of therapy may be effective at posttherapy. Longer periods of therapy appear to be associated with better longer term outcomes, particularly in the case of psychodynamic/

interpersonal therapy. In addition, more severely distressed individuals have a greater risk of relapse, and, while there is no clear indication as to why, there is some evidence from the CPP that clinic-sample patients may be more at risk of relapse than those usually found in research populations.

The Impact of Maintenance Therapies on Relapse: University of Pittsburgh Study

Though the forgoing trials suggest that short-term psychotherapies can successfully impact on depressive symptomatology, a clear (and fairly consistent) finding is that after 1 year, only about one-fourth of a treated sample will remain well. The issue of relapse is an important one that is explored further later in this chapter. Frank and colleagues' study is unusual in that its primary aim was to examine the impact of maintenance treatment offered after short-term intervention had been completed (Frank et al., 1989, 1990, 1991; Kupfer et al., 1992).

Two hundred thirty patients were selected for inclusion in the trial on the basis of a history of recurrent depression. All had experienced at least three previous episodes of depression, with the preceding episode occurring no more than 2½ years before the index episode (the mean number of episodes was 6.8, with a median of 4). All were selected on the basis of a clear DSM-III-R diagnosis of MDD in the absence of other Axis I disorders. Those with double depression were excluded, as were patients with severe Axis II disorders.

All patients received short-term treatment with imipramine and interpersonal psychotherapy. Psychotherapy sessions were scheduled weekly for 12 weeks, then biweekly for 8 weeks, and then monthly. At whatever point that patients achieved remission (defined as a HRSD score or a Raskin Depression Scale score ≤ 5 for 3 consecutive weeks), a further 17 weeks of treatment was offered, during which Hamilton and Raskin scores had to remain stable. At this point, a third evaluation was carried out, and the 128 patients who had reached the recovery criteria were assigned to one of five maintenance treatments for 3 years, or until the recurrence of depression; treatments were offered monthly and consisted of (1) medication clinic/clinical management and imipramine, (2) medication clinic/clinical management and placebo, (3) IPT and imipramine, (4) IPT and placebo, or (5) IPT alone (see Table 4.3). It should be noted that all patients had been receiving IPT; those assigned to medication conditions alone continued to see their original therapist, though the nature of their interaction changed from one of therapy to clinical management, along the lines of the NIMH study (Frank & Kupfer, 1994).

Unusual both in research studies and probably in clinical practice, imipramine continued to be prescribed at high levels (a mean of 207 mg

TABLE 4.3. Mean and Median Survival Times in Five Maintenance Conditions for 3 Years

Treatment condition	Mean ± SD survival time (in weeks)	Median survival time (in weeks)
Medication clinic and imipramine	124 ± 13	[a]
IPT and imipramine	131 ± 10	[a]
Medication clinic and placebo	45 ± 11	21
IPT	82 ± 13	54
IPT and placebo	74 ± 12	61

Note. Data from Frank et al. (1990).
[a] Since 50% of these subjects did not have a relapse, no median can be calculated.

daily). Attrition from the maintenance phase of the study was relatively low; only 22 (17%) of patients assigned to this phase failed to complete the 3-year protocol.

Results are reported at 3 years for the main trial (Frank et al., 1990) and at 5 years for a further group of patients maintained on imipramine or placebo alone (Kupfer et al., 1992). At 3 years, and contrasted with patients receiving placebo, medication or the combination of medication with IPT resulted in a significant reduction in the relapse rate ($p < .0001$). Maintenance therapy with IPT or IPT and placebo also resulted in a significant though less marked reduction in relapse ($p < .043$). There was no advantage to combination treatment over imipramine alone.

Overall, over 3 years, patients treated with imipramine had a 22.6% recurrence rate contrasted with 78.2% for those on placebo. Patients treated with IPT (with or without placebo) had a 44.2% recurrence rate over the same period. Further analysis suggests that when the quality of treatment delivered was high, relapse rates with IPT were equal to those achieved with imipramine. Frank et al. (1991) examined audiotapes of 38 of the 52 patients receiving maintenance IPT (either alone or in combination with placebo) and used rating scales of therapy adherence to determine the degree to which this therapy was implemented as intended. Therapies were defined as high quality if the patients received IPT above the median of adherence ratings, or low quality if delivered below the median. Results were striking; patients receiving high-quality therapy had a median survival time to relapse of approximately 2 years, while those receiving low-quality therapy had a median time of only 5 months.

The quality of therapy delivered was not a reflection of "good" or "bad" therapists, since individual therapists implemented IPT accurately with some patients, and with less success with others. Although requiring further study, accuracy of implementation seemed to reflect an interaction between patient and therapist factors.

Patients completing the 3-year protocol who had been receiving active medication (with or without maintenance IPT) were invited to continue a further 2-year randomized trial of active medication against placebo (Kupfer et al., 1992). Twenty patients entered this trial, either continuing to receive the high-dose imipramine regimen, or being transferred to placebo medication. Thirteen patients continued to receive monthly IPT, evenly split across placebo and medication conditions. Again, survival times were significantly greater for patients receiving active medication (99.4 ± 4.4 weeks) than for those assigned to placebo (54.0 ± 14.6 weeks, $p < .006$). Only one-third of patients receiving placebo survived the study period without relapse; 78% of placebo survivors were receiving continuation IPT. Only 11% of patients receiving neither medication nor IPT survived without experiencing a relapse.

Summary

The studies reviewed in this section meet the most stringent criteria of methodological rigor and indicate the efficacy of IPT and CBT; in the single trial in which there was a contrast of dynamic-IPT and CBT, the two modes of treatment were equivalent in their efficacy. This broad equivalence between outcomes from bona fide therapies is an important finding, suggesting, as it does, that depression may be responsive to a range of psychotherapeutic techniques.

Contrast of pharmacotherapy to psychotherapy in these trials is open to interpretation, because the pattern of outcomes is rather complex. In the NIMH trial, a differential response favoring medication was apparent for more severely depressed clients, particularly in the contrast of pharmacotherapy and CBT. However, in both this and the University of Pittsburgh study, the efficacy of IPT was more or less equivalent to medication, though, in the latter trial, this was true only when it was well implemented. The University of Minnesota and University of Pennsylvania–Vanderbilt trials counterbalance findings from the NIMH study, not only indicating an equivalence of action between CBT and medication but also demonstrating this equivalence in samples selected for depression severity. Based largely on the NIMH trial, some commentators have recommended the first-line use of medication in cases of severe depression. Whatever the clinical merits of this approach, this is unjustified by evidence from the four trials reviewed to this point.

Although clinically significant change was observed in as few as eight sessions for less severely depressed patients, at least 16 sessions were necessary for more severely depressed individuals. This suggests that there is usually little justification for considering very brief treatments. However, whatever the immediate benefits, the long-term effectiveness of short-term treatments is relatively poor for the majority of patients: between only one-third and one-fourth of any sample can be expected to be in remission after 18 months. This highlights the critical issue of relapse. The obvious implication of outcomes from these trials is that many patients will need further treatment beyond an initial intervention if they are to maintain optimal levels of functioning and avoid further episodes of depression.

All of these trials delivered therapies at high levels of quality, and there is some evidence (both in these studies and others) that better outcomes were obtained when therapists were more adherent to the planned treatment, and when they delivered therapy more competently. In order to achieve this, all studies ensured that there was extensive monitoring and supervision for therapists, and when practice was found wanting, remedial action was taken. The degree to which supervision contributes to outcome is unclear and largely untested, but because monitoring of fidelity is often seen as reflecting the requirements of research protocols, its potential contribution to achieved outcomes is often overlooked. In this sense, it may be important to remember that outputs from therapies in research contexts represent supervised rather than independent practice, and that this will have implications when implementing research findings into routine clinical settings.

A final methodological point is that even in these very well-controlled trials, there were a number of unexplained sources of variance—an obvious example of which was large treatment-by-site interactions. Inconsistency in outcomes between and within studies cautions against overinterpretation based on single-research cohorts and reinforces the need for methodological standards that enable researchers to identify and to report such unexplained variance.

QUANTITATIVE REVIEWS OF TREATMENTS FOR DEPRESSION

Many quantitative reviews of treatments for depression examine the relative efficacy of psychological treatments, as well as their efficacy when contrasted with adjunctive medication, or with medication alone. Three early reviews focus on contrasts between psychotherapy and pharmacotherapy (Conte et al., 1986; Quality Assurance Project, 1983; Steinbruek et al., 1983); these reviews excluded research examining the benefits of psychotherapy alone. Dobson (1989) and Neitzel et al. (1987) restricted their analyses to trials using the BDI as an outcome measure. Robinson et al.'s (1990) review is more comprehensive, examining a wider range of studies of psychotherapy and pharmacotherapy using multiple outcome measures and more diverse forms of therapy. The U.S. Public Health Service's Agency for Health Care Policy and Research (AHCPR) also reviews psychopharmacological and psychotherapeutic treatments, but with the more specific aim of developing clinical practice guidelines for primary care and other health care practitioners

(Depression Guideline Panel, 1993a, 1993b, 1993c). There is a tendency for more recent reviews to be concerned with specific issues. Gaffan et al. (1995) focus on the impact of researcher allegiance on reported outcomes, Cuijpers (1997) on bibliotherapy (discussed below), Gloaguen et al. (1998) on studies of CBT, Westen and Morrison (2001) on manualized psychotherapies, McDermut et al. (2001) on group treatments, Leichsenring (2001) on a contrast of CBT and psychodynamic therapy, and Churchill et al. (2001) on contrasts of psychotherapies. Though not formal meta-analyses, three "mega-analyses" aggregate data from previously published trials and examine outcomes for psychotherapy alone and combined with pharmacotherapy (Casacalenda et al., 2002; Thase et al., 1997), and for CBT and pharmacotherapy (DeRubeis et al., 1999).

Aggregating information across these meta-analyses is complicated by the fact that each uses different inclusion and exclusion criteria, and sometimes employs different metrics for the analysis. In some cases, they do not include a full list of included studies (Neitzel et al., 1987; Quality Assurance Project, 1983; Steinbruek et al., 1983), making it hard to be clear about the degree of overlap between reviews (though this is indicated where feasible). Earlier meta-analyses also inevitably include a number of studies with serious methodological problems, necessarily weakening their conclusions.

Because of clinical implications, the relative and adjunctive benefits of medication and psychological therapies have long been debated by researchers. However, this debate is hampered by the limited evidence on which it rests: There is a relative paucity of large-scale trials, ands some earlier trials have been appropriately criticized for inadequate provision of medication, further reducing the pool of studies from which conclusions can safely be drawn. Reasonable expectations that trials ensure adequate dosage, and monitoring of drug compliance and prescriptions by adequately trained pharmacotherapists have not been met in many earlier trials, meaning that their inclusion in meta-analyses contributes confusion rather than clarity. Few trials contrast each treatment modality alone and in combination; given the number of possible combinations of psychotherapy and pharmacotherapy, it is inevitable that only some of the possible permutations have been explored. Furthermore, rather few trials include a contrast of active psychological therapy with pill placebo, a state of affairs that has led to some debate as to whether this does, or does not, weaken interpretation of current trials (e.g., Jacobson & Hollon, 1996a; Klein, 1990, 1996). All this hampers the inferences that meta-analysis can make about the relative and combined efficacy of these approaches.

Earlier reviews do not disaggregate particular types of psychotherapy, often contrasting any form of therapy against pharmacotherapy. The Quality Assurance Project (1983) largely focused on the efficacy of medication; of 200 trials in this review, only 10 involved the use of psychotherapy. On the

basis of this (limited) sample, an effect size of 0.69 was found for psychotherapy of any type, contrasted with a mean effect size of 0.55 for tricyclics and
0.39 for monoamine oxidase inhibitors (MAOIs). Conte et al. (1986)
reviewed 17 studies published between 1974 and 1984, in which psychotherapy in combination with medication was contrasted with another treatment
(all except two are included in Robinson et al.'s [1990] review). A statistical
weighting procedure was used to reflect methodological adequacy, the results
of which were used in the assessment of treatment effects. This procedure
makes a number of assumptions about the link between methodological quality and outcome that have not been supported by more conventional meta-
analyses (Smith et al., 1980), and its use may be questioned. No distinction
among different types of therapy was made. Conte et al. (1986) conclude that
there is some limited evidence for the greater effectiveness of combination treatments compared to psychotherapy or pharmacotherapy alone.
Steinbruek et al. (1983) examined 56 studies published between 1962 and
1981, in which psychotherapy alone or pharmacotherapy alone was contrasted with a control group. A significantly larger mean effect size was found
for psychotherapy (1.22) contrasted with medication (0.61). Although an
effect size for tricyclic medications was derived (0.67), no separate analyses
are given for the differing categories of psychotherapy. Furthermore, contrasting therapies against waiting lists would be expected to give a different
result than comparison with placebo; in this study, both groups are subsumed
under a single heading ("control group"). These considerations undermine
the usefulness of this review.

Neitzel et al. (1987), and Dobson (1989) restricted their coverage to trials that used the BDI as an outcome measure, aiming to increase the uniformity of comparisons. Neitzel at al. (1987) analyzed data from 31 studies, concluding that the type of therapy, whether classified as cognitive, behavioral,
or combination treatment, did not influence outcome and that individual
therapy produced larger effect sizes than group treatment. To determine the
clinical significance of treatment effects, they contrasted the mean pre- and
posttreatment BDI scores of treated and control patients with the mean scores
of two "reference groups" for which normative data for the BDI are available. The first set of norms is derived from individuals selected for the
absence of pathology (a nondistressed group); the second set is norms derived
from general population surveys. Contrasting outcomes against the former
group is a more stringent (but perhaps less relevant) test of recovery than
comparison with the latter sample. Using these contrasts, the average treated
client moved from 4.79 standard deviations (*SD*) above the mean for the
nondistressed group to 1.62 *SD* posttreatment; using general population
norms, the comparable figures are 2.9 and 0.71 *SD*. Control subjects had
similar pretreatment scores to those of treated patients but showed little gain
posttreatment. (Their posttreatment scores were 3.97 and 2.96 *SD* when

contrasted with the nondistressed and general population samples.) Gains were maintained at follow-up, though it is worth noting that the mean follow-up period was only 16 weeks (range 4–52).

These figures can be expressed, perhaps more meaningfully, in terms of percentiles. On this basis, the average treated client moves from a pre-treatment level at the 99.9th percentile to the 94.7th percentile of the nondistressed group at posttreatment. Contrasted to the general population, sample the gains are more striking—from the 99.8th percentile to the 76.1th percentile. Although there may be some debate about the clinical significance of these scores, they do indicate that the average treated client will have an approximate posttreatment BDI score of 10, which would place him/her at the boundary between a normal and a mildly depressed level of functioning.

Dobson's (1989) review was based on 28 studies published between 1976 and 1987, in which cognitive therapy was contrasted with other thera-pies, and (as with Neitzel et al., 1987) in which the BDI was included as an outcome measure. Given that Neitzel et al. did not cite the studies included in their review, the degree of overlap between the two analyses cannot be readily ascertained (though it is likely to be considerable). However, in con-trast to Neitzel et al., Dobson (1989) found mean effect sizes favoring cogni-tive therapy contrasted with pharmacotherapy (0.53), behavior therapy (0.46), and other psychotherapies (0.54). Comparing cognitive therapy to wait–list or no-treatment controls gave a mean effect size of 2.15, indicating that the average treated client did better than 98% of control subjects. All effect sizes were based on posttherapy outcomes, with no analysis of follow-up data.

Robinson et al. (1990) reviewed studies published between 1976 and 1986, including 58 trials of outpatient psychological therapies and a further 15 in which psychological and pharmacological interventions were con-trasted. Therapies were classified as behavioral, cognitive (in which treat-ments focused on the evaluation and modification of cognitive patterns), cognitive-behavioral, or general verbal. Only nine trials recruited patients through standard clinical channels; around half recruited using media an-nouncements; in a quarter, the samples were students, and 12% did not report on the source of their patients. In addition, only 35% of investigations had inclusion criteria specifying that patients should meet formal diagnostic crite-ria for depression. The analysis is further weakened by the fact that most of the results are reported using posttreatment rather than follow-up data, on the basis that the figures for each data point were very similar (34 of the 58 studies had follow-up, but the mean length of follow-up was only 13 weeks, with a range of 2–52 weeks).

Contrasting therapy of any kind against no therapy (defined as wait list or placebo) gives an effect size of 0.73 at posttherapy and 0.68 at follow-up. As might be expected, effect sizes are higher when contrasted with a wait list (0.84); when compared to placebo, the effect size is nonsignificant (0.28).

Overall, behavioral, cognitive, and cognitive-behavioral treatments showed moderate effect sizes (1.02, 0.96, and 0.85, respectively). Verbal therapies showed a more modest effect size (0.49), though this figure is based on only six studies.

Within–study treatment contrasts afford a more robust assessment of the relative efficacy of different classes of therapy. Using data from such trials, there is evidence of a modest superiority for cognitive-behavioral over behavioral treatment (effect size = 0.24), and a moderate superiority of cognitive and cognitive-behavioral treatments over verbal treatments (effect size = 0.47 and 0.27, respectively). Fifteen studies examined the implementation of these therapies in group or individual settings, finding equal efficacy for all approaches.

Longer treatment or the number of sessions did not contribute to a greater effect size, though the mean length of treatments was only seven sessions, and this may not be sufficient to test this variable. There was little evidence of any specific client characteristics that influenced treatment outcome. Effect sizes did not vary reliably when outcomes in relation to the initial severity of depression (as measured by BDI), the presence or absence of diagnosed depression, or the source of referral of the client were examined.

To examine the clinical significance of the gains made by patients (Jacobson et al., 1984), Robinson et al. (1990) identified 39 studies reporting data on the BDI, in order to contrast the level of depression after treatment with that obtaining in the general population (the same strategy followed by Neitzel et al. [1987]). On this basis, therapy appears to shift the average client from 2.4 SD above the mean for the general population to 0.8 SD. Comparison with a nondistressed population gives an equivalent pre- to posttherapy shift (from 3.4 to 1.4 SD above the mean) but does suggest some residual distress. Nonetheless, the clinical effect of treatment is clear.

Robinson et al. (1990) also examined 15 studies comparing the effectiveness of psychological interventions alone, medication alone, and the combination of these treatments. The majority of these studies employed cognitive-behavioral or behavioral psychotherapies. However, basic methodological requirements were not always met. Not all studies ensured that therapeutic levels of medication were prescribed, and although most trials utilized antidepressants, two (surprisingly) employed benzodiazepines. When contrasted with the use of tricyclic antidepressants, psychotherapy showed a significant though small advantage (effect size = 0.12). There was no evidence of a significant advantage to combination treatments contrasted with psychotherapy alone or medication alone. However, if the effect of investigator allegiance is controlled statistically (as discussed earlier), the advantage to psychotherapy disappears.

The AHCPR review (Depression Guideline Panel, 1993a, 1993b, 1993c) aimed to develop clinical practice guidelines for use by primary care practitioners and other health care professionals. However, most studies included in the analysis were conducted in tertiary care units, and it is unclear how research in these settings generalizes to treatment of the milder depressive conditions frequently seen in primary care. A later follow-up review by Schulberg et al. (1998, discussed below) considers this issue further.

The panel conducted an extensive review of studies published between 1975 and 1990, identifying a subsample for meta-analysis. Inclusion criteria specified that patients met DSM-III-R criteria for MDD, that the research design was a randomized controlled trial, and that treatment effects were measured using a standardized method that permitted assessment of depressive and/or functional status before and after treatment (Jarrett & Maguire, 1991; summarized in Jarrett & Rush, 1994). The number of included studies was further reduced by the decision to use Bayesian models rather than conventional meta-analytic methodology. Bayesian statistical methods can be described as a formal framework within which data from available studies are used to produce the best fit to a hypothetical, perfectly performed study. Existing data form a "prior distribution," which describes our present state of knowledge about, for example, outcomes for a particular therapy. The addition of further studies describes a "posterior distribution," representing our new state of knowledge as a consequence of the addition of further evidence. The application of Bayesian statistics results in a series of probability functions, which in essence describe the likelihood of a particular intervention having a particular result—for example, the probability that a treatment will be successful in resolving depression. It is argued that these methods are more sensitive and appropriate than conventional statistical techniques, and allow more scope for the management of possible bias in the studies forming the meta-analysis. Although the Confidence Profile Method (CPM) used in the AHCPR review (described fully in Eddy et al., 1990) can be undertaken using continuous data (e.g., differences in BDI scores), a categorical scoring system was used, because it has the advantage of indicating whether patients have reached a recovery criterion, hence making results more meaningful for practitioners.

Jarrett and Maguire (1991) identified 22 randomized controlled trials of cognitive therapy, 13 of behavioral therapy, 4 of interpersonal therapy, 8 of brief dynamic therapy, and 1 of marital therapy. Some of these studies were excluded because data were reported in a form that made it inimical to the CPM approach. Trials included in the analysis involved treatment of both adult and elderly populations, and used both individual and group formats for behavioral and cognitive therapy. Data were analyzed using "intention-to-treat" samples (contrasting outcomes for all patients entered into the trial, regardless of whether a full course of therapy was given).

All therapies combined yielded an estimated overall efficacy of 50%; contrasted to waiting list, there was a 26% advantage to therapy, and contrasted to placebo, a 16% advantage. The overall efficacy of behavioral therapy was 55%. Contrasted to all other forms of psychotherapy, it was 9% more effective (six studies), and compared to wait list (five studies), 17% more effective. Cognitive therapy was found to have an overall efficacy of 47%, with approximately equal efficacy to the other therapies (−4.5%, six studies). Brief dynamic therapy had an overall efficacy of 35%, though, contrasted to other therapies, it was slightly less effective (−8%, eight studies). For IPT, only the NIMH study provided data appropriate for meta-analysis; on this basis, it had an overall efficacy of 52% and exceeded the efficacy of cognitive therapy by 13%.

Comparison of all psychological therapies alone to medication showed an advantage to psychological therapy of 14% (based on eight studies). In all comparisons, specific therapies delivered alone showed advantage over medication alone: for behavioral therapy alone (24% more effective, based on two studies), cognitive therapy alone (15% more effective in three studies), brief dynamic therapy alone (8.5% more effective in two studies), and IPT alone (12%, based on the NIMH study). Combination treatment showed an advantage over behavior therapy alone (7% based on two studies) but was less effective than cognitive therapy alone (−6.5%, based on 6 studies).

The statistical sophistication of the CPM is both its strength and its weakness, because relatively few studies are appropriate for inclusion in this form of analysis. Studies meeting the inclusion criteria for conventional meta-analysis may not be representative of either clinical work or even of research trials, a criticism that may apply even more strongly to the CPM technique. This may lead to the emergence of misleading conclusions. Thus, few clinicians would accept that behavior therapy alone was the most effective treatment method for depression. Although achieving a high ranking in the meta-analysis of the depressions guidelines panel, this is most likely an artifact of sampling and of the six contrasts performed. Although CPM meta-analysis is an exciting development, it will require a considerable extension of the database to ensure that specific contrasts of therapies with one another can be interpreted reliably.

Gloaguen et al. (1998) located 78 controlled trials published between 1977 and 1996, in which cognitive therapy for depression or dysthymic disorder was contrasted to wait list, placebo, behavior therapy, or an alternative psychological treatment. Of these, 48 met inclusion criteria for methodological quality and were included in the review. Meta-analysis ostensibly demonstrated an advantage to cognitive therapy over wait list or placebo (20 comparisons, effect size = 0.82), over antidepressants (17 comparisons, effect size = 0.38), and over other therapies (22 comparisons, effect size = 0.24), and equivalent impact against behavior therapy (13 comparisons, effect size = 0.05).

Though this appears to offer evidence of a strong advantage to CBT in contrast to other interventions, Gloaguen et al. (1998) noted significant heterogeneity across studies and further analyses. Wampold et al. (2002) suggest that this relates to a failure to separate contrast therapies into bona fide and non-bona fide therapies. This distinction relates to Wampold's (1997) observation that control treatments fall into two classes: bona fide treatments (which are expected to work) and non-bona fide interventions (whose impact is predicted to be negligible); clearly, contrasts between "active" treatments and non-bona fide interventions will overestimate relative treatment efficacy. Wampold et al. (2002) reanalyzed Gloaguen et al.'s (1998) data and found that separating bona fide from non-bona fide treatments restored homogeneity across studies. Crucially, when CBT was contrasted to bona fide interventions, outcomes were equivalent (effect size = 0.16).

The efficacy of group therapies has been evaluated by McDermut et al. (2001), who identified 48 trials published between 1970 and 1998. Most reports were of behavioral or cognitive-behavioral interventions, but eight were based on psychodynamic and/or interpersonal principles. Control conditions usually included wait list or delivery of the therapy on an individual basis. Contrast to no treatment (15 studies) yielded a mean posttreatment effect size of 1.03 in favor of group therapy. Comparing the same therapy delivered in individual and group formats (nine studies) yielded an effect size of −0.15, suggesting equivalence of outcome. Although dropout rates from individual and group therapies were very similar, there is evidence from two of the trials in the review that dissatisfaction with the group format was associated with greater attrition. This suggests that in routine clinical settings, it may be important to take into account patient preferences regarding the format of therapy delivery.

Westen and Morrison (2001) located 12 studies, published between 1990 and 1998, that met inclusion criteria for methodological quality, and included a comparison of an active psychological therapy with wait-list control, an alternative psychological therapy, or pharmacotherapy. Results are aggregated rather than identifying the specific benefits of specific approaches. Though this reflects Westen and Morrison's focus on broader issues relating to the presentation of outcome data, it limits the utility of the analysis for the present discussion. Though the mean pre- to posttherapy effect size for psychological therapies was large (effect size = 2.23) contrasted to control conditions, the median effect size at termination was small (effect size = 0.3).

Though 54% of patients who completed treatment met criteria for improvement, this dropped to 37% of the "intention-to-treat" sample; in line with other analyses, this raises issues about the proportion of patients who can expect to benefit from therapy. Furthermore, in those studies that report relevant data, there may be cause for concern about the extent and stability of change. Although patients showed substantial gains, posttreatment mean scores on the HRSD and BDI remained above the conventional cutoff scores applied to these measures. These are usually set at ≥ 6 and ≥ 9, respectively; mean scores from Westen and Morrison's analysis (2001) were 8.68 and 10.98, respectively. Very few studies reported long-term follow-up data— only two at 12–18 months, and one at 2 years. At 18 months, only 36% of patients who completed treatment improved and remained improved; among the "intention-to-treat" sample, this figure drops to 28.5%.

Although only a preliminary finding, there was a suggestion that studies with higher exclusion rates prior to randomization to treatment tended to report better patient outcomes and lower rates of treatment seeking after therapy had ended. This raises a central dilemma for researchers. Setting clear inclusion criteria is a necessary and indeed helpful research strategy, but it has consequences for external validity. This is not a straightforward issue, however. Some exclusion criteria can be seen as enhancing external validity. For example, excluding patients who are only mildly depressed is both common and reasonable (though it also has the consequence of reducing information about treatment response in individuals whose depression lies below diagnostic thresholds). However, excluding patients with comorbid presentations, which is common in clinical settings, inevitably raises questions about generalization of results. Ultimately, this is an empirical rather than a philosophical issue, and one that will only be answered by more effectiveness trials, and particularly by more extensive use of benchmarking studies in routine clinical settings (e.g., Barkham et al., 2001).

Leichsenring (2001) reviewed evidence for the comparative efficacy of short-term psychodynamic psychotherapy (STPP) and CBT, restricting analysis to studies with more than 13 therapy sessions (a cutoff based on assumptions about the period required for psychodynamic therapy to show efficacy). Six studies were identified, though two of these employed therapies that may not best be described as either STPP or CBT. One of these was the NIMH trial, whose IPT arm is classified by Leichsenring as a psychodynamic intervention on the (accurate but contentious) basis that it was delivered by therapists whose background training was in psychodynamic therapy. In the second, Hersen et al. (1984) employed social skills training, a behavioral (rather than a cognitive-behavioral) treatment with unproven efficacy in relation to depression. Given these problems of definition, it is not quite clear that all trials contrast equivalent interventions. A final concern is that analysis of the Sheffield trials (Barkham et al., 1996a; Shapiro et al., 1994) is restricted to the 16-session arm, reflecting the dosage criteria described earlier. Broadly, in all but one trial, CBT and STPP (as defined by Leichsenring, 2001) were of equal efficacy. Gallagher-Thompson and Steffen (1994; reviewed elsewhere in this chapter and in Chapter 15) looked at the impact of therapy on care-givers, finding some advantage to CBT for longer term (as opposed to shorter term) caregivers. Although the evidence from this meta-analysis is best taken to indicate an equivalence of action between CBT and STPP, this conclusion is based on only a small sample of direct contrasts of these approaches, itself enlarged by questionable inclusion criteria.

Churchill et al. (2001) reviewed brief psychological treatments for depression (defined as interventions of less than 20 sessions), contrasting each treatment with another and with TAU or wait list. Of 63 identified studies published between 1973 and 1998, 50 were suitable for meta-analysis. The authors noted that most samples were relatively small, with a range of 18–276 (median = 44), and a median arm size of 13. On this basis, few trials would have sufficient statistical power to detect differences between interventions. Only 60% of studies monitored adherence, and while 37% of trials requested that patients desist from medication, 20% allowed "naturalistic" prescribing—all trends that introduce ambiguity about the treatments received by patients. Only one-third of trials reported follow-up data, and those with follow-up of more than 6 months had high rates of attrition over this period. Although intended, a cost-effectiveness analysis was not undertaken, because only five trials reported relevant data.

Classes of therapy contrasted were variants of CBT (behavioral, cognitive, and cognitive-behavioral), psychodynamic therapy, IPT, and supportive therapy. The latter clustering included a mix of approaches, most of which were humanistic in orientation. Analysis was based on the proportion of patients recovered at posttherapy and (where available) follow-up. Compared to TAU or wait-list controls, there was significant benefit to psychological intervention. For all variants of therapy, the odds ratio (OR) was 3.01; significant benefit was apparent for CBT (OR = 3.42; 12 trials), IPT (OR = 3.52; one trial), and supportive therapy (OR = 2.71; 4 trials). Contrasts of CBT to commonly practiced alternative forms of therapy suggested equivalence with IPT (2 trials) but greater efficacy compared to psychodynamic therapy (OR = 2.23; 6 trials) and supportive therapy (OR = 3.45; 10 trials). CBT delivered in individual rather than group format was more effective in the short term (OR = 1.98; 6 trials), though this advantage was not evident at follow-up. No differences were found for the contrast of CBT and behavior therapy (3 trials). Based only on one trial, psychodynamic therapy showed equivalent efficacy to supportive therapy. Overall, while this analysis suggests consistent benefit to CBT, the number of available contrasts limit conclusions when contrasting the relative benefits of other specific therapies.

Several cautions are appropriate. Where follow-up data were available, between-therapy differences reported earlier were no longer evident. Studies in which patients were self-selected or volunteers tended to have larger effect sizes than those in which they were clinic attenders, and higher quality trials also had lower effect sizes. It is also worth noting that there was significant heterogeneity in the data set contrasting CBT and other therapies; further analysis suggested that trials with more severely depressed patients showed fewer differences between therapies, and trials with fewer sessions favored CBT. Critically, there is overlap between this review and that of Gloaguen et al. (1998; reviewed earlier), and inclusion of contrasts of CBT and non-bona fide therapies may account for this heterogeneity, as well as inflating apparent between-therapy differences (Wampold et al., 2002). Finally, the reviewers inappropriately include the Sheffield trial in the contrast of CBT and IPT; although its presence or absence does not alter the significance of the odds ratio, its removal makes this comparison reliant solely on the NIMH trial.

"Mega-Analyses"

Thase et al. (1997) presented a "mega-analysis" of six studies contrasting the impact of psychological therapy alone or in combination with medication. All trials in the analysis were conducted completely or partially at the University of Pittsburgh (hence, including the NIMH and Frank studies reviewed earlier). In total, 243 patients received psychological therapy alone (CBT or IPT), and 352 received IPT in combination with antidepressant (imipramine or nortriptyline). Less depressed individuals (those having an initial HRSD score of ≤ 19) had equivalent outcomes with either treatment modality, but for more severely depressed patients, there was a significant advantage to combination treatment over psychological therapy alone (with respective recovery rates of 43% and 25%). For patients with recurrent depression, this advantage was even more marked (60% vs. 19%). A sensitivity analysis indicated that this pattern of results was consistent across all studies, further supporting the contention that patients with severe and recurrent depression will benefit from combination therapy.

DeRubeis et al. (1999) examined a different set of contrasts—the relative benefits of CBT alone and pharmacotherapy alone (imipramine or nortriptyline). The analysis combined data from four trials—the NIMH study (also included in Thase et al., 1997), the University of Minnesota trial, Rush et al. (1977) and Murphy et al. (1984). Data were reanalyzed to include only the more severely depressed patients (those with an initial score > 20 on the HSRD or > 30 on the BDI). Comparing CBT and medication using the HRSD yielded a small effect size of 0.22 in favor of CBT; when the BDI was used, there was no difference in efficacy between treatment modalities (effect size = 0.07). Unlike the Thase analysis, there is some variation in the pattern of results across studies, with better outcomes for medication and poorer outcomes for CBT in the NIMH trial when contrasted to the pooled outcomes from the other trials (though the effect size of approximately 0.5 was not significant). In contrast, the Rush et al. (1977) study showed an inverse pattern, with outcomes for CBT being markedly better than those for medication (though, as detailed below, this study has been criticized for poor medication delivery).

Casacalenda et al. (2002) identified six studies that contained direct contrasts of medication, psychotherapy, and a control condition, and that contained data on remission (defined as a score on a depression scale within the normal range) (Elkin et al., 1989; Herceg-Baron et al., 1979; Jarrett et al., 1999; Mynors-Wallis et al., 1995; Schulberg et al., 1996; Scott, 1992). Medications in these trials were either tricyclics or phenelzine, and psychotherapies were usually CBT or IPT; most patients had mild to moderate levels of depression. Remission rates with active treatment were equivalent at approximately 46% of the intent-to-treat sample in contrast to 24% for control conditions.

A critical issue in these analyses is the relative impact of treatments for more severely depressed patients. In this respect, it seems reasonable to conclude that while the evidence for differential efficacy of each modality delivered alone is not strong and appears mixed, the evidence for the benefit of combination treatment over therapy alone appears both stronger and more consistent.

Researcher Allegiance and Outcome

Robinson et al. (1990) employed a 5-point scale to estimate the degree to which researchers displayed an allegiance to the therapy under examination and found a significant correlation between this measure and the results of direct comparisons between treatments ($r = .58$). Using a regression analysis to partial out this effect reduced the effect sizes almost to zero. Gaffan et al. (1995) explored this important issue further by reanalyzing the same sample of studies examined by Dobson (1989), and extending their sampling by including a further 37 studies published between 1987 and 1994. Their analysis of Dobson's original sample yielded similar effect sizes and conclusions, though controlling for sample size reduced the magnitude of the effect sizes. The allegiances of researchers were strongly biased in favor of cognitive therapy, and regression analysis suggested a significant association between this measure and estimations of outcome. Although controlling for this reduced the effect size markedly, the superiority of cognitive therapy over other treatments claimed by Dobson remained (corrected effect size = 0.17). Analysis of the second (more recently published) sample yields a set of conclusions similar to Dobson's sample. Though effect sizes are smaller, sample sizes are larger, and weighted and unweighted effect sizes are not significantly different. Strikingly, regression analysis suggested no association of investigator allegiance and reported outcome. Considering the complete sample of trials, year of publication emerges as a significant factor in mediating the link between effect size and allegiance, with early trials (most obviously those published up to 1985) showing the strongest influence of allegiance. Under-standing this shift is not easy: It would seem that both the effect size favoring cognitive therapy and allegiance have declined with time.

Summary

Summarizing quantitative reviews of outcomes for MDD, it seems clear that psychological therapy has benefit over no therapy, though when active thera-pies are contrasted, differences between them are less clear. Although there are indications that CBT is superior to less structured forms of psychothera-peutic intervention, it is worth noting that this conclusion appears less robust when the contrast treatment is credible and theory-grounded. There are few well-structured studies of psychodynamic therapy, though in the one, per-haps limited review in which this approach was explicitly contrasted to CBT, reasonably similar outcomes were evident. Group therapies appear to have comparable effect sizes when individual and group-based forms of the same approach are compared. Though persons with depression are vulnerable to relapse, relatively few studies include adequate follow-up data, making it dif-ficult for reviews to derive conclusions about the robustness of change. When they do, they confirm the lack of stability of posttreatment gains.

Estimates of effect sizes differ across meta-analyses as a function of the sampling frame of the original studies, the dependent measures used, the sta-tistical principles of the meta-analysis, and the original date of the investiga-tion. Broadly speaking, larger effect sizes are observed when trials include less severely impaired and more highly selected patient samples assessed on clini-cian ratings as opposed to self-report measures, when they employ shorter rather than longer follow-up, and (though perhaps less obviously in more recent studies) when they are carried out by the proponents of techniques. A critical methodological concern should be to distinguish between bona fide or non-bona fide control treatments, since contrast of an active therapy to plausible and theoretically grounded techniques appears to reduce effect sizes.

Though a critical clinical issue, judging the relative benefits of medica-tion and psychological therapy offered either alone or adjunctively is difficult. There is no consistent evidence that psychotherapeutic treatment is more effective than pharmacological treatment, but there is less certainty as to whether medication has benefit over psychological therapy, and especially whether there is an advantage to combination treatment. In general, there has to be concern that at least some studies included in reviews are fundamentally flawed in their implementation of medications. It is also the case that few of the trials available to reviewers employed newer, more specific antidepres-sants (with fewer side effects and probable greater acceptability to patients) that are likely to have lower rates of attrition.

While the strength of meta-analytic reviews is their capacity to identify trends that individual studies do not, aggregation of data often relies more on methodological than clinical considerations. This can result in contrasts that disguise important clinical differences between studies, obscuring clinically pertinent issues and yielding erroneous or misleading conclusions concerning treatment effectiveness. Examples of this would be the comparison of active treatments to ones that are not expected to be effective (hence boosting apparent efficacy), or when effect sizes for an intervention are based on trials where it was implemented as a control treatment rather than an "active" therapy (in this way probably reducing its impact).

SPECIFIC TREATMENT APPROACHES

Pharmacotherapy and Psychotherapy in Combination and Alone

This section supplements the quantitative reviews already discussed with qualitative reviews, and considers individual studies because they have either been published since these reviews or they illuminate the current status of an approach.

A number of methodological concerns complicate interpretation of trials that contrast these two modalities.

1. *Inadequate implementation of medication.* Though recent trials are more attentive to the need to implement pharmacotherapy in a manner that its proponents would recognize as appropriate, earlier researchers sometimes failed to ensure that patients received adequate dosages, did not conduct checks on compliance, and in some cases used inappropriate medications (such as anxiolytics), creating non-bona fide contrasts and almost certainly enhancing psychotherapy treatment effects. Meterissian and Bradwejn (1989) examined 11 studies carried out between 1977 and 1987, finding that only around half employed optimal levels of antidepressants, and only three measured drug plasma levels. Two widely cited studies illustrate the problems of inadequate prescription of medication. Rush et al. (1977) employed low doses of medication, which were then rapidly withdrawn before outcome measures were taken. Blackburn et al.'s (1986) study was carried out in both an outpatient and a primary care setting; patients in primary care showed an unusually low response to medication, against which therapy inevitably showed a superior outcome.

2. *Inadequate representation of newer antidepressants.* Many studies of medication utilize "older" medications—usually tricyclics—rather than SSRIs. The import of this is unclear. Although SSRIs have relatively fewer side effects and are hence likely to be better tolerated by patients, evidence that they are more effective than older medications is equivocal (e.g., Barbui & Hotopf, 2001).

3. *Influence on outcome of "blindness" to medication status.* Detecting the impact of medication requires control for patient and researcher expectancies, since these are known to influence outcomes. Although most medication trials attempt to ensure that all parties are "blind" as to the medication received, this is hard to achieve. Patients receiving placebo are less likely to experience side effects or other indicators that they received active medication, and this will impact on their expectancies of outcome. Whether consciously or not, clinicians making judgments about outcome will also use the presence of side effects as a way to determine treatment allocation. There is also good evidence that patients, as well as therapists, are able to detect whether they were allocated to drug or placebo, despite attempts at "blinding" (e.g., Margraf et al., 1991). More subtle effects are also apparent. Greenberg et al. (1992) identified 22 trials in which both new antidepressants were contrasted to placebo, with older antidepressants also used as a control treatment, arguing that researchers would have less investment in the older antidepressants and (because two active treatments were under test) would find it harder to distinguish between the two. Under these conditions, there was a marked reduction in effect size relative to control: Effect sizes for medication fell to between one-half and one-fourth of those usually reported, suggesting that—in some way—expectations of their efficacy influenced apparent outcome. Further evidence for expectancy effects comes from studies employing "active" placebos (which mimic drug side effects). Of nine such trials, only two showed effect sizes significantly favoring active medication (Moncrieff et al., 1998). These reports raise questions about the potential for overestimating drug effects and—perhaps more pertinent to this review—the possibility of bias when contrast of medication and psychotherapy is undertaken by researchers with an allegiance to either modality. These points also reinforce Hollon and DeRubeis's (1981) argument that psychotherapy alone is not equivalent to psychotherapy plus placebo, largely because of the expectancy effects associated with the latter combination. On this basis, they suggested a nine-cell design for medication and psychotherapy comparisons in which all possible combinations of drug, placebo, and nonintervention could be tested. While this represents an ideal rather than a practical suggestion, it does point to the difficulty of interpreting the more usual restricted set of contrasts.

4. *Depression subtype and response to placebo control.* There is an ongoing (and at points contentious) debate regarding the classification of depression, with the suggestion that the "endogenous" subtype reflects a biological etiology responsive to medication but not to psychological intervention (e.g., Feinberg, 1992; Thase & Friedman, 1999). It is also argued that patients with milder and, hence (at least potentially), more transient cases of depression show a greater response to most nonspecific interventions. On this basis, no active therapy would be expected to show benefit over another, leading to an erroneous conclusion that all therapies have equal efficacy.

Reflecting these concerns, some researchers (e.g., Klein, 1996) have argued that studies contrasting psychotherapy and medication should include a placebo control to demonstrate that the sample was (as it were) medication-responsive—by implication more severely distressed, with a low rate of placebo response, and therefore likely to be treatable only with the application of specifically effective therapies. However, there is a risk that these arguments become self-fulfilling, drawn on selectively to critique trials in relation to outcomes rather than criteria for trial entry. Though, on this basis, the specific argument may be overstated, there is merit in this position, though not simply in relation to contrast of medication and psychotherapy. It seems reasonable to question the degree to which maintaining diagnostic homogeneity protects researchers against predictable variations in treatment responsiveness within any sample of depressed individuals. However, the challenge is to derive a reliable and valid system for factoring any such differences into clinical trials.

5. *Controlling for the impact of attention.* When contrasted with patients receiving medication alone, psychotherapy patients are likely to receive three or four times more time with their therapists (typically, three or four times as much time), making it hard to distinguish the relative benefits of attention as opposed to therapeutic interventions. Again, this issue is managed better in at least some recent studies, where regular medication clinics ensure regular (if nonspecific) therapeutic contact.

Three qualitative reviews cover the period up to the early 1990s, inevitably including rather few contrasts of psychotherapy and newer medications. Meterissian and Bradwejn's (1989) review (described in part earlier) identified 11 studies, of which five were considered to have offered adequate doses of medication. Of these, one reported psychotherapy to be superior to medication; the remainder found it equivalent. In those studies using inappropriately low doses of medication, two studies indicated that psychotherapy was superior, one that it was equivalent, and one that a combination treatment was best.

Wexler and Cicchetti (1992) examined outcomes from eight treatment studies; Manning et al.'s (1992) review is rather larger, including 17 trials (six of which were included in Wexler and Cicchetti).

All studies in Wexler and Cicchetti's (1992) review used the BDI as a measure of outcome and employed broadly similar criteria for recovery. Psychological treatments included behavior therapy, CBT, psychodynamic therapy and IPT; medication was invariably a tricyclic. Three trials compared psychotherapy alone, pharmacotherapy alone, and the two in combination. Two of these (Blackburn et al., 1981; Murphy et al., 1984) suggested that combination treatments had the greatest efficacy, with intermediate efficacy for psychotherapy, and the lowest for medication. The third (Hersen et al., 1984) showed a nonsignificant trend favoring psychotherapy over combination, with medication showing the least efficacy. Combined data from these studies suggested a trend indicating that combination treatments were the most effective, followed by psychotherapy alone and medication alone. Overall, however, there was no statistically significant evidence demonstrating the greater efficacy of any one treatment over the other two.

In three studies comparing psychotherapy alone to medication alone (Elkin et al., 1989; McLean & Hakstian, 1979, 1990; Rush et al., 1977). two showed an advantage to psychotherapy, while in the NIMH trials, similar response rates were obtained. Finally, Beck et al. (1985) contrasted psychotherapy alone to combination treatment, producing results favoring psychotherapy over medication. However, these studies may form a poor basis for comparison of medication and psychotherapy. The Rush et al. (1977) study has been criticized for poor implementation of medication regimens; Beck et al. (1985) employed relatively low doses of amitriptyline for short periods; and in the NIMH (Elkin, 1994) trial, medication was offered in combination with clinical management.

Overall, Wexler and Cicchetti (1992) estimated that of 100 patients treated, the success rate will be 29% for medication contrasted with 47% for both psychotherapy alone and combination treatments. These figures suggest a strong advantage for psychotherapy or its combination with medication. However, it is clear that each therapy modality shows a high rate of partial or nonresponse—42% with psychotherapy alone and 52% with medication alone, suggesting that treatment strategies based exclusively on either modality will show little benefit to a significant number of patients.

Manning et al.'s (1992) review included contrast of psychoanalytic, behavioral, cognitive, interpersonal, and marital therapies, usually contrasted with tricyclic medication, though in two cases with benzodiazepines. The reviewers note that no studies were conducted by investigators with a primary allegiance to pharmacotherapy. Small sample sizes (hence, low statistical power) were identified as a problem by these reviewers: Only two studies had more than 30 patients per treatment cell. In addition, all but two trials focused on the acute phase of antidepressant treatment. Only seven included follow-up data (varying from 3 to 24 months), and four focused on maintenance therapy.

The efficacy of therapies was examined using a "box score" method contrasting the relative outcomes associated with each treatment modality rather than their absolute impacts. Although some advantage was found to combination treatment, no clear superiority was evident; however, in no study was combined therapy less effective than its component treatments. Summing across studies, combined treatments outperformed medication alone in 4 of 10 instances (40%) and outperformed psychotherapy alone or with placebo in 7 of 18 instances (39%). Not enough trials were available to examine the impact of specific psychotherapies.

Data from a number of studies have suggested that both treatment failure and rate of dropout were highest for patients receiving medication. Given that the cited success rate of most studies usually reflects treatment completers, these factors are important to any consideration of clinical effectiveness. There is some evidence to suggest that dropout reflects dissatisfaction with treatment rather than clinical improvement. Weissman et al. (1979) reported that 92% of patients drop out because of dissatisfaction with treatment; in the NIMH study (Elkin et al., 1989) 77% of dropouts did so for similar reasons. Fawcett et al. (1989) reported that 98% of dropout was because of problems with medication side effects or dissatisfaction with treatment. Wexler and Cicchetti (1992) estimate the rate of dropout at 52% for medication, 30% for therapy alone, and 34% for combination treatments. Casacalenda et al. (2002) reported attrition at 37% and 22%, respectively, for medication and psychotherapy. In contrast, Manning et al. (1992) reported that of 11 studies reporting attrition rates, only one study found that attrition rates varied between single and combined treatments.

Psychodynamic Therapy and Medication

Two recent studies examined the impact of adding psychodynamic therapies to medication, though both are somewhat problematic. de Jonghe et al. (2001) contrasted pharmacotherapy alone or in combination with "short-term psychodynamic supportive therapy." Psychotherapy was delivered in 16 sessions over 6 months, but although described as psychodynamically informed, the protocol emphasized supportive and problem-solving elements, and excluded the use of transference interpretations (raising questions about the best description for the therapy being conducted). Pharmacotherapy employed fluoxetine in the first instance; dependent on patients' responses, the protocol allowed for them to be switched to amitriptyline or (finally) to moclobemide. Of the 167 patients randomized to treatment, high initial refusal rates meant that 57 started pharmacotherapy and 72 started combined therapy. At the end of the 6-month treatment period, and with remission defined as an HRSD score ≤ 7), combined treatment showed significant advantage over pharmacotherapy alone (21% and 44% of the completer sample achieved remission at posttherapy), with evidence that more rapid remission was achieved with the combined treatment. However, at later stages of the trial, there was significantly greater attrition from pharmacotherapy alone contrasted to combined treatment, which may have contributed to this finding.

Burnand et al. (2002) assigned 95 patients with HRSD scores ≥ 20 to 10 weeks of either psychodynamic therapy in combination with clomipramine, or the same period of treatment with clomipramine alone. In practice, clomipramine was combined with "supportive care" offered at the same intensity as psychodynamic therapy, and comprising "empathic listening, guidance support, and facilitation of an alliance." Psychotherapy was offered by nurses working under the supervision of a psychoanalyst. Both groups evidenced equivalent gains at 10 weeks, though the proportion meeting criteria for MDD was lower among those receiving psychodynamic therapy. In contrast to the rate of response found in most trials, improvements were unusually marked and rapid for such a brief period of intervention: HRSD means in both treatment groups reduced from a mean of approximately 24 to 9 at posttherapy, perhaps raising questions about the sample under study. After this acute treatment phase, patients were rereferred to routine outpatient treatments, though at clinicians' discretion, some continued in the original treatment condition to which they had been randomized (Burnand, personal communication, 2003). Monitoring continued until clinicians discharged patients (based on clinical rather than research criteria), though variations in the length and type of additional treatment make it difficult to attribute longer term outcomes to the original treatment received. With this important caveat, there was some evidence that patients who received psychodynamic therapy had fewer inpatient admissions, suggesting some modest advantage of psychodynamic therapy in combination with medication when contrasted to medication combined with counseling and support.

Cognitive-Behavioral Therapy and Medication

In a trial that also examined the impact of maintenance therapy, Blackburn and Moore (1997) allocated 75 patients to one of three combinations of acute–continuation treatments—pharmacootherapy in both phases, CBT in both phases, or acute-phase pharmacotherapy followed by CBT. Acute treatment lasted for 16 weeks and the continuation phase, for 2 years. Patients were relatively unselected contrasted to many trials, and many had both chronic and severe presentations. Medication was prescribed under naturalistic conditions through hospital or primary care doctors (hence, patients received a range of antidepressants), though a research protocol specified minimum dosages. Patients receiving CBT met with their therapists weekly in the acute phase and monthly thereafter; no comparable information on frequency of contacts is available for the medication group, though, on the basis of a naturalistic mode of delivery, it probably varied widely. All three groups showed equivalent gains across both phases of the trial, though (perhaps reflecting the sample) overall response rates were somewhat lower than for comparable trials (using a criterion of an HRSD score $\leq$ 6; rates of remission after the acute phase for (pooled) pharmacotherapy and CBT were 24% and 33%, respectively).

Jarrett et al. (1999) contrasted the efficacy of cognitive therapy, phenelzine, and placebo in 108 patients with "atypical" depression (a subclass of DSM-IV-TR MDD usually associated with a chronic and recurrent course). The choice of an MAOI was based on evidence of greater efficacy of this medication with this population. Over 10 weeks of treatment, cognitive therapy and phenelzine appeared to have equivalent efficacy, and both were more effective than placebo. A recovery criterion of an HRSD score ≤ 9 was met by 58% of patients in both the cognitive therapy and phenelzine groups contrasted to 28% of those receiving placebo.

A large multicenter trial conducted by Keller et al. (2000) randomly assigned 681 patients to one of three conditions—nefazodone alone, a variant of CBT, or a combination of the two treatments. Although the psychotherapy employed—cognitive behavioral analysis system of psychotherapy (BCASP)—contains many standard elements of CBT, it has a strong interpersonal focus, emphasizing social problem solving and making use of interpersonal themes arising in the therapeutic relationship. Patients were recruited on the basis that they had a chronic condition, with their current episode of MDD lasting for at least 2 years. Psychotherapy was delivered twice weekly for the first 4 weeks, and weekly thereafter to 12 weeks. Remission was defined as an HRSD score ≤ 8 at weeks 10 and 12. On this basis, psychotherapy alone and medication alone had equivalent outcomes (33% and 29%, respectively), but combination therapy showed significant advantage both in terms of remission (48%) and in the speed of recovery.

Interpersonal Psychotherapy and Medication

Reynolds et al. (1999a) reported on outcomes in 187 patients over 60 years of age, recruited over a 7-year period on the basis that they presented with a current episode of MDD, had a HRSD score ≥ 17, and had experienced at least one prior episode of MDD. In the first acute phase of the trial, all patients received a combination of nortriptyline and weekly sessions of IPT, until they achieved remission (defined as an HRSD score ≤ 10). Following remission, patients received 16 weeks of continuation treatment; 107 patients met criteria for a stable recovery and entered a maintenance phase (which lasted for 3 years, or until they relapsed). At this point, they were randomized to receive one of four possible treatments: medication clinic and nortriptyline alone; medication clinic and placebo alone; monthly maintenance IPT with nortriptyline, or monthly maintenance with IPT alone. Survival analysis over 3 years indicated a clear benefit to all active treatments over placebo, and for the combination of nortriptyline and IPT over other active treatment options. Recurrence rates for the combination of nortriptyline and IPT were 20%; for nortriptyline alone, 43%, for IPT with placebo, 64%, and for placebo, 90%.

A second report by the same research group (Reynolds et al., 1999b) focused on the efficacy of nortriptyline or IPT on later life depression associated with bereavement. Eighty patients over 50 years of age were recruited on the basis that their depression began close to the death of a partner (either 6 months prior to the death or in the year following it), and randomly assigned to one of four treatments: IPT combined with nortriptyline, IPT combined with placebo, nortriptyline alone or placebo alone. Reflecting trial entry requirements, patients were largely self-referrals and most were female. The protocol allowed for 8 weeks of acute treatment under double-blind conditions; at this point, patients in remission (defined as having an HRSD score ≤ 7 over 3 consecutive weeks) were entered into a 16-week continuation phase. The trial protocol allowed clinicians to break the blinding conditions if they were concerned about patients' progress during the acute phase, effectively compromising the initial randomization; there was a marked difference in the mean length of the acute phase in each "arm" of the trial. Patients receiving nortriptyline and IPT completed a mean of 76 days of treatment contrasted to (approximately) 50 days in each of the other contrasts (patients in IPT combined with nortriptyline received a mean of 9 sessions and 6 when IPT was combined with placebo). Remission rates for the combination of nortriptyline and IPT were 69%; for nortriptyline alone, 56%; for placebo, 45%; and for placebo plus IPT, 29%. At face value, this provides robust evidence for the benefits of active medication and at best suggests some benefit to its combination with IPT. However, some caution seems appropriate because of the methodological problems discussed earlier: the small sample sizes in each treatment cell and the unusually high placebo response rate.

Frank et al. (2000) described the use of two different strategies for implementing IPT and medication in a successive cohort design that recruited women in their second or greater episode of MDD. In the first (sequential treatment) condition, 158 women received IPT alone for between 12 and 24 weeks until remission, followed by a further 17 weeks of IPT. If continued remission was not evident at this point, IPT was combined with an SSRI. In the second (combination) condition, IPT and medication were offered together from the outset, with a broadly similar pattern of psychotherapy. Remission rates in 159 women offered sequential treatment were 50% with IPT alone, boosted to 79% with the addition of medication. In 180 women offered combination treatment, remission rates were 66%. Lack of randomization and small differences in delivery of IPT caution against over-interpretation, particularly because a theoretical rationale for the observed differences in remission rate is not obvious. Nonetheless, this does suggest that the manner in which combination treatment is initiated may be pertinent to outcome.

Couple Therapy and Medication

Based on evidence that the degree of criticism expressed by a partner toward a patient is associated with a poorer prognosis, Leff et al. (2000) recruited depressed patients living in a stable relationship with a critical partner. Seventy-seven patients were stratified into those with and without a previous history of significant depression, and were then randomized either to receive couple therapy or pharmacotherapy. Though desipramine was prescribed initially, nonresponders were prescribed trazodone or fluvoxamine; blood testing was used to check adherence. Alongside medication, psychoeducation and 12–20 outpatient sessions were offered over 1 year, after which medication was tapered. Couple therapy was conducted using a flexible protocol that identified and attempted to remedy problematic patterns of interaction, and was delivered by experienced clinicians over 12–20 sessions. At 1 and at 2 years, intention-to-treat analysis showed gains for patients in both groups, though whether mode of therapy impacted differentially was dependent on the form of measurement: The BDI indicated a significant advantage to couple therapy, but on the HRSD, both therapies showed equivalent outcomes. This rather ambiguous outcome is difficult to interpret, but a conservative interpretation suggests that couple therapy is of equivalent efficacy to medication for individuals with histories suggesting that relationship issues may be relevant to their presentation.

"Problem-Solving" Treatment and Medication

Problem-solving treatment has a psychosocial, here-and-now focus, and encourages patients to specify and work toward resolving areas of functioning that they identify as problematic. Most trials examine the impact of this approach for individuals with mild to moderate depression in primary care settings.

Mynors-Wallis et al. (1995, 2000) recruited patients through primary care centers in Oxfordshire. They (1995) allocated 91 patients to one of three treatments—amitripyline and clinical management, placebo and clinical management, or six sessions of problem solving delivered over 12 weeks. Setting a recovery criterion as HRSD scores ≤ 7 at 12 weeks, the recovery rate in patients receiving amitripyline and problem-solving therapy was equivalent (60% and 52%, respectively), but was significantly greater than for patients receiving placebo (27%). A later study by the same research group (2000) randomized 151 patients to receive problem solving therapy alone, fluvoxamine or paroxetine alone, or problem solving combined with one or the other of these medications. Over 12 weeks, all treatments showed equivalent efficacy. It should be noted that entry criteria for these studies are lower than in most trials reported in this section (patients needed to meet research diagnostic criteria for depression and have an HRSD score ≥ 13, usually an indicator for mild depression). On this basis, it may be inappropriate to generalize these results beyond benefit to patients with mild to moderate depression.

Brief Dynamic Therapy

There continue to be fewer controlled trials of brief dynamic therapy than would be expected given its widespread use in clinical practice. Unfortunately, of those studies available, few have been carried out by proponents of the technique, and often dynamic therapy has been employed as a contrast to alternative therapies with which the investigators were professionally identified. Treatment periods are usually short [a mode of 12 sessions (range = 12–36) in the studies reviewed in this chapter], which may be too short for this technique. Therapists in these trials were unlikely to administer dynamic therapy appropriately because of their lack of commitment to the method. These methodological problems, together with the likely bias introduced by investigator allegiance, suggest that results from these studies should be viewed with caution.

Many studies of psychodynamic therapy suggest that dynamic therapy is significantly less effective than other forms of intervention. Thus, Steuer et al. (1984) found it less effective than cognitive therapy; McLean and Hakstian (1979) found that it performed more poorly than behavior therapy; and Covi and Lipman (1987) found that it was less effective than both cognitive therapy alone and cognitive therapy combined with medication. Kornblith et al. (1983) contrasted behavioral self-control methods against dynamic therapy; all treatments were administered in groups and were found to be equally effective. However, small sample sizes and variations in sample size across treatment conditions make interpretation of this study difficult. Bellack and colleagues (1981; Hersen et al., 1984) treated 50 depressed women with amitriptyline, social skills training and medication, social skills training and placebo, or dynamic therapy with placebo (designated as a "nonspecific therapy"). All treatments resulted in equivalent gains. Thompson et al. (1987, 1990) contrasted dynamic therapy, cognitive therapy, and behavioral therapy against a wait-list control; all treatments were delivered in group formats and with elderly depressed patients. Dynamic therapy was more effective than a wait-list control, and all three treatments were equally effective both posttherapy and at 1- and 2-year follow-up.

Although outcomes from the Sheffield psychotherapy study (Shapiro et al., 1994) are a more robust demonstration of the potential efficacy of this technique, it remains the case that, overall, support for brief dynamic therapy is sparse and at best equivocal. No study favors dynamic therapy over other therapies, and some suggest that it performs more poorly. Firm conclusions regarding the efficacy of brief dynamic techniques still require further and better designed research.

Interpersonal Psychotherapy

An unusual—indeed, probably unique—trial reports on the application of IPT in rural Uganda (Bolton et al., 2003). Using a cluster randomized design, 30 villages were selected for study. Because therapy was conducted in gender-specific groups, in 15 of these villages participants were male, and in the remaining 15 they were female. Half the "male" and "female" villages were assigned to the intervention, with half acting as a control. Potential participants were identified by local leaders and screened using appropriately adapted standardized measures. Trial entrants were also required to meet DSM criteria for MDD, though these were slightly relaxed, allowing entry for individuals who fell short of MDD diagnosis by one symptom criterion. In each village, IPT was offered in a group format over 16 weeks, with 116 villagers receiving this intervention and 132 acting as controls. Therapists were locally recruited and trained, and appear not to have had prior psychotherapeutic expertise. Contrasted to controls, IPT resulted in a significant reduction in symptoms and a marked reduction in rates of diagnosed MDD (which fell from 86% to 6.5% in the IPT group, and from 94% to 55% in controls). This carefully constructed study demonstrates the benefits of a psychosocial intervention (though not necessarily the specific benefits of IPT) despite clear cultural differences between villagers' conceptualizations of depression and those of the patients for whom IPT was originally developed.

Couple Therapy

Baucom et al. (1998) and Beach et al. (1998) reviewed four studies that contrasted individual IPT and couple-based IPT (Foley et al., 1989), behavioral marital therapy, individual cognitive therapy or a combination of both approaches (Jacobson et al., 1991), behavioral marital therapy, individual cognitive therapy or a wait-list control (Beach & O'Leary, 1992), and individual cognitive therapy and "communication-focused marital therapy" (Emanuels-Zuurveen & Emmelkamp, 1996). These trials were consistent in indicating that, for depressive symptoms, there was an equivalence of action between individual and couple therapies, and between variants of couple therapy. However, when the focus of the therapy lay more with discordant marital relationships, there was evidence that couple therapies were more effective than individual therapy. A caution on the generalizability of these results is in order, because all trials had relatively small sample sizes, and the majority of index patients were female. Leff and Everitt (2001, reviewed earlier) found that pharmacotherapy and couple therapy were of equivalent efficacy for couples selected for marital distress. Current evidence does not provide robust indicators for couple therapy as contrasted to individual therapy. Nonetheless, there is some support for the clinically intuitive notion that couple-based approaches are preferable when relationship stress is a prominent feature of the presentation, because of their differential impact both on the quality of the relationship and on symptoms.

Bibliotherapy and Computer-Aided ("Self-Help") Therapy

These interventions involve little or no direct therapist–client contact, and the usual contrasts are to the efficacy of a similar intervention offered by a therapist. Only behavioral and CBTs have been adapted to this form of delivery; these modalities have a clear rationale that can be presented in a systematic and structured manner. Nonetheless there are significant variations in the way the "self-help" version of the therapies is delivered; at one end of the scale, studies examine the impact of reading recommended texts; at the other, patients interact with a sophisticated, computer-aided therapy package that tailors itself to individuals' needs. Because there is relatively little research in this area, the heterogeneity of approaches suggests that conclusions about the efficacy of self-help approaches need to pay due regard to the specific interventions employed. Cuijpers (1997) conducted a meta-analysis, and Williams and Whitfield (2001), a qualitative review, of bibliotherapy and computer-based treatments.

Bibliotherapy

Cuijpers' (1997) meta-analysis identified seven trials of bibliotherapy for depression, of which six met criteria for methodological quality. Bibliotherapy materials employ a behavioral or cognitive-behavioral approach, and all included at least some therapist contact, though the extent of this varied widely from trial to trial (three had weekly contact, one had contact at the beginning and end of the "session," one at the start and finish of the trial, and one at the start, middle, and end point). Against wait-list control, there was a mean effect size of 0.82; against individual therapy (four studies) the effect size was 0.1. Although this suggests that there may be utility to this approach, all patients were nonclinical populations recruited through media announcements.

Scogin et al. (1989) used media announcements to recruit 67 mildly to moderately depressed older adults randomized to receive one of two forms of bibliotherapy or to be placed on a wait list. The two bibliotherapy texts set out either a behavioral or a cognitive-behavioral model of depression management; participants read the books over a period of 4 weeks, with a research assistant phoning at weekly intervals. Both forms of bibliotherapy resulted in a significant reduction in BDI scores contrasted to the wait list; after treatment, the wait-list group showed improvements equivalent to those receiving immediate treatment. Two-year follow-up (Scogin et al., 1990) suggested that gains were maintained.

Using a similar research design but with a younger sample, Jamison and Scogin (1995) randomized 80 patients solicited through newspaper advertisements to bibliotherapy or to a wait-list control. Bibliotherapy employed a book setting out a CBT model of depression; again, a research assistant phoned at weekly intervals over the 4-week intervention period. Posttherapy patients receiving bibliotherapy showed a significant reduction in BDI scores; at this point, only 30% of patients met DSM criteria for depression, contrasted to 97% of wait-list controls. After the wait-list group received bibliotherapy, their outcomes were equivalent to the immediate treatment group. Three-year follow-up (Smith et al., 1997) found that gains were maintained, although 44% of those followed up had either sought further help for depression or met criteria for depression at the time of follow-up. This result, though impressive, exceeds the usual epidemiological pattern of relapse in depression; hence, it raises some question about the representativeness of the sample.

Beutler et al. (1991) randomized 63 patients to receive 20 weeks of group CBT, group experiential therapy, or a self-directed form of bibliotherapy (patients were asked to read a number of self-help texts, none of which were based on CBT or experiential models; each patient was contacted for about 30 minutes a week by a researcher (indicating that this would be better described as a minimal contact therapy). At 3-month follow-up, all three treatments had equivalent outcomes.

Computer-Aided Therapy

Selmi et al. (1990) solicited 36 patients with mild or moderate depression through newspaper announcements, randomizing them to one of three conditions. The two active conditions both involved a 6-week structured CBT intervention, delivered either by a therapist or through an interactive computer program; the remaining patients were allocated to wait-list control. At posttherapy and at 2-month follow-up, patients receiving both forms of CBT showed equivalent gains over those placed on the wait list; at follow-up, around two-thirds of those receiving CBT met criteria for remission, contrasted to only one wait-list patient. Although the active solicitation of patients limits generalizability, the majority of participants in this study had a depressive episode meeting research diagnostic criteria for more than 6 months, suggesting that their difficulties did not reflect transient distress.

In a small trial, Bowers et al. (1993) allocated 22 depressed inpatients to 2 weeks of CBT delivered by a therapist, 2 weeks of a computer-based therapy, or to treatment as usual. At discharge, those receiving the computerized therapy were unimproved. The computer program has been criticized for relying only on cognitive rather than behavioral techniques (Marks, 1999), though whether this is the basis for differential outcomes is not clear.

A large-scale trial (Proudfoot et al., 2003) randomized 167 patients to receive an eight-session, computer-based CBT program for depression, or TAU from their primary care physician. The package was standardized but became customized to patients as they interacted with the program. Inclusion criteria did not restrict the sample to those with depression alone—nearly half were diagnosed with mixed anxiety and depression. Recruitment was by both referral from a primary care physician and screening in general practitioners' waiting rooms, using the General Health Questionnaire (GHQ-12). (The broad inclusion criteria and the use of screening [which would lead to patients entering the trial who may not have otherwise come forward for help] raises at least some question about contrast of results from this to other trials of treatments for depression.)

Though patients receiving computer-aided therapy received pharmacotherapy and any nonspecific support associated with TAU, they were precluded from receiving any form of concurrent psychological therapy. In addition, the treatments received by all patients were monitored. At posttherapy and through to 6-month follow-up, patients receiving the CBT program compared to TAU evidenced a significant reduction in BDI scores; mean pretreatment scores for CBT and TAU, respectively, were 25.5 and 24.0, and at 6-month follow-up, 9.5 and 16.0. Post hoc analysis suggested that CBT patients evidenced equivalent gains whether or not they were in receipt of medication, and that while initial severity did not predict outcome, duration of illness did: Patients who had been depressed for more than 6 months prior to trial entry showed significantly greater impairment at assessment points. This study provides a helpful pointer to the potential utility of computer-aided packages but is at present unique and requires replication.

Summary

Although a number of recent studies add to our knowledge of the relative impacts of pharmacotherapy and psychotherapy, there is continuing variability in outcomes from individual trials. Nonetheless, there is good evidence of the superiority of either active treatment over placebo. In relation to each modality offered alone, psychotherapy does not appear superior in efficacy to medication; only rarely does medication show clear advantage over psychotherapy and, on the whole, a reasonable conclusion would be that psychotherapy is of equivalent efficacy to medication. While there is some suggestion of benefit to combination treatment, this is hard to demonstrate. It is possible that the impact of combination treatment (which is widely practiced in routine settings) is less in its additive impact than in facilitating the acceptability of treatment—for example, better accommodating issues, such as the slower speed of change for psychotherapeutic interventions with more severely depressed individuals, or the attrition associated with the impact of side effects in pharmacotherapy.

Although most medication–psychotherapy contrasts are to CBT, there is some diversity in terms of psychotherapeutic approach studied. As yet, there are not enough trials to detect whether there are variations in the way specific therapies interact or contrast with pharmacological approaches, though, on the basis of limited evidence, patterns of outcome seem similar.

Though rather limited, information on the relative acceptability of medication and psychotherapy suggests that psychotherapy or combination treatment is associated with lower attrition rates than pharmacotherapy alone. Definitive conclusions about pharmaco- and psychotherapies are hampered by methodological issues of both a specific and a conceptual nature. A lack of rigor and therapeutic equipoise in earlier trials almost certainly acted to enhance the relative benefits of psychotherapy, while problems with blinding may have led to overestimation of medication effects. More recent trials seem better designed and, hence, less susceptible to basic problems of interpretation.

Brief dynamic therapy, while widely practiced, continues to have a limited evidence base. Where good-quality trials have been conducted, outcomes are equivalent to alternative psychotherapies, but the paucity of trials represents a serious concern and severely limits conclusions that can be drawn about this approach. This position contrasts the increasing evidence base for a range of approaches—in particular CBT, IPT, couple therapy, problem-solving therapy, bibliotherapy, and computer-aided therapy, all of which show evidence of efficacy, though not necessarily of advantage relative to other approaches.

A pertinent observation is that all structured psychotherapeutic approaches show short-term efficacy in around 50–60% of cases. While this could reflect the impacts of specific elements of each therapy, it also raises the possibility that nonspecific responsiveness of many patient samples, together with regression to the mean, could account for this equivalence of action. In this respect, the concerns expressed by Klein and others (discussed earlier) may have some force. This does not imply accepting all their arguments, but without greater control for nonspecific effects, it is hard to be certain that short-term outcomes can be attributed to the technical ingredients of therapies. It is possible that an alternative explanation for the consistency of outcome is that this reflects a maximum treatment effect imposed by the nature of research samples and the lengths of treatment. If this were so, the important difference between treatments would be sought not in immediate treatment effects but in their capacity to delay relapse, a measure of outcome that more closely maps to the chronic nature of depression in many individuals.

MANAGING RELAPSE AND RECURRENCE

Though predicting relapse in individual patients is difficult, there is consistent evidence that the probability of experiencing a further episode of depression is greater if patients have achieved only partial remission after treatment. A number of trials (e.g., Paykel et al., 1995; Thase et al., 1992; Van Londen et al., 1988) reported that the presence of residual symptoms was associated both with higher levels of relapse and with shorter intervals between the previous and subsequent episodes. Residual symptoms were associated with more severe initial illness and with a history of previous depressive episodes but not with other indicators such as duration of depression or the presence of dysthymic disorder. Contrasted to patients who were asymptomatic after treatment, relapse appears to be about three times as likely in patients with residual symptoms, and to occur about three times more quickly (Judd et al., 1998a, 2000).

A claim often made for CBT is that it acts prophylactically against recurrence of depression, in part because the therapy addresses the dysfunctional cognitions thought to contribute to depressed states. There is little evidence of such specificity of action. For example Gortner et al. (1998) contrasted the impact of three treatments: (1) exclusively cognitive, (2) exclusively behavioral, and (3) both elements. Posttherapy data on 137 patients suggested that all three treatments were of equal efficacy, and relapse rates and survival time to relapse at 2-year follow-up were equivalent. Although there are now a number of trials suggesting that CBT lowers relapse rates, the contrast is often against no treatment or against patients withdrawn from medication. Since there is little research into the potential efficacy of other forms of psychological therapy, it is not clear that these reduced relapse rates are specific to CBT. Finally, though a reduction in relapse can be demonstrated, this is better seen as relative rather than absolute, since a significant number of patients suffered a further episode of depression.

Kovacs et al. (1981) followed up patients in the Rush et al. (1977) study; after 1 year, treatment gains with both CBT and medication were maintained, though patients treated with CBT had significantly lower levels of depression than those treated with medication, and there was a trend for more of them to be judged as being in remission. Beck et al. (1985) found improvement to be stable over 6- and 12-month follow-up in patients who had received CBT, or CBT in combination with medication. There was a trend for the combination group to do better than the CBT group at 12 months. Simons et al. (1986), reporting follow-up data from a study by Murphy et al. (1984), found that at 12 months, patients who had received CBT had a significantly lower relapse rate than those receiving medication. Blackburn et al. (1986), reporting follow-up data of Blackburn et al. (1981), found significantly greater relapse in patients who received medication than in patients receiving CBT at 6 months, though this reduced to a trend at 2 years. Rotzer–Zimmer et al. (1985, cited in Williams, 1992) and Evans et al. (1992) also found a significantly reduced rate of relapse in patients treated with CBT compared to those receiving medication. In contrast, the follow-up phase of the NIMH study (Shea et al., 1992a) suggested no significant advantage to CBT over other interventions.

Though there is evidence for (at least a limited) prophylactic effect of short-term CBT, the evidence from most of the trials reviewed above is clear: Individuals with MDD are at risk of relapse following circumscribed interventions. Despite this, rather few trials examine the impact of adding a continuation phase to short-term interventions. Frank et al.'s (1990) seminal study was described in detail earlier; briefly, this study found some benefit to monthly IPT over 5 years for individuals with recurrent depression, defined as three or more episodes of MDD, with the most recent being no more than 2½ years prior to the present episode.

Blackburn and Moore (1997; reviewed earlier) followed patients over 2 years, though attrition makes it inappropriate to consider data beyond 12 months. All patients were defined as suffering "recurrent" depression, though the criterion for "recurrent" was set at one previous episode of MDD (a somewhat less rigorous marker than that used by Frank et al. [1990]). All received active maintenance treatment (either medication or monthly CBT); both treatments showed equal efficacy in terms of subsequent relapse. Of the 49 patients in this trial initially treated with medication, 13 failed to respond at the end of the acute phase of treatment. Seven of these patients were randomized to continue on medication, and six, to receive CBT. In the continuation phase, attrition further reduced this already small sample (Moore & Blackburn, 1997), and though more of those receiving CBT were categorized as showing a full or partial response than those receiving medication, the difference was not statistically significant.

Fava et al. (1998b) reported a seminaturalistic design that followed the progress of 40 patients with recurrent depression (defined using Frank et al.'s [1990] criterion) treated between 3 and 5 months with a range of antidepressant medications. At this point, patients were randomized to receive ten 30-minute sessions of CBT or clinical management, and medication was tapered and discontinued. Immediately after this phase, patients with CBT showed a significantly lower level of residual symptoms, and at 2-year follow-up had a significantly lower relapse rate (25% contrasted to 80% for clinical management). It should be noted that the therapy applied was a modification of standard CBT (though it retained recognizable elements of this approach) conducted by one therapist for all patients.

Fava et al. (1998a) reported outcomes over 6 years following an initial phase of treatment (Fava et al., 1994), in which 40 patients with MDD who had been successfully treated with antidepressants were randomly assigned to

10 sessions of either fortnightly CBT or clinical management; in both groups, medication was tapered and discontinued. Over the length of follow-up, relapse rates in the CBT groups were lower than those in clinical management, though this difference was only statistically significant at 4-year follow-up (at 2 years, respective relapse rates were 15% and 35%; at 4 years, 35% and 70%; and at 6 years, 50% and 75%).

Paykel et al. (1999) recruited 158 patients whose MDD had only partially remitted following an initial phase of treatment with appropriate levels of antidepressant medication. Patients were then assigned either to clinical management alone, or to clinical management combined with 16 sessions of cognitive therapy over 20 weeks (with two further booster sessions 6 and 14 weeks later). Unlike Fava et al. (1994, 1998a) they continued to prescribe medication throughout this phase. Patients in receipt of cognitive therapy showed a significantly reduced cumulative relapse rate. Based on the intent-to-treat sample, at 68-week follow-up, relapse rates were 29% contrasted to 47% for controls. Though relatively few patients met criteria for remission (stable subclinical scores on the HDRS and BDI over 4 weeks), significantly more experimental than control subjects achieved this status (at 20 weeks, 25% and 13%, respectively). Scott et al. (2003) reported a cost–benefit analysis of this study, which suggests that the additional cost of providing CBT was somewhere between £4,000 and £5,000 per relapse prevented (despite evidence of a marked reduction of in- and day-patient services). In this respect, it can be concluded that the addition of CBT is more costly but also more effective (particularly if it impacts on the longer term course of the disorder).

In contrast to these studies, Jarrett et al. (1998, 2001) did not include pharmacotherapy in any arm of their trial. On the basis of earlier promising outcomes from a nonrandomized pilot trial, 156 patients were entered into an acute phase of cognitive therapy comprising 20 sessions over 12–14 weeks. After this initial intervention, 84 patients agreed to be randomized either to receive 10 further sessions of therapy over 8 months or to a control condition in which they were monitored but no further intervention was offered. At this point, relapse rates for patients in receipt of continued therapy were significantly lower than in controls (10% and 31%, respectively). Stratifying the sample in relation to age of onset (before or after age 18) suggested that earlier onset was associated with greater vulnerability to relapse; 67% of control patients with onset prior to age 18 relapsed over 8 months contrasted to 36% of those with later onset. Though continuation therapy was especially beneficial for "early onset" patients, with significant reduction in relapse rates compared to controls (16% and 67%, respectively), it showed less impact for patients with later onset (relapse rates of 50% and 36%, respectively). This pattern was maintained at 24-month follow-up. A further subanalysis confirmed that individuals who failed to achieve stable remission in the later phases of acute treatment were also vulnerable to relapse. Contrasted to controls, at 24 months, relapse rates for patients with unstable remission were significantly reduced by continuation therapy (62% and 37%, respectively).

Mindfulness-based cognitive therapy (MBCT) has developed as a way of conceptualizing vulnerability both to depression and to relapse in patients with a history of MDD (Teasdale, 1999). The conventional CBT model assumes that vulnerability to depression arises from dysfunctional beliefs or attitudes, which are modified by successful intervention. MBCT assumes that it is not so much the dysfunctional content of beliefs or attitudes that lead to depressive states as the facility with which patterns of negative thinking can become activated when individuals become dysphoric, and the ease with which these can rapidly escalate into a ruminative cycle. Vulnerability to depression arises not only because of the accessibility of negative thoughts but also because individuals find it difficult to gain a sense of perspective from which to appraise themselves. In practice, MBCT aims both to help patients increase awareness of their patterns of thought and to foster their capacity to appraise their cognitions from a "decentered" or disidentified position. On this basis, there is no direct challenge to cognitions (as in conventional CBT), but an attempt to alter the degree to which individuals react to these cognitions as if they were isomorphic with their sense of self.

Teasdale et al. (2000) explored the utility of MBCT in a multicenter trial based at three treatment sites (in the United Kingdom and Canada). Inclusion criteria required patients to have a history of two or more episodes of MDD within the past 5 years, with at least one of these episodes in the 2 years prior to the study. One hundred forty-five patients in recovery or remission from MDD were randomly assigned either to MBCT (delivered in a group format over nine weekly sessions) or to TAU. Analysis of relapse patterns over the 60 weeks of the study period suggested different outcomes for patients with three or more previous episodes of depression (who constituted 77% of the intention-to-treat sample), compared to those with two previous episodes. In the former group, significantly fewer of those in receipt of MBCT relapsed contrasted to those given TAU (66% and 40%, respectively). Among patients with two prior episodes of depression, relapse rates across treatment conditions were statistically equivalent (56% of MBCT and 31% of TAU group). Further analysis suggested that for TAU, there was a linear relationship between the number of prior episodes and the risk of relapse (31% for patients with two prior episodes, 56% for three, and 72% for four). This pattern was not present for patients in receipt of MBCT. Subanalyses suggested that the reduction in relapse rate was not attributable to increased medication prescription (which was comparable across treatment conditions). Patients with more than three episodes of depression experienced their first episode of depression at a significantly younger age than those with two prior episodes. This observation suggests the utility of identifying a subgroup of especially vulnerable individuals for whom MBCT might be especially beneficial, and echoes Jarrett et al.'s (2001) suggestion that age of onset may be an important marker of vulnerability. Furthermore, both trials only demonstrated differential effects on relapse for individuals with a significant history of depression; if replicated by other trials, this would be a helpful marker for clinical intervention.

Summary

Medication, CBT, and IPT have shown efficacy in reducing relapse in patient samples selected on the basis of their vulnerability to relapse, usually using "booster" or maintenance sessions. There is evidence of the efficacy of maintenance psychotherapies combined with medication and also when offered alone in the context of discontinuation of medication.

Provision of maintenance sessions appears to be effective, but it is also costly. In view of this, it is helpful to have some preliminary indications of differential benefit for individuals with early onset and a history of previous relapses. This finding does not suggest that maintenance therapies should be restricted to this group; though they might be privileged for such an intervention, their higher response rate presumably rests on their known excess vulnerability to relapse.

Whether some therapies are better than others at reducing relapse is, as yet, a moot point. While it is encouraging to see the development of therapies (such as MBCT) that have developed from theoretical ideas about the nature of relapse, their benefit over standard technique is, as yet, unclear.

STUDIES OF EFFICACY IN DIFFERENT TREATMENT CONTEXTS
Inpatient Treatment

Although many trials of CBT with inpatients have been reported, five studies are of particular interest in that they examine the use of CBT with patients with more severe depression, and with associated behavior likely to exclude them from other treatment trials, such as suicidal behavior.

Thase et al. (1991) treated 16 unmedicated inpatients characterized by an HRSD score of ≥ 15 and with an index episode of MDD of less than 2 years' duration. All were drug-free for at least 7 days before the trial commenced. Twenty-six patients were assessed as suitable for the trial; 16 of these completed treatment, while the remainder had electroconvulsive therapy (ECT) or medication, either because of noncompliance with therapy or the emergence of severe symptomatology before therapy commenced. Intensive CBT was offered five times a week over 4 weeks; on average patients received 13 sessions of therapy. Response was defined by reduction in HRSD scores of at least 50% and a final score of ≤ 10, and 13 patients (81%) reached this criterion. Follow-up therapy was offered, but only seven patients received more than 1 month of outpatient CBT; though the follow-up period is not specified, Thase et al. (1991) report that of these patients, only one relapsed, compared to three out of four patients who refused further therapy and whose progress was monitored.

Thase and colleagues (1993) reported an extension of this work to larger samples in three research trials (Nofzinger et al., 1993; Simons & Thase, 1992; Thase et al., 1991). In total, 142 unmedicated patients were treated either as outpatients ($n = 110$) or inpatients ($n = 32$). Outpatients received up to 20 sessions of CBT over 20 weeks; inpatients received more intensive therapy—20 sessions over 4 weeks (as reported in detail earlier [Thase et al., 1991]). Across all three patient samples, significant reductions in HRSD scores were found, though higher initial levels of depression were associated with poorer response rates. This effect was most marked for patients with HRSD scores above 20.

Bowers (1990) conducted a comparative trial of nortriptyline alone, relaxation in combination with nortriptyline, or CBT and nortriptyline, offered to 30 inpatients in addition to the usual hospital milieu. Therapy was conducted in groups, and 12 therapy sessions were offered. Forty-one patients were approached, eight declined, and one patient per group dropped out "because of violation of the protocol."

Patients were moderately to severely depressed; the mean pretreatment BDI scores for the CBT, relaxation, and medication groups were 24.2, 25.8, and 31.2, respectively (giving a nonsignificant trend toward greater initial severity in the medication group). All therapies were offered by the same therapist.

Symptoms were assessed using the BDI, the HRSD, and measures of cognitive adjustment at sessions 1, 6, and 12, and at discharge. All groups improved, but patients receiving CBT or relaxation had significantly fewer depressive symptoms and negative cognitions than patients in the medication-alone condition. In addition, patients receiving CBT were less likely to be judged depressed at discharge than those in the other treatment conditions. A recovery criterion of an HRSD score of ≤ 6 was achieved by 8 of 10 patients in the CBT group, compared with 1 of 10 and 2 of 10 patients receiving relaxation or medication alone.

The degree to which this result reflects the specific impact of CBT is not clear. Using a criterion based on a BDI score of ≤ 9, patients receiving relaxation showed similar gains to those in the CBT group. Interpretation of this study is also made more difficult by the fact that there was no control for the additional attention psychotherapy patients received in contrast to those on medication alone.

Miller et al. (1989) assigned 47 patients to one of three conditions—standard treatment (hospital milieu, medication, and medication management), CBT and standard treatment, or social skills training and standard treatment. All patients had BDI scores $\geq$ 17 and HRSD scores $\geq$ 17. Therapies were conducted daily while the patients were in the hospital, and continued weekly after discharge. CBT was offered daily while patients were in the hospital and weekly after discharge. All therapies led to significant gains on a range of measures. At discharge, there was a trend for patients receiving combination treatments to be categorized as responders; after outpatient treatment, the trend reached significance. However, there were significant differences in the dropout rate between conditions—41% from standard treatment, 31% from CBT, and 14% from social skills. In addition, all patients from the standard treatment group had dropped out by week 8 of follow-up, leading to problems in interpreting the follow-up data.

Scott and colleagues in Newcastle present data from two open trials of combined medication and CBT, offered to chronically depressed inpatients who had previously failed to respond to standard antidepressants and had been depressed for at least 2 years. Pharmacotherapy comprised phenelzine, L-tryptophan, and lithium. In the first trial (Barker et al., 1987), 20 patients were randomly assigned either to pharmacotherapy alone or to combination treatment with CBT (delivered biweekly for 3 weeks, followed by nine weekly sessions). Though 11 patients showed a 50% reduction in HRSD scores (all within the first 6 weeks), there was no evidence for an additional benefit from CBT. In a second trial with a similar population (Scott & Freeman, 1992), 24 patients were divided into two cohorts. The first ($n = 8$) received 12 weeks of combined pharmacotherapy and CBT as described in Barker et al. (1987), with similar outcomes to those described earlier. The second ($n = 16$) was offered a modified CBT package with a "milieu" treatment; patients were admitted to a dedicated inpatient unit, and therapy was more intensive and prolonged—approximately 26 inpatient sessions followed by at least 6 months of outpatient treatment. Percentage change scores on the BDI and HRSD were greater for patients receiving the modified package (52% and 57%, respectively) than for those receiving standard CBT (42% on both measures), and significant change was observed in 69% of patients. Although suggestive, small sample sizes and nonrandom allocation limit the conclusions that can be drawn.

Treatment in Primary Care

Most research focuses on patients referred to specialist services, and though outcomes from this work are almost certainly applicable to those seen in primary care, it is not safe to assume that the same outcomes will be achieved. Patients seen by primary care physicians probably represent a broader range of presentations than those seen in secondary care, and the clinical picture is often complicated by somatic presentations. For many patients, their first (and sometimes only) port of call is primary care; on this basis, this section considers whether specific interventions have greater efficacy than TAU offered by primary care physicians. TAU is a nonspecific comparison, potentially containing a number of uncontrolled elements—not only interventions offered by the physician but also treatments offered by specialists to whom the patient is referred. This means that TAU can vary significantly in relation to the treatments offered to individual patients, and in relation to the practices of different family physicians, reducing internal validity. In addition, any differences that emerge between TAU and a comparator treatment will reflect the quality of local primary care services and the services to which it has access. Although contrast to TAU is ecologically appropriate, care is needed in interpreting results from these studies.

Teasdale et al. (1984) treated 17 patients with BDI scores ≥ 20, contrasting them with 20 patients receiving TAU. Although CBT led to a significant difference in the number of patients judged recovered posttreatment (indicated by a BDI score ≤ 10), at 3-month follow-up the TAU group had also improved, leading to no between-group differences at this point. Ross and Scott (1985) treated 51 patients with BDI scores ≥ 14; patients continued to receive TAU from their family physician but were additionally allocated either to individual or group CBT, or to a 3-month wait-list control group (that subsequently received CBT). A 64% reduction in BDI scores was found for the CBT group, contrasted to a 13% reduction in the wait-list group. However, no figures using a recovery criterion are given in the study, and relapse was defined as a BDI score ≥ 16, which is markedly less stringent than that usually adopted. Partial data from a 12-month follow-up suggested that no patients receiving CBT relapsed on this criterion.

Scott and Freeman (1992) requested that 63 family physicians from 14 primary health care practices refer patients with a depressive disorder. One hundred ninety-four patients were referred and 121 were accepted into the trial. The study design was such that some patients would be assigned to treatment with medication; of some interest is the fact that most patients who declined to take part in the study cited as a reason a reluctance to take medication. Patients were randomly assigned to one of four conditions for 16 weeks of treatment. Help was offered by a psychiatrist (for amitriptyline), a clinical psychologist (for CBT), or a social worker (for supportive counseling). In the remaining condition, patients were reassigned to their family physicians for TAU. One difficulty in this study is that randomization of patients to treatment conditions was not successful; only 11 of 29 (38%) of patients seeing the social worker had HRSD scores ≥ 16, suggesting that most clients in this group did not achieve a level of "caseness" for depression (contrasted to 22 of 30 [73%] patients in the family physician group). In addition, only 2 of 29 (7%) patients seeing the clinical psychologist had a previous episode of depression. At the end of treatment, only social work counseling

showed a greater reduction in depressive symptoms when contrasted to care
from the physician. It has already been noted, however, that patients in each
of these groups differed markedly in their initial levels of depression, which
makes it difficult to interpret this result. Patient satisfaction was greatest with
social work counseling, though the fact that only one therapist offered each
treatment modality increases the likelihood of therapist-specific effects.

Schulberg et al. (1996) randomized 276 patients with a diagnosis of
MDD to receive nortriptyline, IPT, or TAU. A very large number of
patients (7,652) attending primary care services were screened for depression,
and further filters ensured that all patients met DSM-III criteria for depression
and had an HRSD score ≥ 13. For both active treatments an acute phase
determined whether patients were treatment responders; for medication, this
phase continued over 6 weeks, and for IPT, over 16 weeks, with improvement defined as a 33–50% reduction in initial BDI score. Those who met
these criteria entered a 4-month continuation phase (with sessions at monthly
intervals). There was significant attrition from both phases of the trial. Only
50% of patients completed the acute phase; in the continuation phase, 40% of
patients receiving medication and 20% of those in receipt of IPT dropped
out. Though symptom levels in the intent-to-treat sample reduced across all
interventions, the active treatments showed equal efficacy, and both resulted
in significantly greater gains over TAU. A similar pattern was evident for
patients who completed the continuation phase. At 8 months, a recovery criterion of an HRSD score ≤ 7 was met by 48% and 46%, of patients receiving
medication and IPT, and by 18% of those receiving TAU.

Scott et al. (1997) contrasted the efficacy of brief CBT plus TAU to
TAU alone. Forty-eight patients with a BDI score ≥ 20 and a depressive episode of less than 2 years were randomized to treatment. CBT was delivered
in six sessions and followed a systematic but flexible protocol that was adapted
to each patient; all therapies were offered by the same therapist. At 7 weeks,
BDI scores in the CBT group were significantly lower than those for patients
receiving TAU. Although data from the follow-up period suggest greater
gains for CBT at 1 year, significantly greater attrition from TAU, combined
with a low sample size, suggests that this result should be interpreted cautiously.

Corney (1987) contrasted 80 depressed women receiving either routine
treatment from their family physician or social work counseling. No clear
model of counseling was followed, though counselors reported using exploration, practical help, and some behavioral goal setting. Overall, there was little difference in outcome among treatment groups. The sample was stratified
according to the degree of severity of depression and its chronicity. Patients
with more acute and less severe problems improved regardless of treatment
received, with more moderate outcomes in more severely distressed patients.
There were some indications that, contrasted with equivalent controls, those

patients with acute but more severe problems had better outcomes when in receipt of counseling.

Raphael (1979) examined the efficacy of counseling for bereaved women considered to be at risk of delayed or pathological grief reactions. In an initial pool 200 women were interviewed. On this basis, 64 patients were selected who demonstrated either marked ambivalence in their relationship to their husbands and/or had poor social support for their grieving. The subgroup of 64 patients was randomly allocated either to counseling or no-treatment groups. Counseling was based on psychodynamic/exploratory methods, focused on the bereavement, and was offered for the 3 months following the death. At 13-month follow-up, 77% of the counseled group had good outcomes, contrasted with 41% of controls.

Holden et al. (1989) reported a trial of counseling for women with acute postnatal depression, delivered by health visitors who had been given a brief (3 week) course in nondirective methods. Forty-eight women were allocated either to eight weekly sessions of counseling, in addition to standard health visitor support, or to standard health visitor support alone. Approximately 3 months after treatment started, 69% of the counseled patients no longer met criteria for depression, contrasted with 38% of the control group.

It may be significant that in both Holden et al. (1989) and Raphael (1979), interventions were targeted, were specific to a client group with acute difficulties, and were delivered by therapists who would have been familiar with their patients' presentation. This draws attention to these specific characteristics of both counselors and patients, and may suggest that counseling interventions may be more likely to be successful when they are focal and focused.

Ward et al. (2000) undertook an ambitiously designed large-scale trial, aiming to examine the relative efficacy of TAU contrasted to 12 sessions of nondirective counseling or CBT, including a patient-preference arm, along with randomization. Four hundred sixty-four patients met entry criteria, which included a BDI score ≥ 14; only 62% of patients were diagnosed as depressed, and the sample is perhaps best characterized as mildly to moderately depressed. While randomization was encouraged, the choices of patients who expressed a strong treatment preference were honored. Monitoring of this strategy suggested that patients were reluctant to be randomized to TAU, though they had few preferences about the type of psychological therapy they received. Since this resulted in rapid recruitment to the two active treatments, a second tranche of patients was offered randomization to CBT or counseling (a two-way rather than a three-way randomization). Although—appropriately—results are reported in way that reflects this complex pattern of sampling, the overall pattern of outcomes for randomized and patient preference arms was not significantly different: At 4 months, both active treatments showed equivalent and significant advantage over TAU, though at 1 year, there were no differences in outcome.

Simpson et al. (2003) carried out a trial of psychodynamic counseling, identifying patients from a number of primary care sites partly through screening of attenders using the BDI, but also through referral from family physicians. On this basis, 143 patients were randomized to counseling or TAU; active treatment comprised 6–12 sessions of nonmanualized therapy. At 6- and 12-month follow-up, no differences between active treatment and control were evident, and while there was evidence that individuals with milder depression showed some benefit, this was not the case for patients with more severe depression (defined as an initial BDI score greater than 24). In addition, many of those who fell into this latter category continued to have scores classifying them as "cases" at follow-up. A parallel report (Simpson et al., 2000) suggests that results were similar for two additional counselors who used CBT rather than psychodynamic techniques. While a number of interpretations are possible, it is worth observing that the pattern of outcomes conforms to evidence from other trials indicating that more severely depressed individuals are unlikely to respond to therapy of this brevity (and that allocation of patients to therapies needs to attend to likely dose–response relationships).

Studies reviewed to this point contrast the impact of individual therapists delivering an intervention. Sherbourne et al. (2001) reported a different strategy, whereby primary care settings as a whole were randomized to receive one of two quality improvement (QI) programs, in which nurse specialists were trained to assess patients and to formulate a treatment plan. In the first (QI-meds), nurses informed patients that medication and therapy were of equal effectiveness, and offered them the option of receiving medication (delivered through the nurse) or counseling (offered in the context of the usual services available in the practice). The second program (QI-therapy), was directed by the family physician, who used the nurse's assessment to decide which patients were appropriate for psychological therapy; if they were, he/she referred them to local psychotherapists, who delivered 12–16 sessions of individual or group CBT, or (for patients whose symptoms were milder) a brief four-session CBT intervention. Medication was available from the primary care setting. The program was monitored every 6 months over 2 years, and the sample comprised 1,299 patients from a total of 27,332 consecutive attendees screened for depression and 3,918 patients identified as potentially eligible for the program.

Four hundred five patients received QI-meds, 464 received QI-therapy, and 430 received TAU. Of these, about half had a diagnosis of MDD or double depression, one-fourth, depressive symptoms in the context of a history of MDD, and one-fourth had depressive symptoms without a previous episode of depression. In the first and second 6 months of QI-meds, 51% and 43% of patients took medication; for QI-therapy, the equivalent medication rates were 39% and 35%, and 38% and 34% received at least four sessions of therapy.

Over the first year, patients receiving QI-meds or QI-therapy had a significantly reduced probability of depression contrasted to those receiving TAU. The trajectory of change was greater for patients in the two QI groups; at 6 months, the rate of probable depression was 51% for TAU, contrasted to 41% in both QI groups. At 1 year, depression rates in both QI groups remained stable, but the rate in TAU had declined (to 48%). The trajectory of this group was a slow improvement, with the result that, by the end of the second year, rates of depression in all groups were equivalent (at approximately 43%). Examining the trajectory of change over time for all three groups, there was evidence that patients receiving QI-therapy had a more stable pattern of change, and a lower probability of poor outcomes, than those receiving QI-meds or TAU.

Summary

There is good evidence that CBT, particularly when delivered intensively, can be a useful adjunct to treatment in inpatient settings and with more severe cases of depression. However, trials usually offer CBT in combination with other treatments, such as social skills training, bibliotherapy, and relaxation. Though this means that the specific effects of CBT are not well established, the effect of therapy is to reduce the severity of depression on discharge and follow-up, and lead to better levels of adjustment.

In primary care, CBT, IPT, and nondirective counseling all seem reasonably effective, though the usual contrast is to TAU, and any advantage is short term rather than long term. Outcomes suggest that interventions are transportable, in that what seems efficacious in secondary or tertiary care also seems to work in primary care. Although it might be expected that briefer treatments would be effective in primary care, the duration of therapies employed in many trials is similar to that in more specialist contexts. While the efficacy of shorter and longer treatments appears equivalent, no trials directly contrast treatment length and, overall, there are too few trials to allow us to draw reliable conclusions.

TREATMENTS FOR DYSTHYMIC DISORDER

Prior to reclassification in DSM-III, patients with dysthymic disorder were seen as suffering a problem of personality rather than a mood disorder. However conceptualized, there is a clinical need to understand the most effective way of managing such patients. Though their depressive symptomatology may be mild (making them appear less needy), the chronicity of their condition appears to result in greater social incapacity than that experienced by many individuals with MDD (Klein & Hayden, 2000; Klein et al., 2000). Furthermore, they are at enhanced risk of suffering an episode of MDD (at which point their condition would be described as "double depression"). Many present in a primary care context, but until recently, there has been little substantive research into the management of individuals who present as dysthmymic (as contrasted to the treatment of such individuals once they enter into a depressive episode).

Markowitz's (1994, 1996) reviews of psychological therapy for dysthymic disorder noted that, at this point, there were no available psychodynamic studies, some small-scale open trials of IPT (Markowitz, 1994; Mason et al., 1993), and seven open trials of CBT. Subsequently, a number of controlled trials have been published, though most contrast the relative impacts of medication and psychotherapy in various combinations. The absence of studies of the efficacy of psychotherapy alone is striking.

Cognitive-Behavioral Therapy

Gonzales et al. (1985) treated 113 patients with 12 two-hour individual or group "psychoeducational" sessions over 2 months, with follow-up at 1 month and at 6 months. Results varied according to diagnosis, with more improvement for those with acute MDD (75% reaching a recovery criterion) than for those with chronic intermittent depression (43%) or double depression (27%). De Jong et al. (1986) treated 30 unmedicated inpatients over 3 months. A combination of activity scheduling, social competence training, and cognitive restructuring achieved a higher response rate (60%) than cognitive restructuring alone (30%) or a wait list (10%). However, data from dropouts from treatment were not analyzed. At 6-month follow-up of half the sample, gains were maintained. One problem with this study is that response was defined as a BDI score ≤ 14, or as a 50% reduction in pretreatment BDI scores. The clinical significance of gains defined in this way is arguable.

Five very small-scale studies were identified by Markowitz (1994); in all cases, the sample size renders them exploratory. Fennel and Teasdale (1982) treated five patients with long-term depression, all of whom had failed to respond to previous treatment; only one patient showed clear improvement. Harpin et al. (1982) reported the treatment of 12 patients who failed to improve with medication. Patients either received 10 weeks of twice-weekly CBT ($n = 6$) or were allocated to a wait-list control group ($n = 6$). A significant drop in HRSD scores was found in the active treatment group as contrasted to the control group, though results were poorer with more severe levels of depression. Two of the six treated patients showed significant pre- to posttreatment improvement, but only one maintained this at 6 months. Stravynski et al. (1991) treated six patients with 15 weekly sessions of CBT; significant improvements in HRSD scores were obtained, and four patients no longer met criteria for dysthymic disorder following treatment. McCullough (1991) treated 10 patients with dsythymic disorder over a rather longer period than the above-mentioned studies, with a range of 14–44 weekly sessions. All reached the recovery criterion of a BDI score ≤ 10, and nine remained in remission at 2-year follow-up. These results are perhaps less promising than they appear, in that in an original cohort of 20 patients treated, four did not complete treatment and six were unavailable to follow-up. Mercier et al. (1992) reported a 12- to 16-week trial with 15 patients with chronic dysthymic disorder; four booster sessions were offered over the 6-month follow-up period. Three of eight patients with dysthymica and three of seven patients with double depression responded, and of the six responders, four remained well over the follow-up period. Given that all responders had been depressed for 7 years or longer, this is an impressive result.

Contrasts of Psychological Therapy and Medication Alone and in Combination

Cognitive-Behavioral Therapy

Becker et al. (1987) allocated 39 patients either to social skills training or to crisis–supportive psychotherapy, along with either nortriptyline or placebo. After 16 weeks of treatment, gains were evident in all conditions. Dunner et al. (1996) contrasted the short-term treatment with CBT or fluoxetine in 24 patients randomized to 16 weeks of either treatment. Though at 8 and 16 weeks more patients receiving fluoxetine met criteria for recovery (7 of 13, contrasted to 2 of 11 receiving CBT), this was not statistically significant, and no follow-up data were collected.

Interpersonal Psychotherapy

de Mello et al. (2001) contrasted the impact of moclobemide alone and moclobemide combined with IPT. Thirty-five patients were randomized to each treatment; group therapy comprised 16 weekly sessions followed by monthly maintenance sessions over 6 months. Outcomes for both treatments were equivalent, though small initial sample sizes and consequent high levels of attrition limit interpretation of results from this trial.

Brown et al. (2002) conducted a large trial in primary care, allocating 707 patients to sertraline alone, to 10 sessions of IPT alone, or to the combination of these treatments. Patients were identified on the basis of epidemiological screening and advertisement. No information is given regarding therapist qualifications for conducting IPT, but random adherence checks were conducted (though it should be noted that the dosage of IPT is lower than in most trials). The acute phase of this trial took place over 6 months, with a further 18-month naturalistic follow-up. At posttherapy, sertraline alone and

combined treatment showed equivalent outcomes, and both were superior to
IPT alone, with respective response rates of 60%, 58%, and 47%. At 2-year
follow-up, there was evidence of lower health care utilization by patients in
the combined group, but an obvious potential confound is that all patients
were offered sertraline over follow-up, an offer taken up by about 60% of
those receiving medication in the acute phase, but only 12% of those receiving IPT.

"Problem-Solving" Treatment

Problem-solving treatment has a psychosocial, here-and-now focus, and
encourages patients to specify and work toward resolving areas of functioning
that they identify as problematic. Most trials examine the impact of this
approach for individuals with mild to moderate depression in primary care
settings.

Mynors-Wallis et al. (1995, 2000) recruited patients through primary
care physicians in Oxfordshire. They (1995) allocated 91 patients to one of
three treatments—amitripyline and clinical management, placebo and clinical
management, or six sessions of problem-solving treatment delivered over 12
weeks. Adopting a recovery criterion of an HRSD score ≤ 7 at 12 weeks, the
recovery rate in patients receiving amitripyline and problem-solving therapy
was equivalent (60% and 52%, respectively), but was significantly greater than
for patients receiving placebo (27%). A later study by the same research group
(2000) randomized 151 patients to receive problem-solving therapy alone,
fluvoxamine or paroxetine alone, or problem-solving therapy combined with
one or the other of these medications. Over 12 weeks, all treatments showed
equivalent efficacy. It should be noted that entry criteria for these studies are
lower than in most trials reported in this section (patients needed to meet
research diagnostic criteria for depression and have an HRSD score ≥ 13—
usually an indicator for mild depression). On this basis, it may be inappropriate to generalize these results beyond benefit to patients with mild to moderate depression.

Dowrick et al. (2000) report a multicenter, multinational study conducted in the United Kingdom, Ireland, Spain, Finland, and Norway, identifying suitable participants on the basis of a community survey. Four hundred
fifty-two people were recruited (though it is unclear how this number differs
from the potential pool of participants) and randomized to one of three conditions—six sessions of problem-solving therapy, one of two variants of
group psychoeducation (over 8 weeks), or a no-treatment control. The
design is complicated by the fact that only one site offered both interventions,
that both rural and urban centers were included, and (relatedly) that
problem-solving sessions were usually offered in the patient's home, whereas
psychoeducation involved travel: Attrition for psychoeducation was signifi-

cantly greater than for problem solving (less than half the sample completed the course). At 6 months (though not at 12 months), the two active treatments showed gains over controls, with approximately 58% no longer meeting criteria for depression, contrasted to approximately 42% of controls. Though methodologically problematic, this study is unusual in describing the delivery of interventions in a community-based context.

Barrett et al. (2001) reported outcomes from a multicenter trial based in primary care, which randomized 241 patients with dysthymic disorder (127) or minor depression (114) to problem-solving therapy, paroxetine, or placebo. All patients had six scheduled treatment sessions over 11 weeks, with follow-up over 6 months. The criterion for remission was set at an HRSD score ≤ 6 at 11 weeks. For patients with minor depression, there was a high rate of remission (at around 64%) and no differences between interventions (though whether this speaks to the high level of contact for all patients or the tendency toward patient responsiveness is not clear). For patients with dysthymic disorder, there was a differential treatment effect: paroxetine and problem-solving therapy achieved a significantly higher remission rate than placebo (80%, 57%, and 44%, respectively). Though at 6 months no between-treatment differences were observable (Oxman et al., 2001), follow-up was complicated by the fact that (in effect) patients received treatment as usual posttherapy, making it inappropriate to attribute changes to the original randomization.

A second report from this group (Williams et al., 2000) followed the same research strategy as had Barrett et al. (2001) but focused on a sample of older adults (over age 60, with a mean age of 71); 211 patients presented with dysthymic disorder and 204 with minor depression. Again, problem-solving therapy was contrasted to paroxetine alone or to placebo over 11 weeks of treatment. On intent-to-treat analyses, patients with dysthymic disorder showed significant benefit from paroxetine but not from problem-solving therapy. However, marked site differences were found in remission rates for patients who received four or more sessions of either treatment; rates for problem-solving therapy ranged from 33 to 80%, and for paroxetine, from 27 to 67%. Though the authors note site-specific variations in therapist expertise in problem-solving therapy, there is no formal analysis of factors that might have contributed to this pattern of outcomes.

Group Therapy

Two trials have examined the impact of combining group therapy with medication for individuals with dysthymic disorder. Hellerstein et al. (2001) randomized 40 patients who had responded to 8 weeks of treatment with fluoxetine either to continue with medication alone, or to receive medication combined with 16 sessions of a manualized group therapy (which included both a cognitive and interpersonal focus). An equivalent proportion of patients in each therapy met the recovery criterion, an HRSD score ≤ 7.

Ravindran et al. (1999) randomized 97 patients with dysthymic disorder to receive either sertraline alone, placebo alone, sertraline in combination with group CBT, or placebo in combination with group CBT, with group therapies conducted over a 12-week period. With response defined as an HRSD score ≤ 10 and at least a 50% decline in HRSD score at posttherapy, there was a higher (but nonsignificant) response rate for the combination of setraline and CBT contrasted to setraline alone (71% and 55%, respectively). There was also no difference in the response rate between CBT combined with placebo and placebo alone (33%), suggesting that, in this trial, CBT not only failed to enhance the benefits of medication but it also achieved no more benefit than placebo.

Summary

In recent years, there has been an increase in research focusing specifically on dysthymic disorder, with most of this increased attention contrasting the efficacy of psychological treatment against medication. Available contrasts suggest that adding psychological therapy to medication confers little advantage, and in some trials, medication alone showed greater efficacy than psychological therapy alone. Our earlier review of this area (Roth & Fonagy, 1996) was based on the small-scale trials extant at that point and tentatively concluded that there was some evidence of the efficacy of IPT and CBT. Since that time, there has been increased interest in problem-solving therapy but no equivalent focus on the use of therapies with proven benefit in more serious depressive disorders. In some ways, this is surprising; 79% of individuals with dysthymic disorder will eventually present with MDD (McCullough et al., 1992), and there is a natural course of remission and recurrence (Keller & Shapiro, 1982; Keller et al., 1983). After intervention for MDD, they are almost certainly at enhanced risk of subsequent relapse. From this vantage point, greater knowledge about the most effective management of patients with subthreshold symptoms would be an advantage; at present, the focus of researchers makes it harder to derive clear guidelines.

PROCESS FACTORS

Relating patterns of outcome to process factors is a difficult task. The effect sizes attributable to process factors are usually small, as are the sample sizes on which they are based. Only rarely do designs include process factors as main effects. Post hoc analysis can only look for associations between variables, but the success of this strategy is based on an assumption that these relationships will be linear—an assumption that is almost certainly erroneous (e.g., Stiles & Shapiro, 1989; discussed further in Chapter 16). A further concern is that although analysis of any one data set may suggest process–outcome links, these may be findings that are specific only to the sample—a risk that is heightened by multiple analyses of the same data set. To some degree, the volume of research into depression offers the possibility of more robust research, but even here it is probably fair to say that there remain more questions about process factors than there are answers.

Therapeutic Alliance

As discussed in Chapter 16, most analyses find a significant association between measures of the therapeutic alliance and outcome. Krupnick et al. (1996) found that the quality of the therapeutic alliance (and especially measures of the patient-related alliance) predicted outcome in all arms of the NIMH trial, including pharmacological interventions. Castonguay et al. (1996) reexamined the University of Minnesota trial, taking measures of both the quality of the alliance and the degree to which therapists challenged dysfunctional assumptions (a core aspect of CBT technique). Importantly, they found that in the context of a positive alliance, greater cognitive challenge was associated with better outcomes, but that this technique exerted a negative impact if the alliance was negative. Stiles et al. (1998) found that, broadly speaking, a positive alliance was associated with positive outcomes in the Sheffield trial, though the detailed pattern of associations with particular aspects of the alliance was complex. Across a number of different therapeutic approaches, the influence of the alliance is well established. This raises important, but unresolved, questions about the interplay between the techniques embedded in "brand-name" therapies and the common therapeutic factors implied by the alliance concept.

Patient Characteristics and Outcome

Of these, initial severity, age at first onset, number of episodes, and chronicity at presentation have all been discussed earlier. In line with clinical observation, most (but not all) research suggests that each of these factors makes it more likely that patients will be less responsive to therapy, and this will be reflected by both a poorer outcome after short-term intervention and a greater probability of subsequent relapse. A combination of greater chronicity, severity, and earlier first onset tends to predict higher residual symptoms at the end of therapy (e.g., Agosti & Ocepek-Welikson, 1997), which in turn increases the risk of subsequent relapse (Hamilton & Dobson, 2002). Of course, this general observation may not apply in the individual case, and undue therapeutic pessimism may be inappropriate, but such findings should at least alert clinicians to plan for likely patterns of treatment response.

Personality Disorder

Although there is a broad clinical consensus that the presence of a personality disorder leads to poorer outcomes (e.g., Department of Health, 2001), evidence to support this belief is not strong. Methodological issues are pertinent here. How personality disorder is defined, and perhaps more crucially, how it is measured, seems to impact on the degree of support for this assertion, and it appears that the better the quality of study design the less likely it is that a relationship will be found (Mulder, 2002). There is also the risk that assessments of personality disorder made while the patient is depressed may be unreliable (e.g., Stuart et al., 1992). Results from individual studies are not always consistent. In the NIMH trial, some 74% of patients received a diagnosis of personality disorder. Contrasted to individuals without personality disorder, mean depression scores were equivalent at termination, though there were poorer outcomes in relation to social functioning and a higher probability of residual symptoms—a pattern consistent across all clusters of personality disorder (Shea et al., 1992b). Analysis of outcomes for 27 patients who met criteria for DSM Cluster C (anxious–fearful) in the Sheffield trial (Hardy et al., 1995b) suggested that these patients had higher initial symptom levels but that those who received CBT improved to the same degree as patients without personality disorder. However, those treated with psychodynamic therapy had poorer outcomes. This later finding is echoed by two studies of psychodynamic treatments; both Diguer et al. (1993) and Hoffart and Martinsen (1993) reported that although individuals with personality disorder improved, they made smaller gains. Tyrer et al. (1993) reported on a cohort that included dysthymic (but not depressed) patients; they found that people with personality disorders tended to be less receptive to psychological therapies (in their trial, CBT), but were more responsive to medication. Kuyken et al. (2001) conducted a post hoc analysis of 162 depressed patients treated under naturalistic conditions. Fifty-nine percent of this sample was diagnosed with a personality disorder; though their initial symptom levels were higher, outcomes were equivalent to those without this comorbidity. Despite this equivalence of action, there was some evidence that some types of beliefs linked to personality disorder—specifically, avoidant and paranoid beliefs—were associated with poorer outcome. It is hard to discern a definitive pattern in these results, though more structured therapies appear to have greater capacity to produce an equivalence of action in the face of comorbidity. It is also relevant that differential impact appears not to be located in the domain of symptomatic change, but in relation to aspects of presentation that intertwine with the notion of personality disorder itself, such as interpersonal functioning and the level of background symptomatology both pre- and posttherapy.

Personality Type

Barber and Muenz (1996) suggest that avoidant patients will be more responsive to CBT (because it will encourage them to confront feared situations), while obsessive (hence, unexpressive) patients will benefit from more expressive therapies (such as IPT) that facilitate emotional expression. Though 32 completer patients met DSM–III criteria for these two categories, sample sizes across the four "arms" of the analysis were inevitably low. Nonetheless, their results were intriguing, complicated by the fact that nonmarried patients had better outcomes with IPT, and married patients, with CBT (a result that may make sense in the context of IPT's focus on interpersonal gains, and that there may be less potential for gains in this area for married patients). Holding this factor constant, the predicted relationship between personality type and outcome was found. A somewhat different picture emerges from the Sheffield trial (Hardy et al., 2001), in which patients who tended to distance themselves from relationships (in this sense, avoidant) did less well in CBT than those who were more interpersonally engaged, though the presence of a positive alliance mitigated the impact of this factor.

Perfectionism

Sotksy et al. (1991) found that, overall, higher levels of perfectionism were associated with poorer outcomes. Blatt et al. (1996) found that in both CBT and IPT, outcomes for patients low and high in perfectionism were effectively unrelated to the development of the alliance. It may be that those low in perfectionism are able to tolerate therapeutic imperfections, while those high in perfectionism are relatively impervious to anything other than a negative view of self and other. However, outcomes for patients in the midrange of perfection were significantly related to the strength of the alliance, suggesting that these patients will be sensitive and potentially responsive to variations in therapist style. There are indications that these patients do not show the usual pattern of an increasing engagement as therapy progresses (Zuroff et al., 2000), suggesting that therapists may need to be focused on strategies to enhance patients' capacity to be active collaborators in their own therapy.

Summary

Although most trials are organized in relation to interventions, there is evidence that a positive therapeutic alliance is associated with better outcomes. The temporal relationship between alliance and symptomatic improvement is

probably rather complex (a matter discussed further in Chapter 16). However, it seems reasonable to suggest that in the absence of a positive alliance,
specific technical interventions are unlikely to be effective.

Patients who present the greatest therapeutic challenge can be described
fairly clearly: They are more likely to have had an early onset of depression
and many previous episodes. It needs to be borne in mind that while these
statistical associations are reasonably consistent across studies, there is considerable variability in the response of individual patients, even within studies.
Importantly, severity of depression is not necessarily a negative indicator, presumably because the intensity of symptoms may be a poor guide to their
underlying determinants.

While there is reasonably consistent evidence that personality disorder
(more than personality type) impacts negatively on outcome, it should not be
assumed that the presence of Axis II comorbidity necessarily attenuates treatment effects, in part because it is conceptually and methodologically difficult
to disentangle deficits that relate to personality disorder from those attributable to depression. Persons with personality disorder may make therapist
adherence to technique more difficult and, hence, require therapists to be
more competent in their delivery of technique and their management of the
alliance. In this sense, variations in findings may reflect the capacity of trialists
to apply the treatment protocol—a particular test of alliance–technique interactions.

SUMMARY AND CLINICAL IMPLICATIONS

Depression is both common and chronic; reflecting this, a large body of
research addresses its treatment. DSM-IV-TR makes an important distinction
between patients presenting with acute episodes of depression and those who
suffer from depression in a less intense but more chronic form (dysthymic disorder). Although (at least potentially) the latter represent a greater clinical
challenge than the former, relatively few studies focus on their treatment.

Evidence from meta-analytic review combined with consideration of
individual studies demonstrates short-term efficacy for structured psychological therapies offered in brief formats (usually around 16 weeks), with no clear
evidence of advantage to any particular approach. Although these initial gains
are clinically significant, rather few trials have extended follow-up, and where
this exists, there is a clear tendency for patients to relapse. A number of studies (using IPT or variants of CBT) have investigated the benefits of maintenance or "booster" therapy, and there is evidence for the efficacy of this
approach in reducing the recurrence of depression.

Although there is an increasing amount of research on dysthymic disorder, nearly all major trials focus on the adjunctive use of psychological ther-

apy and medication, with little evidence that psychotherapy either adds benefit to pharmacotherapy or is effective when offered alone. The inappropriate
characterization of dysthymic disorder as a minor form of depression has
probably contributed to this lack of research. This is unfortunate, partly
because we know less than we should about how therapies commonly used
to treat MDD would perform if applied to dysthymic disorder. Equally,
knowing more about how best to manage individuals with subthreshold and
chronic depressive symptoms would be helpful when considering the treatment of MDD, since we know that individuals who continue to have
subthreshold symptoms after treatment are at elevated risk of relapse.

Trials contrasting pharmacotherapy and psychotherapy suggest an equivalence of action between the two approaches, and it has been difficult to
demonstrate that their combination is more effective than either offered alone
(though studies conducted in inpatient contexts and with dysthymic disorder
may be an exception to this conclusion). The reliability of studies contributing to this comparison is not as robust as we might wish, both in terms of the
quality of pharmacotherapy and the management of "blinding" to medication
effects.

Though review does not imply any necessary benefit from combining
medication with psychological interventions, ensuring access to both seems
warranted on pragmatic grounds. Clinically, it is not unusual for individuals
who might benefit from psychological intervention to receive exclusively
medical treatment; equally, patients receiving psychological treatment may be
undermedicated or have received no psychiatric assessment when this might
have been indicated. Better integrated treatment provision has a number of
advantages. It would not only facilitate greater patient choice but greater efficacy is also likely, since it should ensure that patients are not treated over long
periods with methods to which they are not responsive, or to which their
response could be optimized.

The pattern of results for a structured therapy (and for pharmacotherapy)
is quite consistent; a simple rule of thumb would be that, in around 50% of
cases, symptoms will have remitted posttherapy, but that over 1 year of
follow-up, around half of those who recovered will relapse. On this basis,
only about one-fourth of patients treated using a brief therapy remain well. It
is possible that the consistency of outcome reflects the fact that within any
research sample, a proportion of patients will be responsive to almost any
intervention. One strategy would be to screen out such individuals on the
basis of their response to therapy, and to examine outcomes in those who
appear to be treatment-resistant. Without this, there may be little to learn
about the impact of specific techniques or, indeed, the differential impacts of
medication and psychotherapy. However, this approach has the obvious
drawback that defining a sample in terms of failure to respond to treatment
does not necessarily guarantee its homogeneity: Treatment failure is under-

pinned by an admixture of biochemical and psychological factors, and without a hypothesized mechanism, we risk reifying what is only a description of outcomes into a unitary category. One approach to this problem is entirely pragmatic: broadly, a form of stepped care in which those who do not respond to one treatment are offered another, with the intent of maximizing outcomes. While this makes clinical sense, it is worth observing that developments in the field require a better understanding of the ways that different pathways to and presentations of depression contribute to outcome, something that can only be done in the context of hypotheses about the nature of the problems confronting depressed individuals.

Concerns about the limitations of brief intervention should not obscure its short-term benefit, but it is clear that treatment planning for individuals with depression should consider the need for maintenance therapy. In this respect, chronicity and age of onset appear to be more relevant factors to consider than severity. There is a risk that because the literature largely examines brief therapies delivered in single episodes of care, service provision will reflect this. A cascade or stepwise model may be more appropriate, with patients who fail to respond to brief (or even computerized) treatments offered alternative therapies, with the delivery of maintenance therapies seen as normative rather than unusual. The near-uniformity of treatment length in trials makes it very difficult to be clear about the duration of therapy. On this basis, there is little that can be said about the value of long-term therapy, though it is clear that very brief treatment regimens (of around 10 sessions) may not be adequate for more severely depressed individuals.

In summary, while treatments for depression are effective in the short term for at least a proportion of patients, longer term impacts are limited. Given the nature of the disorder, this is a creditable achievement, but it is clear that there needs to be a focus on the most pernicious aspect of life with this disorder—the tendency to relapse. Hand in hand with this, there may be a need to adopt a more complex framework for classifying depression. In this respect, greater consideration of developmental pathways, as well as personality variables, may be relevant factors for future research to consider.

CHAPTER 5

BIPOLAR DISORDER

DEFINITIONS

Bipolar disorder—sometimes referred to as manic–depression—is characterized by one or more manic episodes, usually alternating with one or more major depressive episodes. Depressive episodes have been defined in Chapter 4, which discusses treatments for depression.

DSM-IV-TR defines the essential diagnostic features of a manic episode as a period lasting at least 1 week (or any period, if hospitalization is required or psychotic symptoms are present), during which the predominant mood is either elevated, expansive, or irritable, and there are associated features of the manic syndrome. The disturbance is sufficiently severe to cause marked impairment in social and occupational functioning or to require hospitalization to prevent harm to self or others. At least three of the following characteristic symptoms should be present: inflated self-esteem or grandiosity (which may be delusional), decreased need for sleep, pressure of speech, flight of ideas, distractibility, increased involvement in goal directed activity, psychomotor agitation, and excessive involvement in pleasurable activities that may have a painful outcome that the person does not recognize.

Only when the severity of symptoms is such that there is a marked impact on functioning can a diagnosis of manic episode be made. Individuals without delusions and with milder symptoms, who are able to function socially and occupationally without a need for hospitalization, would receive a diagnosis of hypomanic episode.

DSM-IV-TR distinguishes bipolar I disorders and bipolar II disorders, as follows:

Bipolar I Disorders

There are four variants of bipolar I disorder, each of which relates to the history of previously diagnosed manic or depressive episodes: (1) most recent episode hypomanic (but where there has been at least one previous manic episode), (2) most recent episode manic, (3) most recent episode mixed, and (4) most recent episode depressed. A further category of bipolar I disorder, single manic episode, is characterized by only one manic episode and no past major depressive episodes.

Bipolar II Disorders

This diagnosis is reserved for individuals who present with major depressive disorders accompanied by hypomanic episodes, in the absence of any previous manic episode.

Cyclothymia

Some individuals show a pattern of chronic mood disturbance characterized by numerous hypomanic episodes and depressive episodes that do not meet criteria for a major depressive episode. To meet diagnostic criteria, such a pattern should be present for more than 2 years, and the individual should not have been without hypomanic or depressive symptoms for more than 2 months at a time. It is worth noting that the boundaries between cyclothymia and bipolar disorder are not well specified.

Bipolar Disorder Not Otherwise Specified

These are disorders with manic or hypomanic features that do not meet the criteria for any specific bipolar disorder. Examples might include patients showing rapid alternation between manic and depressive symptoms, which never reach the minimal duration criteria for a manic episode or major depressive episode, or recurrent hypomanic episodes without intercurrent depressive symptoms.

PREVALENCE, COMORBIDITY, AND NATURAL HISTORY
Prevalence

Data from the Epidemiologic Catchment Area survey (ECA; Weissman et al., 1988) suggest a 1-year prevalence rate of 1.0%, with men and women almost equally affected. Angst (1992) cites 1-year prevalence rates of bipolar disorder in community samples at between 1.0% and 1.7% in the adult population.

Comorbidity

Data from the ECA survey (Regier et al., 1990) indicate that approximately half of patients with bipolar illness have comorbid alcohol or drug abuse at some point during their lifetime. Since substance abuse is associated with a significantly poorer prognosis (Feinman & Dunner, 1996), this an important finding. A significant subset of patients meet criteria for schizoaffective disorder, borderline personality disorder, panic disorder, obsessive–compulsive disorder, or generalized anxiety disorder (Elkin, 1994).

Natural History

Bipolar disorder is usually a recurrent disorder (Goodwin & Jamison, 1990), with more than 80% of individuals presenting with one manic episode going on to have further episodes. Both the manic and depressive episodes are more frequent than the major depressive episodes in major depressive disorder. Frequently, a manic episode is followed by a short depressive episode, or vice versa. In 5–15% of individuals with bipolar I disorder, there are four or more mood episodes within a year; such cases of rapid cycling are associated with a poorer prognosis.

Although the majority of individuals with bipolar disorder return to a functional level between episodes, some 20–30% of patients continue to display some lability, and interpersonal and occupational difficulties. Untreated, there is significant mortality associated with bipolar disorder; Müller-Oerlinghausen et al. (1992) estimate that without treatment, mortality rates are two to three times higher than that in the general population.

TREATMENT APPROACHES

Psychological interventions for bipolar disorder will almost certainly be adjunctive to medication (which has a primary role in ameliorating symptomatology). A recent review concludes that lithium provides a prophylactic response in about two-thirds of patients with bipolar disorder only (Goodwin, 2002). Newer mood stabilizers are generally of equivalent efficacy to lithium (Moncrieff, 1995; Solomon et al., 1995). Carbamazepine and Valproate appeared to prevent relapse as monotherapy even though there is still a paucity of data from randomized placebo-controlled trials (Keck & McElroy, 2002). Lamotrigine has been found to have a long-term role in delaying or preventing the recurrence of depressive episodes, but lithium and divalproex sodium remain the first-line treatment (Calabrese et al., 2002). Other antipsychotics such as clozapine and olanzapine are also used clinically, but more research is needed, because the adverse side effects associated with these antipsychotics may outweigh the benefits (Kusumakar, 2002). Although standard antidepressant medications also show efficacy during depressive phases of the disorder (Gelenberg & Hopkins, 1993), their use is potentially complicated by the risk of provoking a manic episode or accelerating cycling (Peet, 1994).

Despite the efficacy of medication, it is estimated that, even if maintained on appropriate medication, between 41 and 60% of patients will experience a manic or depressive relapse over a 2-year period of follow-up (Prien et al., 1984). Furthermore, the clinical effectiveness of medication is reduced by nonadherence, estimated at between 25 and 50% of bipolar patients (Prien & Potter, 1990), and even with adequate adherence and optimal treatment response, the impact of medication on social functioning is usually limited (Clarkin et al., 1990).

Interest in the efficacy of psychological interventions for bipolar disorder links to (but lags behind) the development of therapies for people with a diagnosis of schizophrenia (reviewed in Chapter 10). Both client groups appear vulnerable to similar psychosocial stressors (Johnson & Roberts, 1995). There is specific evidence that families of people with bipolar disorder experience considerable burden related to the disorder (Perlick et al., 1999) and that the expression of family stress increases vulnerability to relapse. Miklowitz et al. (1988) followed up 23 patients and their families for 9 months after discharge from the hospital after an acute episode of bipolar disorder. Using a measure that combined an estimate of expressed emotion (EE),[1] together with an assessment of the family's affective style, they found marked differences in relapse rates. Families rated low on the combined measure had a relapse rate of 17% compared to a rate of 94% in families with high ratings. Perlick et al. (2001) examined a larger cohort of 264 patients and found that caregiver burden reported both at the time of a relapse and during a period of stabilization predicted subsequent relapse, again suggesting the relevance of a focus on these sort of factors. It follows that research has examined the impact psychoeducation and the reduction of marital and family stress; in addition, techniques have been developed that are based on conceptualization of the disorder itself, and hence aim to help patients stabilize their lifestyle, cope better with specific stressors, and react more appropriately to prodromal signs.

Other emergent areas of research specific to bipolar disorder have direct application to treatment development. These include evidence of the importance of patterns of social rhythm and disruption (e.g., Malkoff-Schwartz, & Andersen, 1998), the relevance of early indicators for relapse (e.g., Lam &

---

[1] EE is a measure of family functioning, most thoroughly researched in relation to people with a diagnosis of schizophrenia, and more fully discussed in Chapter 10. In brief, a number of studies indicate that relapse is more likely if patients live with, or have extensive contact with, relatives who are excessively critical and/or overinvolved.

Wong, 1997; Lam et al., 2001), and the pertinence to relapse of dysfunctional assumptions that may incline patients to more 'risky' behaviors (e.g., Lam et al., 2004; Scott & Pope, 2003)

To date, most trials are small scale, but larger trials are in progress both in the United Kingdom and in the United States. The largest of these is the Systematic Treatment Enhancement Program for Bipolar Disorder (STEP-BD), a multicenter, longitudinal trial, initiated in 1998, which aims to recruit 5,000 patients in 20 treatment centers in the United States over a 5-year period (Sachs et al., 2003). The design of the trial allows for "standard care pathways," as well as "randomized care pathways," creating the opportunity to examine both the effectiveness of pharmacological and psychosocial interventions in routine practice and their efficacy under research conditions. Within randomized pathways, participants are offered one of three psychosocial treatments—cognitive-behavioral therapy (CBT), family-focused therapy, or interpersonal social rhythms therapy (all approaches considered further below). As this and other trials publish their results, more authoritative statements about efficacy will become possible.

At this stage of development, it may be appropriate to signal some caution regarding implementation of these approaches. Engaging and holding bipolar patients within therapy is challenging, partly because (by definition) their mood can be labile, and many have an unstable lifestyle. It follows that therapists will need sufficient expertise not only to hold patients in therapy but also to apply the therapies competently. Attrition rates even from trials can be quite high, though this may vary in relation to the point at which patients are recruited. (For example, Frank et al. (1999) and Miklowitz et al. (2000) recruited patients during or shortly after bipolar episodes, and had quite high attrition rates of 35% and 22%, respectively; in contrast, Lam et al. (2001) recruited patients between bipolar episodes and report attrition rates of 15%.) Any application of these approaches to routine practice may need to recognize the level of therapist training required to minimize likely refusal and attrition rates.

A number of reviews have been published, including Callahan and Bauer (1999), Huxley et al. (2000), Meyer and Hautzinger (2000), Rothbaum and Astin (2000), Swartz and Frank (2001), Miklowitz and Craighead (2001), Patelis-Siotis (2001), and Scott (2001).

Group Therapies

Though there have been no controlled studies of the adjunctive benefits of group therapy in addition to lithium, there have been a number of open trials (which, it should be noted, utilize a variety of therapeutic approaches). Shakir et al. (1979) and Volkmar et al. (1981) reported on outcomes at 4 years from 20 participants in a Yalom-style group (Yalom, 1975). All patients were responsive to lithium and had been on medication for a mean of 21 months. Significant differences in functioning were found by contrasting the 2 years prior to and the 2 years subsequent to entry into the group. In particular, medication adherence was improved and there was a decrease in hospitalization rates.

Cerbone et al. (1992) treated 43 outpatients in weekly group therapy, with a focus on education about the disorder and interpersonal problems. Using the year prior to group entry as a baseline, patients evidenced lower rates of hospitalization and shorter inpatient stay, and reported higher levels of functioning. There were, however, no reported changes in medication usage.

Kripke and Robinson (1985) described a group of 14 bipolar patients (13 of whom were male) conducted over 12 years; eight members stayed in the group over this time. The group contained both psychodynamic and problem-solving elements, and there was some evidence of reduced hospitalization and better social functioning. Wulpsin et al. (1988) conducted a group run in a community mental health center (CMHC) for 22 bipolar patients over 4 years. Though there was some reduction in hospitalization, attrition was high, with almost half the group members dropping out.

Patelis-Siotis et al. (2001) recruited 49 patients to an open trial of group CBT, of whom 38 completed the 14-week program. Although there were indications of improved social activity, there was no symptomatic change at posttherapy. However, patients were recruited at a point when they were only mildly depressed or euthymic, making it unlikely that substantial symptomatic change would occur.

Psychodynamic Therapy

There are few studies of psychodynamic therapy with bipolar patients. Benson (1975) describes a case series of 31 patients who received psychodynamically oriented individual, group, or couple therapy. Over 41 months in an open trial, 24 patients were reported to have a good clinical outcome, of whom 19 continued with the maintenance treatment, and five discontinued medication but continued psychotherapy. Though Benson suggests that this level of functioning is higher than that usually found in follow-up studies of medication alone, measures of functioning were determined by the author acting alone, a procedure open to bias. In a problematic but widely cited study, Davenport et al. (1977) contrasted outcomes in 65 hospitalized patients meeting research diagnostic criteria (RDC) for bipolar disorder, all of whom had intact marriages at the start of the trial. Patients were randomly assigned for follow-up either to psychodynamic couple group therapy (12 patients), a lithium clinic (11 patients), or the patients' local CMHC (42 patients). However, there were significant differences in the ages of couples assigned to each group, with those receiving couple therapy being significantly older and married longer than those in the other treatment conditions. In addition, while patients in the first two conditions were treated by the researchers, those seen in the CMHCs were not. Relatedly, though lithium was prescribed and adherence was monitored in patients seen by the researchers, it is not clear what treatment was given within CMHCs. Patients were studied retrospectively 2–10 years after hospitalization; those who had received the couples group therapy were functioning best in terms of social and family functioning, and reported no rehospitalization or marital failure. In contrast, the CMHC group had the poorest outcomes, with 16 readmissions and 10 marital failures. However, this group was not significantly different from the lithium clinic. It should be noted that though the researchers found no association between length of illness and outcome, the significant differences between the groups noted earlier are likely to have selected for marital stability. Hence, though the results of this study appear to demonstrate the benefits of psychological therapy, poor control of both patient assignment and subsequent treatment makes interpretation problematic.

Psychoeducation

A number of trials of psychoeducation have been published, though earlier trials are smaller scale, usually uncontrolled, and interventions tend to be brief or focus on general knowledge about the disorder rather than on strategies that will aid responsiveness to prodromal signs. Outcomes are modest and inconsistent (Rothbaum & Astin, 2000), but this may reflect variations in the type and intensity of the approach taken. Van Gent and Zwart (1994) reported outcomes for 26 patients in receipt of lithium prophylaxis, treated in group psychoeducation therapy over 10–13 sessions. Group content was largely psychoeducational, together with some interpersonal focus. Contrasted with the period before group therapy and following up patients for 5 years after intervention, there appeared to be some increase in medication adherence and some reduction in hospital admission. Perry et al. (1999) assigned 69 patients either to routine care, or to routine care plus a median of nine individual sessions of psychoeducation, which identified prodromal signs and discussed stressors associated with previous episodes and management of indicators of relapse. The intervention significantly delayed relapse of manic episodes (the 25th percentile time to relapse was 65 weeks in the experimental group, and 17 weeks in controls). However, there was no significant delay in time to relapse for depressive episodes. Colom et al. (2003) randomized 120 patients to 21 sessions of group psychoeducation or to 21 sessions of unstructured group meetings. All received standard care, had been in remission for at least 6 months, and were compliant with their medication regimen. Over 2-year follow-up, 67% and 92%, respectively, of the psychoeducation and control groups experienced a relapse. Though the rate of depressive and hypomanic relapses was reduced, this was not the case for manic episodes.

Cognitive Therapies

Cochran (1984) examined the impact of six sessions of cognitive therapy on lithium adherence rates and outcomes for 28 newly diagnosed patients meeting RDC for bipolar disorder (Spitzer et al., 1978). Patients were randomly assigned either to therapy or to treatment as usual (TAU); adherence both at 6 weeks and 6 months was significantly better in patients receiving the intervention. There were problems in the criteria adopted for rating adherence, which depended both on measurement of serum levels and (potentially highly reactive) ratings by the patient and treating physician. Poor inter-correlations between these ratings suggest that the reliability of the overall measure of adherence is poor. Nonetheless, only three (21%) cognitive therapy patients discontinued medication, and two (14%) were hospitalized; in the control group, eight (57%) discontinued medication and eight (57%) were hospitalized.

In a small study, Palmer et al. (1995) examined the impact of Newman and Beck's (1993) manualized CBT for bipolar disorder. Four patients received 17 weekly sessions of group therapy; sessions contained psychoeducational elements but largely focused on strategies for managing and coping with the various manifestations of bipolar disorder. Although all patients attended psychiatric outpatient clinics, medication use was not monitored. Symptom status and social adjustment were assessed weekly, while the group was running, and monthly for five follow-up visits after the end of active treatment. In addition, the use of outpatient clinics and inpatient facilities in the 12 months prior to the group was contrasted with their use during the period of active treatment and follow-up.

Overall, there was some evidence of improvements during the active treatment phase, though the pattern of change varied among individuals and across measures. Though generalization from such a small sample is inappropriate, three of the four participants showed gains on measures of symptomatic status, greater stability in their condition, and better social adjustment; however, there was evidence of some loss of gains during the follow-up phase. There were no changes in the use of outpatient clinics, and changes in hospital stay were difficult to assess, since only one participant had been an inpatient in the year prior to the trial.

Zaretsky et al. (1999) contrasted the impact of 20 sessions of CBT for 11 patients with bipolar disorder against outcomes for 11 patients with recurrent unipolar depression, matched for demographic and some clinical variables. No patient received antidepressant medication, though those participants with bipolar disorder received either lithium or carbamazepine. Similar reductions in depressive symptomatology were observed in both groups, though there are no data on subsequent rates of relapse. However, the clinical validity of using a control group of unipolar patients is questionable, even though the authors' logic (that CBT has shown efficacy with this group) is accurate.

Lam et al. (2000, 2003) reported a pilot and a larger scale trial that suggest benefits of CBT in patients recruited for a history of relapse. In the pilot study, 25 patients were allocated to standard clinical care or standard care combined with 12–20 sessions of CBT (which included psychoeducation, emphasized building an alliance with the patient, and focused on a range of strategies for relapse prevention) over a 6-month period (Lam et al., 1999). Contrasted to controls, over 1 year, the CBT group had fewer bipolar episodes (83% had no episodes compared to 18% of controls), showed more stability in mood, and had higher levels of social functioning. Lam et al. (2003) examined these same treatment contrasts in 103 patients. Treatment was offered over 12 months, with an average of 14 sessions in the first 6 months and two booster sessions in the second 6 months. CBT appeared to significantly reduce relapse rates during the treatment period (43% and 75% for the CBT group and controls, respectively), number of hospitalizations (15% vs. 33%) number of days spent in hospital, if admitted, and the duration of manic or depressive episodes (a mean of 27 days contrasted to 88 days). Though mean mood levels (as measured monthly on the Beck Depression Inventory [BDI]) did not differ between groups, there were indications of a trend for depression scores for the CBT group to decline over time, while those for controls increased. Finally, the CBT group showed less lability in manic symptoms. As in the pilot study, the CBT group coped with manic prodromes significantly better than did controls over the year. Though this was true of depressive prodromes at 6 months, at 1 year, the CBT group and controls were equivalent. Medication compliance was higher in the CBT group, though results remain robust after statistical control for this factor. While the impact of better adherence to medical regimen requires further investigation, the benefits of CBT in this trial appear clear.

J. Scott et al. (2001) reported a pilot study that contrasted outcomes in 42 patients (all of whom were in receipt of standard psychiatric care) allocated to a 25-session CBT intervention either immediately or after a 6-month wait. The intervention included CBT similar to that used for treating unipolar depression, tailored to a formulation of each individual, along with three additional elements: (1) a package of psychoeducation based on an exploration of the individual's cognitive representations of the disorder, (2) incorporation of key elements of the self-regulation model (as used in interpersonal and social rhythm therapy, discussed below) and management of prodromes, and (3) exploration of attitudes and beliefs toward the disorder, including consideration of high-risk behaviors (such as substance misuse and non-adherence). Over the period of treatment, the CBT group showed significant reduction in depressive symptoms and measures of functioning, and a reduction in frequency of affective relapses and inpatient admissions. Although the intervention appeared to reduce manic relapses, it did not prevent the occurrence of isolated manic symptoms. Scott (personal communication, 2001) has suggested that the program might help patients better manage their prodromal symptoms, with the result that they do not cascade into a relapse. A larger trial of this approach is in progress.

"Interpersonal and Social Rhythm Therapy"

The rationale for interpersonal and social rhythm therapy (IPSRT) assumes the importance of a stable lifestyle, improved interpersonal functioning, and explicit consideration of strategies for maintaining treatment gains. Hence, it includes a focus on both social and circadian rhythms, techniques adapted from interpersonal psychotherapy (IPT; which has known efficacy in treating unipolar depression), and an extended maintenance phase prior to termination. Frank et al. (1997, 1999) reported on an ongoing trial in which 91 patients received either IPSRT or routine clinical management (CM). The trial had two phases: (1) acute management (the period during which patients achieve remission), and (2) a subsequent preventive, or maintenance therapy phase. While some patients had received the same therapy throughout, a crossover design meant that others switch to the alternative therapy between the acute and maintenance phases (giving four possible "routes" through the trial). Interim reports on progress over 2 years suggest that while IPSRT contributed to a more stable lifestyle than did clinical management (Frank et al., 1997), there were no statistically significant differences between treatments in speed of remission from manic or depressive episodes. Nonetheless, there is some evidence that IPSRT is more effective than clinical management at reducing fluctuations in depressive symptoms, suggesting at least some impact on stability of mood (Swartz & Frank, 2001). Furthermore, of the 22 patients recovering from depressive episodes, the median time to recovery was 21 weeks with IPSRT, contrasted to 40 weeks with clinical management (Hlastala et al., 1997). Frank et al. (1999) reported on outcomes in 82 patients who had completed the acute management phase, followed by 1 year of maintenance treatment. At this point, *consistency* of treatment appeared to be more important than *type* of treatment—regardless of therapy administered. Over 1 year, those maintained on the same intervention had lower levels of recurrence and lower levels of symptomatology than those who were switched from one treatment to the other between the acute and maintenance phases. This result is difficult to interpret given that patients continued to see the same therapist whether or not they switched treatment modality.

Further information about the efficacy of this approach should emerge from ongoing reports and from the STEP-BD program (discussed earlier).

Couple Therapy

Davenport et al.'s (1977) trial of couple therapy was discussed earlier. Clarkin et al. (1998) assigned married patients either to routine psychiatric care (*n* = 23) or to routine care plus 25 marital psychoeducational sessions over approximately 11 months (*n* = 19). Though only data for the completer sample are reported, the addition of marital therapy significantly improved medication adherence and levels of functioning, but there was no difference between treatments in symptom levels.

Family-Based Interventions

Clarkin et al. (1990) reported data from a large trial of inpatient family interventions. Patients with a range of diagnoses were randomly assigned to receive family intervention in addition to TAU, with TAU acting as a control condition. Family intervention comprised psychoeducation, identification of family stress, exploration of likely precipitants for current and future episodes, and consideration of problem-solving strategies for managing future stress.

Outcomes for a subsample of 21 individuals with a diagnosis of bipolar disorder, were reported separately. At admission, 13 of these patients were manic, seven depressed, and one presented with a mixed episode. Seventeen were psychotic, and 14 had had previous episodes; 14 (66%) of the sample were female. Twelve received family interventions, and nine TAU, with outcome monitored at 6 and 18 months. For female patients, outcome was better following family intervention, with improvements in social and work functioning, and improved family attitudes toward treatment; it should be noted that over 18 months, this effect diminished. No benefit to family intervention was seen in males. Statistical analysis of the gender-by-treatment effect suggests that it is robust. However, the small number of male patients in the sample and, indeed, the small overall sample size cautions against overinterpretation of what the authors themselves considered to be an exploratory study. Although they speculate that male patients may be particularly sensitive to interpersonal stimuli, and hence may find family interventions more stressful, gender differences in outcome from family intervention are not notable in comparable studies of outcome with patients diagnosed as schizophrenic (reviewed in Chapter 10). As such, the clinical implications of the interaction effects noted in this study are unclear in the absence of replication in a larger scale study.

Miklowitz and Goldstein (1990) described an adaptation of Falloon's behavioral family management technique (Falloon et al., 1984). Nine recent-onset patients with bipolar disorder were treated with 21 family sessions spread over 9 months. Sessions were held weekly for the first 3 months, tapering to biweekly and monthly, and comprised family education, communication skills training, and problem-solving skills training. Outcomes in this group were contrasted with 23 patients who participated in a naturalistic study of outcomes conducted by the same authors (Miklowitz et al., 1988). These patients received lithium alone and were followed up over 9 months. Among the treatment group, one out of nine patients relapsed over 9 months (11%), a significantly lower rate than that found in the contrast group (14 of 23, a 61% relapse rate). A larger trial (Miklowitz et al., 2000) used the same treatment type and intensity in 31 patients and their families, whose outcomes were contrasted with a control treatment in which 70 patients were offered two sessions of psychoeducation and follow-up crisis management. At 1 year, depressive relapses were significantly lower for patients receiving family interventions, though the treatment condition did not influence the number of manic relapses. One potential criticism of this trial is the marked difference in the amount of therapy contact time in each intervention. On this basis Rea et al. (2003) matched the number of therapy contacts (though not the amount of therapy contact time) by offering 21 sessions of family or individual therapy over 9 months, followed by 3 months of medication management. Individual therapy was problem-focused, supportive, and psychoeducational. Fifty-three patients were randomized to treatment, with outcomes monitored for 1 year posttherapy. While the relapse rate did not differ between groups during the treatment year, those who received family therapy showed a significantly decreased probability of relapse in the follow-up period (28% vs. 60%), and a reduced rate of rehospitalization throughout the study period. Medication compliance was equivalent and high in both groups. Despite randomization, patients in individual therapy had an earlier age of onset and worse premorbid functioning. Age of onset did not impact differentially on outcomes; while patients with good adjustment had equivalent relapse rates in both conditions, those with poor adjustment had significantly lower rates of relapse with family therapy.

A further report from this group (Miklowitz et al., 2003) contrasted 31 patients allocated to family treatment with 70 patients allocated to crisis management. Active treatment lasted 9 months, and all patients received appropriate pharmacotherapy. Family intervention was broadly administered as described above; crisis management comprised two sessions of family psychoeducation, followed by community intervention in response to indicators of relapse and/or family crisis. Over 2-year follow-up, significant benefit to family intervention was observed; among this group, 35% experienced a relapse or serious exacerbation, contrasted to 54% in those treated with crisis management. Differences in the stabilization of mood between treatment groups was more evident in relation to depressive rather manic symptoms.

Honig et al. (1995, 1997) conducted a multifamily psychoeducational intervention of six biweekly sessions, consisting of education about the disorder and coping strategies. Outcomes in 29 patients and family members (usually a partner) were contrasted with a control group of 23 patients on a wait list. Measures of expressed emotion taken pre- and posttherapy suggested that reductions from high to low EE were more likely in the intervention group than in the control group. Though there is no direct evidence of the benefits on relapse of this form of intervention, and the trial is in many ways a pilot study, participants with high-EE relatives had histories of a higher rate of admission than those from low-EE environments. To some degree this echoes outcomes from Miklowitz et al. (2000, reviewed earlier). Although they found only weak support for an association of high pretreatment EE and relapse, post hoc analysis suggested that patients from high-EE families had the highest depression scores at entry to the study, and also the greatest symptomatic improvement.

Interventions for Comorbid Substance Abuse

Although the rate of comorbid substance abuse among patients with bipolar disorder is high, in most studies, the presence of this comorbidity is an exclusion factor. In an exception to this pattern, Weiss et al. (2000) presented data from a pilot study of a group program that used CBT techniques to enhance relapse prevention in relation both to bipolar disorder and substance abuse. Forty-five patients were recruited to the study following hospital admission, 21 of whom received 12 or 20 weekly group therapy sessions. Group attenders showed some reduction in substance abuse over a 6-month monitoring period and improvement in manic (but not depressive) symptomatology. A larger scale randomized trial of this approach is in progress.

Impact of Interventions on Different Phases of the Disorder

Manic and depressive states present very different challenges both to individual patients and to their therapists, and the studies reviewed earlier suggest that interventions can differentially impact on one phase or the other. While some interventions aim at improving adherence and sensitivity to prodromal signs (e.g., Perry et al.'s [1999] psychoeducational approach) and appear to impact on rates of manic but not depressive relapse, this is not the case for other approaches (Colom et al., 2003). CBT, family interventions, and IPSRT seem to improve depressive episodes but not the rate of manic relapse. This makes clinical sense: Depression is known to be tractable to the various elements included in these latter interventions and is unlikely to improve in the absence of specific interventions aimed at its management. Although psychological models for depression are well advanced, we lack a similar conceptualization of psychological processes in mania, and manic states appear to be inimical to the sort of collaborative effort associated with psychological therapies. Indeed, evidence suggests that the impact of psychotherapeutic strategies during manic episodes is negligible. This suggests that psychological interventions may need to be implemented during euthymic or depressive phases, with strategies restricted to symptom management during manic phases. However, some caution in switching treatment modality to match the phase of the disorder is appropriate given the suggestion that consistency of management may be critical (Swartz & Frank, 2001).

SUMMARY AND CLINICAL IMPLICATIONS

The application of psychosocial treatments for people with bipolar disorder mirrors the application of a range of techniques for patients with schizophrenia, though the field is at an earlier stage of development. As in schizophrenia, interventions for bipolar disorder are invariably adjunctive to medication and aim to reduce relatively high relapse rates through psychoeducation about the disorder, increased responsiveness to prodromal signs, promotion of better regulation of lifestyle, and management of depressive episodes.

To date, many trials have been small, but results from larger trials are now available. Although this makes it possible to consider the efficacy of different approaches, and outcomes are promising, the field needs to develop further before conclusive statements are possible. With this caveat, there is evidence that psychoeducation (which focuses on identifying prodromal signs) shows some efficacy in delaying manic (though not so obviously depressive) relapse. Cognitive-behavioral techniques utilize a number of strategies for relapse prevention and for the management of depressive symptomatology, with some variations across studies in specific techniques and emphasis. Both smaller and larger trials indicate that this approach yields superior outcomes contrasted to clinical management in terms of depressive symptoms and, in some studies, in reduction of bipolar episodes. Cognitive techniques often attempt to stabilize patients' lifestyles; IPSRT focuses on this explicitly, and employs IPT techniques to manage depressive symptoms. Initial results from a single (but large-scale) trial have shown positive outcomes in terms of speed of remission from a bipolar episode relative to clinical management, but long-term efficacy is as yet unknown. Family interventions also show promise, with some evidence of reduced rates of relapse, most obviously from families with higher levels of EE.

Reduction in relapse rates sometimes seems to impact differentially on manic or depressive relapses. At this stage, it is not clear whether this is a meaningful pattern; there are few available studies, and within trials, significant improvement in one form of relapse can be mirrored by a trends toward improvement in the other. Differential improvement in rates of manic relapse might make some clinical sense, because manic prodromes may be more obvious to patients, and therefore more readily acted on by themselves or their significant others. However, clinicians are more familiar with the psychosocial management of depressive presentations than they are with manic symptoms, and patients are more likely to be tractable to interventions while in a depressive state than while they are manic. On this basis, further trials may be appropriate before we draw any conclusions regarding this issue.

As more research programs develop and report, the research base will enable more robust conclusions about efficacy. There remain some basic questions. It is not yet clear whether observed improvements with this group relate to specific psychological changes or to improved adherence and responsiveness to pharmacological interventions. Critically, the significance of commonalities and variations in technique across effective programs is hard to appraise at present.

All approaches require the careful construction of a collaborative relationship between patient and therapist, but the particular challenge for work with this client group is that, at different points in patients' clinical presentation, different treatment strategies may be required, especially because patients are (in a sense) psychologically unavailable when in a manic phase. There is some evidence that consistency of approach may be as important as technique to outcome. This suggests the importance of establishing a sense of shared purpose and expectation between patient and therapist that can "bridge" necessary shifts in approach as the therapist responds to the needs of the patient. These considerations suggest that these therapies may be better conceived of as specialist treatments rather than as applications of a generic approach.

CHAPTER 6

ANXIETY DISORDERS I

Specific Phobia, Social Phobia, Generalized Anxiety Disorder, and Panic Disorder with and without Agoraphobia

DEFINITIONS

DSM-IV-TR identifies a number of anxiety disorders but begins by describing panic attacks, on the grounds that (though not a distinct disorder) their ubiquity across anxiety disorders justifies separate definition. A panic attack is characterized by the sudden onset of feelings of intense apprehension, dread, fear, or terror, often associated with feelings of impending doom. During this period, at least four of a possible 13 symptoms, such as palpitations, sweating, shaking, shortness of breath, choking, nausea, dizziness, derealization, fear of losing control, or dying, must be present.

Specific Phobia

Specific phobias are characterized by a persistent fear of a specific stimulus. Though the person invariably recognizes that his/her fear is excessive, exposure to the phobic stimulus provokes an immediate anxiety response.

Social Phobia

This is defined by a persistent fear of one or more social situations in which the person is anxious that he/she may act in a way that may be embarrassing or humiliating. This includes concerns about being judged by others; worry about displaying anxiety symptoms can often compound the person's difficulties. Exposure to feared social situations invokes anxiety and can pro situationally bound panic attacks. Despite the fact that the person recognizes that his/her fear is excessive, avoidance is common and can lead to disruption of social and occupational functioning. A distinction is made between those people whose social phobia is specific (e.g., restricted to a fear of public speaking) or generalized to a broad range of social contexts.

Generalized Anxiety Disorder

The essential feature of generalized anxiety disorder (GAD) is persistent and excessive anxiety, and worry that the person finds difficult to control, and that is of a sufficient level to cause clinically significant distress or impairment in functioning. The focus of anxiety is on events that are overvalued in relation to their likely actual impact, and the intensity of worry is out of proportion to the actual probability or impact of the feared event.

To meet criteria for this diagnosis, the focus or origin of concern should not be related to another Axis I disorder—for example, it should not arise as part of a mood disorder, or be better classified within alternative diagnoses (e.g., worry about being embarrassed in public would be an indicator for a diagnosis of social phobia rather than GAD). Worry needs to have been present on most days over a period of 6 months or more. At least three of the following six symptoms also need to be present: restlessness, easily fatigued, difficulty concentrating, irritability, muscle tension, and sleep disturbance.

Panic Disorder without Agoraphobia

The essential feature of this condition is the presence of recurrent and unexpected panic attacks, accompanied by a month or more of persistent concern and worry about the possibility of additional attacks. These attacks are, at least initially, unexpected; in other words, they do not reflect exposure to a situation that always causes anxiety (as in *specific phobia*). In addition, they are not triggered by social attention (as in *social phobia*). Later in the course of the disturbance, certain situations, such as driving a car or being in a crowded place, may become associated with panic. These situations then increase the likelihood of panic occurring. Arguably, many patients in this group could be seen as nonsevere agoraphobics within ICD-10 (World Health Organization, 1992), since they manifest panic mainly in public places, even if avoidance is not always present.

Panic Disorder with Agoraphobia

In clinical settings, most cases of panic disorder present with agoraphobia (and to this degree, the distinction between panic disorder with and without agoraphobia may be somewhat artificial). This is defined in DSM-IV-TR as a fear of being in situations from which escape might be difficult or embarrassing, or in which help might not be forthcoming in the event of a panic. This results either in restrictions on travel or in endurance of situations outside the home in spite of high anxiety. Typical agoraphobic situations include being outside the home alone, being in crowded situations, waiting in queues, and travel by train, bus, or car.

PREVALENCE, COMORBIDITY, AND NATURAL HISTORY
Prevalence

Kessler et al. (1994), reporting data from the U.S. National Comorbidity Survey (NCS), suggest a lifetime prevalence for specific phobia of 11.3% and a 12-month prevalence of 8.8%.

Six-month prevalence of social phobia, as estimated from two sites in the National Institute of Mental Health's Epidemiologic Catchment Area (ECA) survey, was 1.2% and 2.2%, respectively (Eaton et al., 1991); surveys in New Zealand estimated 6-month prevalence at 2.6% (Wells et al., 1989). Angst and Dobler-Mikola (1983) cite rates of 1% from their survey.

Wittchen et al. (1991) and Kessler et al. (1994) suggest that GAD is a relatively rare current disorder, with a current prevalence of 1.6%, but a more frequent lifetime disorder affecting 5.1% of the population between ages 15 and 54 years; 12-month prevalence is estimated at 3.1%. Other community surveys produce a wide range of estimates; Breslau and Davis (1985), using the DSM-III definition of GAD in a sample of 375 women surveyed from the general population, found prevalence rates of 2.4% and 11.5% for 1 month and 6 months, respectively. One-year prevalence rates of GAD have been reported as 6.4% (Uhlenhuth et al., 1983), 2.3% (Angst et al., 1985), 2.6% (Dean et al., 1983), and 3.8% (Blazer et al., 1991).

Data from the ECA study give 6-month prevalence rates of 0.8% for panic disorder and 3.8% for agoraphobia. Rates for these disorders vary slightly from study to study: Although those quoted seem reasonably representative of a number of investigations (Oakley-Brown, 1991), some authors suggests rather higher prevalence—for example, Reich (1986) suggests that the 6-month prevalence rate for agoraphobia is 6%, and for panic disorder, 3%. Angst and Dobler-Mikola (1983), using a community sample of 19- and 20-year-olds in Zurich, found 4-week prevalence rates of 2.8% for panic disorder and 1.0% for agoraphobia.

The prevalence of all these disorders is significantly higher in women than men—60% higher for panic, 30% higher for agoraphobia, and 50% higher for social phobia and for GAD (Myers et al., 1984; Weissman et al., 1985; Wittchen et al., 1994).

In many of the community surveys just reported (United States, many, and Switzerland), a relatively large proportion of identified cas _ ᵤₑ untreated for their complaint (in excess of 50%). Although a pattern not unique to this group of disorders, it is perhaps more marked in the case of phobias, panic disorder, and GAD than in many other conditions.

Comorbidity

Comorbidity within the Anxiety Disorders and with Depression

Between 30 and 80% of patients with a principal diagnosis of anxiety have at least one other anxiety disorder (Lesser et al., 1988; Weissman et al., 1986). Brown et al. (2001) found that of 1,127 patients attending an anxiety disorders unit for assessment, 43% had another current anxiety disorder and 28% had a mood disorder, with GAD being the most frequently assigned additional diagnosis (at 25%). Comorbidity rates were particularly high for individuals with a primary diagnosis of social phobia and GAD.

The highest rates of comorbidity with a current mood disorder were for GAD (26%) and panic disorder with agoraphobia (24%); somewhat lower rates were evident for panic disorder (8%) and social phobia (14%). If lifetime comorbidity is considered, these rates are much higher (64% for GAD, 50% for panic disorder with agoraphobia, 44% for social phobia, and 36% for panic disorder), indicating that these disorders rarely occur in isolation. Estimates of comorbidity within clinical samples are probably higher than those based on community surveys; Wittchen et al. (1991) reported that 53.8% of anxiety disorders in community surveys are "pure," contrasted to only 37.1% in clinical samples.

Comorbidity with Personality Disorder

Four reviews (Friedman et al., 1987; Green & Curtis, 1988; Mavissakalian & Hamann, 1988; Reich et al., 1987), suggested that 40–63% of persons with agoraphobia have associated DSM-III-R personality disorders, usually in the avoidant or dependent cluster. Chambless et al. (1992), studying a clinical sample of persons with agoraphobia using the Millon Clinical Multiaxial Inventory, found rates of 91%, again, usually in the avoidant or dependent personality disorder cluster.

Comorbidity of Social Phobia with Avoidant Personality Disorder

Patients with avoidant personality disorder (APD) are characterized by long-standing, pervasive, and active withdrawal from social relationships; they are devastated by disapproval and are vigilant for signs of ridicule. There is some overlap between the description of social phobia and APD, and while there are high levels of comorbidity between the two, there is evidence that patients who receive both diagnoses are the most severely disordered (Heimberg, 1996; Rettew, 2000). Whether or not there is a meaningful diagnostic distinction between the two, it is the case that, whereas social phobia can be triggered by a specific social context (e.g., public speaking anxiety), the same seems unlikely for APD.

Comorbidity of Generalized Anxiety Disorder with Other Disorders

The high comorbidity of GAD with other disorders—especially with major depressive disorder (MDD)—has led to some disagreement as to whether it is best conceptualized as a separate disorder or regarded as a residual or prodrome of other disorders (e.g., Kessler, 2000). Data from the NCS (Wittchen et al., 1994) suggested that 66.3% of patients with current GAD report at least one other disorder in the previous 30 days, and lifetime comorbidity between GAD and other disorders is 90.4%—most usually with affective disorders (MDD and dysthymia), panic disorder, and (for current comorbidity only) agoraphobia. Only in one-third of current cases of GAD was there no additional diagnosis. Borkovec et al. (1995) reported that of 55 patients entered into an outcome study for GAD, 78% had received at least one additional diagnosis pretherapy, and 31% had more than one comorbid diagnosis. Approximately half of the sample also met criteria for past major depressive episodes.

Although estimates of comorbidity vary, there is some consensus that many patients are likely to have concurrent Axis I and II disorders. This suggests that, to be fully informative about effectiveness in everyday practice, trials will need to include and to identify such patients. Such conditions are not usually seen in clinical trials.

Natural History

Anxiety disorders are usually chronic and persistent. Wittchen (1988) defined "remission" as an absence of relevant symptoms in the 6 months preceding survey. On this basis, remission rates for panic disorder were 14.3%, for agoraphobia, 34.6%, and for social phobia, 21.9%. Blazer et al. (1991) found that among patients with current GAD, 40% had suffered for more than 5 years, and 10%, for more than 10 years.

Summary

Overall prevalence rates for anxiety disorders suggest that they are relatively common within the general population; the most frequently occurring one is panic disorder with agoraphobia, followed by GAD, social phobia, and panic disorder without agoraphobia. Prevalence rates are between one-third and two-thirds higher in women than men. Anxiety disorders represent problems with a wide range of chronicity and severity, and are frequently comorbid with other anxiety disorders, affective disorders (particularly depression), and personality disorders. Prevalence figures for individuals who would require treatment for anxiety alone are approximately 50% of those cited earlier.

TREATMENT APPROACHES

The sections following cover evidence for treatment efficacy derived from meta-analyses, general reviews, and specific trials for each anxiety syndrome in turn. As noted in the earlier discussion of meta-analyses for depression, lists of the studies included in analyses are not always available. Without this information, the overlap between reviews and the degree to which they supplement or repeat one another are difficult to determine. Where possible, the degree of overlap is reported.

Treatments for Specific Phobia

Emmelkamp (1994) and Antony and Barlow (2002) reviewed behavioral treatments for specific phobia. The efficacy of systematic desensitization and exposure techniques has been widely researched, with strong evidence that the latter is more effective than the former, particularly when exposure is prolonged to the point at which anxiety is markedly reduced (e.g., Marshall, 1985, 1988). Clinically significant improvement is achieved in 70–85% of cases (e.g., Emmelkamp, 1982; Jansson & Öst, 1982; Marks, 1987).

There is good evidence for the efficacy of exposure in relation to a wide variety of phobias—for example, fear of animals (e.g., Öst et al., 1997b), claustrophobia (e.g., Öst et al., 2001a) or flying phobia (e.g., Öst et al., 1997a). Where fears are specific and circumscribed, fairly brief interventions can be helpful, and there is some indication that prolonged exposure carried out over one or a very few sessions can be as effective as shorter periods of exposure over longer periods (e.g., Liddell et al., 1994; Öst et al., 2001b; Smith et al., 1990). Therapist-directed exposure appears to be markedly more effective than self-directed exposure (e.g., Öst et al., 1991b).

Person with blood–injury phobias appear to require additional treatment measures when exposed to feared stimuli, because there is evidence that, in contrast to the usual anxiety response, these individuals show bradycardia and a decrease in blood pressure (Connolly et al., 1976; Öst et al., 1984) that may result in fainting. Öst et al. (1984, 1989, 1991a) have trained such phobics to recognize early signs of a drop in blood pressure and to apply tension techs at this point. Combining this with exposure gives better results than simple exposure; in Öst's (1989) trial, 73% of patients were clinically improved posttreatment, and 77% at follow-up.

Developments in technology make it feasible to expose patients using a variety of virtual reality techniques, ranging in sophistication from videotape to computer-generated images. This has the potential advantage of making phobic stimuli more available for exposure, and there is evidence that this approach can be of equivalent efficacy to *in vivo* exposure—for example, for flying phobias (Rothbaum et al., 2000), height phobias (Emmelkamp et al., 2002), dental phobias (Thom et al., 2000), and spider phobias (Garcia-Palacios et al., 2002b).

The efficacy of exposure may explain why few studies have explored any potential benefit from cognitive therapy. De Jongh et al. (1995) showed some benefit of cognitive restructuring in preparation of dental phobics for dental treatment, though it is not clear how this impacted on subsequent attendance for treatment.

Though evidence regarding the relative impact of pharmacotherapy and psychological therapy is sparse, there is some suggestion that any immediate benefit conferred by anxiolytics is not sustained, even in the short-term. Thom et al. (2000) randomized 50 dental phobic patients to receive either benzodiazepines, a stress management package (which combined relaxation, exposure, and cognitive restructuring), or no treatment. Though both active treatments led to marked reduction in anxiety, relapse with benzodiazepines was marked; only 20% of patients from this group completed dental treatment, contrasted to 70% of those receiving psychological treatments. Wilhelm and Roth (1997) randomized 28 flight phobics to receive either alprazolam or placebo while undertaking a first flight, finding that active medication resulted in greater levels of anxiety during a second flight, suggesting that medication had rendered exposure less effective.

Summary

Phobic symptoms respond well to exposure treatments. A very high percentage of specific phobics—perhaps as many as 70–85%—show clinically significant improvement when treated by this method, and when fears are specific and circumscribed, interventions can be quite brief. The addition of cognitive techniques appears to add little to efficacy, and there is some evidence that the use of adjunctive anxiolytics reduces the impact of exposure. Therapist-directed exposure is more effective than self-directed exposure. An increasing number of studies have examined the use of virtual reality techniques; while the technical investment may be beyond that available to most clinical settings, this approach may have the advantage of creating the conditions for clinic-based exposure to a wide range of phobias.

Treatments for Social Phobia

A number of behavioral and cognitive-behavioral therapy (CBT) approaches have been developed to manage social phobia. Variants of CBT focus on cognitive restructuring, relaxation training, and social skills training. Most studies include exposure to feared social situations. This is entirely justifiable from a clinical perspective but makes it harder to distinguish the mutative elements of treatment packages. There are almost no studies of alternative approaches—indeed, there appears to be only one small-scale open trial of IPT (Lipsitz et al., 1999), and no trials of psychodynamic therapy.

Meta-Analyses

Chambless and Gillis (1993), Feske and Chambless (1995), Gould et al. (1997), and Taylor (1996) reviewed the efficacy of psychological treatments, and Fedoroff and Taylor (2001) reviewed psychological and pharmacological approaches. Chambless and Gillis (1993) reviewed 10 trials of behavioral therapy and CBT for patients with social phobia, including anxiety management, exposure, and social skills training. Contrasted with control subjects, they derived a weighted average effect size of 0.68 for measures of social phobia and 0.7 for fear of negative evaluation. Results were maintained at follow-up varying between 1 and 6 months. Feske and Chambless (1995) contrasted the relative benefit of CBT (which includes exposure) and exposure alone in 10 and 9 studies, respectively, and found that both approaches were of equal efficacy. A subanalysis explored the possibility that some forms of cognitive therapy (such as those developed at the time of the review specifically for social phobia) might be more effective than less specific forms. This hypothesis was not supported; both were of equal efficacy, and each was no more effective than exposure.

Gould et al. (1997) identified 24 studies of both CBT and pharmacological interventions, deriving a mean social anxiety effect size of 0.74 for the former and 0.62 for the latter. Exposure or exposure combined with cognitive restructuring yielded the largest effect sizes (0.89 and 0.80, respectively). Taylor (1996) reviewed 25 trials that employed exposure alone, cognitive therapy alone, exposure combined with cognitive therapy, and social skills training. Four trials included medication-placebo and two attention-placebo; arguably, these were combined on the basis of their equivalent efficacy. All psychological approaches showed equivalent efficacy relative to wait-list control, though only the combination of cognitive therapy and exposure yielded a significantly larger effect size than placebo. Benefits were maintained at 3-month follow-up. A later review (Fedoroff & Taylor, 2001) focused on both psychological and pharmacological interventions, slightly extending the number of available trials of psychological interventions, and confirming the pattern of efficacy of psychological interventions identified by Taylor (1996). Although posttherapy effect sizes for benzodiazepines and selective serotonin reuptake inhibitors (SSRIs) were greater than those for psychological interventions, too few pharmacotherapy trials supplied follow-up data to ascertain longer term outcomes.

Qualitative Reviews and Individual Studies

Several qualitative reviews of interventions for social phobia have been undertaken (e.g., Heimberg, 2001, 2002; Heimberg & Juster, 1994; Stravynski & Greenberg, 1998).

EXPOSURE

A number of studies have demonstrated significant effects of *in vivo* exposure for social phobia (e.g., Butler et al., 1984; Mattick & Peters, 1988; Mattick et al., 1989; Turner et al., 1994a) and APD (Alden, 1989; Renneberg et al., 1990; Stravynski et al., 1982, 1994). There is evidence for the stability of gains: Fava et al. (2001a) conducted a naturalistic follow-up over 2–12 years of a consecutive series of 45 patients. At 2 years, the cumulative percentage of patients in remission was 98%, stabilizing at 85% at both 5 and 10 years. The clear benefits of exposure need to be borne in mind when evaluating the treatments, especially when an exposure component is implicit rather than explicit (as is the case in social skills training and many pharmacological interventions, the protocols of which often encourage social engagement [Heimberg, 2002]).

COGNITIVE-BEHAVIORAL THERAPY

There is good evidence that packages based on CBT can be effective, particularly when offered in small groups, an approach extensively researched by Heimberg and colleagues. Heimberg et al. (1990) contrasted cognitive-behavioral group therapy (CBGT) with an educational–supportive therapy (comprising education on topics relating to social phobia (e.g., social skills and models of anxiety) together with opportunities for mutual support. Forty-nine patients were randomly assigned to either therapy over 12 weeks of treatment. At 6-month follow-up, 81% of patients receiving cognitive therapy were judged improved, contrasted with 47% of those receiving the educational package, with maintenance of gains at 4–6 year follow-up (Heimberg et al., 1993).

Cottraux et al. (2000) contrasted CBT with supportive therapy in 67 individuals, 89% of whom met criteria for generalized social phobia, and 75% for APD. The CBT group received eight sessions of individual CBT over 6 weeks, followed by six sessions of group social skills training. Those allocated to supportive therapy were given six half-hour sessions of therapy over 12 weeks, after which they were switched to the CBT program. At 6 weeks and 12 weeks, CBT showed gains over supportive therapy; after switching to CBT, patients who originally received supportive therapy made gains equivalent to the CBT group. Although this suggests some specificity of action to CBT, this interpretation is moderated by the fact that supportive therapy was delivered at a lower "dosage" than CBT.

Clark and Wells (1995) and Rapee and Heimberg (1997) attempted to explain why social phobics do not benefit from naturalistic exposure, focusing on factors that maintain social phobia, such as excessive self-focus and monitoring, negative appraisal of performance in social situations, and the use of "safety behaviors" that are intended to promote security but often increase anxiety. At this point, there is good experimental support for this model (Clark & McManus, 2002) and some evidence for efficacy. Wells and Papageorgiou (2001) reported a single-case series of six patients treated using a package that aims to reduce the level of self-focus in social situations and utilizes exposure as a form of behavioral test of negative expectancies. After 14–18 individual sessions, all patients demonstrated marked gains, sustained at 6-month follow-up. The model also suggests that social phobics engage in "safety behaviors" (e.g., conscious rehearsal prior to a conversation), which they experience as anxiolytic, but which can be construed as maintaining their fears. Morgan and Raffle (1999) contrasted 14 patients who received standard CBGT with 16 who received additional instruction aimed at reducing reliance on safety behaviors. While both groups made significant pre–posttherapy gains, the additional instruction conferred a significant benefit over standard CBGT. Clark et al. (2003) assigned 60 patients to receive 16 weeks of cognitive therapy, fluoxetine combined with self-exposure instruction, or pill-placebo plus self-exposure; at the end of this period, patients receiving active treatment had three booster sessions over 3 months. At posttherapy and 12-month follow-up, cognitive therapy showed significant advantage over fluoxetine and placebo. On a composite measure of social phobia (based on seven scales), there was significant advantage to CBT at all time points, with good maintenance of gains. Posttherapy effect sizes for the contrast to placebo were 1.31 for CBT, and 0.21 for fluoxetine. In a further replication of this approach Stangier et al. (2003) allocated 71 patients to individual or group-format CBT; a subgroup was initially assigned to a wait list and to one of the two treatments after 10 months. At posttherapy, individual therapy showed clear gains over group therapy; 50% and 13% of patients, respectively, no longer met diagnostic criteria, with gains in individual treatment maintained at 6-month follow-up.

Lincoln et al. (2003) conducted a large-scale effectiveness study, enrolling 217 patient selected for a primary diagnosis of social phobia, but in other respects applying no exclusion criteria. Patients were treated in one of four outpatient anxiety clinics, using a CBT program that initially comprised intensive *in vivo* exposure combined with cognitive intervention over 1 week, followed by a 6-week period of patient-directed self-exposure. Therapists were largely psychologists in training. Outcomes were equivalent to those reported in research trials; at 6-week follow-up, 56% of patients showed reliable change; the effect size on measures of social phobia was 0.82, close to those reported in meta-analyses reviewed earlier. This suggests the transportablility of this approach to routine clinical settings, the more so because post hoc analysis stratifying the sample using standard exclusion criteria suggested that outcomes were not influenced by these factors.

BENEFIT OF ADDING COGNITIVE-BEHAVIORAL THERAPY TO EXPOSURE

The degree to which cognitive techniques enhance outcome when combined with exposure, rather than being effective *sui generis,* is unclear. Though Emmelkamp et al. (1985) have demonstrated the efficacy of self-instructional training and rational–emotive therapy in the absence of directed exposure, most studies are less conclusive. Mattick and Peters (1988) and Mattick et al. (1989) contrasted the effects of cognitive restructuring alone, exposure alone, and cognitive restructuring in combination with exposure, and found that the combination was more effective than either treatment alone on some measures. The effect of combined treatment was more apparent at 3-month follow-up than at posttreatment, particularly on measures of fear of appraisal. Mattick and Newman (1991) raise the possibility that self-directed exposure, facilitated by cognitive treatment, resulted in these gains. Butler et al. (1984) found that exposure alone was inferior to its combination with an anxiety-management package, which included relaxation, distraction, and rational self-talk; effects were particularly marked at 1-year follow-up. At this point, 40% of patients receiving exposure alone had requested further therapy, whereas none from the group receiving exposure and anxiety management had done so. However, other researchers have failed to find any additional benefits for CBT or for packages of intervention over gains attributable to exposure-based techniques alone. Scholing and Emmelkamp (1993) and Hope et al. (1990) found no evidence that cognitive therapy and exposure was more effective than exposure alone. Similarly, Mersch (1995) contrasted 34 patients assigned either to exposure alone or to a treatment package comprising rational–emotive therapy, social skills training, and exposure. Equal gains were found for both treatments posttherapy and at 3- and 18-month follow-up. Hope et al. (1995a) assigned 43 patients either to exposure-alone, to CBGT, or to a wait-list control. On measures of clinically significant change (based on clinician ratings of severity), rates of response in each of these conditions were 70%, 36%, and 0%, respectively (though low statistical power makes these differences suggestive rather than conclusive).

Relatively small cell sizes in many of these studies make it difficult to draw substantive conclusions regarding the benefits of cognitive procedures alone or in combination with exposure. Though there is limited support for cognitive procedures offered without exposure, it may be premature to draw firm conclusions regarding their additive value.

INDIVIDUAL VERSUS GROUP DELIVERY OF COGNITIVE-BEHAVIORAL THERAPY

Although a number of programs are designed to be delivered in group format, there are few direct contrasts of these approaches. While Stangier et al. (2003) found individual therapy superior to group therapy, Scholing and Emmelkamp (1993) found them to be equivalent. The logic of group formats is that they allow sharing of problems and vicarious learning; the potential disadvantage is a loss of focus on individual needs. At present, there is no clear evidence of relative advantage or disadvantage, and it may be that interventions designed and manualized for individual or group delivery do not necessarily translate across formats.

PHARMACOTHERAPY AND PSYCHOLOGICAL THERAPY

Trials of medication alone suggest short-term efficacy for some medications—particularly SSRIs, monoamine oxidase inhibitors (MAOIs), and benzodiazepines—but indicate that others are ineffective, particularly reversible MAOIs such as moclobemide (Fedoroff & Taylor, 2001). Unfortunately, at least some trials that contrast the relative benefits of psycho- and pharmacotherapies do so using ineffective medications, rendering them uninformative. Studies by Turner et al. (1994b) (using atenolol) and Clark and Agras (1991) (using buspirone) fall into this category. Oosterbaan et al. (2001) assigned 82 patients to individual cognitive therapy, moclobemide, or placebo conditions. Cognitive therapy showed greater efficacy than both medication conditions, but moclobemide was no more effective than placebo (confirming its lack of efficacy for this condition).

Gelernter et al. (1991) contrasted cognitive therapy with phenelzine, alprazolam, and pill placebo in 65 patients. However, all patients were encouraged to expose themselves to feared situations; more accurately, the study is a contrast of these treatments in combination with exposure. All treatments conferred some gains; though patients treated with phenelzine showed greater gains than those in other treatment groups, these were not significant. In addition, only patients treated with phenelzine and cognitive therapy maintained their gains at follow-up.

Heimberg et al. (1998) contrasted CBGT and phenelzine; this study controlled for allegiance effects, because patients were treated at two sites, each of which had particular expertise in one or the other treatment approach. One hundred thirty-three patients were randomized to 12 weeks of CBGT, phenelzine, pill placebo, or an educational–supportive group (acting as an attention placebo). At posttherapy, both active treatments showed significant gains contrasted to control conditions, though response to medication was more rapid (response rates for phenelzine, CGBT, pill-placebo, and attention placebo at 12 weeks were 65%, 58%, 33%, and 27%, respectively). There were no between-site differences, indicating allegiance effects were minimal in this study. Treatment responders were enrolled to a further 6 months of treatment in whichever modality they had shown benefit, with a subsequent 6-month follow-up (Liebowitz et al., 1999). Patient-responders who had received medication continued to demonstrate somewhat greater gains through the maintenance phase, and those who did not relapse continued to show this advantage. However, though the relapse rate among this group was higher than for CGBT, this observation should be tempered by the small cell sizes in this phase of the study.

Otto et al. (2000) contrasted 12 weeks of CGBT and clonazepam in 45 patients; at posttherapy, both treatments were of equivalent efficacy, with no differences in speed of response. Attrition among patients receiving clonazepam was high (at 40%), though effect sizes were comparable with those of other studies.

Blomhoff et al. (2001) conducted a multisite, primary care trial in Norway and Sweden, allocating 387 patients to sertraline or to placebo. In addition, half the patients were further randomized to receive exposure, which comprised eight 15-minute sessions delivered by family physicians (who received some training in the technique; Haug et al., 2000). At posttherapy, patients treated with sertraline showed greater benefit than those who received placebo, but the addition of exposure was of only marginal benefit, and exposure in combination with placebo was not significantly more effective than placebo alone. At 1-year follow-up (Haug et al., 2003) there were indications of continued improvement in the exposure group and some decline in patients treated with setraline.

SOCIAL SKILLS TRAINING

The rationale for using social skills training (SST) with persons with social phobias rests on the assumption that they are deficient in social skills. Whether this is so is unclear, since social phobics do not seem to lack behavioral competence in social situations (e.g., Rapee & Lim, 1992) and (as discussed earlier) it may be that bias in their appraisal of social situations is more pertinent to their difficulties.

There are relatively few studies of SST. Earlier trials suffered from methodological problems: One difficulty is that patients in some studies were selected as much for social skills deficits as for social phobia. Mersch et al. (1989, 1991), Öst et al. (1981), and Wlazlo et al. (1990) found SST equivalent in outcome to rational–emotive therapy (RET) and applied relaxation and exposure, respectively. Alden (1989) allocated patients who met criteria for APD to one of three active group treatments or a wait-list control. Active intervention included successively more elements (exposure alone, exposure combined with SST, and exposure and SST combined with discussion of intimate relationships), but all interventions were of equal efficacy.

Stravynski et al. (1982) found that addressing cognitions did not improve outcomes with SST. Mersch (1995) contrasted exposure alone to a package that combined exposure, RET, and SST, and found both approaches to be of equivalent efficacy. Turner et al. (1994a, 1995) conducted an open trial of a package that combined SST, exposure, and psychoeducation, and found evidence of gains at posttherapy and 2-year follow-up. van Dam Baggen and Kraaimaat (2000) contrasted the efficacy of group SST and group CBT; 48 patient were assigned to treatment on the basis of matching rather than randomization. Although patients receiving SST evidenced significantly greater benefit than those treated with CBT, SST included an exposure element, whereas this (potentially mutative) element was specifically excluded from CBT.

INTERPERSONAL PSYCHOTHERAPY

There is only one small-scale open trial of IPT (Lipsitz et al., 1999), in which nine patients received 14 weeks of treatment with a modified form of IPT. At posttherapy, seven patients were rated as treatment responders by independent clinicians. Although a promising result, larger comparative trials are needed to appraise the benefits of IPT for social phobia.

IMPACT OF SUBTYPES OF SOCIAL PHOBIA AND OF PERSONALITY DISORDER ON OUTCOME

Most studies suggest that though individuals with generalized social phobia make gains at the same rate as those with specific social phobia, their lower levels of pretherapy functioning are mirrored by poorer posttherapy outcomes (e.g., Brown et al., 1995; Hope et al., 1995b; Mersch, 1995; Turner et al., 1996). Though the overlap between APD and more severe forms of social phobia makes this a questionable form of comorbidity, it is reasonable to ask whether its presence impacts on outcome. Evidence is mixed; some studies (e.g., Hofmann et al., 1995; Hope et al., 1995b; van Velzen et al., 1997) found no differential outcome for individuals with or without APD. Most studies reported a pattern of outcome similar to that for generalized social phobia, with rate of gain similar to those without APD, but lower end point functioning (e.g., Chambless et al., 1997; Feske et al., 1996; Scholing &

Emmelkamp, 1999), though some report a slower rate of change (e.g., Oosterbaan et al., 2002). Massion et al. (2002) reported a 5-year prospective study examining the impact of personality disorders in 514 patients in the Harvard–Brown anxiety research program. The presence of a personality disorder reduced the probability of remission in social phobia by 39%. Much of this was explained by the presence of APD. Finally, while Erwin et al. (2002) found that the presence of comorbid anxiety disorders did not impact on treatment response, comorbid depression predicted poorer outcome, an issue that may benefit from further research.

Although trials suggest that gains are possible for social phobics, relatively few studies address the issue of clinically significant improvement. Using a criterion of high end-state functioning to determine the clinical significance of change in CBT, 37% and 33%, respectively, of patients in Mattick and Peters (1988) and Mattick et al. (1989) achieved high or very high end-state functioning. Of the 58 treatment completers in Gelernter et al.'s (1991) study, 34% achieved scores below the mean for the general population on the fear questionnaire (Marks & Mathews, 1979). Alden (1989) found that while there were significant improvements on a range of measures, only 9% of patients treated for APD rated themselves as completely improved. However, other trials report more encouraging rates; as cited earlier, Heimberg et al. (1998) reported a response rate of 58% for CBGT.

Summary

Most trials of social phobia focus almost exclusively on behavioral and cognitive-behavioral approaches. Inevitably, most procedures employ some form of exposure, and this makes it difficult to disaggregate the impact of specific technical elements. Both cognitive therapy and exposure show good evidence of efficacy; their combination is associated with the largest effect sizes in meta-analytic reviews. Some manualized procedures—such as CBGT—have been subject to a number of trials and show good evidence of efficacy.

Direct contrast of exposure, alone and in combination with cognitive techniques, does not show clear evidence of additional benefit, though whether this reflects issues of statistical power or a true equivalence of action is as yet unclear. Despite this lack of clarity, the question of additive benefit from cognitive techniques remains an active area of enquiry, with an increasing focus on attentional processing in social phobics. Initial trials have applied treatment strategies that reflect greater experimental understanding of these issues, with results suggesting that this is a promising development in terms of effectiveness and efficiency. This attempt to link emergent models of cognitive processing with treatment promises to be a productive approach to increasing treatment efficacy.

There are rather few good-quality trials of SST, and those available suggest an equivalence of action to CBT. In some respects, this may not be surprising, since both approaches include exposure—whether implicitly or explicitly. Since the assumption that social phobics are deficient in social skills may be inappropriate, SST might best be reserved for those with demonstrated problems in social performance.

Because, by definition, problems related to social phobia arise in a social context, some programs that have been developed employ group therapies, on the grounds that this enables both direct exposure and social support and vicarious learning. Equally, a number of approaches are intended for delivery as individual therapy. Both formats show efficacy, but there is little evidence suggesting that one is to be preferred over the other. However, one of the few direct contrasts of these approaches indicated that a program originally designed for individuals showed markedly reduced efficacy when delivered in a group. This suggests that implementation of these therapies should pay attention to the contexts within which they have been tested under research conditions. Though there are few studies of the effectiveness of exposure and CBT, available evidence does suggest that these therapies are applicable with standard clinical populations.

Trials contrasting pharmacotherapy and psychological interventions have not always employed effective medications or dosages, reducing the number of available trials. There appear to be no studies of combination treatments, and direct comparison of psychological approaches with medication (specifically, MAOIs, SSRIs, and benzodiazepine) has yielded mixed results. Some trials suggest an equivalence of action; others suggest greater benefit to medication, though there is evidence of better retention of gains with psychological therapy.

The overlap between APD and more severe, generalized forms of social phobia is a source of much debate. By definition, individuals with either presentation are more disabled than those whose social phobias are more restricted. Nonetheless, both groups are likely to make the same rate of gains from therapy, though the higher level of initial severity means that the former group is likely to achieve lower end point functioning. This being so, it may be productive to consider the degree to which diagnostic distinctions among individuals with social phobia reflect similar or different underlying mechanisms, since this has the potential to create more specific, and, hence, more effective intervention strategies.

Treatments for Generalized Anxiety Disorder

Treatments developed for GAD include various relaxation techniques; as implied by its name, "applied relaxation" helps patients to apply relaxation techniques in everyday life, and in response to anxiogenic thoughts or situations. Anxiety management techniques also include relaxation, along with other elements (such as positive self-talk). Cognitive therapy focuses directly on identification and modification of worrying thoughts. Because avoidance of worrying thoughts or situations is common, approaches often include exposure techniques. In practice, many treatments include various combinations of these elements.

Meta-Analyses and Systematic Reviews

Chambless and Gillis (1993) identified seven trials that contrasted CBT against a control condition; these included pill placebo, nondirective therapy, or wait list conditions. Presumably because of the small number of studies, these were collapsed into one variable, though this range of controls means that expected effect sizes could be expected to vary across trials. Against control there was a pre- to posttreatment effect size of 1.69 for CBT, and a pre-treatment follow-up effect size of 1.95 (though follow-up was only reported in four studies, and was either 6 months or 1 year). Gould et al. (1997) identified 22 trials of pharmacotherapy and 13 of CBT published between 1974 and 1996 (extending by six studies Chambless and Gillis's sample). Post-treatment effect size for CBT was statistically equivalent to that of pharmacotherapy (0.7 and 0.6, respectively). Though the largest effect sizes were for treatments that combined cognitive and behavioral techniques, other than for the contrast of CBT and relaxation training, there were no statistical differences in effect size across the various forms of CBT. Many individuals entering trials are already in receipt of medication; while some protocols restrict drug use, most do not. Contrasting 16 studies of CBT that allowed concurrent medication with six trials that did not yielded effect sizes of 0.69 and 0.88, respectively, a nonsignificant difference.

Borkovec and Ruscio (2001) reviewed 13 studies (eight of which are included in Gould et al. [1997]); in two trials, patient samples included those with mixed GAD and panic disorder. On measures of anxiety and depression, there was some advantage to CBT against treatments offering only behavioral or cognitive components (effect size = 0.26 at posttherapy and 0.54 at follow-up). Against a category of interventions identified by Borkovec and Ruscio as "placebo and nonspecific" therapies (psychodynamic therapy, "supportive listening," and subthreshold doses of valium), CBT again showed advantage (effect size = 0.71 at posttherapy and 0.3 at follow-up). A similar pattern of effect sizes was found on measures of depression.

Westen and Morrison's (2001) analysis is restricted to trials published since 1990, and identifies five trials that inevitably overlap with the previous analyses but also, and uniquely, includes one study of supportive–expressive therapy (Crits-Christoph et al., 1996). A median effect size of 0.9 was derived at posttherapy, with 52% and 44%, respectively, of completer and "intention-to-treat" patients improved, but the analysis did not address differences in efficacy across therapy type.

The clinical significance of change has been examined in two reviews— Durham and Allan (1993) and Fisher and Durham (1999)—covering the periods 1980–1991 and 1990–1999, respectively. Both restricted coverage to studies that used a common outcome measure, and both applied Jacobson et al.'s (1984) criteria to delineate categorical criteria that indicate when clinically significant change has occurred. The earlier review identified 14 studies that measured change using the Hamilton Anxiety Scale (HAS) and the State–Trait Anxiety Inventory (STAI-T; Speilberger et al., 1983), and the latter review identified six that employed the STAI-T. Studies by Durham and Allan included cognitive and behavioral therapies, relaxation, biofeedback, and nondirective therapy. Across trials, there was wide variation in posttreatment gains; overall, there was a 54% reduction for somatic symptoms on the HAS (range across studies 20–76%) and a 25% reduction in "general tendency to worry" on STAI-T (range 6–50%). Usually, but not consistently, the best results were obtained by CBT. Though these improvements are modest, they compare well with results for anxiolytic medication and placebo (which show an average reduction in HAS scores of 47 and 30%, respectively [Barlow, 1988]). Only half the studies followed up patients; where this was reported, follow-up was between 3 and 12 months (mode = 6) and gains were maintained. Five studies (all contrasting cognitive therapy and behavior therapy) employed cutoff points on anxiety scales or a reduction of 2 standard deviations from pretreatment scores to gauge clinically significant change. On average, 57% of patients who had received cognitive therapy were in the normative range, compared to 22% of behavior therapy patients. There was some limited evidence of better outcomes when studies included more patients with a first episode of anxiety, though only three studies gave information about this.

Fisher and Durham (1999) reviewed a further six trials (Barlow et al., 1992; Borkovec, 1997; Borkovec & Costello, 1993; Butler et al., 1991; Durham et al., 1994; White et al., 1992); therapies used included CBT, behavior therapy, psychodynamic therapy, applied relaxation, and nondirective therapy. Their rationale for basing analysis on the STAI-T is that it measures general vulnerability to anxiety, low mood, and poor self-esteem, hence capturing something of the complexity of GAD. Again using Jacobson's methodology to determine cutoffs for clinical change, they calculated the proportion of patients recovered at posttherapy, the proportion who remained in remission at 6 months, the proportion who were not recovered posttherapy but had recovered at 6 months, and, finally, the overall recovery rate (the combination of the last two categories). Across all forms of intervention, at posttherapy, 3% were worse, 45% showed no change, 20% had improved, and 32% had recovered. At 6-month follow-up, there was some evidence of gradual improvement, with 2% worse, 36% unchanged, 24% improved, and 38% recovered. Disaggregating type of therapy, individual applied relaxation and CBT had the highest rates of recovery (rates at 6 months were 60% and 51%, respectively). Individual nondirective therapy, group CBT, and group behavior therapy had moderate outcomes (6-month recovery rates of 38%, 33% and 31%, respectively). Very few patients were classified as recovered after treatment with individual behavior therapy and psychodynamic therapy (11% and 4%, respectively). Overall, this suggests that a substantial proportion of patients will not benefit from therapy, and though there is evidence of differential efficacy across therapies, the reliability of this observation is threatened by the small number of trials included in the analysis (which necessarily results in limited replication of therapy type across studies).

COGNITIVE-BEHAVIORAL THERAPY VERSUS BEHAVIOR THERAPY

Butler et al. (1991) contrasted CBT and behavior therapy with a wait-list control group. Fifty-seven patients participated in the trial; the mean duration of the index episode of GAD was 3 years. Both treatments were superior to wait-list control, but CBT was more effective than behavior therapy across a range of symptoms. Clinical significance of change was assessed using as a criterion scores ≤ 10 on the HAS, ≤ 10 on the Beck Anxiety Scale, and ≤ 6 on the Leeds Anxiety Scale. Thirty-two percent of patients receiving CBT and 16% of those receiving behavior therapy met this target posttherapy. At 6-month follow-up, the advantage to CBT was more marked; 42% of CBT, but only 5% of behavior therapy, patients met the criterion.

Durham and Turvey (1987) treated 51 patients with GAD of at least 1 year's duration, assigning them to 16 sessions of either CBT (modification of maladaptive thoughts and assumptions) or behavioral treatment (relaxation, distraction, and exposure). On global ratings by independent assessors, posttreatment gains were similar in each treatment condition; overall, 25% of patients showed no change, 20% showed moderate gains, and 55% had greatly improved. However, the stability of these gains varied across treatment groups; at 6-month follow-up, 62% of CBT patients were rated as greatly improved, contrasted with only 30% of those treated with behavior therapy.

COGNITIVE-BEHAVIORAL THERAPY VERSUS APPLIED RELAXATION

Barlow et al. (1992) contrasted 15 sessions of three active interventions (applied relaxation, cognitive therapy, or applied relaxation combined with cognitive therapy) to a wait-list control. Sixty-five patients were randomized to treatment; against wait list, all three treatments resulted in significant and equivalent gains, which were sustained at 2-year follow-up. Borkovec and Costello (1993) examined the relative efficacy of 14 sessions of CBT, applied relaxation, and nondirective counseling in 55 patients (though it should be noted that CBT largely focused on applied relaxation, with limited additional time given to cognitions). At posttherapy, patients treated using applied relaxation and CBT improved to an equivalent extent, and significantly more so than those who received nondirective counseling. At 12-month follow-up, the percentage of patients defined as having a high response to treatment was 58% for those receiving CBT, 33% for applied relaxation, and 22% for nondirective counseling.

Öst and Breitholtz (2000) assigned 36 patients to 12 weeks of cognitive therapy or applied relaxation, with equivalent outcomes at posttreatment and 1-year follow-up; at these assessment points, the proportion of patients meeting Jacobson's criteria for clinically significant change was (respectively) 53% and 67% for applied relaxation and 62% and 56% for cognitive therapy. Arntz (2003) contrasted the same treatments used by Öst and Breitholtz (2000), though in a sample of 45 patients recruited from a CMHC, and with higher rates of comorbidity. Both treatments showed equal efficacy, with gains maintained at 1 and 6 months, and comparable to those in research trials with stricter exclusion criteria. Fisher and Durham's (1999) cutoffs on the STAI-T were used to determine clinically significant change; on this basis, 55% and 53%, respectively, of patients were deemed to have recovered at 1-year follow-up.

Borkovec et al. (2002) contrasted cognitive therapy, applied relaxation, and a combination of these approaches (effectively, CBT). Seventy-six patients were randomized to 15 sessions of treatment, and followed up at 6 months and 2 years. There were no differences between treatments; overall, patients improved, and at 2 years, an average of only 17% of patients met diagnostic criteria for GAD.

COGNITIVE-BEHAVIORAL THERAPY VERSUS OTHER TREATMENTS

Durham et al. (1994, 1999) contrasted the efficacy of CBT, analytically based psychotherapy, and anxiety management training (AMT) in 99 patients. Mean duration of GAD was 30 months (range, 6–60 months); 80% of patients had comorbid Axis I disorders; 46% also received an Axis II diagnosis. Though CBT and analytic therapy were delivered by experienced therapists, AMT was offered by therapists relatively inexperienced in this approach. Treatment was offered over 6 months, with analytic therapy and CBT delivered either at "high" frequency (essentially weekly) or "low" frequency (essentially fortnightly). AMT was delivered at low frequency. This study has been subject to methodological critique (e.g., Borkovec & Newman, 1998). Most critically, failure of randomization led to lower pretreatment scores for CBT patients in the low-frequency condition, though this is recognized and controlled for in later statistical analyses (Durham et al., 1999).

Overall, patients receiving CBT showed significant and consistent gains across a range of measures, with improvements maintained at 6-month and 1-year follow-up. While patients receiving analytic therapy and AMT also showed significant gains on some measures, these were not maintained through follow-up. Using the STAI-T as an index, the percentage of patients meeting Jacobson et al.'s (1984) criteria for recovery at posttherapy, 6 months and 1 year, respectively, was 37%, 60%, and 58% for CBT, 31%, 25%, and 10% for AMT, and 10%, 7%, and 14% for analytic therapy. Though at 6 months, equivalent results were found for patients treated at both high and low frequency, at 1 year, higher frequency of contact was associated with better maintenance of gains both for CBT and analytic therapy. The percentage of patients meeting Jacobson criteria at high and low frequency, respectively, for CBT were 67% and 50%, and for analytic therapy, 30% and 0%, signaling a clear advantage to CBT when delivered more intensively. However, very long-term follow-up of 61 individuals at between 8 and 10 years (Durham et al., 2003a) suggests that about half of those who had achieved recovery status at 6 months maintained their gains. At this stage, there were no differences in outcome between CBT and non-CBT-treated patients.

White et al. (1992) and White (1998) described a large-group format for delivering therapy in a primary care setting. One hundred nine patients were allocated to one of five groups—cognitive therapy, behavioral therapy, CBT, wait list, or a placebo-control "subconscious retraining" (SCR). Therapy was delivered in six 2-hour sessions, with group size in the active therapy conditions ranging from 20 to 24 patients, and was didactic in approach. At posttherapy and at 6-month and 2-year follow-up, there was no differential impact of therapies, though the small numbers allocated to SCR (10 patients) precluded statistical analysis beyond posttherapy.

Though there have been developments in the conceptualization of worry that focus on metacognitions and attentional processes (e.g., Wells, 1995), there are few trials of therapies utilizing these ideas. Ladouceur et al. (2000) conducted a small trial that solicited 26 patients through advertisement, assigning them to treatment or to a wait-list. Therapy focused exclusively on the management of uncertainty, beliefs about worry, orientation to problem solving, and cognitive avoidance related to worry, and was delivered over 16 sessions, with follow-up at 6 and 12 months. At posttherapy, 77% of patients no longer met diagnostic criteria for GAD, and 46% met criteria for both high-responder status and high end point functioning; at 12 months, this figure remained stable at 54%. A further study from the same group (Dugas et al., 2003) assigned 52 participants to the same therapy delivered in group format, with similar outcomes. Though clearly a promising result, and a potentially interesting development, within-study contrast to other treatments is required to indicate whether this approach represents an advance over other, more commonly practiced interventions.

PSYCHODYNAMIC THERAPY

There appear to be only two trials of psychodynamic thera
ham et al. (1994) was reviewed earlier. A second study (
al., 1996) was an open trial in which 26 patients were o
supportive–expressive therapy, followed by three monthly booster sessions.
Posttherapy patients showed evidence of improvement (at this point, 79% no
longer met diagnostic criteria for GAD), and effect sizes for outcome were
comparable to those from other trials. However, the lack of a control group
and absence of follow-up data limit interpretation of this result.

PHARMACOTHERAPY AND PSYCHOLOGICAL THERAPY

There are rather few contrasts of medication and CBT. Lindsay et al. (1987)
contrasted 40 patients assigned to lorazepam, CBT, AMT, and a wait list.
Although lorazepam showed a rapid response, this effect diminished over the
4 weeks of the trial. Patients in both the CBT and AMT groups showed
improvements, though this was greatest for CBT. Power et al. (1989) showed
that CBT and relaxation training was superior both to diazepam and pill-
placebo treatment, both at posttreatment and at 12-month follow-up. Power
et al. (1990) treated 101 patients recruited from primary care and assigned to
diazepam or placebo alone, and also in combination with CBT. Ten weeks
of treatment was offered, with control for therapist attention for those
patients receiving medication alone. Defining recovery as an HAS score of
more than 2 standard deviations from the pretreatment range, at posttreatment, between 83 and 86% of patients in the three groups receiving
CBT recovered, contrasted with 68% and 37%, respectively, in the diazepam
and placebo-alone groups. At 6-month follow-up, patients receiving CBT
tended to maintain their gains, while those receiving medication relapsed; at
this point, around 70% of those receiving CBT had maintained their recovery and had no further treatment. In contrast, this status was achieved by 40%
and 21%, respectively, of the diazepam and placebo groups. Very long-term
follow-up of around 30% of this sample (between 11 and 14 years) indicated
that just under half of those followed up, who had been classified as recovered at 6 months, had maintained their gains (10 of 23). Dependent on measures used, between 33 and 48% met criteria for recovery, though around
70% had no diagnosable disorder (Durham et al., 2003a). However, at this
point, there were no significant differences between CBT and non-CBT
patients.

Bond et al. (2002) randomized 60 patients to received either buspirone
or placebo and (nested within this allocation) seven sessions of either AMT or
nondirective therapy. At posttherapy, there were no differences between
treatment groups, though this may reflect the low statistical power of the
study (with initially low cell sizes further reduced by high levels of attrition

or patients receiving buspirone). In the absence of any follow-up data, this result is rather difficult to interpret; across all treatment arms, there was evidence of a significant response to rather short-term treatment, even with interventions (placebo and nondirective therapy) that would not usually be expected to show benefit in GAD.

GENERALIZED ANXIETY DISORDER IN OLDER ADULTS

Although the incidence of GAD appears to increase with age, unlike most anxiety disorders, there are rather few trials exploring the impact of therapies for older adults (Stanley & Novy, 2000b).

Stanley et al. (1996) contrasted CBT and nondirective therapy in 48 patients (ranging in age from 55 to 81 years); treatment was delivered in small groups over 14 weeks. A high rate of attrition (at 33%) limits interpretation of outcomes, though among completer patients, the percentage of patients classified as responders at 6-month follow-up was statistically equivalent in both therapies (50% in CBT, and 77% in nondirective therapy). Stanley et al. (2003) contrasted the same form of CBT to a minimal contact control in 85 patients over 60 years of age; minimal contact comprised a weekly phone call. At both posttherapy and at 1 year, there was significant advantage to CBT: At this latter point, 45% of patients were classified as responders, contrasted to 8% for minimal contact. Wetherell et al. (2003) assigned 75 older adults (ages 55 and older) to 12 sessions of CBT (offered in a group format), a discussion group (which focused on topics "known to be worry-provoking for older adults," or to a wait list. In contrast to trials with younger adults, a rather smaller treatment response was evident, and both active treatments appeared to be of equal efficacy. On a composite measure of anxiety, at posttherapy and 6-month follow-up, the percentage of patients classified as treatment responders was 23% and 50%, respectively for CBT, and 27% and 53%, respectively for those in the discussion group. These studies offer reasonable support for the use of CBT in older adults, though its benefit over credible alternative therapies remains uncertain. Further discussion of this issue can be found in Chapter 15.

PREDICTORS OF OUTCOME

Post hoc analysis of the Durham et al. (1994) study suggests that Axis I, but not Axis II, comorbidity predicts relapse (Durham et al., 1997). Sanderson et al. (1994) examined the impact of one or more personality disorders on immediate outcome, and found no relationship to outcome. Two reports from the Harvard–Brown anxiety research program (a 5-year prospective study) indicate that a concurrent Axis II disorder reduces the likelihood of remission (Massion et al., 2002; Yonkers et al., 2000). The former examined the clinical course in 167 patients and found a reduced likelihood of remission in patients with a comorbid cluster B or C personality disorder. The latter study, following 514 individuals, found that the presence of either APD or dependent personality disorder reduced the probability of remission in GAD by 30%. Evidence of poor relationships also appears to be associated with poorer outcomes (Borkovec et al., 2002; Durham et al., 1997; Yonkers et al., 2000).

Summary

Although the impact of a variety of approaches has been explored, meta-analytic reviews and examination of individual studies indicate that both CBT and applied relaxation show the greatest efficacy. Dependent on the criteria used, between 50 and 65% of patients show clinically significant improvement using these methods, with reasonable maintenance of gains over follow-up. Other approaches—such as psychodynamic therapy, behavioral methods, and nondirective counseling—show markedly lower levels of efficacy in controlled trials, and on this basis, it would be difficult to recommend their use. However, it is also clear that the impact of treatment is less marked than in other anxiety disorders, and many patients will continue to exhibit residual symptoms.

There are very few contrasts of pharmacological and psychological treatment, and this makes it inappropriate to reach conclusions regarding their relative efficacy, or the degree to which maintenance of gains differs between trials.

Given the prevalence of GAD in older adults, there are regrettably few studies of treatment efficacy in this age group. Available studies suggest that CBT is an effective treatment, though the absence of tests against alternative therapies weakens arguments for its specific impact. The impact of CBT in this age group is somewhat lower than that for younger adults.

A common observation is that around 50% of participants enter trials maintained on medication. If uncontrolled, this represents a threat to internal validity, though it could be argued that since many patients with GAD are in receipt of medication, the external validity of outcomes from the treatment of medication-free patients is questionable. Researchers adopt different strategies for managing this issue, and although there is some evidence that effect sizes are not impacted by continuing or discontinuing medication during concurrent psychological treatment, this factor complicates conclusions. On this basis, it may be helpful to devise trials that systematically manipulate this variable.

The presence of extensive comorbidity with anxiety disorders or depression complicates the picture with GAD; as yet, there is only limited evidence on the degree to which treatments impact on these comorbid conditions.

resents a greater treatment challenge to clinicians than do other ..ιy disorders. This may reflect the fact that psychological models of GAD are still relatively unfocused, and hence poorly geared to the management of patients' presenting difficulties. As yet, there are rather few tests of emerging "metacognitive" models, but the specificity of this approach represents a helpful development.

Treatments for Panic Disorder with and without Agoraphobia

Behavioral and cognitive-behavioral approaches are the most widely researched. These include exposure (in earlier studies imaginal exposure, in later *in vivo*), anxiety management techniques, and cognitive interventions aimed at managing anxiety-provoking thoughts related to panic or phobia. Panic control therapies focus on the catastrophic thoughts which accompany the somatic manifestations of anxiety and panic, aiming to combine cognitive challenge of these thoughts with 'interoceptive' exposure to the somatic sensations.

Quantitative and Qualitative Reviews

A number of reviews consider the efficacy of treatments for panic disorder with agoraphobia (PDA) and without agoraphobia (PD). Drawing conclusions from these reviews is complicated by the fact that differences in their focus and in their inclusion and exclusion criteria do not always account for the lack of overlap between them (and in some cases, the extent of overlap cannot be determined, because there is no list of included trials). In addition, variations in the basis for effect-size calculations make it harder to contrast meta-analytic reviews. Furthermore, the long history of research in this area means that some studies antedate development of the DSM, raising questions about the diagnostic fidelity of patient samples.

A number of reviews focus on both psychological therapy and pharmacotherapy (Clum & Surls, 1993; Cox et al., 1992; Gould et al., 1995; Mattick et al., 1990; van Balkom et al., 1995, 1997). A smaller set of studies contrasts the benefits of behavioral and cognitive-behavioral interventions (Chambless & Gillis, 1993; Oei et al., 1999; Trull et al., 1988).

One caution is that many patients with PD and PDA enter trials on medication, or start new medications either during or after intervention. This has led some to question the reliability of efficacy studies that do not control for this (e.g., Power & Sharp, 1995). Although Otto et al. (1996) found no difference in effect sizes for studies that prohibited or allowed concurrent medication use, it would clearly be desirable for studies to monitor this factor closely.

Meta-Analyses

Trull et al. (1988) examined outcomes for patients with PDA treated with behavior therapy in 19 trials carried out between 1975 to 1987. As discussed below, analysis was restricted to studies that used the Fear Questionnaire (FQ) as an outcome measure in order to determine the clinical significance of change (though a list of studies examined is not given in the review). Therapy was usually *in vivo* exposure carried out either individually or in groups, though, in some studies, imaginal exposure was used, and in a small minority, no exposure. Larger effect sizes were found for *in vivo* exposure contrasted with imaginal exposure, and better results were found for more experienced therapists (though the magnitude of these effect sizes is not given).

The clinical significance of treatment effects was computed by contrasting treated patients to two reference groups on whom normative data for the FQ had been obtained. The first of these reference groups was specifically selected as a nondistressed group; the second was a general population sample. Using these contrasts, and using the Agoraphobia subscale of the FQ, the average treated client moved to within 2.2 *SD* units above the mean for the nondistressed group and to within 0.47 *SD* units of the mean for the general population sample. Seventy-five percent of studies included follow-up data; of these, the median length of follow-up was 18 weeks (range = 4–96), which is perhaps rather brief. Effect sizes at follow-up were very similar to those obtained posttreatment.

Oei et al. (1999) adopted the same procedure for determining clinical significance of change as Trull et al. (1988), identifying 35 studies of CBT for PDA published between 1969 and 1996. Studies employed *in vivo* exposure, relaxation techniques, and cognitive therapies, and contrasted these approaches to medication, placebo, alternative therapies, and to varying versions of CBT itself (though the review aggregates outcomes across these contrasts). On the FQ agoraphobia subscale, the average client moved from 3.9 to 1.7 *SD* units from the mean for the nondistressed sample at posttreatment and at follow-up (which varied from 1 to 16 months); in relation to the general population sample, the average client moved from 1.4 to 0.17 *SD* units at posttherapy and 0.24 at follow-up.

Chambless and Gillis (1993) contrasted the impacts of cognitive and cognitive-behavioral treatments. Comparing cognitive treatments against cognitive treatment combined with exposure for PDA (five studies), combination treatments were more effective than control groups, but no more effective than exposure alone; overall, 66% of clients treated using these methods were panic-free at the end of treatment. Contrasting interventions using combined treatment with control patients receiving pill-placebo or wait-list control, effect sizes between 0.40 and 1.07 were found. On average, of clients receiving these treatments were panic-free posttherapy, contrasted with 25% of subjects in control groups. Cognitive therapy for PD using the Salkovskis and Clark (1991) model (discussed further below) is examined in six studies, with effect sizes of 1.0–1.73. On average, 85% of clients were panic-free at posttest, contrasted with 12% of control subjects, and 88% were panic-free at follow-up (though figures for length of follow-up are not given).

Qualitative Reviews and Individual Studies

BEHAVIORAL TREATMENT

There has been extensive investigation of the efficacy of exposure in treating PDA, with evidence both of short- and long-term efficacy (Marks & O'Sullivan, 1988; O'Sullivan & Marks, 1990). In 10 studies reviewed by O'Sullivan and Marks, patients were followed up at between 1 and 9 years (mean, 4 years). Combining data from these trials, 76% of patients were judged improved or much improved, with 24% rated as unimproved. This suggests that considerable gains are possible with this treatment, though when patients in this sample were followed up over the longer term, many of them evidenced residual symptoms, albeit with diminished handicap. Fava et al. (1995, 2001b) examined outcomes from 200 patients with PDA treated with exposure. One hundred thirty-six were panic-free after 12 sessions, and of these, 132 were followed up over a median of 8 years. Over this time, 23% of the sample had relapsed; the cumulative proportion of patients remaining well was 93% over 2 years, dropping to 62% over 10 years. The presence of depression at intake and failure to overcome agoraphobic avoidance were associated with greater risk of relapse. The latter observation is reinforced by other studies (e.g., Michelson et al., 1996), which also found the presence of residual panic attacks at posttherapy to be associated with an increased probability of relapse.

Though an effective technique, the degree to which exposure alone results in symptom remission of both panic and phobic avoidance is unclear. Jacobson et al. (1988) reanalyzed data from 11 studies, applying criteria for clinical significance developed by Jacobson et al. (1984). All employed *in vivo* or imaginal exposure, flooding, or cognitive restructuring in various combinations, contrasted against a control condition, which was usually one of the aforementioned treatments (in 10 of 11 cases), with follow-up between 3 and 6 months. Although a statistically significant percentage of cases improved (a weighted mean of 58% pre- to posttreatment) and gains were maintained (60% pretherapy to follow-up), the proportion reaching a criterion of recovery was lower (a weighted mean of 27% posttreatment and 34% at follow-up). In a representative study Michelson et al. (1996) note that while patients treated with exposure in their study improved, some 30–60% of clients reported continuing panic posttherapy and through follow-up. It seems reasonable to conclude that while there is good evidence for the efficacy of exposure-based treatments, there may be scope for improving their efficacy, especially through the addition of cognitive techniques—an issue considered further below.

Self-Exposure and Therapist-Aided Exposure. Exposure-based treatments may be administered either by therapists accompanying the patient during exposure or by patient-directed ("self-directed") exposure. Although decisions about which method to use reflect technical and clinical concerns, it is obvious that the two modes of delivery have very different costs. If the two methods are of equivalent efficacy, self-directed exposure would clearly be the preferred method. At least four controlled trials by Marks and colleagues suggest this to be so (Al-Kubaisy et al., 1992; Ghosh & Marks, 1987; McNamee et al., 1989; Park et al., 2001).

A number of studies examined whether outcomes vary with the extent of therapist contact. After assessment, Ghosh and Marks (1987) assigned 46 patients with agoraphobia to receive exposure instructions from a therapist, via computer instruction, or with reference to a book detailing the management of anxiety using self-exposure. All patients were instructed in the rationale for exposure but received different amounts of therapist contact. The mean contact time for each mode of delivery was 4.6, 2.7, and 1.5 hours, respectively; equivalent results were obtained for each treatment condition.

McNamee et al. (1989) assessed 37 housebound patients with agoraphobia over the telephone; 23 agreed to treatment and were assigned either to telephone-guided self-exposure or telephone-guided self-relaxation. Exposure subjects were given a self-exposure manual. Patients using self-exposure improved significantly more than those using relaxation, though they remained somewhat symptomatic and improved more slowly than in other trials in which therapists guided exposure. Swinson et al. (1995) administered telephone-based therapy for patients in rural communities, finding this to be effective contrasted with wait-list controls. Their patients were less severely disabled than in the McNamee et al. (1989) study, and their results were more robust. This may suggest that chronicity and severity of presentation should influence the choice of therapist or self-directed exposure.

Al-Kubaisy et al. (1992) examined the efficacy of (1) therapist-assisted exposure combined with self-exposure, and (2) self-exposure and relaxation with no exposure. Of the 80 patients with mixed phobias who completed treatment, 30% were agoraphobic, 30% had social phobia, and 40% had a specific phobia. Both exposure conditions resulted in significantly greater ₗs than did relaxation; the addition of therapist–assisted exposure did not add to efficacy, though there was some evidence that social phobics showed some additional gains from this procedure.

Applied Relaxation. Applied relaxation has been evaluated in a series of studies reviewed by Öst (1987). This technique focuses on generalizing the patient's ability to apply progressive relaxation techniques. Though essentially a behavioral technique, it does contain cognitive elements in the rationale it offers to patients. In nine studies with populations containing mixed anxiety diagnoses, applied relaxation was contrasted to alternative behavioral techniques such as *in vivo* exposure, social skills training, progressive relaxation, and self-instructional training. Applied relaxation was equivalent in efficacy to these techniques in most studies, though superior to progressive relaxation in patients with PD. Öst (1988) reported a trial of 18 patients, the majority of whom had PD (14) or GAD (4), contrasting applied and progressive relaxation. At posttreatment, 75% of the applied relaxation group and 38% of the progressive relaxation group met a recovery criterion based on a number of anxiety scales. At follow-up (mean length 19 months), 100% of the applied relaxation group were judged recovered, contrasted with 25% of those receiving progressive relaxation. The efficacy of this technique was somewhat poorer in the study conducted by Clark et al. (1994), which is discussed further below. However, these authors made some modifications in the rationale offered to patients, which may have influenced outcome.

COGNITIVE AND COGNITIVE-BEHAVIORAL THERAPIES

CBT approaches include cognitive restructuring, breathing retraining, and interoceptive and *in vivo* exposure. Cognitive restructuring aims to correct a tendency to misinterpret bodily cues as evidence of an imminent catastrophe. Breathing retraining is used to manage hyperventilation, and interoceptive exposure aims to reduce reactance to physical sensations associated with anxiety (which are therefore avoided). *In vivo* exposure is usually added for patients showing agoraphobic avoidance. Across studies, there is some variation in the emphasis placed on cognitive and behavioral elements across studies, and the extent to which all elements are included. Panic control treatment (PCT; developed by Barlow and Craske), includes all these elements, whereas Clark's cognitive therapy for panic largely focuses on cognitive restructuring.

The efficacy of PCT has been studied in a number of studies, contrasted against other psychological interventions or against medication (with the latter reviewed below). Usually, patients in these trials have only mild or moderate levels of agoraphobic avoidance. Barlow et al. (1989) allocated patients with panic disorder alone or with mild or moderate agoraphobia to PCT alone, relaxation alone, relaxation and PCT in combination, or a wait-list control group. Data are presented for 56 completers from an original sample of 72 patients. All treatments were superior to the wait-list control, but PCT and PCT in combination with relaxation were superior to relaxation alone in reducing panic frequency but not generalized anxiety. Posttreatment, 85% and 87%, respectively, of patients receiving PCT alone and in combination were panic-free, contrasted with 60% of those receiving relaxation alone, and 36% of those on the wait list. At 2-year follow-up (Craske et al., 1991), the percentages of panic-free patients were 81% for PCT alone, 43% for PCT with relaxation, and 36% for relaxation alone. However, if measures of general anxiety are adopted, rather less impressive results are obtained, largely accounted for by continuing agoraphobic avoidance in the absence of panic. As discussed below, this may reflect a need for separate procedures to alleviate symptoms of panic and avoidance.

Beck et al. (1992) allocated 33 patients (80% with panic disorder without agoraphobia) to either 12 weeks of cognitive therapy or 8 weeks of client-centered supportive therapy, attempting in this way to control for nonspecific effects of therapy contact. Patients who received supportive therapy were then given the opportunity to cross over to cognitive therapy for 12 weeks. When assessed at 8 weeks, cognitive therapy patients were significantly more likely to be panic-free than those receiving supportive therapy (71% and 25%, respectively). Nearly all the patients receiving supportive therapy subsequently received cognitive therapy; at 1-year follow-up 87% of the cognitive therapy group and 79% of the crossover group were panic-free.

Beck et al. (1994) contrasted cognitive therapy, relaxation training, and a minimal contact control group in 64 patients with panic disorder with mild or moderate agoraphobia. Both active treatments were significantly more effective than control, and cognitive therapy was more effective than relaxation. At posttherapy, 82% of those receiving cognitive therapy were classified as treatment responders, in contrast to 68% of those receiving relaxation and 36% of the controls.

Öst and Westling (1995) contrasted the efficacy of cognitive therapy with applied relaxation in a sample of 38 outpatients, 30 of whom had a diagnosis of PD; the remainder showed mild agoraphobic avoidance. After 12 weeks, patients treated with cognitive therapy showed greater gains than those treated with applied relaxation; the proportion considered to have "high end-state functioning" (no panic attacks over a 3-week period and an independent assessor rating them to have low severity of PD) was 74% and 47%, respectively. However, over 12-month follow-up, patients treated with applied relaxation continued to improve, such that 82% were rated as having high end-state functioning, contrasted to 79% of those receiving CBT.

Role of Cognitive Techniques in Managing Agoraphobic Avoidance Though there is good evidence for the efficacy of behavioral techniques in managing agoraphobic avoidance, and for the benefits of cognitive techniques in managing panic, the additive impact of cognitive techniques in managing agoraphobic avoidance is less clear, especially since there is evidence that panic and agoraphobic avoidance improve independently (e.g., Basoglu et al., 1994; van den Hout et al., 1994). A small number of studies directly examined this issue. Though some suggest there is little benefit from adding cognitive techniques to exposure procedures (e.g., Burke et al., 1997; de Ruiter et al., 1989; Ito et al., 1996; Öst et al., 1993; van den Hout et al., 1994), others suggest a clear benefit (e.g., Marchione et al., 1987; Michelson et al., 1996). Ito et al. (2001) found that exposure to interoceptive cues was as effective as exposure to external cues in managing agoraphobic avoidance, and that the combination was no more effective than either modality alone. Craske et al. (2003) found that PCT alone was as effective as PCT combined with exposure (though the possibility that patients receiving PCT engaged in self-exposure was not controlled for). Taken together, these studies suggests that intervention at various points in the cycle of panic and avoidance may have benefit. However, it seems reasonable to conclude that patients with moderate to severe agoraphobia may not be well served by cognitive treatment that does not include exposure.

Effectiveness Trials. A small number of studies examined the impact of CBT in nonresearch settings. Robinson et al. (unpublished) reported on outcomes from 45 patients receiving group cognitive therapy in a PD clinic; most patients had moderate or severe agoraphobic avoidance. At the end of 11 weeks of treatment, 73% of the treatment group was panic-free, contrasted with 5% of a wait-list control group, with gains maintained at 9-month follow-up. However, measures of agoraphobic avoidance suggested gains only when the patients were accompanied, with no significant differences for agoraphobic avoidance when unaccompanied. Wade et al. (1998) treated 110 patients with PD or PDA in a community unit, with all patients receiving 15 sessions of manualized CBT, with two major research trials (Barlow et al., 1989; Telch et al., 1993) used to benchmark outcomes. In contrast to the research samples, community unit patients were less well educated, more likely to be taking concurrent medication, more symptomatic, and more likely to display agoraphobic avoidance. The magnitude of reductions in panic and agoraphobic avoidance were equivalent to research trials, though poorer outcomes were observed for less well-educated individuals. At 1-year follow-up (Stuart et al., 2000), gains were maintained. Martinsen et al. (1998) reported a case-series of 83 consecutively admitted patients, the majority of whom were diagnosed with PDA and treated with group cognitive therapy over 11 weeks (though there were variations in treatment approach across the sample). Outcomes at posttherapy and at 1 year suggested a significant reduction in agoraphobic avoidance. Garcia-Palacios et al. (2002a) conducted a small-scale contrast of 14 weeks of group CBT applied in a research setting or in a community clinic. Twenty-five patients with PD or PDA were treated; outcomes were equivalent in both sites and consistent with the benchmarking studies by Wade et al. (1998). Hahlweg et al. (2001) reported outcomes from 416 patients treated in three outpatient clinics; although there was loss of data from one site, the majority of patients were consecutive admissions receiving "high-density" exposure over 4–10 days. About 80% of patients competed treatment; of these around 55% met criteria for clinically significant improvement. Though not a direct test of effectiveness, Williams and Falbo (1996) found that higher levels of agoraphobic avoidance were associated with lower levels of treatment efficacy, though this does not temper the overall conclusion that results from studies of routine practice appear to be broadly equivalent to those obtained in research settings. This may be pertinent when considering likely outcomes for individual patients.

Impact of Brief Therapies. The usual length of CBT therapies is between 12 and 15 sessions, though a small number of studies have examined their efficacy when delivered in briefer formats. Clark et al. (1999) contrasted the impact of 14 sessions of cognitive therapy for PD against seven sessions in 43 patients with panic disorder with little or no agoraphobic avoidance. The briefer intervention included self-study modules that the patients read prior to sessions, and which introduced many of the ideas used in sessions. At posttherapy and at 3- and 12-month follow-up, both forms of treatment were of equal efficacy. Other researchers have had poorer results using abbreviated forms of therapy. Craske et al. (1995) contrasted a four-session version of PCT against four sessions of nondirective therapy. Though this form of PCT was more effective than nondirective therapy, its efficacy was less than that usually obtained for standard-format PCT. Newman et al. (1997) conducted a small study in which 18 patients with PD or PDA were assigned either to standard PCT or to a four-session computer-assisted version of PCT. Though standard-format therapy showed greater gains at posttherapy, at 1-year follow-up, outcomes were equivalent. Interpretation of this study is difficult not only because of small sample size but also because it potentially conflates both duration and the form of treatment delivery. Black et al. (1993) developed an eight-session form of CBT for panic; though not contrasted against a longer form of the therapy, it was no more effective than placebo medication.

Dismantling Studies. A small number of studies of CBT have examined the utility of its various components. Schmidt et al. (2000) assigned 77 patients with PD or PDA to CBT with or without breathing retraining, or to a

.-list control. Although outcomes for both active treatments were statis-
ally equivalent at posttherapy, and at 6- and 12-month follow-up, there
were indications that those who received CBT without breathing retraining showed greater and more robust change. Craske et al. (1997) contrasted versions of CBT that included either interoceptive exposure or
breathing retraining in 38 patients with PDA. Though both variants
showed efficacy, interoceptive exposure appeared to be more effective at
posttherapy and at 6-month follow-up. These results contrast reports of the
efficacy of breathing retraining (e.g., Clark et al., 1985; Salkovskis et al.,
1986), but two factors may be pertinent. Differences in patient characteristics (in particular, the presence or absence of symptoms related to hyperventilation) may impact on overall outcomes. In addition, the possibility of
an iatrogenic impact is raised by both Craske et al. (1997) and Schmidt et
al. (2000), who note that breathing retraining has the potential to become
a "safety" behavior that could inhibit rather than facilitate improvement
(because it becomes part of the patient's coping behavior rather than a
strategy for disconfirming fearful cognitions, as originally intended by Clark
and Salkovskis).

Bibliotherapy. There is rather limited evidence regarding the effectiveness of
bibliotherapy (as contrasted to the impact of self-directed exposure, considered earlier). Gould et al. (1993, 1995) conducted small-scale trials with a
self-help manual and found that bibliotherapy was as effective as a wait-list
condition. Though it was also as effective as an imaginal coping procedure,
this may not represent an optimal contrast intervention. This same research
group conducted a multiphase trial for patients with PD in which bibliotherapy alone was initially contrasted against bibliotherapy in combination
with self-monitoring, self-monitoring alone, and a wait-list control (Febbraro
et al., 1999). Outcomes suggested no significant impact of these interventions. In a subsequent phase of the trial, a subset of participants was offered
further bibliotherapy, though with the addition of brief contact by telephone
(Wright et al., 2000). In this phase, significant differences were apparent
when telephone contact was contrasted to a wait-list control, raising the possibility that therapist contact was relevant to outcome. Lidren et al. (1994)
employed the manual used in the Gould studies (1993, 1995), administering
it to 36 patients with PD or PDA, either as self-directed bibliotherapy or in
the context of a group intervention (in which a group leader introduced the
manual and led discussion on it). In contrast to a wait-list control, both interventions were of equal efficacy. Sharp et al. (2000) allocated 104 patients
with PD or PDA to receive manualized CBT in one of three conditions—
standard therapist contact, minimal contact, or bibliotherapy. The greatest
efficacy was found for standard therapist contact. Overall, though studies suggest a possible role for bibliotherapy, further research is needed to demon-

strate its relative efficacy compared to a robust intervention, and in populations usually seen in clinical contexts.

Although outcomes for various forms of CBT are broadly positive, a methodologically important paper by Brown and Barlow (1995) has broad implications for this and other fields. They reanalyzed outcomes from a dismantling study of PCT conducted by their own research group, in which 63 patients with PD with no or mild agoraphobia were assigned to one of four conditions: cognitive restructuring, cognitive restructuring and breathing retraining, cognitive restructuring and interoceptive exposure, or a combination of all four components. Little difference was found among treatment conditions, and 3-month and 2-year follow-up data appeared to indicate continued improvement with time. High end-state (HES) status was defined by the absence of panic attacks in the month prior to evaluation; this criterion was met by 68% of the sample at 3 months and 75% at 2 years. However, these aggregated data obscure shifts in HES status by individual patients. Thus, 19 patients who failed to meet the HES criterion at 3 months met it at 2 years; equally, eight patients rated as panic-free at 3 months failed to meet this criterion at 2 years. Similarly, some patients started and others discontinued medication, such that the population of medication users was not the same at each evaluation point. Finally, the HES criterion itself proved misleading in some cases. Thus, 34% of patients classified as having HES status at 2 years nonetheless reported having had one or more panic attacks in the previous year.

Brown and Barlow (1995) show that outcome for patients in this study varies markedly dependent on the stringency with which the criterion for HES status is set. Using aggregated data and the original criterion, at 2 years, 75% of patients achieved HES status. However, if HES is defined by no panic attacks in the previous month and no treatment over 2 years, this percentage falls to 48%, and to 21% if a further requirement of no panic in the past year is added. It may be relevant to add that though the presence of comorbid diagnoses was not strongly predictive of outcome (Brown et al., 1995), patients with more severe pretreatment symptomatology were more likely to have poorer outcomes at 2 years, despite evidence of gains at 3 months. Thus, although responsive to treatment, this group showed poor maintenance. Overall, these results confirm the fact that PD tends to be a chronic disturbance, and suggest that, over time, outcomes in clinical settings with individual patients may not reflect those achieved in research using shorter follow-ups and aggregated data.

EYE MOVEMENT DESENSITIZATION AND REPROCESSING

Feske and Goldstein (1997) carried out a partial dismantling study of eye movement desensitization and reprocessing (EMDR), assigning 43 patients with PDA to six sessions of EMDR, EMDR without eye movements, or to wait list. At posttherapy, EMDR showed greater impact than the wait list or the modified version of EMDR, though overall gains were modest, and at 3-month follow-up, EMDR clients showed some loss of gains. Goldstein et al. (2000) contrasted EMDR against attention placebo (essentially relaxation) and wait list in 46 patients with PDA. Although there was some (but inconsistent) evidence of superiority to wait list, EMDR was equivalent in efficacy to attention placebo. Although both trials are modest in size (raising some questions about statistical power), they do not offer support for the efficacy of EMDR.

OTHER PSYCHOLOGICAL THERAPIES

Clinicians commonly employ therapies other than CBT for anxiety disorders (Goisman et al., 1999), despite the paucity of research into these methods.

As noted earlier, nondirective therapies have been used as control treatments in several trials (e.g., Beck et al., 1992; Craske et al., 1995), and have been found less effective than experimental therapies. In a small number of studies, there is more of a sense of therapeutic equipoise, with a greater likelihood that therapies are presented as credible and conducted at an appropriate level of expertise. Shear et al. (1994) contrasted 15 sessions of manualized CBT with a "nonprescriptive" therapy (NPT). The study was designed as a test of the efficacy of CBT against a credible control therapy (NPT), in which the therapist's role was largely restricted to reflective listening. The first three sessions for all patients were given over to education about anxiety, together with the identification of stressors that might trigger panic. Forty-five patients with PDA completed the treatment; no significant differences were found between treatments, either posttherapy or at 6-month follow-up. Because this result challenges the specificity of the CBT model, Shear et al. (2001) extended and partly replicated this study, using a similar form of therapy (labeled "emotion-focused"), but applying it to patients with PD, with no more than mild agoraphobia. Patients were allocated to one of four groups—emotion-focused therapy (n = 30), CBT (n = 36), imipramine (n = 24) or pill-placebo (n = 23). Therapies were delivered weekly for 12 weeks, followed by a maintenance phase comprising six monthly visits. On a clinician-based rating (in the completer sample), response rates across conditions at 12 weeks were 82% and 93%, respectively, for CBT and imipramine, in contrast to 52% and 64%, respectively, for emotion-focused and pill-placebo groups, with rates at 6 months showing the same pattern. On this basis, results are comparable to those reviewed earlier, when a nondirective therapy has been used as a control intervention. Teusch et al. (1997) randomized 40 patients with PDA either to client-centered therapy alone or to client-centered therapy combined with exposure. Unusually, treatment took place in an inpatient setting, using both individual and group formats. Exposure (either alone or in combination) led to a more rapid decrease in ratings of anxiety about exposure to phobic situations, though at 1 year, equivalent outcomes were apparent.

Although numerous case reports have been published (Milrod & Shear, 1991), there appear to be only two trials of psychodynamic therapy. Wiborg and Dahl (1996) randomized 40 patients with PD or PDA to receive clomipramine alone (prescribed by patients' general practitioners), or clomipramine combined with 15 weekly sessions of brief psychodynamic therapy. Although outcomes at posttherapy were equivalent, relapse rates were significantly higher among those receiving medication alone (at 18-month follow-up, 75% vs. 20%). Milrod et al. (2001) conducted an open trial of a manualized "panic-focused psychodynamic therapy" for 21 patients with PD and PDA. Therapy was twice weekly over 12 weeks, with follow-up at 6 months; 16 participants experienced remission of panic and agoraphobic symptoms. Although this is a promising result, the study is both unique and unrandomized, and replication and extension of this work is required.

Psychological Therapy versus Pharmacotherapy

META-ANALYSES

Mattick et al. (1990) reviewed 54 trials of treatments for PD and PDA published between 1973 and 1988; therapies included *in vivo* exposure, a range of alternate psychological techniques, and medication. On measures of panic, patients in wait-list conditions or placebo treatments had low rates of improvement; mean effect sizes for measures of panic were 0.32 and 0.29, respectively. Forty studies of *in vivo* exposure (in various contrasts with other techniques) yielded a substantial effect size on measures of phobia (1.7), while that for panic was lower, at 0.96 (a pattern that is consistent across all reviews). On measures of anxiety and depression, effect sizes were more moderate (0.68 and 0.69, respectively). Improvements were maintained at a mean of 16 months' follow-up. Although most studies utilized *in vivo* exposure, nine trials did not use this technique. Interventions used were imaginal exposure, relaxation, assertion therapy, or cognitive therapy, with somewhat lower effect sizes than for *in vivo* exposure (on measures of phobia, effect size = 0.96; on measures of panic, effect size = 0.47).

In 16 studies that employed cognitive anxiety management along with exposure, smaller effect sizes were found on measures of phobia (1.43). However, effect sizes were greater on measures of panic (1.29), anxiety (1.04), and depression (0.84), suggesting a broader impact of treatment. Mattick et al. (1990) noted that in these studies, less time was given to exposure, which may account for these differences in effect sizes.

A smaller number of studies (12) combined imipramine and psychological treatments. Although the effect of combined treatments on measures of
phobia is greater than that produced by imipramine alone, combination treatments are no more effective than exposure alone. Benzodiazepines showed
some effect on symptoms, though this was more marked for alprazolam than
for diazepam; on measures of panic, effect sizes were 1.04 and 0.56, respectively. Imipramine showed an effect similar to that of alprazolam on panic
measures (1.01) but had a greater impact on depression (0.89 vs. 0.41 for
alprazolam).

Cox et al. (1992) reviewed trials carried out between 1980 and 1990, in
which the majority of patients presented with PDA rather than PD, and
treatment comprised *in vivo* exposure, imipramine, or alprazolam. Thirty-
four studies were reviewed (but are not identified in the paper), excluding
combination treatments and studies that included agoraphobia without panic.
Pre- to posttherapy effect sizes were calculated for a range of outcome measures; overall, the most consistent benefit was evident with exposure and
alprazolam, and the least with imipramine; for example, on a measure of
agoraphobic fear, effect sizes for each treatment were 3.32, 1.21, and 0.91,
respectively.

Two further meta-analyses (Chambless & Gillis, 1993; Clum & Surls,
1993) contain full lists of studies examined. There is little overlap between
these reviews; though the two are focused on the same diagnostic group,
each uses different study selection criteria. In addition there is only limited
(and inconsistent) overlap with reviews discussed earlier.

Clum et al. (1993) identified 29 studies of treatments for PD and PDA
published between 1964 and 1990. Studies were selected on the basis that
they include a control group, which was sometimes a wait list, placebo, or
comparison between treatments; active treatments included behavioral and
cognitive-behavioral interventions, medication, and combination treatments.
Effect sizes were given for "psychological coping techniques" and "expo-
sure/flooding," though the former category includes interventions that
employed an element of exposure. Compared to psychological techniques or
drug placebo, these interventions yielded effect sizes of 1.41 and 1.36, respectively, and antidepressant and benzodiazepine treatment effect sizes of 0.82
and 0.29 (with the latter result contrasting with results reported by Cox et al.
[1992]).

Further effect sizes were calculated to determine the relative efficacy of
each treatment modality against another, rather than defining overall effect
sizes for treatments per se. Multiple comparison indicated that psychological
interventions such as relaxation training, cognitive restructuring, and exposure produced the highest effect sizes, followed by combination treatments.
When medication was used alone, antidepressants had the highest effect sizes;
benzodiazepines performed poorly. Combination treatments using antide-

pressants also performed well; medication makes a small, additional contribution to exposure treatments (comparison of exposure alone to combination treatment gives an effect size of 0.34). Few of the studies reviewed included follow-up data (12 of 29), and treatment gains were not mentioned. Studies were divided into those that included more than or less than 75% of patients with agoraphobic symptoms; no significant difference in effect size was found (though in only six studies were there less than 75% of participants with agoraphobia).

Van Balkom et al. (1995) critically review the preceding three meta-analyses, noting the relatively small overlap consequent to their different sampling frames, and the fact that they disagree about the relative efficacy of imipramine, alprazolam, exposure and panic control therapies, and the benefits of their combination. In an attempt to resolve this issue, they restricted their own review to studies that afforded within-study contrasts, in order to avoid confusing confounding variables for true between-treatment effects. They identified 25 such contrasts of treatment for PDA, published between 1964 and 1993. Many of these directly compared imipramine and high-potency benzodiazepines ($n = 9$) or contrasted the combination of exposure and PCTs against exposure alone or PCT alone ($n = 11$). The remaining studies contrasted cognitive therapy against alprazolam ($n = 1$) and against fluvoxamine ($n = 1$), exposure in combination with alprazolam against alprazolam alone or exposure alone ($n = 1$), and exposure in combination with imipramine against imipramine alone ($n = 2$). It should be noted that the Mattick et al. (1990), Cox et al. (1992), and Clum et al. (1993) meta-analyses each included some of these studies (eight, nine, and seven, respectively); among them, 15 of the 25 studies were examined, though between- and within-study contrasts were not presented separately.

Contrast of imipramine and high-potency benzodiazepines (usually alprazolam) yielded a mean between-treatment effect size of 0.0 for both completer and intention-to-treat samples (though the dropout rate for imipramine was 27%, versus 13% for alprazolam). Comparison of *in vivo* exposure and panic management techniques (which included paradoxical intention, applied relaxation, cognitive therapy, breathing retraining, and flooding in imagination) consistently favored exposure *in vivo*, and suggested that the addition of panic control techniques did not enhance efficacy. Thus, exposure alone was more effective than panic management alone. Panic management and exposure in combination was more effective than panic management alone, but no more effective than exposure alone. The remaining contrasts, based on a single trial and sometimes with rather small sample sizes, suggest that cognitive therapy showed superiority over alprazolam. The contrast between cognitive therapy and fluvoxamine was complex. Outcomes varied between intent-to-treat and completer samples; overall, there appeared to be no difference between cognitive therapy and fluvoxamine on measures of panic, though fluvoxamine appeared more effective if measures of anxiety and depression were employed. Alprazolam in combination with exposure appeared more effective than exposure alone; exposure alone was more effective than alprazolam alone. Two studies examined the combination of imipramine and exposure in contrast to imipramine alone and found large between-treatment effect sizes favoring the combination treatment.

Gould et al. (1995) identified 43 studies that employed medication alone, CBT alone, or their combination for patients with both PD and PDA (though the great majority of studies focused on people with PDA). Overall, the highest posttherapy effect sizes were found with CBT (0.68; 19 studies), contrasted to medication (0.47; 16 studies, including 9 contrasts of antidepressant and 13 of benzodiazepines) and their combination (0.56; eight studies, six of which employed antidepressants). In relation to medication, no significant differences were found between benzodiazepines and antidepressants. Analyses of specific forms of CBT were hampered by small numbers of studies and variations in the control groups used to assess between-treatment differences. To examine longer term outcomes, they calculated effect sizes that contrasted mean gains at follow-up and posttherapy, with follow-up ranging from a minimum of 6 months to 2 years. For CBT, the effect size = 0.06, for combination of medication and exposure, effect size = −0.07, and for medication, effect size = −0.46, suggesting stability of outcomes for CBT and combination treatment but loss of gains for medication. Attrition rates with CBT appeared to be lower than for pharmacotherapy—5.5% contrasted to 20% for medication alone, and 22% for combination treatment.

van Balkom et al. (1997) identified 106 studies of treatments for PD or PDA published between 1964 and 1995, contrasting the efficacy of high-potency benzodiazepines, antidepressants, panic management (as defined earlier), control therapies, *in vivo* exposure, and *in vivo* exposure in combination with panic management, pill–placebo, or antidepressants. Separate posttherapy effect sizes were computed for measures of panic and for agoraphobia. Though all active interventions showed significant gains over control treatments (which included wait list, attention control, and pill–placebo), the largest effect size was found for the combination of antidepressants and exposure. While exposure alone impacted on agoraphobic symptoms, it was not effective for symptoms of panic. Curiously, panic management alone showed significant gains over control treatments on measures of both panic and agoraphobia, but when combined with exposure, it had a significant impact only on agoraphobic symptoms (a result that van Balkom et al. suggest is related to the more limited time available to apply both behavioral and cognitive methods in the combination treatment). Of the 106 trials, 59 had follow-up data; mean follow-up was at 62 weeks (though the range was very wide at 4 weeks to 8 years). Analysis of these studies (Bakker et al., 1998) suggests that gains evident at posttherapy are maintained.

QUALITATIVE REVIEWS AND INDIVIDUAL STUDIES

Clum (1989) reviewed 67 studies of treatments for PD and PDA conducted between 1964 and 1988. The meta-analysis by Clum and Surls (1993) (discussed earlier) has some overlap with this review but is more focused, including only trials with placebo or wait-list control groups. The relative merits of psychological and psychopharmacological interventions were determined using as criteria dropout rates, treatment outcome rates, and relapse rates. Success rates were defined by the absence of panic attacks or a 50% reduction in their frequency; relapse was defined as an increase in panic frequency above 50% of the pretreatment baseline, or a return to treatment.

Behavioral interventions have a significantly higher aggregate success rate (71%) than that shown by placebo controls (40%); propanolol and low-potency benzodiazepines show no greater efficacy than placebo, with success rates of 30% and 45%, respectively. The success rate of antidepressants and high-potency benzodiazepines is equivalent to that of behavior therapy. Combining medication and behavior therapy has little impact on outcome, though there is a trend toward reduced efficacy, a finding that is more marked with high-potency benzodiazepines (where success rates of 57% were obtained). Wardle (1990) has suggested that benzodiazepines may interfere with the therapeutic process, and there is direct evidence of this from Marks et al. (1993b). This issue is discussed further below.

Patients with PDA have somewhat lower rates of success (59%) than those who have PD (66%). Although this effect is consistent regardless of treatment modality, it is more marked for behavioral therapies and high-potency benzodiazepines.

Only 23 of the 67 studies followed up patients to estimate relapse rates; length of follow-up is not detailed by Clum (1989). However, on the basis of available figures, aggregated relapse rates were lowest with behavioral therapy (12%), contrasted with 28 % for high-potency benzodiazepines and 55% for MAOIs. The paucity of data in this review makes firm conclusions difficult.

Dropout rates were higher with medication, particularly tricyclics, than with psychological treatment (28% and 14.5%, respectively) and for PD with agoraphobia as contrasted to panic disorder without agoraphobia (24% and 14%, respectively).

Milrod and Busch (1996) considered the long-term outcome of interventions for PD and PDA, identifying 31 studies published between 1980 and 1995, in which follow-up continued for at least 6 months. The review notes a number of methodological problems in trials, such as failure to use DSM criteria and lack of clarity about treatment technique. More critically— and a general concern in the field—is that many patients enter trials in receipt of medication. It could be argued that their symptomatic status at trial entry makes it possible to relate any improvement to the experimental treatment, but this does not allow for the possibility of an adjunctive effect. A related concern is the fact that, over follow-up, many patients receive various additional treatments, but these are not always identified or tracked. Milrod and Busch considered only five studies to meet all criteria for methodological adequacy, only three of which included psychological interventions (Marks et al., 1993b; Nagy et al., 1993, 1989). On the basis of this limited set, they concluded that short-term gains were maintained through follow-up. This review helpfully identifies methodological criteria to which studies should aspire, and acts as a cautionary comment on the current review. However, outcomes from studies that control for issues of concurrent treatment are equivalent to those from trials that are well-controlled in all other respects.

EXPOSURE VERSUS ANTIDEPRESSANTS

Five controlled studies have directly examined the relative efficacy of imipramine and exposure (Marks et al., 1983; Mavissakalian & Michelson, 1986; Telch et al., 1985; Zitrin et al., 1980, 1983). Marks et al. (1983) contrasted therapist-assisted *in vivo* exposure and relaxation in combination with either imipramine or placebo, and found that imipramine did not have an effect beyond exposure either posttreatment or at 1-year follow-up. In contrast, the remaining four studies suggest a facilitative effect for imipramine and exposure in combination. Mavissakalian and Michelson (1986) contrasted imipramine and placebo in combination with either therapist-aided exposure or self-exposure in 62 patients over 12 weeks of treatment, finding that the addition of imipramine significantly increased response at termination. However, at 6-month follow-up, there were no between-treatment differences, largely attributable to significantly greater relapse rates in the patients receiving imipramine and continued improvement in those receiving placebo. Zitrin et al. (1980, 1983) treated patients with imipramine or placebo for 4 weeks, followed by 10 weeks of *in vivo* exposure and a further 12 weeks of maintenance drug treatment. *In vivo* exposure was conducted in groups, and it is not clear that individual programs were constructed for patients. Global ratings of improvement made by the patient and by an independent evaluator favored patients receiving imipramine, though on therapist ratings there were no differences between imipramine and placebo. At 2-year follow-up, there were no indications of differential relapse between treatment groups.

Further studies have examined whether exposure enhances the effects of imipramine. Mavissakalian et al. (1983) contrasted imipramine alone with imipramine and exposure; after 12 weeks of treatment, the combined treatment showed statistically greater gains. Using a broadly similar design, Telch et al. (1985) controlled for the possibility that patients receiving medication alone might self-expose by including an additional antiexposure condition. The patients receiving the combination of imipramine and exposure improved significantly more than those receiving medication alone, or medication and antiexposure. Posttreatment, patients who had been receiving antiexposure showed significant improvement when given exposure instructions.

These studies suggest that the combination of imipramine and exposure may have beneficial effects, though there is some evidence from follow-up data that the addition of imipramine is at best neutral in relation to exposure; at worst, there is some tentative evidence of greater relapse with medication (Mavissakalian, 1993; Mavissakalian & Michelson, 1986).

EXPOSURE VERSUS BENZODIAZEPINES (ALPRAZOLAM AND DIAZEPAM)

Although there is evidence that psychological treatments can combine well with tricyclic antidepressants (though, as discussed above, with mixed evidence as to their differential efficacy), there has been concern that benzodiazepines may interfere with exposure through the mechanism of state-dependent learning (e.g., Wardle, 1990). Spiegel and Bruce (1997) reviewed the combination of exposure and benzodiazepines treatments for PDA. Most studies suggest that there is no significant benefit—or disbenefit—to combining exposure with moderate doses of diazepam (Hafner & Marks, 1976; Hegel et al., 1994; Wardle et al., 1994).

Marks et al. (1993a) reported a cross-national study (carried out in London and Toronto) of *in vivo* exposure in combination with alprazolam. Four treatment conditions contrasted alprazolam with exposure, alprazolan with relaxation, placebo with exposure, and placebo with relaxation. Patients were given active outpatient treatment for 8 weeks, followed by a drug taper from weeks 8–16 and a follow-up at 10 months. One hundred fifty-four patients entered treatment. The mean duration of agoraphobia was 8 years; 10% of participants also met criteria for a current episode of major depressive disorder (MDD), and 30% had had a previous episode. However, those patients with a current history of MDD that predated the agoraphobia or predominated over it were excluded from the trials. Attrition was relatively consistent across conditions; 16% dropped out before the end of active treatment, and 50% were followed up at 10 months.

All four conditions resulted in posttreatment improvements on a range of measures of phobias, mood, and adjustment. At 10 months (using a clinician-rated measure of global improvement), the rate of relapse in patients who had shown improvement during treatment was significantly different across treatment conditions. The proportion of patients who both responded to treatment and stayed well was 62% for placebo and exposure, 36% for alprazolam and exposure, 29% for alprazolam and relaxation, and 18% for placebo and relaxation. This suggests that not only does withdrawal of alprazolam result in higher levels of relapse, as contrasted with exposure, but also that exposure is less effective when combined with alprazolam. Speigel et al. (1993) have criticized Marks et al.'s study on the grounds that excessively high doses of medication were employed, a factor disputed in turn by Marks et al. (1993a). Given that Marks et al. imply that certain medication combinations are contraindicated, further research may be required to clarify this issue.

Though this pattern of results suggests little advantage to combining benzodiazepines and exposure, Spiegel and Bruce (1997) note that exposure or CBT administered as part of drug taper from benzodiazepines has reduced subsequent relapse in a small number of trials (e.g., Otto et al., 1993), suggesting that there may be some benefit to this strategy.

COGNITIVE-BEHAVIORAL THERAPY VERSUS PHARMACOTHERAPY

Klosko et al. (1990) contrasted PCT to alprazolam, a drug placebo, and a wait-list control in a sample of 57 patients. PCT was significantly more effective than placebo (87% panic-free) and wait list (33%), but was not significantly more effective than alprazolam (50%), which, in turn, did not differ significantly from placebo (36%).

Clark et al. (1994) described a controlled trial of cognitive therapy contrasted with applied relaxation, imipramine, or a wait list. Sixty-four patients participated. All had panic disorder with mild or moderate agoraphobia; those with severe agoraphobia were excluded. Twelve sessions of treatment were offered over 3 months, with up to three booster sessions over the subsequent 3 months. Imipramine was withdrawn after 6 months. All three treatments were effective, though cognitive therapy was markedly more effective than both imipramine and relaxation, both 3 months after treatment and at 1 year. At this point, 85% of patients receiving cognitive therapy were panic-free, contrasted with 47% and 60%, respectively, for relaxation and imipramine. It is worth noting that 26% of the relaxation group and 40% of those receiving imipramine sought further treatment over the follow-up period, contrasted with 5% of the cognitive therapy group.

Sharp et al. (1996) assigned 190 patients with PD or PDA to receive CBT alone, CBT combined with fluvoxamine or with placebo, fluvoxamine alone, or placebo over 13 weeks, with a 6-month follow-up. All active treatments showed equivalent and clinically significant gains at posttherapy, with some evidence that patients receiving CBT and fluvoxamine showed the greatest and most rapid gains. However, at 6 months, maintenance of gains was greatest for those patients who had received CBT as part of their intervention.

Loerch et al. (1999) assigned 55 patients with PDA to 10 weeks of treatment with CBT combined with either moclobemide or placebo, moclobemide combined with clinical management, or placebo combined with clinical management. Followup was naturalistic and took place at 1, 3, and 6 months. At posttherapy, there was a clear advantage to CBT over medication conditions; on measures of agoraphobic avoidance, 71% of patients in both CBT conditions met categorical criteria for response, contrasted to 31% and 27% for moclobemide and placebo, respectively. On measures of panic, differences were less clear; though the percentage of CBT patients achieving panic-free status was greater than that for medication condition, this did not achieved statistical significance. Though gains were maintained by those receiving CBT, at 6 months, these group differences were no longer evident, which is attributable to the fact that 70% of patients received further help over follow-up and also continued to show improvement. One problem with this study is that initially small cell sizes were further reduced by high levels of attrition. This was most marked for moclobemide alone, where 44% of patients did not complete therapy, limiting the interpretation of any between-treatment differences.

In the largest study of this issue to date, Barlow et al. (2000) reported on outcomes in 326 patients with PD randomized to receive CBT alone, CBT combined with imipramine or with placebo, or imipramine alone. Study design meant that investigators were committed to both pharmacotherapy and CBT, instating a degree of equipoise. Patients received 11 sessions of treatment over 12 weeks, and those who responded to acute intervention entered a maintenance phase comprising six monthly sessions in the same modality (without breaking the study bind). At posttherapy, all active treatments showed superior gains to placebo. A categorical system was established to delineate treatment response; on this basis, posttherapy response rate on the Panic Disorder Severity Scale were 49% for CBT alone, 60% for CBT combined with imipramine, 57% for CBT combined with placebo, 46% for imipramine alone, and 22% for placebo. There was evidence that among responders, those who received imipramine had the best outcomes. Over the maintenance phase, combined CBT and imipramine showed an advantage over other active treatments. After a 6-month no-treatment follow-up, there was evidence of loss of gains from imipramine; as in Sharp et al's (1996) study, this suggests that although gains from medication are initially more striking, they are not as durable as those from CBT.

Impact of Personality Disorders on Outcome

Dreessen and Arntz (1998) identified 16 trials for PD or PDA in which patients were treated with psychological therapy or medication, of which eight met a number of criteria which reduce the risk of methodological confound—perhaps most critically, diagnosing personality disorders prospectively rather than post hoc, and establishing the diagnosis using interviews rather than questionnaire methods. The review attempted to answer two questions—

whether the presence of a personality disorder led to poorer response to treatment, and whether it led to poorer end-state functioning. Of the eight trials, six included psychological therapies (Black et al., 1994; Chambless et al., 1992; Dreessen et al., 1994; Hoffart & Martinsen, 1993) and two tracked naturalistic outcomes (Mellman et al., 1992; Noyes et al., 1990). Chambless et al. (1992) and Hoffart and Martinsen (1993) found that though short-term outcomes were equivalent, the presence of APD was associated with poorer outcomes at follow-up. In Black et al. (1994) personality disorder, as assessed by self-report, but not as assessed by the Structured Clinical Interview for Diagnosis (SCID), impacted on outcomes. The remaining trials found that outcomes were uninfluenced by the presence of personality disorder. However, Dreessen et al. (1994) reported two trials examining the impact of personality disorders on CBT with 31 patients with panic disorder and 57 patients with mixed anxiety diagnoses. In both samples, the presence of a personality disorder was associated with more severe Axis I pathology, with the consequence that though such patients evidenced rates of improvement parallel to the rates of those without personality disorders, their outcomes were poorer. In this respect, end-state functioning may be a critical measure.

A later review by Mennin and Heimberg (2000) examined the impact of personality disorder on outcome in trials that employed exposure or CBT. They identified nine relevant trials (six of which were also included in Dreessen and Arntz (1998), though three were excluded because they did not meet the methodological concerns noted earlier). Six of the nine studies found that the presence of a personality disorder was associated with poorer outcome. In one further trial, Rathus et al. (1995) reported that while personality disorder did not influence outcomes, better outcomes were associated with lower scores on the Millon Clinical Multiaxial Inventory.

Two trials postdating both reviews came to different conclusions. Marchand et al. (1998) found that the presence of any personality disorder led to poorer outcomes, and that progress in therapy was slower. Massion et al. (2002) found that the presence or absence of a personality disorder did not predict time to remission in 514 participants in the Harvard–Brown anxiety research program. The absence of consistent findings may relate to methodological variations across trials and to low sample sizes (especially in relation to individual subtypes of the personality disorders). More research is required to clarify this issue.

Summary

This field has been particularly well covered by meta-analytic studies and qualitative reviews. These yield unusually consistent findings and suggest that applied relaxation, exposure, and variants of CBT are effective treatments of choice for PD and PDA. Relatively brief treatments (of around 12–15 sessions) appear to be effective, with some attempts—not all successful—to reduce this still further.

Whereas some treatment approaches to panic disorder incorporate a mix of behavioral and cognitive elements, others focus more specifically on cognitive restructuring. Though there is little evidence to favor one specific package over another, there are clear indications that in individuals with PDA, exposure is important in managing agoraphobic symptoms; adding cognitive techniques does not appear to confer additional benefit. This reflects the fact that two separate, and to some degree independent, therapeutic processes appear pertinent to efficacy—behavioral techniques focused on agoraphobic avoidance, and cognitive techniques aimed at managing panic. Since there is good evidence that panic and avoidance improve independently, the application of both therapeutic processes in combination is probably more effective than either alone. Hence, though there is some evidence that cognitive therapy can contribute by intervention at other points in the cycle of anxiety, patients with agoraphobic avoidance probably require exposure.

On the basis of available studies, there is little evidence to support the use of EMDR, psychodynamic, or client-centered approaches. The status (indeed, the utility) of therapeutic approaches to panic other than those rooted in cognitive or behavioral methods is unclear, essentially because so little research is available to assess their efficacy.

The relative impacts of psychological therapies and pharmacotherapy have been explored by a number of meta-analyses. Though they are somewhat inconsistent in their conclusions regarding specific medications (usually SSRIs, tricyclics, or benzodiazepines), effect sizes for cognitive and behavioral interventions are usually larger than those for pharmacotherapy. Evidence for the benefit of combination treatment is variable, and, indeed, there are suggestions that some medications—particularly benzodiazepines—may reduce rather than enhance outcomes. Though some trials suggest an equivalence of posttherapy outcome, there is consistent evidence that the stability of gains over follow-up after psychotherapy is greater than for pharmacotherapy.

The application of these techniques in the field has been demonstrated to a greater degree than in most areas, with effectiveness trials showing their applicability in routine clinical settings. Though benchmarking trials suggest that outcomes in these contexts can match those obtained in research trials, it is worth observing that the presence of agoraphobic symptoms appears to decrease efficacy. Unfortunately, the exclusion of moderately or severely agoraphobic individuals from many studies makes it more difficult to be certain about the benefits of treatment strategies that systematically combine behavioral and cognitive techniques, despite the obvious benefit that this would bring when applying research findings to clinical populations where PDA is more usual than PD.

SUMMARY AND CLINICAL IMPLICATIONS

...ito the treatment of anxiety disorders is extensive, though perhaps ...n its representation. Whereas panic disorder, with and without ago-
....a, and specific phobias have received considerable attention for some decades, work on social phobia and GAD is somewhat more limited and more recent. Overall there is good evidence for the efficacy of behavioral and cognitive-behavioral approaches in the treatment of these disorders. Despite this generally positive picture, it is important to note that even after effective treatments, many patients with anxiety disorders continue to show some degree of impairment relative to a nondistressed sample. In this sense, therapies are not necessarily "curative." This is particularly important, since studies of efficacy are performed largely by those who are responsible for these innovative treatment methods, and the effectiveness of treatment can be expected to be more modest in clinical practice.

Pharmacological treatments for anxiety disorders are common in clinical practice. On the whole, they tend to be no more effective than psychological approaches, even for chronic and severe conditions, and discontinuation is associated with relapse. Evidence for the benefits of combination treatment is not strong, especially when longer term outcomes are considered. However, it needs to be recognized that choices about treatment modality reflect a range of resource issues as much as evidence for efficacy, but factors such as the acceptability and risks of medication (and in particular long-term dependence) are pertinent. Broadening access to psychological therapies is in part dependent on the availability (and cost) of suitably trained therapists, and incorporating bibliotherapy and computer-aided techniques into a stepped-care approach has obvious application, enabling better use of, and access to, therapeutic resources.

The striking absence of research into interventions other than behavioral, cognitive, and cognitive-behavioral therapies makes it difficult to recommend the first-line use of alternative techniques. In practice, clinical judgment may indicate that these are warranted—for example, when treatment failure has occurred in all the therapeutic modalities for which efficacy has been demonstrated, or when prominent aspects of the patient's presentation (particularly personality disorders) threaten to complicate the implementation of brief, structured treatments.

Whatever view is taken of the relative hegemony of cognitive-behavioral approaches in this area, the development of effective treatments using these techniques represents a powerful interplay between theory and practice, with models of anxiety continuing to be developed and tested, and translated into therapeutic interventions that are themselves subject to further appraisal. Modeling of disorders increasingly attempts to determine the nature of underlying dysfunctions or deficits, and to increase the specificity of the interface between treatment and the nature of the problem. While it is tempting to suggest that this approach would be beneficial in many areas of clinical investigation, it is worth noting that, at root, anxiety is an adaptive neurobiological response, albeit one that is maladaptive in the context of anxiety disorders. On this basis, conditions such as phobias and panic disorder are potentially more encapsulated than other presentations, because they are less likely to represent a disorder of the self, making them potentially more tractable to strategies that enable reappraisal of the relationship between the individual and his/her environment. Extending this approach may be challenging when the experience of distress is more diffuse, though there are already models for this in the extension of cognitive models to treatments for GAD.

CHAPTER 7

ANXIETY DISORDERS II

Obsessive–Compulsive Disorder

DEFINITION

Obsessions are defined in DSM-IV-TR as recurrent, persistent, and distressing ideas, thoughts, impulses, or images; these do not reflect worry about real-life problems and are experienced (at least at sometime in the disturbance) as intrusive and senseless. An example would be a parent having repeated thoughts about harming a loved child or a religious person having blasphemous thoughts. The person attempts to suppress or to neutralize such thoughts or impulses with another thought or action. There is clear recognition that the obsessions are the product of the person's own mind and not imposed from without.

Compulsions are repetitive and intentional behaviors (such as hand washing, ordering, or checking) or mental acts (such as praying, counting, or repeating words silently). These are performed in response to an obsession, according to certain rules that have to be applied rigidly and are aimed at preventing or reducing distress, or preventing a dreaded event or situation. However, the behavior is either not connected in a realistic way with what it is designed to neutralize or prevent, or it is clearly excessive. The act is performed with a sense of subjective compulsion that is (at least initially) combined with a desire to resist. Diagnostic criteria also specify that the obsessions and compulsions cause marked distress, are time-consuming, or significantly interfere with the person's functioning.

Depression and anxiety are commonly associated with obsessive–compulsive disorder (OCD), together with phobic avoidance of situations that involve the content of the obsession (such as dirt or contamination).

PREVALENCE, COMORBIDITY, AND NATURAL HISTORY
Prevalence

Six-month prevalence rate of OCD in the Epidemiologic Catchment Area survey (ECA) was 1.5% (Karno et al., 1988); very similar rates of 1.5% and 1.6% were found in Canadian and New Zealand studies (Oakley-Brown, 1991). The disorder appears to be chronic; lifetime prevalence rate is estimated at 2.5% in the ECA study, and at 3.0% and 2.2% in the Canadian and New Zealand studies, respectively.

These prevalence rates stand in contrast to the rate at which individuals with OCD present clinically, and prior to community surveys OCD was thought of as a relatively uncommon disorder. The ECA survey found that only 34% of individuals with OCD had ever mentioned their symptoms to a health professional. Mayerovitch et al. (2003) found that whereas treatment seeking was associated with the total number of OCD symptoms, and with violent or unpleasant obsessional thoughts, there was no such association with compulsions alone, and this group had a very low prevalence of treatment seeking (17%).

Comorbidity

Data from the ECA survey (Karno et al., 1988) indicate that there is high comorbidity of OCD with other Axis I disorders: 46.5% of patients diagnosed with OCD had an additional diagnosis of phobic disorder; 31.7%, an additional diagnosis of a major depressive disorder; and 24.1% were substance abusers (usually alcohol abuse).

Natural History

Data from the ECA survey indicate that OCD has an early age of onset and a prolonged duration (Karno & Golding, 1991). Twenty percent develop the disorder in childhood, 29% in adolescence, and 74% before the age of 30. A similar pattern was found in the Edmonton study (Bland et al., 1988; Kolada et al., 1994), in which 46% of men and 58% of women developed the disorder before age 20. One-year recovery rates were low; the percentage of people who had met DSM-III-R criteria but had not had symptoms in the past year was 36% in the ECA study and 38.7% in the Edmonton study. Skoog and Skoog (1999) followed up 251 patients approximately 45 years after they had first presented with a diagnosis of OCD. Although about 80% had improved by this point, only 20% had obtained full remission. Two-thirds continued to suffer clinical or subclinical symptoms, 10% showed no improvement, and 10% had deteriorated. Those with compulsive rituals and "magical" obsessions were significantly less likely to recover than those with other forms of symptomatology.

TREATMENT APPROACHES

Exposure and response prevention (ERP) is the most common psychological technique used to treat OCD. The two components of this approach require patients to expose themselves to factors that would usually elicit obsessions, but under conditions that prevent them from responding to these obsessions by performing compulsions. Exposure techniques include systematic desensitization, paradoxical intention, flooding, and satiation, either *in vivo* or in imagination. Blocking interrupts ruminations or rituals through response prevention, distraction, or thought stopping (though the latter is sometimes seen as a cognitive rather than a behavioral technique). A number of cognitive models of OCD have been advanced (Beck, 1976; Creamer, 1987; Reed, 1983; Salkovskis, 1985), which suggest that symptoms develop and are maintained by anxiety consequent on the appraisal of intrusive thoughts or actions. There is evidence that people with OCD tend to have a heightened sense of responsibility, and that it is their tendency to appraise obsessional thoughts through this "filter" that makes them vulnerable to developing symptoms (Foa et al., 2001; Salkovskis et al., 2000). These models have their origins in theory, but there are also pragmatic reasons for exploring their utility. Although there is good evidence for the efficacy of ERP, the procedure can pose a challenge to patients. For example, they may be unable to confront their symptoms directly, perhaps because they hold very fixed beliefs, or they believe that their symptoms represent a realistic way of managing their concerns (both factors linked—at least in some studies—to poorer outcomes (Steketee & Shapiro, 1995; discussed further below). Cognitive therapy techniques focus on challenging obsessional thoughts, challenging negative automatic thoughts which are precipitated by obsessional thoughts, or thought stopping (which attempts to disrupt obsessional thoughts). Researchers have examined the effect of employing cognitive strategies alone, or of supplementing ERP with cognitive interventions.

Meta-Analyses

Three meta-analyses have reviewed outcomes from psychological and pharmacological treatments (Christensen et al., 1987; van Balkom et al., 1994; Kobak et al., 1998). Christensen et al. (1987) reviewed studies of exposure therapies, nonspecific treatments (such as relaxation), tricyclic medication, and psychosurgery carried out between 1961 and 1984. Twenty-seven studies contained enough pre- and posttreatment data to permit calculation of an effect size, but a further 44 lacked sufficient information to make these calculations directly and, in these cases, probit transformations were used to derive effect sizes. Considering only trials from which effect sizes could be derived directly, effect sizes for exposure treatments and tricyclic medications were not significantly different (1.22 and 1.4, respectively); in contrast, nonspecific treatments gave an effect size of 0.21. Treatment of any kind is more successful when compulsions are present than when they are absent (effect size = 1.13 and 0.41, respectively; though this latter figure is based on only 6 trials). Ten trials had follow-up data. For exposure therapies, the mean effect size at posttreatment did not differ significantly from that at follow-up (at an average of 82 weeks posttreatment). No follow-up data were available from medication trials. Effect sizes based on observer ratings were higher than those derived from self-report measures; because medication trials were more likely to use observer ratings, and psychological interventions to use self-ratings, this has the potential to bias interpretation of results.

van Balkom et al. (1994) reviewed 86 trials carried out between 1970 and 1993, of which 58 were controlled studies. The majority of trials focused on antidepressants, behavior therapy, and combination treatments, with a very small number of studies ($n = 4$) examining the efficacy of cognitive therapy. Effect sizes associated with serotonergic antidepressants (clomipramine, fluoxetine, and fluvoxamine) were significantly higher than other antidepressants, which had effect sizes equal to or smaller than placebo. As discussed further below, there is consistent evidence for the efficacy of serotonergic antidepressants in OCD.

Because results from analyses using self- and observer ratings gave different results, they were reported separately (as in Christensen et al. [1987], observer ratings tended to yield larger effect sizes than self-ratings). Using self-ratings, and contrasting serotonergic antidepressants alone, behavior therapy alone, and their combination, behavior therapy had a larger effect size than antidepressants alone. Combination treatment had a greater effect than medication alone but was equivalent to behavior therapy alone. Effect sizes based on observer ratings showed no differences among treatments. Follow-up for the majority of studies was conducted at between 3 and 6 months, with effect sizes tending to remain stable over this period.

All behavioral therapies employed exposure *in vivo*, with variations in technique such as therapist or self-controlled exposure, spousal involvement, therapist modeling, or the addition of cognitive strategies such as thought stopping. No differences in effect size were found among these variants, a finding most reasonably attributed to the common element of exposure *in vivo*.

Kobak et al.'s (1998) meta-analysis covered the period from 1973 to 1997, and as a consequence, has broader coverage of serotinergic agents. The review examines 77 studies in which medication was used alone or in combination with ERP. Kobak et al. also reviewed meta-analyses of pharmacological trials, noting that their own and other reviews consistently suggest the greatest efficacy for clomipramine. Despite evidence of its statistical superiority, they caution against recommending clomipramine as a first-line treatment, given its potential side effects and lethality in overdose, and good evidence for the efficacy of fluoxetine and fluvoxamine. Effect sizes for ERP were 0.99 (36 comparisons), for all medication, 0.87 (64 comparisons), and for combination treatment, 1.07 (6 comparisons), though controlling for methodological differences suggested an equivalence among all three modes of intervention.

Though these meta-analyses are consistent in providing evidence for the efficacy of exposure treatments, they differ in their assessment of the relative efficacy of medication and behavior therapy. This may be attributable to methodological issues that require resolution. The superiority of behavioral therapies over medication indicated in van Balkom et al.'s (1994) review rests on self-report rather than observer ratings. While this may reflect different assessment strategies adopted by behavior therapists and pharmacotherapists, Kobak et al. (1998) found that effect-sizes based on observer ratings were *lower* than those for self-ratings (though whether there is an association between assessment method and treatment strategy is not made clear). Overall, it seems reasonable to conclude that ERP and serotinergic agents are of equivalent efficacy.

Three meta-analyses by Abramowitz (1996, 1997, 1998) focus on the impact of ERP alone or contrasted to other psychological procedures. Abramowitz (1996) examined outcomes from 24 trials; overall ERP yielded a large effect size (on patient self-rating of obsessive–compulsive symptoms the pre- to posttherapy effect size = 1.2), with outcomes stable over a mean of 18 weeks' follow-up (pretherapy to follow-up effect size = 1.1). Considering the impact of variations in the delivery of ERP, therapist-supervised exposure was more effective than self-exposure (pre- to posttherapy effect size = 1.6 contrasted to 0.8), and total response prevention was more effective than partial (indicating that complete abstention from rituals during the treatment period is an important part of the technique; pre- to posttherapy effect size for full response prevention = 1.67 and for partial = 1.11) A dose–response relationship with outcome was apparent, though complicated by the difficulty of coding variations in duration of exposure to anxiety-provoking stimuli (e.g., through homework exercises). Length of sessions was positively correlated with effect sizes at posttherapy (r = .47) and follow-up (r = .64).

Abramowitz (1997) examined outcomes from eight trials that compared the impact of ERP to an alternative psychological procedure. Using self-ratings, they found a small but nonsignificant effect size in favor of cognitive therapy (effect size = −0.19); compared to exposure alone or response prevention alone, there was a moderate but nonsignificant effect size = 0.59. ERP contrasted to relaxation yielded an effect size = 1.18 (though this figure is based on clinician ratings). A correlation of .87 was found between outcome and the number of hours of therapist-guided exposure.

In an attempt to gauge the clinical significance of outcomes with ERP, Abramowitz (1998) meta-analyzed 10 trials published between 1983 and 1995, all of which used the Maudsley Obsessive–Compulsive Inventory (MOCI) as a measure of efficacy. The analysis is weakened by the inclusion of multiple reports of the same study populations, and the fact that Paul Emmelkamp and colleagues conducted the majority of the trials. Furthermore, the MOCI has some well-known deficiencies (it is a better indicator of compulsions than obsessions, and is somewhat insensitive to cognitive, counting, and hoarding rituals). Notwithstanding these concerns, overall, patients receiving treatment showed a clinically significant improvement in MOCI scores; their mean scores shifted from 2.0 to 0.8 standard deviation units from the mean of general population following treatment. Though this would meet the standard criteria for clinically significant change (Jacobson et al., 1984), posttreatment scores remained significantly higher than those found in normative studies, suggesting that some level of impairment remained.

Specific Interventions and Treatment Issues

Exposure and Response Prevention

Early studies indicated that exposure alone or response prevention alone was associated with poor outcomes and high rates of relapse (e.g., Foa et al., 1980, 1984), and more recent trials almost invariably examine imaginal or *in vivo* exposure combined with response prevention. Emmelkamp (1994), in an overview of the clinical implementation of this technique, suggests that gradual exposure *in vivo* is as effective as flooding (Boersma et al., 1976; Marks et al., 1975), that modeling by the therapist has no greater effect than self-exposure (Boersma et al., 1976; Marks et al., 1975), and that exposure sessions of long duration (around 2 hours) are more effective than short sessions (Foa & Kozac, 1996; Rabavilas et al., 1979).

The relationship between chronicity and severity of symptoms and outcome is unclear; while some studies have suggested that patients with more chronic and more severe symptoms have poorer outcomes (e.g., Cottraux et al., 1993; Foa et al., 1983b), others find either no or only weak associations between these variables (e.g., Basoglu et al., 1988; Hoogduin & Duivenvoorden, 1988; Hoogduin et al., 1989; Visser et al., 1992). A more complex picture emerges from Castle et al. (1994), who reviewed outcomes from an audit of 178 patients receiving ERP in an inpatient setting. For women, lower initial severity predicted better outcome, though, for men, the only predictor was living alone (leading to a poorer response). In reviewing this issue, Steketee and Shapiro (1995) noted that patients with more severe symptoms may also present with associated comorbid conditions and poorer functioning, a combination that was indeed predictive of poorer outcomes in Basoglu et al.'s (1988) study.

While some studies suggest that patients with compulsions have better outcomes than those with checking rituals or ruminations (Basoglu et al., 1988; Boulougouris, 1977), others find that the type of symptom is only weakly or not predictive of outcome (Castle et al., 1994; Foa et al., 1983b; Rachman et al., 1973). The form of the symptom may relate to outcome; Merckelbach et al. (1988) found that patients with fears that related to more "realistic" anxieties (such as checking for fires) showed fewer gains. The influence of fixity of belief on outcomes is discussed below.

EXPECTED OUTCOMES WITH ERP

Cottraux (1989), Perse (1988), and Steketee and Cleere (1990) reviewed an overlapping sample of approximately 20 studies of ERP alone, carried out between 1974 and 1989. Perse (1988) suggests that 70–80% of patients who accept and comply with treatment will improve. In the Steketee and Cleere (1990), review, an average of 85.8% of clients were rated as improved/much improved posttreatment (range, 67–98%). Follow-up (range, 3 months to 3 years) showed good maintenance of gains, with 77.8% of patients retaining this rating.

Foa and Kozac (1996) reviewed studies examining outcomes for over 300 patients presenting with rituals, treated by ERP. Defining improvement as an improvement over pretreatment symptoms of over 30%, the response rate was 76% (range, 60–100%) at 3–6 years posttreatment. In seven studies of the long-term effects of exposure, reviewed by Öst (1989), 85% of patients maintained their gains 1–3 years posttreatment. In the same study, more than half the patients required no further therapy. These relatively low relapse rates are particularly impressive when compared with the relatively low proportion (10%) of patients who retained their gains after withdrawal from clomipramine (Pato et al., 1988).

IMPACT OF SETTING AND FREQUENCY OF DELIVERY

Many earlier studies were carried out in hospital settings using daily treatment (e.g., Hodgson et al., 1972; Marks et al., 1975; Rachman et al., 1971, 1973; Roper et al., 1975), but most recent trials are conducted on an outpatient basis, and outpatient treatment appears to have equivalent outcomes to inpatient treatment (e.g., Emmelkamp et al., 1989; van den Hout et al., 1988).

The frequency of ERP sessions varies from study to study; for example, Kozac et al. (2000) employed 15 daily sessions over 3 weeks, Fals-Stewart and Lucente (1993), twice weekly ERP for 12 weeks, and van Balkom et al. (1998), 16 sessions over 16 weeks. Many research trials favor the more intensive form of delivery, though this may not be easy to transport into clinical settings. Although the variation in frequency of delivery across trials does not seem to impact on outcome, there is little direct evidence on this point, and the range of frequencies is not wide. In one of the few trials to consider this issue directly, Abramowitz et al. (2003) matched two groups of 20 patients on initial OCD and depression severity, assigning them to receive either 15 sessions of ERP twice weekly over 8 weeks, or daily over 3 weeks, with follow-up at 3 months. Essentially, outcomes were equivalent; though a significantly greater proportion of patients in the intensive group met criteria for recovery at posttherapy (85% and 70%), at follow-up recovery rates were comparable (55% an 60%), in part because of greater relapse among the intensively treated patients.

GROUP VERSUS INDIVIDUAL TREATMENTS

Although there are a number of examples of ERP offered in a group context, rather few trials directly examine the impact of mode of delivery on outcome. Fals-Stewart and Lucente (1993) contrasted outcomes for 62 patients allocated to receive 24 sessions of ERP over 12 weeks either in a group or individual format; a further control group of 32 patients received relaxation therapy. At posttherapy, both forms of delivery were equivalent and showed clear gains compared to the control group, though patients receiving individual therapy showed more rapid change. Van Noppen et al. (1997) presented an uncontrolled trial of group-based therapy delivered over 10 sessions; 17 patients received ERP in a group comprised only of fellow patients, and 19 in a multifamily group that included the patients' partners and parents. Participants in both types of group showed significant gains; however, on measures of clinical significance, there was some advantage to multifamily groups at posttherapy and 1-year follow-up. The lack of random assignment makes this a difficult result to interpret, however, given that those assigned to standard group therapy either had no partner or a partner who refused to participate. Himle et al. (2001) reported outcomes from an open trial of 113 patients, 89 of whom participated in a 7-week group program; 24 patients received a similar program extended to 12 weeks; duration of the program did not impact on efficacy, with equivalent gains in both groups being maintained at 3-month and (on average) 4-year follow-up.

OUTCOMES IN CLINICAL SETTINGS

Although there is little direct evidence of effectiveness in standard clinical settings, Franklin et al. (2000) contrasted outcomes from 110 patients receiving ERP on a "fee-for-service" basis with results from four previously reported randomized controlled trials (RCTs) (Fals-Stewart & Lucente, 1993; Kozac et al., 2000; Lindsay et al., 1997; van Balkom et al., 1998). All the patients were either unsuitable or unwilling to be entered into an NIMH trial of treatments for OCD, and from this perspective are probably more representative of clients in standards settings (46% had a comorbid diagnosis, most usually of depression or an Axis II disorder). Although interventions were conducted in a specialized clinical research unit, therapists varied in their level of experience (though the service setting meant that they received unusually expert supervision). Clinically significant improvements were achieved for both obsessional and depressive symptoms, and outcomes were comparable with results obtained in the four efficacy trials. Consistent with accumulating evidence, multiple regression suggested that pretreatment depression and OCD severity predicted outcome (though this analysis was restricted by the limited range of posttreatment scores). Two smaller scale trials that recruited patients in a manner equivalent to routine practice both reported outcomes equivalent to research populations. Kirk (1983) treated 36 patients in a specialized anxiety disorder unit; 76% were moderately improved or better posttherapy. Warren and Thomas (2001) reported on 26 consecutive patients referred to a private anxiety disorders clinic; of the 19 patients who completed treatment, 16% were classified as treatment responders. Wetzel et al. (1999) reported on 85 unselected inpatients with OCD treated by daily ERP for between 2 and 3 weeks; at 1 year, improvement rates were equivalent to those reported in research contexts.

Cognitive-Behavioral Therapy

James and Blackburn (1995) reviewed 15 trials of cognitive therapy up to the mid-1990s, noting that many investigations are single-case or uncontrolled trials, often using more than one treatment modality, hence making it difficult to discern the relative importance of cognitive and behavioral components.

COGNITIVE THERAPY VERSUS ERP

Hiss et al. (1994) reported a small controlled study of a relapse prevention program following an intensive, 15-day ERP package. Half the sample then received relapse prevention, and the remainder, a control placebo treatment ("free-association therapy"). Relapse prevention combined training in self-exposure with anxiety management, goal setting, recruitment of social support, and some additional interventions addressing anticipated sources of stress, maladaptive patterns of interpersonal interactions, and unrealistic expectations of treatment results. A core part of the program was cognitive restructuring, identifying and challenging cognitive distortions. Although sample sizes were small (a total of 18 patients), those receiving relapse prevention maintained their posttreatment outcome, whereas those receiving control placebo treatment ("free-association therapy") showed a tendency to relapse at 6-month follow-up. This small study is additionally interesting because it suggests that the combination of effective followed by ineffective treatment may have detrimental effects on long-term outcome.

Emmelkamp and colleagues carried out a series of controlled studies that contrast the efficacy of behavioral and cognitive-behavioral interventions in OCD. Emmelkamp et al. (1980) compared the effects of exposure therapy alone with exposure therapy combined with self-instructional training. Fifteen patients were treated (eight and seven, respectively per group); both groups improved and both maintained their gains at 6-month follow-up. Emmelkamp et al. (1988) contrasted nine patients receiving rational–emotive therapy (RET) to nine patients treated with *in vivo* exposure; treatments were of equal efficacy, though there was a slight trend for better outcomes with *in vivo* exposure. Both earlier studies used young, well-educated, and non-chronic participants; in contrast, Emmelkamp and Beens (1991) used a more clinically representative pool of subjects, with 10 subjects receiving RET and self-directed exposure, and 11 receiving *in vivo* exposure. Again, the treatments gave equivalent outcomes.

In a larger study of 71 patients, van Oppen et al. (1995) contrasted the efficacy of exposure therapy and cognitive therapy. In the latter treatment, patients were initially encouraged to identify negative automatic thoughts regarding their symptoms and to challenge them—for example, by noting that they were overestimating danger or the degree of their own personal responsibility. After six sessions, patients were encouraged to carry out behavioral experiments to test their beliefs and assumptions (in itself, of course, a form of exposure). While the two treatments led to significant improvements, using Jacobson and Truax's (1991) criteria for clinically significant change, there was evidence (on some but not all measures) that patients in receipt of cognitive therapy had better outcomes than those receiving exposure. This suggests some additive benefit for cognitive therapy (including an element of exposure) over exposure alone.

McLean et al. (2001) contrasted ERP against cognitive therapy (which aimed to modify beliefs and attitudes, and which included behavioral experiments designed to test beliefs rather than to achieve habituation). Both therapies were conducted in a group format over 12 weeks. Seventy-six patients were assigned to treatment, 38 of whom were wait-listed for 3 months before being assigned to one of the two treatments. Patients waiting for treatment showed no gains; at posttreatment, both active treatments showed equal efficacy, though at 3-month follow-up, significantly more patients treated with ERP met recovery criteria.

COGNITIVE THERAPY IN COMBINATION WITH ERP

Enright (1991) reported on 24 patients treated in four groups over 9 weeks using a range of techniques, including thought stopping, exposure, anxiety management, and cognitive therapy. Although significant improvements were found on a variety of measures of OCD symptoms, mood, and anxiety, only 17% of patients improved using the criterion of improvement of at least 1 standard deviation from the group pretreatment mean.

Salkovskis and Warwick (1985) reported the treatment of a patient with fears of contamination and compulsive hand washing, who had relapsed after treatment with ERP. Rather than modifying the intrusive thought ("I'll be contaminated"), attention was directed to modifying the negative automatic thought associated with the intrusive thought ("I'll be rejected"), which often produced low mood and frequently preceded the intrusive thoughts. This, recombined with behavior therapy, produced almost complete recovery. Given the patient's previous history, this single-case study provides evidence of the potential gains to be made by adding a cognitive focus to treatment. Jones and Mezies (1998) reported on an intervention package for individuals with concerns about contamination. The package focused on patients' attitudes and beliefs using a series of educational techniques that address fears of contamination and employed attentional training and cognitive restructuring (but explicitly did not include ERP). Twenty-one patients were randomly assigned either to immediate treatment or a wait list, with treatment conducted in a group format over eight weekly sessions. Contrasted to controls, treated patients showed statistically significant gains, which were sustained over 3-month follow-up. However, the clinical significance of these changes was moderate, and contrasts with more striking improvements found by Jones and Mezies (1997) and Krochmalik et al. (2001), who reported single-case series using this approach on an individual-patient basis. Notably, Krochmalik et al. described outcomes for five patients, all with chronic conditions, and all of whom had failed to respond to intensive treatment with ERP. Four patients showed striking gains after intervention.

Management of Ruminations

Patients who have ruminations without associated rituals present a therapeutic challenge (Rachman, 1983); reflecting this, there have been fewer trials for ruminations than is the case for other obsessional presentations. Historically, the primary intervention strategy has been thought stopping, though more recently, the absence of evidence of efficacy in this approach has focused attention on techniques that permit habituation. Salkovskis and Westbrook (1989) reviewed single-case studies and six small-scale comparative trials of thought stopping. In total, these involved only 50 patients, and though ruminations were the primary problem, a number of patients did have associated rituals. Thought stopping was contrasted with assertiveness training (Emmelkamp & van der Hayden, 1980), with imaginal exposure (Emmelkamp & Kwee, 1977), with flooding (Hackman & McLean, 1975), and with habituation (Likierman & Rachman, 1982). Other trials have compared exposure to ruminations to exposure to irrelevant, fear-provoking scenes. Emmelkamp and Giesselbach (1981) and Stern et al. (1973) contrasted thought stopping to stopping a neutral thought. Approximately 46% of patients in these trials showed a 50% improvement in symptom frequency, though only 12% showed a 50% reduction in subjective distress.

Salkovskis and Westbrook (1989) described the technique of "revised habituation," in which patients record their ruminations onto a tape-loop, taking care to avoid including thoughts that might act to reduce anxiety ("covert rituals"). Listening to the recording then becomes a form of exposure. Initial single-case studies described by Salkovskis and Westbrook and others (Martin & Tarrier, 1992; Roth & Church, 1994; Thyer, 1985) showed promising results. Lovell et al. (1994) carried out a small, controlled trial essentially using the same technique; 12 ruminators listened either to their ruminations or to neutral prose. Though the two groups improved equivalently, there were indications that patients who successfully engaged with the technique by becoming anxious while listening to the tape improved more. More research is required to demonstrate the efficacy of this approach. Freeston et al. (1997) randomly assigned 29 patients either to immediate or delayed treatment that explicitly followed Salkovskis and Westbrook's (1989) procedures. Wait-list patients showed no improvements until treated, at which point their gains were commensurate with those seen immediately. Sixty-seven percent of the total sample showed clinically significant change at posttherapy, reducing to 53% at 6-month follow-up.

Combination Treatments

The efficacy of antidepressant medications has been reviewed by Klerman et al. (1994), Piccinelli et al. (1995), and Kobak et al. (1998), with meta-analyses consistently suggesting the greatest efficacy for clomipramine (as discussed earlier). Though there are rather few trials of exposure in combination with medication, given the clear advantage of serotinergic agents, it is appropriate to exclude trials that use tricyclic medication as a contrast (e.g., Foa et al., 1992).

Neziroglu (1979) treated 10 patients with clomipramine followed by behavioral treatment. Medication reduced symptoms by 60%; behavioral treatment decreased symptoms by a further 20%. Rachman et al. (1979) administered either clomipramine or placebo to 40 patients in a complex multiple baseline design. After 4 weeks on either clomipramine or placebo, patients received either 15 sessions of ERP or relaxation training over 3 weeks. Following this, patients who had received relaxation training were trained in ERP. Analyses immediately after administration of exposure or relaxation training suggested that patients receiving clomipramine fared better than those given placebo, and that exposure was more effective in reducing symptoms than relaxation. The effect of clomipramine was more apparent in more depressed patients and was absent in those with low initial depression scores; it seemed to act more as an antidepressant than against compulsions. Exposure had a significant effect in reducing rituals, though it had no impact on mood. One-year follow-up (Marks et al., 1980) indicated that patients receiving exposure maintained their gains.

Marks and O'Sullivan (1988) treated 49 patients in a complex design that contrasted clomipramine with placebo, and also with three different types of exposure—exposure homework, antiexposure homework, and therapist-aided exposure added to exposure homework. (In antiexposure, the patient is directed to avoid contact with the feared situation.) There were four conditions; in three of these, all patients received clomipramine for 27 weeks, while the fourth received placebo. In the clomipramine conditions, one group received antiexposure and another exposure for 3 weeks; the third received self-directed and therapist-aided exposure. The placebo group received both self-directed and therapist-aided exposure.

Contrasting the impacts of each treatment, clomipramine compared to placebo gave transient benefits in the first 8 weeks only. Self-exposure treatment was markedly superior to antiexposure; the addition of therapist-aided exposure did little to boost improvements. Exposure appeared to be the most effective of the three treatments. Overall, 81% of patients were improved or much improved; there were very similar outcomes with clomipramine and exposure contrasted with placebo and exposure. Gains were maintained at 2 years (Kasvikis & Marks, 1988), though the best outcomes were with patents whose rituals had been less severe initially (Basoglu et al., 1988).

Cottraux et al. (1990), in a trial with 44 patients without major depression, contrasted three groups: fluvoxamine with antiexposure, fluvoxamine with exposure (8 weeks of imaginal exposure followed by 16 weeks of ERP), and placebo with exposure. Some cognitive techniques, such as distraction, were incorporated into exposure instructions, though these are known to interfere with its efficacy (Grayson et al., 1986). After 24 weeks of therapy, all groups showed a decrease in symptoms of OCD; ERP and fluvoxamine were of equal efficacy.

Freund et al. (1991, cited by Abel, 1993) treated 48 patients with 15 daily sessions of ERP ($n = 13$), clomipramine ($n = 7$), fluvoxamine ($n = 14$), or placebo ($n = 14$). Assignment to therapies was nonrandom, in that patients could choose whether to receive exposure. Exposure treatment was superior to placebo on all measures, and both medications were superior to placebo on some measures. Exposure was superior in efficacy to fluoxetine, but not (on all measures) to clomipramine.

Hohagen et al. (1998) assigned 60 patients to eight sessions of CBT (which included exposure and cognitive restructuring) combined with either placebo or fluvoxamine. Though both treatments were of equal efficacy for compulsions, there was significantly greater reduction in obsessions with CBT and fluvoxamine, and severely depressed individuals with obsessions showed significantly better response to this combination.

Most of these studies combine ERP with active medication or placebo but do not examine the impact of ERP alone. van Balkom et al. (1998) randomized 117 patients either to wait list for 8 weeks, or to one of four active treatments. "Psychological therapy alone" was either cognitive therapy or ERP (offered over 16 weeks); "combination treatment" was fluvoxamine offered for the first 8 weeks, supplemented in weeks 9–16 by either cognitive therapy or ERP. Wait-list patients showed no improvements; against wait list, all combinations of treatment showed efficacy, with no advantage to any of the four permutations at the end of 8 or 16 weeks. The absence of a medication-alone condition offered over 16 weeks makes this result somewhat ambiguous, since it potentially confounds treatment length with the manner in which the combination treatment was offered (with pharmacological interventions followed by psychological ones).

O'Connor et al. (1999) conducted a small trial in which 24 patients were allocated to a wait list or to one of three active treatments: medication (in all cases, serotonergic agents) combined with CBT (ERP combined with some cognitive challenge to beliefs regarding the compulsions); CBT alone; or medication alone, administered while patients were on a wait list for CBT. Not all patients were randomized to treatment conditions; some expressed a preference and others were already receiving medication, in itself resulting in uneven distribution of patients. Though this complicates interpretation, results were in line with other studies: Patients on the wait list showed no gains, and all three active treatments showed equal efficacy.

de Haan et al. (1997) randomly assigned 99 patients to receive cognitive therapy alone or ERP alone, or either of these interventions in combination with fluvoxamine. All treatment modalities showed equal efficacy after the 16-week experimental period. At this point, 45 patients were classified as nonresponders; 17 of these had become responders at 6-month follow-up. The majority of these individuals had continued in therapy, but their original treatment regimen had been varied, apparently in line with clinical need. Analysis suggested that late responders tended to have more severe symptoms than early responders, and their pattern of response might suggest that longer interventions are warranted for such individuals. However, given that treatment in the follow-up period was adapted (e.g., to give more exposure for those who had received a cognitive intervention), this might also indicate the benefits of careful review of treatment failures. Thus, Simpson et al. (1999) identified a cohort of seven patients who had not improved despite an adequate trial of SSRI over a period greater than 12 weeks; administration of ERP resulted in a clinically significant decrease in symptoms.

FACTORS INFLUENCING OUTCOME

Depression and Initial Symptom Severity

Though a number of authors have linked poorer outcomes in OCD with the severity of comorbid depression (e.g., Foa, 1979; Foa et al., 1983a, 1983b), this has not been found in other studies (e.g., Basoglu et al., 1988; Hoogduin & Duivenvoorden, 1988; Mawson et al., 1982).

Keisjers et al. (1994) treated 40 patients with ERP, examining the relationship between outcome and depression, OCD symptom severity, and duration of OCD symptoms. Higher levels of depression were predictive of poorer outcomes on posttreatment measures of compulsive behavior. A greater duration of symptoms of OCD, lower levels of patient motivation, and a poorer therapeutic relationship were predictive of poorer outcomes on posttherapy measures of obsessive anxiety.

In a carefully designed study avoiding post hoc analyses, Foa et al. (1992) stratified 38 patients into high- and low-depressed groups (using a cutoff above or below a Beck Depression Inventory [BDI] score of 20). Patients were in- as well as outpatients, and received either imipramine or placebo, followed by intensive daily treatment exposure with response prevention and supportive therapy over 12 weeks. Although imipramine improved mood, it did not impact on OCD symptoms. Psychological treatment with or without medication was highly effective; significant main effects for treatment only occurred once behavior therapy was initiated. Using a categorical system at posttreatment, 44% of patients were rated highly improved, 44% moderately improved, and only 10% or so worse. There was evidence of some relapse at 2-year follow-up, at which point 29% remained highly improved, 50% were moderately improved, and 18% were rated as failures. No differences were found between in- and outpatient groups, nor was the initial level of depression related to outcome. However, a more recent trial conducted by this same research group found that a diagnosis of comorbid major depressive disorder was associated with poorer outcome (Abramowitz & Foa, 2000). Eighty-seven patients were treated with ERP and divided into four groups: nondepressed, or mildly, moderately, or severely depressed. Only in the latter group was there a clear impact of depression on outcome (Abramowitz et al., 2000).

Although research presents a somewhat mixed picture, more recent trials suggest that patients with severe comorbid depression will show reduced, though still clinically significant gains. Indeed, Abromowitz and Foa (2000) classified 73% of their depressed sample as treatment responders (contrasted to 88% of the nondepressed patients). These authors suggest that individuals whose depression is linked to impairments associated with their OCD may be more responsive to exposure techniques than those who show hopelessness and despair, and who may therefore find it difficult to engage in treatment until their depressive symptoms are better managed.

Fixity of Belief

There is mixed evidence regarding the impact of initial fixity of belief on outcome. While some trials support this notion (e.g., Foa, 1979; Foa et al., 1999a) others have found no link (e.g., Basoglu et al., 1988; Foa et al., 1983a, 1983b). Lelliot et al. (1988) found that one-third of a cohort of 49 compulsive ritualizers viewed their obsessive thoughts as rational and believed that their rituals successfully averted a feared event. Though outcome after ERP was not related to initial fixity of belief, there was a significant association between positive outcomes and a shift in the strength of beliefs. Lelliot et al. also noted that the more bizarre the obsessive belief, the more strongly it was defended, with fewer attempts made to resist the urge to ritualize. Tolin et al. (2001) surveyed a cohort of 395 individuals with OCD, finding an association between poorer insight and certain beliefs (persons with fear of harming others or self, and those with religious obsessions). It is possible that the link between beliefs and outcome is nonlinear, such that only very extreme beliefs will impact on outcome, making this a more difficult phenomenon to detect (Steketee & Shapiro, 1995), but more research is required to make a definitive statement.

Personality Disorders

There is limited information about the impact of personality disorders on outcomes, though two reviews (Dreessen & Arntz, 1998; Steketee & Shapiro, 1995) consider the available evidence. Rabavilas et al. (1979) and Vaughan and Beech (1985) suggest a positive impact for OCD, though this may relate more to compliance than to longer term gains. Steketee (1990) found short-term benefit for individuals with dependent personality disorder treated with exposure, though this group also showed more rapid relapse over follow-up. Reports suggest that patients with schizotypal personality disorder have significantly poorer outcomes (Fals-Stewart & Lucente, 1993; Jenike et al., 1986a, 1986b; Minichiello et al., 1987; Moritz et al., 2004). For example, Minichiello et al. (1987) found that only 7% achieved moderate improvement, compared to 90% of patients with no personality disorder. One difficulty with some of these studies is that personality disorder is assessed after, rather than before, treatment. Dreessen et al. (1997) studied 43 patients undergoing CBT, finding no evidence for the impact on outcomes of personality disorders in general, or for any specific personality disorder except schizotypal personality disorder, in which there was a trend for such patients to do more poorly.

Hoarding

Anecdotal clinical experience suggests that people who hoard have poor clinical outcomes, a notion for which there is some limited research support. Black et al. (1998) treated a cohort of 38 patients, noting that hoarders were significantly less likely to show improvements than individuals with other symptoms. A similar result was obtained by Saxena et al. (2002), who reported on a subsample of 20 hoarders from a larger sample of 190 patients, all treated with CBT and medication. Although both samples responded to treatment, the rate of improvement in hoarders was significantly less than in nonhoarders. Frost and Hartl (1996) have developed a cognitive model of hoarding, along with specific treatment strategies. Two single-case studies report outcomes using this procedure (Cermele et al., 2001; Hartl & Frost, 1999), along with a single-case series of work with six patients (Steketee et al., 2000). In all cases, treatment was carried out over long periods (up to 17 months), and though improvements were moderate rather than substantial, this outcome suggests that further research is needed given the usually intractable nature of this problem.

SUMMARY AND CLINICAL IMPLICATIONS

Behavioral and cognitive-behavioral approaches dominate research into treatments for OCD, with exposure and response prevention (ERP) being the most commonly employed technique. Meta-analyses are consistent in indicating large effect sizes at posttherapy and follow-up for ERP alone, though they show some variation in their assessment of the relative efficacy of medication. While nonserotonergic antidepressants appear ineffective, the relative efficacy of SSRIs alone, ERP alone, and the two in combination is less clear, though effect sizes are broadly equivalent. Treatment of any kind is more successful when compulsions are present than when they are absent. Effect sizes may be influenced by the form and completeness of delivery of ERP; therapist-supervised exposure may be more helpful than self-directed exposure, and ensuring complete abstention from rituals during exposure results in better outcomes. There are indications that longer therapies and longer sessions are associated with better outcomes, though both group and individual delivery appear equally effective.

Though ERP is clearly effective, it should be noted that it may result in a reduction rather than a removal of symptoms in a significant proportion of patients, and as a consequence, these individuals may show some degree of continued distress even after treatment. Notwithstanding this caveat, there is good maintenance of gains for many patients; in contrast, those treated with pharmacotherapy tend to relapse unless maintained on medication.

Though evidence is somewhat limited, ERP as practiced in research appears to be effective in routine settings and with patients with comorbid presentations. Variations in its delivery—most obviously in the frequency of sessions—do not seem to impact on its effectiveness.

The benefits of cognitive therapy are somewhat less clear; some studies suggest that when contrasted with ERP, it appears to be somewhat less effective, while others find advantage. Certainly there is evidence that combining cognitive therapy with ERP appears to be helpful to patients who failed to respond to intensive ERP treatments alone. An area in which ERP is more difficult to apply is in managing ruminations, which are less tractable to behavioral intervention. Here, the combination of cognitive and behavioral techniques seems to show advantage.

Patients with comorbid depression present a therapeutic challenge, though this may be less of an issue in individuals whose depression represents a reaction to their OCD symptoms. The extent to which fixity of belief bears on outcome is unclear, though it seems likely that beliefs of an extreme nature may be a negative indicator. Persons with schizotypal personality disorder will have poorer outcomes, as will those whose symptoms include hoarding. These findings present obvious areas for development.

On the basis of research, it would be hard to justify treating an individual with OCD using techniques other than the behavioral and cognitive approaches described in this chapter. This is not to preclude the use of nonspecific techniques addressed to residual or associated distress; in appropriate circumstances, a combination of symptom-oriented techniques with more general supportive or expressive techniques could be justified, and in some cases might be necessary to manage comorbidity.

Given the continuing gap between community prevalence and clinical presentations, many patients with OCD may be unaware that effective treatments for their difficulties are available. This may call for more availability of treatment in primary care rather than specialist clinics, particularly if computerized techniques can be developed and applied.

CHAPTER 8

POSTTRAUMATIC STRESS DISORDER

DEFINITION

DSM-IV-TR describes posttraumatic stress disorder (PTSD) as the development of a characteristic pattern of symptoms in response to personal experience of an extreme traumatic event that involves actual or threatened death, injury, or a threat to the physical integrity of the self or another person. Common examples of directly traumatizing events are rape, military combat, being taken hostage or incarcerated (e.g., in a concentration camp), and natural or accidental disasters (e.g., floods, car accidents, or large fires). Common witnessed events could include observing serious injury or unnatural death due to violent assault, accident, or war, or accidentally witnessing a dead body or body parts.

The disorder is defined by a pattern of three symptom clusters of (1) intrusive and usually vivid reexperiencing of the event (in the form of recurrent and intrusive images and thoughts, or recurrent distressing dreams), (2) avoidance of reminders of the event and numbing of general responsiveness, and (3) physiological reactivity, memory impairment, poor concentration, exaggerated startle responses, and hypervigilance. Symptoms need to be present for more than 1 month for a diagnosis of PTSD to be made, and DSM-IV-TR distinguishes chronic from acute cases, in which the duration of symptoms is greater than or less than 3 months, respectively. Symptoms of anxiety and depression are common and may in some cases be sufficient for an additional diagnosis of anxiety or depressive disorder to be made.

PREVALENCE, COMORBIDITY, AND NATURAL HISTORY
Prevalence

Data from the Epidemiologic Catchment Area (ECA) survey of approximately 2,500 people (Helzer et al., 1987) suggested a lifetime prevalence for PTSD of 1% in the general population. A similar figure of 1.3% for lifetime prevalence was found by Davidson et al. (1991), with a 6-month prevalence of 0.44%. Some surveys suggest higher prevalence rates, though this may reflect sampling differences across studies. Thus, Shore et al. (1986) reported a lifetime prevalence of 2.6%, and Breslau et al. (1991), in a sample of 1,000 adults ages 21–30, estimated lifetime prevalence at 9.2%. However, general population estimates are less pertinent than prevalence rates in individuals exposed to traumatic events, some—but by no means all—of whom can be expected to develop PTSD. In the ECA survey, those who had been physically attacked had a prevalence of 3.5%, and veterans of the Vietnam War, a prevalence of 20%. Curran et al. (1990) reported that 50% of survivors of the Enniskillen bombing in Ireland had symptoms of PTSD. Morgan et al. (2003) found that 29% of survivors of the 1966 Aberfan disaster met diagnostic criteria for PTSD at 33-year follow-up.

Clearly, many individuals exposed to trauma do not develop PTSD. For example, Kilpatrick and Resnick (1993), in a retrospective study, noted that 35% of rape victims and 39% of victims of assault report symptoms of PTSD. Rothbaum et al. (1992), in a prospective study, found higher rates; in the 3 months following a sexual assault, rates of PTSD were 47%, and for nonsexual assault, 22%. Exploring this issue further, Brewin et al. (2000) meta-analyzed 77 studies that examined the sequelae of trauma. The likelihood of developing PTSD was increased to a small but reliable degree by a previous psychiatric history and various forms of prior adverse experience. Certain variables, such as gender, and educational, social, and intellectual disadvantage, were predictive in some but not all samples, and predictive effects were stronger and more homogenous in combat veterans as contrasted to civilian victims. However, the impact of "proximal" markers (such as the intensity of the trauma, and the degree of social support and concurrent life stress) were more strongly and consistently related to the emergence of PTSD.

Comorbidity

Individuals with PTSD often present with other, comorbid psychiatric disorders. Kessler et al. (1995) reviewed a sample of 5,877 individuals with PTSD, seen as part of the National Comorbidity Survey, and found that nearly 50% had three or more additional diagnoses, most usually of affective disorder, anxiety, and substance misuse. The question of primacy of diagnosis is an important one; though comorbid conditions often develop subsequent to

PTSD, many individuals with PTSD have preexisting diagnoses. Perkonigg et al. (2000) studied a German community sample of 3,021 adolescents and young adults, and found that in the subgroup that met diagnostic criteria for PTSD, 87.5% had at least one additional diagnosis, and 85% had two or more. Some diagnoses tend to precede the traumatizing event (e.g., somatoform disorders, specific phobia, or social phobia); others (e.g., panic disorder) appear to develop contemporaneously, and still other conditions (such as depression and substance misuse) emerge after (and perhaps in response to) the onset of PSTD.

Natural History

As noted earlier only a portion of individuals exposed to trauma will develop PTSD; this consequence is not inevitable and probably depends on a number of factors, only one of which is the traumatizing event itself. However, once present, it can be a disabling and persistent condition. Ramsay (1990) examined the natural course of the disorder in 36 survivors of a freighter collision, who were assessed immediately after the accident and again after 4.5 years, with no systematic psychiatric care in the intervening period. Immediately after the incident, most of the group had multiple psychological and psychosomatic complaints. At follow-up, significant deterioration was found; 12 individuals had been hospitalized, and 26 of the men had received psychiatric help. Holen (1990) followed up survivors of an oil rig disaster; contrasted with a comparison cohort of workers not exposed to trauma, significantly enhanced levels of psychiatric morbidity were still evident 8 years after the disaster. A 40-year follow-up of World War II prisoners of war revealed that two-thirds had suffered from PTSD (Kluznik et al., 1986). Of these, 29% had fully recovered, 39% still reported mild symptoms, 24% showed moderate improvement, and 8% had not recovered. There is also some evidence for the reactivation of trauma. Survivors of the Enniskillen bombing, thought to have recovered 6 months after the event, again showed symptoms at the 1-year anniversary (Curran et al., 1990). Thus, available evidence suggests that untreated PTSD has a chronic course in a significant proportion of individuals exposed to trauma.

Some authors (e.g., Resick & Schnicke, 1992; Turner et al., 1996) suggest that the natural history of PTSD (and, by implication, the likely response to treatment interventions) may be complicated by both the nature of the trauma and the person's response to that trauma. Thus, a precipitating trauma might be categorized as *simple* or *complex*, depending on whether it is a one-time event (such as assault or rape), or one that extends over time (e.g., the experience of being taken hostage). The person's response to trauma might also be categorized as simple or complex depending on whether exposure to thoughts about the trauma evoke fear or a mix of fear, shame, and guilt (Lee et al., 2001). In the latter case, simple exposure carried out without strategies to manage, for example, self-blame might be expected to show poor results. Whereas these propositions may be important clinically, they have not been subjected to systematic evaluation as a part of the studies discussed below.

PSYCHOLOGICAL DEBRIEFING

Psychological interventions—usually in the form of a debriefing—are a frequent component of responses to natural or man-made disasters, as well as traumatic events affecting individuals, such as rape or violent crime (e.g., Ramsay, 1990). However, there are problems in evaluating their efficacy, not least because definitions of debriefing vary widely. For example, this term can refer to a specific model (such as critical incident stress debriefing [CISD; Mitchell & Everly, 1994]), to sessions in which clients are given minimal opportunities to feedback their experience, or to generic counseling. Understandable pressures to mount a rapid response mean that there are few controlled trials of these interventions; consequently, the degree to which these responses actually benefit victims is unclear. Furthermore, many trials that do exist are methodologically weak (Rose et al., 2003). Attrition from open trials following disasters makes it difficult to be clear about the effectiveness of these interventions, particularly because there is evidence that survivors who absent themselves from assessment following trauma may represent the most severely affected individuals (Weisaeth, 1989).

van Emmerik et al. (2002), Rose et al. (2003), and Bisson (2003) identify 7, 11, and 13 randomized studies, respectively in which individuals recently exposed to a trauma received a single-session debriefing (combining some form of emotional expression with recall of the traumatic event). All three reviews comment on the variable quality of trials and the heterogeneity of study populations (victims of road traffic accidents and physical trauma, combat veterans, and women who had experienced a miscarriage). Debriefing did not appear to reduce levels of distress or the probability of developing PTSD. This pattern is fairly consistent across studies; for example, in a large-scale trial Rose et al. (1999) randomized 157 victims of violent crime to one session of education about the sequelae of trauma, debriefing plus education, or assessment alone, finding no differences between groups in rates of PTSD at 6 months. Though a lack of impact is the most common finding, it is worrisome that some trials suggest an enhanced rate of psychopathology following debriefing. Bisson et al. (1997) examined outcomes in a group of 133 burn-trauma victims randomly allocated to debriefing or to no intervention. At 1 year, 26% of the intervention group met diagnostic criteria for PTSD in contrast to 4% of the group that received no treatment. Hobbs et al. (1996) studied 106 consecutive hospital admissions following a road-traffic accident, half of whom were offered a 1-hour debriefing within 48 hours of the accident. At 4 months, there was some indication that the treated group was faring less well than controls. At 3-year follow-up of 61 individuals (Mayou et al., 2000), the treated group had significantly higher scores on the Impact of Events Scale (IES) than did controls. Initial severity was an important determinant of outcome: Individuals with high initial IES scores who received the intervention did not recover. In contrast, participants with lower initial IES scores who received a debriefing recovered to the same degree as those who did not receive a debriefing. These findings hint at the possibility that debriefing has the potential to disrupt normal pathways to recovery.

These studies are restricted to single-session interventions following acute trauma; three studies with longer interventions showed more positive results. Bryant et al. (1999) report a five-session intervention delivered to survivors of motor accidents or assault within 2 weeks of the original trauma. Contrasted to a counseling intervention, exposure, or exposure combined with anxiety management, significantly reduced rates of PTSD at 6-month follow-up. André et al. (1997) assigned bus drivers who had been assaulted to 1–6 sessions of cognitive-behavioral therapy (CBT) or to no intervention. At 6 months, the intervention group showed a lower rate of anxiety and intrusion of traumatic memories. Ehlers et al. (2003) adopted a "stepped care" model to identify individuals at most risk of developing chronic PTSD by screening 205 individuals involved in road traffic accidents and excluding those who (after a 3-week wait) no longer met diagnostic criteria. At this point, 85 participants were randomized to 12 weekly sessions of CBT (plus three monthly booster sessions), to a self-help intervention (one session of clinician contact and bibliotherapy), or to repeated assessments for PTSD symptoms. At 6-month follow-up, 14% of the CBT participants had PSTD in contrast to 55% and 75% of patients receiving repeat assessments and bibliotherapy, respectively.

On the basis of these findings, many commentators now advise against routine debriefing (e.g., Bolwig, 1998; Raphael et al., 1995). This does not imply that individuals in distress should not be offered support, nor does this general conclusion contraindicate psychological intervention at some remove from the initial trauma. However, it does suggest that intervention after trauma should be based on clear evidence of clinical need in the individual case, and that there may be no special advantage to focusing therapeutic effort on the immediate aftermath of trauma (Ehlers & Clark, 2003).

TREATMENT APPROACHES

Treatments for PTSD are varied. Psychodynamic approaches usually focus on the meaning of the traumatic event for the person's sense of self and his/her place in the world. Behavioral techniques such as exposure aim to reduce the patient's reactance to traumatic memories; cognitive techniques focus on the management of the patient's appraisal of the trauma. Anxiety management approaches, such as stress inoculation training, often incorporate both behavioral and cognitive elements, and aim to manage anxiety evoked by traumatic memories. Eye movement desensitization and reprocessing therapy (EMDR; Shapiro, 1989b) requires patients to evoke an image of events causing them anxiety, while tracking the therapist's finger as it is moved rapidly and rhythmically from side to side; at the same time, they generate cognitive coping statements. The saccadic eye movements generated by this procedure were originally considered a critical component of the approach, though some current practitioners suggest that this may be but one of a number of important elements (e.g., Spector & Read, 1999). While EMDR has a relatively unique theoretical rationale, as practiced, there is obvious overlap with both behavioral and cognitive approaches. Because its practitioners have made strong claims for its efficacy and routes into training are restricted, the degree to which this approach is truly distinctive is of more than academic interest.

Meta-Analyses

Sherman's (1998) review focused on psychological interventions; Van Etten and Taylor (1998) considered the efficacy of both psychological and pharmacological approaches. There is surprisingly little overlap between their coverage of psychological approaches; Sherman analyzed data from 17 studies, only five of which were included by Van Etten and Taylor (who identified a total of 20 trials of psychological therapy). Considering the overall efficacy of all psychological treatments, Sherman reported a pre- to posttherapy effect size of 0.52 ($n = 16$), and for follow-up at between 3 months and 2 years, an effect size of 0.64 ($n = 11$). Van Etten and Taylor contrasted behavioral therapy, CBT, and EMDR against a range of control interventions (wait list, hypnotherapy, dynamic therapy, and supportive therapy). On a composite measure of self-reported severity of PTSD symptoms, behavioral and cognitive-behavioral techniques showed a mean pre- to posttherapy effect-size of 1.3 ($n = 13$); on the same index, the mean effect size for EMDR was 1.2 ($n = 11$). Five trials of behavioral and cognitive therapy, and six trials of EMDR reported follow-up at up to 15 weeks, yielding effect sizes of 1.6 and 1.3, respectively.

Two meta-analyses focused on the efficacy of EMDR. Davidson and Parker (2001) identified 34 studies of the efficacy of EMDR for various presentations; 12 trials examined outcomes for individuals with PTSD, and eight outcomes for those with "traumatic memories" (the remaining trials focused on other anxiety conditions). Considering interventions for PTSD, there was a moderate advantage to EMDR when contrasted to no treatment (five comparisons; effect size = 0.39), nonspecific treatment (two comparisons; effect size = 0.34) or non-*in vivo* exposure (one comparison; effect size = 0.39). However, compared to *in vivo exposure* (one comparison), there was an effect size of 0.44 in favor of exposure. Dismantling studies yield small effect sizes:

EMDR, with and without eye movements (four comparisons effect size = 0.22), or compared to other dismantling designs (one comparison; effect size = −0.06). A similar pattern of effect sizes is found when treatment relates to traumatic memories. Maxfield and Hyer (2002) reported overall effect sizes for EMDR compared to wait list/no treatment (effect size = 2.17), nonspecific therapies (effect size = 0.81; five trials), and exposure-based therapies (effect size = 0.45). This latter effect size is based on four trials, one of which (Rogers et al., 1999; discussed further below) was excluded by Davidson and Parker because the treatment condition was confounded by the therapist. Based on effect sizes cited in Maxfield and Hyer (2002), removing this trial gives an effect size of 0.21. As noted by Maxfield and Hyer, the wide variation in outcome from studies of EMDR compared to active therapies (and their paucity) reinforces the need for more research.

EMDR practitioners have expressed concerns that low treatment fidelity in the delivery of EMDR reduces its efficacy in contrast to other active treatments (e.g., Greenwald, 1996). Davidson and Parker (2001) tested this proposition by examining effect sizes across all 34 studies, comparing outcomes in which therapists had received an approved EMDR training and those in which they had not; in all cases, effect sizes were equivalent. Maxfield and Hyer (2002) examined the relationship between effect size and methodological quality, using a scoring system based on the Foa and Meadows (1997) criteria for the judging the quality of randomized trials. Overall, the more rigorous the study, the greater the efficacy of EMDR. However, the most usual source of variance in quality across studies was attributable to the presence or absence of independent observers, or questionable treatment fidelity. Although this is apparent evidence in favor of EMDR, it is not possible to ascertain the reliability of the procedures used to derive estimates of quality. This is especially critical in relation to estimates of treatment fidelity, where the criteria for appraisal are not clear.

While both reviews conclude that EMDR shows good evidence of efficacy when contrasted with nonspecific treatments, they differ in their appraisal of its efficacy in contrast to exposure. This may be attributable to the small number of studies available for meta-analysis, differing inclusion or exclusion criteria across analyses, and (less easy to detect from the information within the papers) the choice of measures from which effect sizes were derived. Meta-analysis of this area may be somewhat premature at this stage; firmer conclusions require a larger sample of studies.

General Reviews

The Treatment Guidelines Task Force established by the International Society for Traumatic Stress Studies has published treatment guidelines based on reviews of available evidence for a wide range of psychological and psychopharmacological approaches (Foa et al., 2000). Comprehensive general reviews can be found in Foa and Meadows (1997), Foa et al. (1995), Frueh et al. (1995), Shalev et al. (1996), and Solomon et al. (1992).

Pharmacotherapy

A wide range of medications has been employed in the treatment of PTSD, reflecting the complexity and range of symptoms in this condition. Friedman et al. (2000) reviewed the efficacy of antidepressants (tricyclic antidepressants [TCAs], monoamine oxidase inhibitors [MAOIs], and selective serotonin reuptake inhibitors [SSRIs]), along with anxiolytics (alprazolam), anticonvulsants, and antiadrinergic agents. A detailed review of this area is outside the scope of this volume, but there is good evidence from randomized controlled trials (RCTs) for the efficacy of antidepressant medication, particularly for the value of SSRIs. There is moderate support for the use of MAOIs, but TCAs appear to confer only a modest benefit. There is suggestive evidence from open trials that anticonvulsants may be helpful. In contrast benzodiazepines appear to be of limited use. The fact that PTSD is defined by a number of symptoms clusters suggests that single medications are unlikely to be completely effective, and the evolution of pharmacotherapy may lie in more careful titration of a number of medications. At present, pharmacological and psychological approaches can be seen as adjunctive (Friedman et al., 2000), though this is an assumption that has yet to be directly tested in clinical trials.

Hypnosis

Although there are a number of case studies describing the use of hypnosis (Cardena, 2000), only one trial of its efficacy (Brom et al., 1989; reviewed below) has been conducted; therefore, there is little support for its use.

Psychodynamic Interventions

Although frequently used, there is limited evidence for the efficacy of psychodynamic techniques. Most studies are case reports or open trials, and most of the latter have a number of methodological problems, including lack of control groups, failure to define treatments, no inclusion and exclusion criteria, failure to assign patients randomly to treatments, and absence of objective measures of target symptoms. An equivocal picture emerges from these trials. Three trials report outcomes from group therapy with female victims of sexual assault. Cryer and Beutler (1980) reported mixed results; though a significant reduction in symptoms was found in most of the nine group members, some did not benefit, and one patient showed an increase in symptomatology. Perl et al. (1985) reported positive benefits in 17 patients treated in an open trial, though no quantitative measures were used. Roth et al. (1988) treated 13 individuals in a group format over 1 year, employing Horowitz's model of trauma to guide the intervention, and contrasting outcomes with a control group. Although therapy appeared to show some benefits, methodological problems make interpretation of gains problematic.

Lindy et al. (1983), who treated 30 survivors and rescue workers 6 months to 1 year after a major fire, employed short-term psychodynamic therapy. Patients in the trial were drawn from a self-selected subgroup of 147 individuals who had responded to outreach programs established in the wake of the fire. However, not all participants met diagnostic criteria for PTSD (only nine met DSM-III-R criteria for PTSD alone; a further 10 presented with comorbid depression). Therapy was conducted over 6–12 sessions, and followed a standardized protocol that included encouragement of reexposure. Comparison of treated to untreated patients suggested improvements in symptom ratings, though this was more marked for patients who completed treatment. Patients with a diagnosis of PTSD were less likely to complete treatment than those with a diagnosis of depression alone, though more experienced therapists were more likely to retain patients for the full course of treatment.

Brom et al. (1989) contrasted psychodynamic therapy, hypnotherapy, and systematic desensitization with a wait-list control. All three treatments led to modest improvements, though in different areas of functioning; those receiving dynamic therapy showed most reduction in avoidance symptoms, while hypnotherapy and systematic desensitization led to more reduction in intrusive thoughts. However, though meeting criteria for a diagnosis of PTSD, only 23 of the 112 patients in this sample had experienced a traumatic event; the remainder were bereaved, which limits the conclusions that can be drawn from this study.

Scarvalone et al. (1995, cited in Foa & Meadows, 1997) contrasted a group-based psychodynamic treatment (interpersonal process group therapy) with wait-list controls. The 43 participants had suffered childhood sexual abuse, though not all presented with symptoms of PTSD. After the intervention, 39% of those receiving treatment met criteria for PTSD, contrasted to 83% of the control group. Marmar et al. (1988) randomly assigned 61 recently bereaved women (less than half of whom met DSM-III criteria for PTSD) to 12 weeks of brief dynamic therapy or to a self-help group led by a nonclinician. At posttreatment, there was evidence of modest gains but little difference in outcome between groups.

Cognitive-Behavioral Therapy

CBT for PTSD includes exposure-based approaches (systematic desensitization, and *in vivo* and prolonged exposure), anxiety management, stress inoculation training, and combinations of these techniques.

Systematic Desensitization and Exposure

Both of these techniques call for exposure to anxiety-provoking stimuli related to the traumatizing event. In systematic desensitization, exposure is paired with relaxation. Imaginal or *in vivo* exposure usually employs a graduated approach, beginning with exposure to moderately distressing images or situations. In "flooding," prolonged exposure to maximally arousing stimuli is employed.

SYSTEMATIC DESENSITIZATION

Most studies of systematic desensitization have focused on Vietnam veterans, and most suffer from methodological problems that limit interpretation of their results. Of these, Brom et al. (1989, discussed earlier) is probably the most robust, though Bowen and Lambert (1986) and Peniston (1986) carried out controlled studies of systematic desensitization alone contrasted with a no-treatment control. Although treatment showed efficacy on a range of psychophysiological measures, no direct measures of PTSD symptoms were taken. Hyer et al. (1989), in an open trial of 5 weeks of systematic desensitization in 50 Vietnam veterans, found no improvements on the Millon Clinical Multiaxial Inventory. Frank et al. (1988) contrasted systematic desensitization and CBT in 84 victims of rape, and found both approaches to be of equal efficacy. However, participants were recent victims of trauma, and it is possible that any improvements reflect the natural reduction in symptoms that can be expected over time. There is therefore only limited evidence for the efficacy of systematic desensitization.

EXPOSURE

Three controlled studies of flooding in the treatment of Vietnam veterans showed evidence for the efficacy of this procedure. Keane et al. (1989) assigned 24 patients either to flooding or to a wait-list control, finding improvements in the treated group on many, but not all, symptoms of PTSD. Cooper and Clum (1989) compared outcomes in 16 patients treated either with a combination of imaginal flooding and "standard treatment" (comprising psychotherapy and pharmacotherapy) or standard therapy alone, and found significant benefit for flooding over control therapy. Using a similar design but in a larger study of 58 patients, Boudewyns and Hyer (1990) contrasted exposure and "conventional" psychotherapy, finding no differences posttherapy. However, at 3-month follow-up, the exposure group showed greater improvements in adjustment, and a greater proportion were classified as successful treatments than those who had received psychotherapy (Boudewyns et al., 1990).

There is evidence for the efficacy of exposure in noncombatants with a range of precipitating traumas. Foa and colleagues have examined the efficacy of exposure in female rape victims, employing an imaginal technique in which the client is encouraged to recount her experiences in detail (Foa & Rothbaum, 1988). Data from these trials provide good evidence for efficacy (Foa et al., 1991, 1995, 1999b [reviewed below].

Studies on individuals who had experienced a range of precipitating traumas also show evidence of efficacy; some of these are reviewed below. In an open trial with 10 patients, Vaughn and Tarrier (1992) employed a form of habituation in which patients tape-recorded a description of the traumatizing event, followed by nine sessions of self-directed exposure. Although measures of symptom severity decreased, mean scores remained quite high, suggesting that few patients showed clinically significant improvement. Richards et al. (1994) administered both imaginal and *in vivo* exposure to 14 patients with chronic PTSD. Half the patients received imaginal exposure for four sessions, followed by four sessions of live exposure to situations they had been avoiding; the remaining patients received these treatments in the reverse order. Equal and significant gains were made by both groups. In an open trial, Thompson et al. (1995) offered patients a package comprising one session of CISD (a procedure that in itself involves a major element of imaginal exposure) followed by eight sessions of imaginal and *in vivo* exposure, along with cognitive interventions. Posttherapy results were reported for 23 patients (from a total of 38) who completed the therapy; 16 of these met DSM-III-R criteria for PTSD. Overall, significant reductions in symptomatology related to PTSD were obtained; half of the patients meeting diagnostic criteria for PTSD no longer did so at the end of the trial.

Combining Exposure and Cognitive Treatment

Two trials from the same research group explored the use of cognitive processing therapy (CPT), which includes both cognitive restructuring (especially in relation to guilt and self-blame) and exposure. In a small trial, Resick and Schnicke (1992) treated 19 rape victims over 12 weeks using a group format and a quasi-experimental design with a naturally occurring wait list. Posttreatment, none of the patients met DSM-III-R criteria for PTSD; gains were maintained at 6-month follow-up. Resick et al. (2002) assigned 171 female rape victims to CPT, prolonged exposure, or a minimal attention condition. Both active treatments were offered on an individual basis, delivered in 12 sessions over 6 weeks, and both were significantly more effective than control both at posttherapy and at 9-month follow-up. Although there were no differences in their impact in relation to PTSD symptoms, levels of guilt were lower in those who received CPT.

Marks et al. (1998; reviewed earlier) found that adding cognitive therapy to exposure did not confer additional benefits contrasted to exposure alone or to cognitive therapy alone. Fecteau and Nicki (1999) allocated 20 patients whose PTSD was consequent to a road traffic accident either to CBT or to a wait list. CBT included exposure, anxiety management, and cognitive restructuring, and resulted in significant gains contrasted to the control condition both posttherapy and at 6-month follow-up. Blanchard et al. (2003) also examined outcomes from 78 survivors of road accidents, contrasting a CBT package that incorporated exposure with supportive therapy and a wait list. At 3-month follow-up, CBT was significantly more effective than either contrast condition, and supportive therapy was more effective than the wait-list condition at this point; the number of individuals no longer meeting diagnostic criteria were 76%, 48%, and 24%, respectively. Bryant et al. (1999) allocated 45 individuals with trauma originating from a variety of causes to exposure alone, exposure combined with an anxiety management package that contained significant cognitive component, or supportive counseling. At 6 months, patients receiving exposure or the combined package showed significant gains over those receiving counseling, but, again, the combination treatment was no more effective than exposure alone.

Paunovic and Öst (2001) contrasted the efficacy of exposure and CBT (which included exposure) in a small trial of 20 patients, all of whom were refugees. Mean initial scores on measures of PTSD, depression, and generalized anxiety were higher than in most trials; nonetheless, significant and equivalent gains were evident, with both interventions equally effective. Gillespie et al. (2002) reported an open trial of outcomes for people presenting with PTSD to standard National Health Service (NHS) settings in the aftermath of a bombing in Omagh. Because treatment took place as part of an emergency response to a major public incident, therapists varied widely in their experience, and patients were unselected. All therapists were given training and supervision using Ehlers and Clark's (2000) model, which combines exposure and cognitive techniques. Ninety-one patients were treated by five clinicians over a median of 8 sessions (though the range was from 2 to 73 sessions, with most patients receiving 20 or fewer sessions). Overall, there was a highly significant decrease in PTSD symptomatology; the pre- to posttherapy effect-size (2.47) compares very favorably with that obtained in controlled trials.

Exposure versus Cognitive Interventions

Systematic contrast of these approaches is difficult because of the need to avoid "inadvertent" exposure during cognitive intervention. Nonetheless, five methodologically sound trials have contrasted these approaches. Frank et al. (1988; reviewed earlier) found equal efficacy for systematic desensitization and cognitive interventions in female rape victims. Marks et al. (1998) assigned 87 patients to prolonged exposure and cognitive restructuring alone or in combination, or to relaxation alone. Exposure and cognitive restructuring were of equal efficacy; combining the treatments conferred no additional benefit, and both were superior to relaxation, which showed only modest benefits.

Two trials employed imaginal rather than *in vivo* exposure, on the basis that the latter approach often introduces coping procedures (such as self-talk). Tarrier et al. (1999a) assigned 72 patients meeting diagnostic criteria for PTSD either to exposure (focused only on reevocation of the traumatic incident) or to a cognitive intervention (which focused only on the meaning of the event, rather than the event itself). Both treatments resulted in clinical improvement posttherapy and at 6- and 12-month follow-up (Tarrier et al., 1999b). However, there was evidence of greater attrition from exposure alone. Bryant et al. (2003) contrasted eight weekly sessions of cognitive restructuring, cognitive restructuring combined with exposure, or supportive counseling in 58 individuals who had suffered a nonsexual assault or road-traffic accident. While both active treatments showed benefit over control, greater gains were apparent with the combination treatment than with exposure alone. At posttherapy (and in the intention-to-treat [ITT] sample), the proportion of patients continuing to meet diagnostic criteria in the control, exposure alone, and combination groups, respectively, were 67%, 50%, and 35%. At 6-month follow-up, this pattern was maintained, with respective rates being 78%, 50%, and 40%.

STRESS INOCULATION TRAINING

SIT combines relaxation, role playing, thought stopping, and guided self-dialogue. Veronen and Kilpatrick (1982, cited in Foa & Meadows, 1997) carried out an uncontrolled study of rape victims 3 months posttrauma, showing a decrease in anxiety and depression on multiple measures. Resick et al. (1988) conducted a controlled study of six 2-hour sessions of group therapy for rape-related anxiety, contrasting SIT, assertion training, and supportive psychotherapy against a wait-list control. Compared to control patients, all three treatments were equally effective on measures of rape-related fear, intrusion, and avoidance, with gains related to fears maintained at 6 months. However, other gains were lost at this point.

Foa et al. (1991) treated 45 rape victims (all at least 3 months after the assault), contrasting prolonged exposure, SIT, and supportive counseling against a wait-list control. The treatment package comprised nine biweekly individual sessions, and PTSD symptoms were assessed directly. (Supportive counseling was almost a control condition, focusing on problem solving that may or may not have been assault-related, but avoiding direct discussion of the assault itself in order not to replicate the exposure treatment.) SIT produced better results on PTSD symptoms posttreatment than exposure or counseling; 50% and 40%, respectively, of the SIT and exposure patients no longer met diagnostic criteria for PTSD, contrasted to 90% and 100%, respectively, of the counseling and wait-list groups. However, at 3-month follow-up, between-treatment differences were nonsignificant, with 55% of both SIT and exposure patients and 45% of the counseling group no longer meeting diagnostic criteria for PTSD.

COMBINING EXPOSURE AND SIT

Foa et al. (1999b) treated 96 women who had been victims of sexual or nonsexual assault, allocating them either to SIT alone, exposure alone, or to SIT and exposure in combination. Contrasted to patients on a wait list, all active treatments resulted in equivalent and significant reductions in both PTSD and depressive symptomatology for patients in the completer sample of 64 patients. However, ITT analysis suggested that posttherapy, exposure alone was more effective than SIT or the combination treatment. Patients undergoing the combination treatment were allocated the same amount of time for both anxiety management and exposure (and hence received less exposure than patients undergoing exposure alone). The possibility that this might account for differential effectiveness requires future research.

Pre- to posttreatment effect sizes for exposure in Foa et al. (1991, 1999b), Devilly and Spence (1999), Marks et al. (1998), and Tarrier et al. (1999a) ranged between 0.8 and 2.1. Though there may be room for debate about the best ways to optimize exposure, and for the degree of effectiveness that can be expected in clinical settings (Devilly & Foa, 2001; Tarrier, 2001), studies offer clear support for the view that this is an effective treatment for PTSD. However, there is evidence that not all patients can tolerate exposure (e.g., Scott & Stradling, 1997), not only because of the distress this procedure generates directly, but also because exposure can stimulate affects related to the meaning of patients' experiences during and after the trauma. While there is no compelling evidence for the adjunctive benefits of cognitive therapy and exposure, clinical judgment may be critical in making decisions about the utility of cognitive interventions, especially for those individuals experiencing high levels of guilt or shame (Foa, 2000).

Eye Movement Desensitization and Reprocessing

Though increasingly widely employed, EMDR has been the object of sceptical debate as a consequence both of its unusual theoretical rationale and the strong claims for efficacy made by some of its proponents (Richards, 1999). Although early research into its efficacy was characterized by poor methodology (Acierno et al., 1994), more recent studies provide a better basis for a reasoned appraisal. Detailed reviews can be found in Lohr et al. (1998), Cahill et al. (1999), Spector and Read (1999), and Shepherd et al. (2000).

EMDR versus Wait List

Wilson et al. (1995) assigned 80 patients (only half of whom met full diagnostic criteria for PTSD) either to immediate or delayed EMDR, hence creating a wait-list control. Active treatment showed significant benefit over wait list, and improved patients showed maintenance of gains at 15 months (Wilson et al., 1997). Rothbaum (1997) allocated 21 women who had been raped either to EMDR or to wait list. Treated patients showed significant improvements that were maintained over 3-month follow-up.

EMDR versus Active Nonspecific Treatment

Contrasts of EMDR against treatments of known efficacy for PTSD (e.g., exposure) form a stronger test of differential efficacy than comparisons against "unvalidated" interventions. Four trials utilized as control treatments either an intervention that had no support for efficacy in relation to PTSD or standard care. Scheck et al. (1998) assigned 60 women (around 75% of whom met criteria for a diagnosis of PTSD) to two sessions of EMDR or Rogerian counseling, and found a significantly greater effect size for EMDR. Jensen (1994) allocated 25 combat veterans either to two sessions of EMDR or to treatment as usual (TAU), and found no differences between groups. Silver et al. (1995) described a program for 100 veterans who were offered EMDR, biofeedback, or relaxation training, comparing outcomes to standard treatment. However, assignment was not random, and some patients received more than one treatment, making interpretation of the apparent benefit of EMDR less clear. Carlson et al. (1998) contrasted the impact of 12 sessions of EMDR and 12 sessions of relaxation training or TAU. Nearly all the 35 patients were Vietnam veterans, and EMDR showed some benefit over relaxation and standard treatment. Marcus et al. (1997) assigned 67 patients either to EMDR or to standard care delivered in the context of a health maintenance organization (HMO; which included various psychological therapies). Those receiving EMDR showed significant benefits and utilized fewer treatment sessions.

EMDR versus Exposure-Based Interventions

Shapiro (1989a) contrasted the impact of one session of EMDR with one session of imaginal exposure in 22 subjects. Though significant results were claimed for EMDR contrasted with exposure, assessments were conducted by the therapist, and it is not clear that all patients met DSM criteria for PTSD. A larger controlled trial by this same group (Vaughn et al., 1994) allocated 36 patients to one of three treatments—EMDR, image habituation training (a form of exposure), or applied relaxation (Öst, 1987). No significant differences were found among treatments, though there was some evidence that EMDR was more successful at reducing flashbacks and nightmares. Boudewyns et al. (1993) assigned 20 veterans to EMDR with imaginal exposure and milieu therapy Though therapist ratings suggested that patients receiving EMDR improved more than those receiving the other treatments, no intergroup differences were evident on standardized assessments, nor were there any improvements over baseline on these tests. Rogers et al. (1999) assigned 12 Vietnam veterans to a single session of either EMDR or exposure. Though both groups showed equal improvement on the IES, the clinical significance of this change is not clear. The very short duration of treatment, the fact that each therapy was delivered by a different therapist, and the small sample size limit the conclusions that can be drawn from this study.

Devilly and Spence (1999) allocated 32 patients to either EMDR or a combination of exposure, SIT, and cognitive restructuring (termed trauma treatment protocol [TTP]). Applying Jacobson and Truax's (1991) criteria for clinical significance to four measures of PTSD symptoms, there was a significant advantage to TTP at posttherapy, with this advantage becoming more evident at 3-month follow-up. A clinician-rated measure (which assessed DSM criteria for PTSD) showed a significant benefit for TTP (at posttherapy, 83% of patients receiving TTP no longer met criteria for PTSD, compared to 36% receiving EMDR). However, on a self-rated measure of diagnostic status, there was no significant advantage to TTP over EMDR (on this basis, 58% of TTP patients no longer met diagnostic criteria, contrasted with 27% of those receiving EMDR). Although this appears to be robust evidence in favor of cognitive interventions, there are some difficulties in interpreting this result. First, treatment assignment for the first 20 patients was sequential rather than random (the first 10 patients received TTP, the second 10, EMDR; the remaining patients were alternated between therapies). Second, only two therapists conducted treatments, one of whom administered all the TTP interventions (raising the possibility that differences between treatments are attributable to therapists rather than orientation).

Lee et al. (2002) assigned 24 individuals with PTSD either to EMDR or to exposure combined with SIT. Both procedures showed equal efficacy. The proportion of patients receiving EMDR and exposure, who no longer met criteria for PTSD at posttherapy were 83% and 75%, respectively, and at 3-month follow-up, 83% in each condition. Ironson et al. (2002) assigned 22 patients to up to six sessions of EMDR or exposure, finding equivalent outcomes between treatments at posttherapy and at 3-month follow-up. Though there were some indications that patients showed more rapid response to EMDR (as indicated by reduction in measures of subjective distress), patients receiving exposure were initially more symptomatic than those treated with EMDR. Power et al. (2002) have conducted the largest comparison of EMDR against exposure, with 105 patients assigned to EMDR (40 patients), to exposure plus cognitive restructuring (26 patients), or to a wait-list control (29 patients). Contrasted to wait list, both active treatments were significantly more effective, but there were no significant differences between them at posttherapy or at 15-month follow-up. There were some suggestions that patients treated with EMDR showed more rapid recovery than those treated with exposure, with patients receiving on average 4.2 and 6.4 sessions, respectively.

Taylor et al. (2003) reported a carefully controlled and conducted study that compared outcomes in 60 individuals with chronic PTSD treated with exposure, EMDR, or relaxation. At 3-month follow-up, approximately 85% of those treated with exposure no longer met diagnostic criteria, contrasted to 65% for EMDR and 45% for relaxation. On this basis, although exposure was significantly more effective than relaxation, it was statistically equivalent to EMDR, and EMDR was statistically equivalent to relaxation. This pattern of trends and significance was repeated in relation to speed of change: Session-by-session analysis suggested that (on measures of avoidance) exposure had significantly more rapid impact than relaxation and was equivalent to EMDR, while EMDR exerted its effects the same rate as relaxation.

Dismantling Studies

A number of researchers have examined the mutative value of eye movements in EMDR. Montgomery and Ayllon (1994) reported results for six patients who first received all the elements of EMDR but without eye movements (patients were asked to look at a fixed point). Only when eye movements were instituted was a reduction in anxiety observed (in five of the six patients). Renfrey and Spates (1994) randomly assigned 23 patients (21 of whom met diagnostic criteria for PTSD) to standard EMDR, to a variant in which eye movements were induced by a light tracking task, or to a procedure in which they focused on a fixed stimulus. Though no standardized assessments were employed, all three treatment variants were equally effective in reducing heart rate and ratings of subjective distress.

Three further dismantling studies randomly allocated Vietnam veterans with chronic PTSD to standard EMDR or to procedures that did not employ visual tracking during exposure. Boudewyns and Hyer (1996) assigned 61 patients to standard group treatment alone, or in combination with either EMDR or EMDR in which patients kept their eyes closed during exposure. Although there were no differences in outcome between the variants of EMDR, it is also the case that there was no advantage for these procedures over standard care. Devilly et al. (1998) allocated 51 patients to standard EMDR, to a procedure in which a stationary flashing light was fixated, or to "standard psychiatric care," finding no significant differences between the variants of EMDR, both of which were more effective than standard care at posttherapy (though gains were lost across all groups at 6-month follow-up). In a somewhat methodologically ambitious study, Pitman et al. (1996) assigned 17 patients to a crossover design in which they underwent either standard EMDR or a variant in which the therapist moved her fingers, but patients were asked to tap their fingers rather than engage in visual tracking. In each condition, participants were exposed to one discrete traumatizing event, and all participants received both versions of EMDR. Overall, both groups made modest and equivalent gains (although there was some benefit for the stationary light/finger-tapping condition on avoidance, as measured on the IES). However, at 5-year follow-up, gains had been lost in both groups, and some patients appeared to have deteriorated at this point (Macklin et al., 2000). Examining a different component of the EMDR package, Cusack and Spates (1999) allocated 38 patients either to EMDR or to a variant of EMDR that did not contain some of its cognitive elements (specifically, the requirement for patients to generate a positive cognition during exposure), and found that patients in both groups improved to an equal extent.

Although there is good evidence for the efficacy of EMDR when contrasted to wait-list or nonspecific treatments, within-trial contrasts against exposure do not suggest any gains in relation to efficacy. However, there have been suggestions that EMDR represents a more efficient and better tolerated procedure than exposure (e.g., Chemtob et al., 2000). Many of the trials of EMDR against wait list reviewed earlier employ very brief interventions (ranging between two and three sessions); when trials contrast EMDR against exposure or an alternative therapy, the interventions employed are longer (ranging between 3 and 12 sessions). In fact, evidence for differential efficiency can only come from within-trial contrasts of the two techniques, and where this exists, exposure appears to be more rapid in its effects than EMDR (Taylor et al., 2003). Finally, while dismantling studies do not support the mutative value of eye movements, they all include a distraction task and to this degree do not disprove the notion that there is a benefit to combining exposure with redirection of attention. Although the theoretical argument for eye movements is unproven and unsupported by current evidence, the pragmatic benefits of elements of the EMDR procedure may require further exploration.

SUMMARY AND CLINICAL IMPLICATIONS

Though uncommon in the general population, the prevalence of PTSD among those with a history of acute trauma is markedly elevated. However, PTSD is not an inevitable consequence of trauma, and its development reflects a number of factors, including but not restricted to, the nature of the trauma itself. It is often associated with significant comorbidity. Untreated, it can be a chronic and disabling condition in a significant proportion of survivors of trauma. While earlier studies tended to focus on the sequelae of combat experiences and sexual assault, more recent trials include a broader range of patient samples, aiding generalization from research to clinical populations. Though symptoms of depression are frequently comorbid with PTSD, intervention techniques primarily focus on symptoms of anxiety.

In the immediate aftermath of disaster or trauma, some form of "psychological debriefing" is often made available, usually in the form of single-session debriefing. There is no evidence that this intervention is of benefit and some indication that it may be harmful (perhaps because in some individuals it has the potential to disrupt the development of coping strategies). More extended interventions appear to have more positive results. In the face of major incidents, services are often under some pressure to demonstrate a response, but it may be more appropriate to provide therapeutic input only to those who indicate a wish for it, and to ensure that information about the condition and access to treatment is available for those whose symptoms emerge over time.

There has been active research into the efficacy of behavioral and cognitive-behavioral techniques, EMDR, and (to a lesser degree) psychodynamic approaches. Meta-analytic review suggests that psychological treatments show efficacy; effect-sizes contrasting CBT against control treatments are large, though contrast between variants of CBT and EMDR shows an equivalence of action. The impact of psychodynamic techniques has been explored in a small number of trials, but methodological problems make it hard to discern a clear benefit.

Systematic desensitization was one of the first treatment approaches to be employed, though evidence suggests that it is ineffective. In contrast, a large number of trials offer support for the efficacy of exposure. In many trials, exposure is combined with cognitive treatments. Though this appears to be effective, research evidence for the additive benefit of cognitive technique is mixed and rather limited. However, global contrast of combinations of cognitive technique and exposure in the context of research may be less meaningful than clinical judgment in relation to individual presentations, since it seems reasonable to suppose that cognitive techniques exert impact on the acceptability of treatment. This observation may be especially important when guilt and shame are prominent; unless these feelings are addressed, it is likely that exposure alone will be difficult for patients to tolerate, because it may reevoke strong negative feeling in relation to the self.

There is good evidence for the efficacy of EMDR, and it seems to have equivalent impact to behavioral and cognitive-behavioral techniques. Though some studies have suggested that it is more rapid in its effects, this claim may not be robust. EMDR has attracted controversy, partly because of the manner in which its proponents have advocated for it, and also because its theoretical rationale places it outside conventional psychological science. In practice, many of its techniques are recognizable as part of CBT, and dismantling studies are—at the least—unpersuasive of the necessity of including some of the more controversial elements of this approach.

Some rapprochement between CBT and EMDR theory and technique seems feasible and appropriate. Although eye movements may not be a necessary part of EMDR technique, the potential benefit of a distraction task concurrent with exposure would be consonant with some cognitive neuroscience models of PTSD (e.g., Brewin, 2001), and may warrant investigation. A second point is that EMDR technique allows for exposure to very specific aspects of the traumatizing experience, an approach that is congruent with recent developments in cognitive technique (Grey et al., 2002).

While all effective techniques employ exposure, they vary in the way that they integrate this and allied psychological techniques. There are no clear research indicators as to how this is best done, or whether there are conditions under which efficacy is reliant on combinations of exposure and other approaches. This suggests that clinical judgment will be important in deciding the most appropriate treatment strategy, and that working with this population is likely to require some skillfulness, especially where presentations are complex and chronic. Specialist knowledge of this population may therefore be more critical to outcome than the choice of any specific exposure-based treatment.

CHAPTER 9

EATING DISORDERS

Anorexia Nervosa, Bulimia Nervosa, and Binge-Eating Disorder

DEFINITIONS

DSM-IV-TR assumes a diagnostic primacy for anorexia nervosa; on this basis, a diagnosis of bulimia nervosa can only be applied in the absence of anorexic features.

Anorexia Nervosa

The essential feature of this disorder is a refusal to maintain body weight at or above a minimally "normal" body weight; this is defined as a body weight 15% below that expected for the individual's age and height. To meet diagnostic criteria, there must also be an intense fear of becoming fat, even though underweight; a severe restriction of food intake, often with excessive exercising, in order to achieve weight loss; a disturbance in the way in which body weight or shape is experienced, and an undue influence of body weight or shape on self-evaluation; and (in postmenarcheal women) amenorrhea.

There are two subtypes of anorexia nervosa—binge-eating/purging type, in which there is regular binge eating or purging (self-induced vomiting, or use of laxatives or diuretics), and restricting type, in which these behaviors are not present.

Bulimia Nervosa

The main feature of this disorder is recurrent episodes of binge eating associated with a lack of control over eating behavior during the binges. Self-
induced vomiting, use of laxatives or diuretics, and strict dieting or excessive exercise are often associated features, together with a persistent
preoccupation with body size and shape. At least two binges a week over a
period of 3 months are required to make this diagnosis. As with anorexia
nervosa, self-evaluation is excessively linked to ideas about body weight
and shape.

DSM–IV–TR subtypes bulimia nervosa to purging type, in which vomiting or purging occurs, or nonpurging type, in which excessive fasting or
exercise occurs but without purging.

Eating Disorder Not Otherwise Specified

A significant proportion of individuals who present with eating disorders
meet criteria for eating disorder not otherwise specified (EDNOS). Although
their symptom patterns lie on an anorectic or bulimic spectrum, they do not
meet diagnostic criteria for anorexia or bulimia nervosa. Examples might
include women who meet all the criteria for anorexia but have regular men-
ses, or patients who meet all the criteria for bulimia, but compensatory
behaviors occur at a frequency of less than twice a week, or for less than 3
months. Although individuals with EDNOS are "subthreshold" from a
strictly diagnostic perspective, their clinical need may well be equivalent to
those meeting "full" criteria.

Within EDNOS, DSM–IV–TR also identifies binge-eating disorder, in
which binge eating takes place in the absence of other compensatory behaviors characteristic of bulimia nervosa—notably, purging.

Most research attention has been directed toward anorexia and bulimia,
though, in recent years, there has been an increasing focus on binge-eating
disorder. However, in clinical settings, a high proportion of patients present
with EDNOS; for example, Millar (1998) found that 47% of 531 consecutive
attenders at an eating disorder service met this diagnosis, contrasted to 40%
with bulimia and 13% with anorexia. Since no research studies examine outcomes in EDNOS, and the generalizability of data to individuals with
EDNOS is unclear, a certain degree of clinical judgment is required in determining the relevance of research to the individual case. Although the extent
to which patients' presentations lie along an anorectic or bulimic spectrum is
an appropriate guide, by definition, individuals with EDNOS present with a
varying admixture of symptoms, and as yet it is unclear how these should
influence treatment recommendations.

PREVALENCE, COMORBIDITY, AND NATURAL HISTORY
Prevalence

Anorexia

The prevalence of anorexia among young females varies across surveys. DSM-IV-TR estimates the prevalence of anorexia nervosa among women in late adolescence and early adulthood at between 0.5% and 1.0%. Estimates based on questionnaire alone are higher than those that adopt a two-stage procedure, in which suspected "cases" are followed up by interview. On the basis of the latter methodology, the average figure for point prevalence is rather low at 0.28% (Hoek, 2002).

Bulimia

Fairburn and Beglin (1990) reviewed studies of prevalence rates of bulimia nervosa; most focus on adolescent and young adult women. A consistent finding is a prevalence rate within this group of 1–3%.

EDNOS and Binge-Eating Disorder

Prevalence for EDNOS in young women is estimated at between 2 and 5% (Hay, 1998). Community surveys suggest prevalence rates for binge-eating disorder of 2–3% in the adult population, and 8% among obese people. Individuals with this disorder tend to have an older age profile than that for anorexia or bulimia, with most individuals with binge-eating disorder aged between 30 and 50 (Grilo, 2002).

Fairburn and Beglin (1990) caution that methodologies used to detect cases may result in an underestimation of the prevalence of eating disorders. Including individuals with subthreshold diagnoses greatly increases prevalence rates to between 5 and 15% (Herzog et al., 1991). Similarly, but more cautiously, King (1989, 1991) reports prevalence rates based on combining clear and subthreshold cases, with rates of 3.9% for women and 0.5% for men.

Differences in Prevalence Rates for Men and Women

Prevalence rates for eating disorders are lower in men than in women, though this is more pronounced for anorexia than for bulimia, and less true for binge-eating disorder. On the basis of a community sample, Woodside et al. (2001) reported prevalence rates for full-syndrome anorexia in women and men at 0.66% and 0.16%, respectively (a ratio of 4.2:1.0), and for full-syndrome bulimia at 1.46% and 0.13%, respectively (a ratio of 11.4:1.0).

However, this gender imbalance becomes less pronounced if prevalence of partial syndromes is considered: Rates for partial-syndrome anorexia for women and men are 0.76% and 1.15%, respectively (ratio 1.5:1.0) and for bulimia, 0.95% and 1.70%, respectively (ratio 1.8:1.0). Though binge-eating disorder is somewhat more common in women than in men, prevalence rates are less skewed than in other eating disorders (with a female:male ration of about 1.5:1.0) (Grilo, 2002). There is some evidence that male homosexuals are at somewhat greater risk of developing eating disorders (e.g., Russell & Keel, 2002; Williamson & Hartley, 1998).

Comorbidity

Mitchell et al. (1991) reported lifetime prevalence of comorbid depression at between 24 and 88%, with similar prevalence rates for anorexia and bulimia. Rates of substance abuse were elevated in bulimia (though not in anorexia), with lifetime prevalence rates varying between 9 and 55%. Anxiety disorders are also common; Laessle et al. (1987a) reported that 56% of a sample of bulimics had a comorbid DSM-III-R anxiety disorder, most frequently social phobia. Obsessive–compulsive disorder may be more common in anorexic patients (Holden, 1990). Mitchell et al. (1991) reported that personality disorder is common in both bulimia and anorexia, though estimates vary markedly between studies. Prevalence rates for the DSM-III-R anxious–fearful cluster range from 2 to 75%, and for the borderline, histrionic, or narcissistic cluster, from 16 to 80%. Higher levels of comorbidity are reported by studies using self-report and those that sample patients with higher levels of severity (Rosenvinge et al., 2000). The extent of variation in prevalence rates across studies is notable. This may reflect the impact of high rates of Axis I comorbidity—especially depression—on the accuracy of Axis II diagnoses, a complex issue that requires further examination (e.g., Grilo et al., 2003; O'Brien & Vincent, 2003).

Natural History

There is evidence of considerable heterogeneity in course and outcome across eating disorders, with "migration" across diagnoses being reasonably frequent (e.g., Fairburn & Harrison, 2003). Anorexia typically starts in midteen years; in some, the disorder is short-lived, but it becomes more severe in between 10 and 20% of individuals, with progression to binge-eating disorder or to bulimia in about 50% of cases (e.g., Bulik et al., 1998a). In many cases, individuals no longer meeting criteria for anorexia or bulimia will continue to have an eating disorder of clinical severity, though often this will be classified as an EDNOS. Equally (though less frequently), individuals with EDNOS can present at a later stage with anorexia or bulimia.

Anorexia Nervosa

The mean age of onset is 17 years, with some data suggesting bimodal peaks at ages 14 and 18 (DSM-IV-TR). Long-term follow-up studies are reasonably consistent in suggesting that though a proportion of anorexic patients will recover, many continue to have disordered patterns of eating, with some moving to a more bulimic pattern, or meeting criteria for EDNOS (Pike, 1998). A representative study by Lowe et al. (2001) followed up 84 patients 21 years after initial admission, classifying 51% as fully recovered and 21% partially recovered; 10% still met diagnostic criteria, and 17% had died of causes related to anorexia. Continued low weight was predictive of poorer outcome. Elevated mortality rates are linked to the consequences of anorectic restriction or associated psychiatric difficulties, with suicide a frequent cause of death. Though estimates vary across studies, from 0 to 22% (Herzog et al., 2000), a meta-analysis of 42 studies by Sullivan (1995) derived an overall death rate of 5.6% per decade of follow-up.

Bulimia Nervosa

Bulimia nervosa usually begins in late adolescence or early adulthood (DSM-IV-TR) and appears to be a chronic condition marked by frequent remissions and relapses (Herzog et al., 1991). King (1989, 1991), following progress in a community sample, suggested that untreated patients with full or partial syndromes of bulimia nervosa tend to progress in severity over 1–3 years. A community-based survey by Fairburn et al. (2000) followed up 75% of an initial cohort of 92 participants initially aged between 16 and 35 years. Initially, rates of bulimia declined rapidly, followed by a more gradual reduction (at 15 months and 5 years, rates were 31 and 15%, respectively). However, at 15 months a diagnosis of EDNOS applied to 32% (a proportion that remained stable over the follow-up period), while the combined rates for any DSM-IV-TR eating disorder were 66% at 15 months and 49% at 5 years.

Extended follow-up moderates—at least to some degree—this somewhat pessimistic picture. Collings and King (1994) followed up 50 patients 10 years after they had participated in a medication trial; of 37 patients traced, 62% had recovered. Similarly, Fairburn et al. (1995) found that of 91 patients followed up approximately 6 years after psychological treatment, 54% had recovered. Steinhausen et al. (2000) examined a cohort of 60 adolescents, initially hospitalized between 1979 and 1988, at both 5 and 11 years. The significant levels of eating disorder symptoms present at intermediate follow-up had reduced by 11 years—at this point, an 80% recovery rate was observed. Keel et al. (1999) followed up 80% of 222 participants in two studies conducted in 1981 and 1987, finding that diagnosed rates of bulimia reduced as follow-up periods increased. However, approximately 30% continued to engage in bingeing or purging behaviors.

Most information regarding the natural history of these disorders is derived from patients seen in tertiary care settings; the prognosis for individuals with subthreshold symptoms and those seen in primary care or community settings may be more benign.

TREATMENTS FOR ANOREXIA NERVOSA

Though case reports are relatively common, there are few comparative trials of psychotherapies for anorexia nervosa. In routine practice, a range of individual therapies are employed (including behavioral, cognitive-behavioral, and psychodynamic techniques), though not all of these have been researched. Family therapies are also common, usually aiming to ameliorate the disruptions and distortions of family life created by the disorder (without the implication that family patterns are in themselves pathogenic). Most treatments recognize the critical importance of establishing an appropriate dietary regimen, and this is usually a common element across interventions.

Individual and Family Therapies

Inpatient treatment for anorexia nervosa, usually combines medical care with programs aimed at increasing weight. Schwartz and Thompson (1981) reviewed 12 outcome studies of inpatient treatments for such a regimen, finding that on follow-up there was a 6% mortality rate from self-starvation, and that though 49% had recovered from anorexia, 31% continued to have eating disorders and 18% showed no significant change.

Hall and Crisp (1987) treated 30 anorexic patients, contrasting 12 sessions of "dietary advice" with psychotherapy. Psychotherapy included both individual psychodynamic and family therapy, depending on the willingness of families to be involved in treatment. There was some overlap between treatment conditions, since dietary advice included discussion of mood and behavior, and psychotherapy included discussion of dietary matters. Both groups showed improvements at 1-year follow-up, though only the dietary group showed significant pre- to posttherapy weight gain. In the psychotherapy group, weight loss in three patients masked overall weight gain in the remaining clients. Those receiving psychotherapy had better social and sexual adjustment, though global clinical ratings were equivalent between treatment groups.

Russell et al. (1987) contrasted family therapy and individual supportive therapy in 80 inpatients, 57 of whom were anorexic and 23 bulimic. Individual therapy was eclectic, and included cognitive, interpretive, and strategic techniques. Outcome was assessed on a number of symptom measures and on weight gain. Although the mean weight of anorexic patients increased significantly, categorical assignment on the basis of clinical measures indicated only moderate gains; 23% of patients had a good outcome, 16% an intermediate outcome, and 61% a poor outcome at 1-year follow-up. However, there were indications of differential impacts of therapies depending on the age of onset of the disorder. Patients with an onset before age 18 appeared to respond better to family therapy, whereas those whose difficulties began at 19 years or older did better with individual therapy. Eisler et al. (1997) reported 5-year follow-up of this study, classifying participants into three subgroups— early onset (before age 18) with a short or a long history, or late onset (after age 18). At this point, patients presenting with a late onset or with an early onset but a long history tended to have poorer outcomes than patients with early onset and short history. In this latter group, those who had received family therapy had better outcomes than those who received individual therapy.

Channon et al. (1989) contrasted cognitive-behavioral therapy (CBT), behavior therapy, and (as a control) nonspecific support in 24 patients with anorexia; given the medical condition of patients, a wait-list control was felt to be unethical. Both CBT and behavioral treatment included self-monitoring and dietary planning; behavior therapy also included gradual exposure to avoided foods, whereas CBT identified dysfunctional beliefs about eating. No differences were found between treatment groups or between the treatment groups and routine treatment, though the very small number of patients in each treatment arm limits interpretation of this result.

Le Grange et al. (1992) conducted a pilot study of the efficacy two forms of family interventions. Although they share a number of features, in "separated family therapy" (SFT), the parents are seen separately from the child; in the other, conjoint family therapy (CFT), the family is seen as one unit. Eighteen patients (all adolescents, with a mean age of 15, and including two boys) were randomly assigned to therapy; at 1-year follow-up, there were similar benefits from each treatment. Eisler et al. (2000) reported a larger trial of this approach in 40 adolescents. Both interventions took place over 1 year. Recovery was defined as the restoration of $\geq 85\%$ of average body weight (ABW), the return of menstruation, and no bulimic symptoms; this criterion was met by 5 (26%) and 10 (48%) of the CFT- and SFT-treated patients, respectively. Significant improvement was defined as a similar weight gain, but with no menstruation and/or occasional bulimic symptoms; this criterion was met by 4 (21%) and 6 (29%) of the CFT and SFT patients, respectively. Although this trial offers some evidence favoring SFT in relation to measures directly related to eating disorder symptomatology, CFT had greater impact on measures of psychological functioning.

Dare et al. (2001) contrasted standard care with three active treatments: (1) family therapy over 1 year, (2) focal psychodynamic therapy over 1 year, or (3) cognitive analytic therapy (CAT; Ryle, 1990) over 7 months. Eighty-four patients were recruited, with a mean age of approximately 26; two men were included in the sample. Using the same criteria as in Eisler et al. (2000), rates of recovery of significant improvement at the end of treatment were 33% for patients receiving focal therapy, 36% for those treated with family therapy, 27% for those receiving CAT, and only 5% of those in standard care. Although family and focal therapy showed significantly greater gains than standard care, there were no significant differences between treatments. While the majority of patients had relatively poor outcomes, patients in this trial had a long history of illness and of unsuccessful prior treatment, making generalization to the broader clinical population more difficult. It should also be noted that standard care comprised relatively brief outpatient sessions with supervised but junior psychiatrists. This contrasts markedly with the specialist experience available to patients in the experimental conditions; though this suggests that routine care is unlikely to benefit these patients, it is somewhat equivocal as to the degree of specialization required for effective intervention.

Treasure et al. (1995) treated 30 outpatients with anorexia randomly allocated either to CAT or to an educational–behavioral treatment. Behavioral treatment included dietary education, whereas CAT maintained a largely interpersonal focus. Therapies were offered weekly over 20 weeks, and though therapists were supervised weekly, they were inexperienced in the therapies they were delivering. Patients in both treatment groups showed weight gain sustained over 1-year follow-up. Although patients receiving CAT reported greater subjective improvement than those receiving the behavioral intervention, there were no significant differences between treatment groups on measures of weight gain.

Geist et al. (2000) randomized 25 female adolescents to one of two interventions over a 4-month period—family therapy (which contained dietary advice and aimed to facilitate family communication and parental management of the disorder) or group psychoeducation sessions (each of which was attended by up to seven patients and their families). All participants were inpatients in a specialist unit and also received medical interventions aimed at weight restoration, along with a number of psychosocial interventions. Though at 4 months both groups showed significant weight gains, it is not clear whether these were additional to those conferred by routine care. Furthermore, measures of eating disorder pathology showed little change, and a significant proportion of patients were readmitted after the trial ended. While the study population was severely ill, the pattern of outcomes highlights the fact that posttherapy weight gain alone is an inadequate measure of outcome.

Serfaty et al. (1999) allocated 25 largely adolescent patients to 20 sessions of cognitive therapy and 10 to the same number of sessions of dietary advice (with the inbalance in numbers reflecting the number of available therapists in each modality). After 6 months, significant pre- to post improvements were evident in those treated with cognitive therapy. However, all those receiving dietary advice had dropped out, making contrasts between the therapeutic modalities inappropriate, and raising questions about the acceptability of this approach.

The trials described previously focus on adolescents or young adults. Pike et al. (2003) recruited 33 older patients (between ages 18 and 45), representing a unique study of interventions for adults with anorexia. All were recruited as inpatients, and eligibility for trial entry was conditional on successful restoration of weight—in a sense, making this a study of relapse prevention. Participants were randomized to manualized CBT or nutritional counseling, with 50 sessions of therapy offered over 1 year (a longer period than in trials reported earlier). "Relapse" was defined as weight loss below 80% of ideal or reemergence of relevant medical or psychiatric symptomatology. On this basis, there was a significant difference in relapse rates between treatments: 53% of those receiving nutritional counseling relapsed over the treatment period contrasted to 22% of the CBT group. A criterion of good outcome based on weight gain was met by 44% of CBT contrasted to 7% of nutritional counseling patients. More robust recovery criteria, which included assessment of disordered attitudes toward eating and bingeing and purging behaviors, were met by 17% and 0% of the CBT and nutritional counseling patients, respectively.

Inpatient versus Outpatient Treatment

Though questions about how to treat anorexia are more central than where this should take place (Crisp, 2002), the relative cost of in- and outpatient programs makes treatment location a legitimate concern. Meads et al. (2001) identified two randomized controlled trials (RCTs), only one of which (Crisp et al., 1991, discussed below) contained adequate trial data, and seven case series. Unfortunately, the case series was hard to interpret, because allocation to in or outpatient care was not randomized, potentially confusing severity of disorder with outcome. Although Meads et al. concluded that there were no additional benefits to inpatient compared to outpatient treatment, this conclusion is largely based on Crisp et al.'s (1991) study, which reports 1-year outcomes for 90 severe anorexics randomly allocated to one of four treatment conditions. Inpatient treatment comprised a package of behavioral techniques aimed at restoring weight, coupled with weekly individual therapy, group therapy, family therapy, dietary advice, and a range of milieu treatments. On discharge, patients were seen for 12 weeks of outpatient therapy. Two outpatient treatments were also offered (both of which included dietary advice). In the first, patients received 12 sessions of psychodynamic individual or family therapy. In the second, they were given 10 sessions of group therapy, which appear to have been structured and topic-based. The three treatment groups were contrasted with patients seen only for assessment and referred back to their general practitioner or consultant, and who then received a variety of unmonitored treatments.

At 1 year, patients in all treatment conditions showed improvements. However, this was most striking for both outpatient groups, which showed significant gains contrasted to patients who had only received assessment. Though inpatient treatment resulted in greater posttherapy gains than the other conditions, significantly greater relapse was evident at follow-up. Gowers et al. (1994) report a 2-year follow-up of patients treated with outpatient therapy and those receiving only a one-off assessment. Gains were maintained by those treated with outpatient psychotherapy, who continued to show better weight maintenance than those receiving assessment alone.

Though this study suggests that even patients at the more serious end of the anorexic spectrum can be treated as outpatients, it should be recognized that clinicians have little research to guide them when admission is being considered as an option. Although, in practice, the need for medical intervention may act as a driver (e.g., Gowers et al., 1994), further research is needed to clarify the short- and long-term benefits of treatment location.

Adherence to Treatment, Relapse, and Relapse Prevention

Using a psychological intervention with patients with anorexia is a particular challenge, since many patients are poorly motivated to change their eating patterns, and (certainly in younger patients) it is often family members or individuals other than the patients who initiate referral. Attrition from clinical trials is relatively high, though there is considerable variation even within the same research group (e.g., rates in Eisler et al. [2000] and Dare et al. [2001] were 10% and 35%, respectively). Relapse rates after intervention range from 30 to 50%, 1 year after discharge (Pike, 1998). There are only broad indications of factors linked to prognosis: Low weight at referral is associated with poorer outcome (Pike, 1998), and (as noted earlier) also signals a poorer long-term outlook. The pattern of weight gain during treatment may be relevant. Lay et al. (2002) found that better outcomes were associated with the speed of weight increase during inpatient treatment and the duration for which patients maintained their target weight. A number of workers have focused on the relevance of motivation (e.g., Leung et al., 1999) and compliance (Towell et al., 2001) to outcome, and a broader review of treatment approaches (Kaplan, 2002) suggests an explicit role for motivational enhancement. Although some studies have demonstrated that it is possible to enhance levels of motivation for change (e.g., R. Field et al., 2001), this has not yet been linked to outcome.

Most reviewers recognize that more comparative trials are required in order to reach definitive conclusions about the efficacy of interventions (e.g., Kaplan, 2002; Treasure & Kordy, 1998). Those that are available often suffer from inadequate initial sample sizes, further reduced by high levels of attrition. The individuals with anorexia included in trials are skewed toward more serious presentations, often seen in the context of specialized services, making generalizations more difficult. Although the need for randomized trials remains, a helpful and alternative strategy is the European Collaborative Longitudinal Observational Study on Eating Disorders (ECLOS-ED), a multinational, multisite study using standardized outcome measures to assess the effectiveness of interventions in a projected sample of some 5,000 individuals.

TREATMENTS FOR BULIMIA NERVOSA
Meta-Analyses

Given the relatively small set of studies available for review, there are a large number of meta-analyses. Hartmann et al. (1992), Hay and Bacaltchuk (2001), and Thompson-Brenner et al. (2003) reviewed trials of psychological therapies; both Lewandowski et al. (1997) and Ghaderi and Andersson (1999) focused on outcomes for CBT. Laessle et al. (1987b) reviewed both psychological and pharmacological interventions, while Whittal et al. (1999) and Bacaltchuk et al. (2000, 2001) considered the relative impacts of pharmacotherapy and psychotherapy.

Psychological Therapies Alone

Laessle et al.'s (1987b) early review has less rigorous selection criteria than later analyses, and little overlap with them; it includes many studies with very few patients and a number of uncontrolled studies. Most trials were of CBT, and most medication trials employed tricyclic antidepressants. On the single measure of binge eating, an overall effect size of 0.95 was found. Psychological therapies including dietary management had a higher effect size than those without (1.30 and 1.14, respectively). The mean effect size for medications (0.60) was lower than that for either psychotherapeutic technique.

Hartmann et al. (1992) examined 18 studies carried out before 1990, some of which were very small scale. The 18 trials reported on 24 treatment groups (433 patients) and 6 control groups (61 patients). Most studies utilized cognitive or cognitive-behavioral interventions; five studies examined the impact of humanistic and psychodynamic interventions. Pre- to post-treatment change in the control groups was negligible (mean effect size =

0.18), indicating that there is little spontaneous remission for bulimia nervosa. For therapy of any type, the mean effect size was 1.04. Treatments employing 15 or more sessions had larger effect sizes (mean effect size = 1.37); those with less than 13 sessions had a mean effect size of 0.79 (though this effect was restricted to the number of sessions rather than the duration of treatment). As in the earlier review, though most studies cite outcomes for bingeing or purging, fewer report data on changes in weight or on broader indices of psychological status.

Lewandowski et al. (1997) identified 26 studies of CBT, though it should be noted that five of these were very small scale (with less than 10 participants), and some were uncontrolled studies. Significant pre- to posttherapy effect sizes were identified both for behavioral measures of outcome (between-groups effect size = 0.69) and on measures of cognitive or attitudinal change (between-groups effect size = 0.64). However, on both indices, effect sizes at follow-up were small (0.24 and 0.32, respectively). A similar pattern of outcomes was identified by Ghaderi and Anderson (1999), using a more restricted pool of seven RCTs of CBT. On measures of bingeing and purging, respectively, between groups pre- to posttherapy effect sizes were 0.47 and 0.58.

Hay and Bacaltchuk (2001) reviewed 27 trials of psychological therapy; most studies employed CBT, with only seven available contrasts to alternative psychological interventions. On a categorical measure of rates of abstinence from binge eating, CBT showed significant advantage to wait-list control (relative risk reduction = 0.64) but was equivalent in action to alternative active psychological interventions (relative risk = 0.80), both on this measure and on most measures of psychological functioning. However, there was significant advantage to CBT over other therapies on measures of depression. On the basis of data from four studies, therapist-guided CBT was as effective as self-help.

Thompson-Brenner et al. (2003) identified 26 trials published between 1980 and 2000. The majority of these employed CBT or behavioral techniques; only eight trials had follow-up data of 12-month or greater duration. As in earlier meta-analyses, posttherapy effect sizes were large: Contrast of treatment versus control on measures of binge eating and purging were 0.88 and 1.01, respectively. Effect sizes for CBT and behavior therapy did not significantly differ; on measures of purging, respective effect sizes were 0.79 and 0.90. Across all treatments, the percentage of patients classified as recovered was 40% in the treatment-completer sample and 33% in the intent-to-treat (ITT) sample. There was a significantly higher recovery rate from individual as opposed to group therapies (46% and 27%, respectively, in completers, and 37% and 21% in the ITT sample).

Although there were clear indications of improvement, at termination patients still exhibited significant symptomatology, with an average of 1.7

bingeing and 2.3 purging episodes per week. Of the eight available follow-up studies, all employed CBT or behavioral techniques. At follow-up 44% of patients met criteria for recovery. Four studies identified patients who met criteria for recovery both at posttherapy and at follow-up, a status met by just 32% of patients.

Subanalyses suggested that later publication is associated with larger effect sizes (suggesting that treatments are becoming more effective), and with smaller treatment–control effects (with increasing use of placebo rather than wait-list control).

Psychological Therapies Alone and in Combination with Medication

Whittal et al. (1999) contrast the efficacy of antidepressants (nine trials), CBT (26 trials), or (in four trials) the combination of the two. Effect sizes for CBT alone were higher than for medication alone on measures of bingeing, purging, and depression. Combined treatment was more effective than medication alone on these measures, and more effective than CBT on measures of bingeing but not on measures of purging. Bacaltchuk et al. (2000, 2001) considered the same contrasts in seven studies. All employed individual or group CBT; pharmacotherapy comprised fluoxetine, desimipramine, or imipramine, and "remission" was defined as the absence of binge eating at posttherapy. Contrasting antidepressants alone to psychological treatment alone (three studies) yielded statistically equivalent remission rates of 20% and 39%, respectively; contrasting combination treatment to medication alone (four trials) remission rates were 42% versus 23% (NNT [number needed to treat] = 5), and combined treatment to psychological treatment (seven trials), 49% versus 36% (NNT = 8). In these studies, attrition was higher when medication was employed. In the contrast of psychotherapy to antidepressant, dropout rates were 18% and 41%, respectively, and for combination therapy versus antidepressant, 35% and 41%, respectively. Though this appears to suggest an advantage to combination over unitary-mode therapy (a conclusion that needs to be balanced by the apparent reduction in acceptability of the combination intervention to patients), these analyses are based on a small number of trials, each with few participants. Without further trials, any conclusion should be viewed as tentative.

Individual Treatment Approaches

Behavioral Approaches (Exposure and Response Prevention)

As is clear from meta-analytic reviews, CBT is the most frequently researched approach, though this can contain behavioral procedures that are analogous to ERP, in which patients are exposed to food and encouraged to delay vomiting and purging. Carter and Bulik (1994) review studies of ERP, noting that, within the literature, distinctions are made between exposure to purging cues and exposure to prebingeing cues. However, in practice, procedures often seem to expose patients to both sets of cues, and this may be more a theoretical than a practical issue.

Leitenberg et al. (1988), with a sample of 47 women with bulimia, contrasted ERP conducted either in a single or in multiple settings, CBT, and a wait-list control All three treatments resulted in significant gains, though multiple-setting exposure resulted in the lowest rates of purging at 6-month follow-up, followed by single setting and CBT. However, cognitive techniques were employed in the exposure treatments (e.g., patients were taught to identify and challenge distorted thoughts during exposure), and this study might be best viewed as demonstrating the benefits of adding exposure to CBT.

In contrast, Wilson et al. (1986) found only limited, nonsignificant benefit for the addition of CBT, Wilson et al. (1991) found that it had no effect, and Agras et al. (1989) found that it had a deleterious effect. These differences in outcome may be accounted for by differing emphases on CBT and exposure in each study—Agras et al.'s (1989) trial, for example, devoted less time to exposure sessions than the other trials reported here, perhaps leading to inadequate implementation of the technique.

There are few studies examining the efficacy of exposure alone as a treatment for bulimia; most are very small-scale or single-case studies (Jansen et al., 1989; Rossiter & Wilson, 1985; Schmidt & Marks, 1988). In two slightly larger trials (Jansen et al., 1992; Schmidt & Marks, 1989), reductions in bingeing and purging were evident. However, only Jansen et al.'s (1989) study included a control treatment. There is therefore little reliable evidence for the efficacy of exposure and response prevention alone.

Bulik et al. (1998b) assessed the incremental benefit of ERP to CBT (rather than directly contrasting these approaches). One hundred thirty-five patients were assigned to one of two forms of exposure after they had received eight sessions of CBT—either to cues that usually triggered bulimia, or to cues associated with purging. A third treatment arm acted as a control, with CBT followed by relaxation training. At the end of first phase of treatment with CBT, there were significant improvements in eating behavior, but the addition of ERP did not appear to enhance the treatment effect; though there was some evidence of further improvement with the addition of more therapy sessions, there were no differences in outcome across groups. Three-year follow-up of 113 participants (F. A. Carter et al., 2003) found good maintenance of gains across all conditions but, again, no indication of advantage to the addition of exposure. Interpretation of this study is difficult, since it sets out to examine additive benefits (of which there is little evidence) rather than directly contrast ERP to CBT.

Cognitive-Behavioral Therapy

Cognitive therapies typically contain an educational component, self-monitoring and self-regulatory strategies, the examination of dysfunctional attitudes toward eating, the management of purging, and the reestablishment of control over eating. Relapse prevention strategies are usually a part of this package.

Craighead and Agras (1991), Mitchell (1991), and Wilson and Fairburn (1993) reviewed among them 18 controlled studies of CBT for bulimia nervosa; unsurprisingly, there is considerable overlap among these accounts. Most trials contrast highly structured therapies that contain techniques from CBT or behavior therapy. Around half the studies employ group approaches, with the remainder using either individual therapy or, more rarely, a mix of group and individual therapy.

Craighead and Agras (1991) reviewed 10 studies of CBT for bulimia nervosa; using the average of mean reductions in binge eating and purging, across studies there was a mean reduction in purging of 79%, with 59% of patients in remission. However, contrasting measures of outcome based on symptom reduction with measures based on a criteria of clinically significant improvement yields somewhat less striking results. In Mitchell's review, the mean percentage reduction in binge-eating frequency pre- to posttreatment across 23 studies is 69.9% (range 40–95%), while the mean percentage of patients found to be free of symptoms at the end of treatment is markedly lower, at 32.8% (0–71%). In four of the most recent controlled trials reviewed by Wilson and Fairburn (1993), the mean percentage reduction in binge eating was 73–93% and for purging, 77–94%. Again however, mean remission rates were lower—from 51 to 71% for binge eating and from 36 to 56% for purging (Agras et al., 1989, 1992; Fairburn et al., 1991; Garner et al., 1993; Mitchell et al., 1990).

COGNITIVE-BEHAVIORAL AND OTHER THERAPIES VERSUS ANTIDEPRESSANTS

All studies tend to involve self-monitoring of eating behavior, a technique that Agras et al. (1989) suggest has some therapeutic benefit in itself. Mitchell et al. (1990) employed four treatment conditions: group therapy using CBT principles combined either with imipramine or with placebo, imipramine alone, and placebo alone. Imipramine alone was superior to placebo but inferior to CBT combined with either medication or placebo. In the two CBT conditions, mean reductions in binge eating were 83% and 92%, respectively, contrasted with 34% and 9% for imipramine and placebo alone. Fifty-one percent of those receiving CBT were in remission posttreatment, contrasted with 16% of those receiving imipramine. Though imipramine had no effect on bulimic symptoms, it did improve mood and anxiety symptoms. All patients who had responded to "treatment" (defined as no more than two purges over the last 2 weeks of treatment) were assigned to a 4-month maintenance program and followed up 6 months after treatment was initiated (Pyle et al., 1990). Relapse was greatest in patients receiving imipramine (67%) or placebo (83%), and lowest for those receiving CBT (22 and 31%, respectively).

Agras et al. (1992) contrasted CBT alone, desipramine alone, and the two treatments in combination. The study design was complex, with medication withdrawn at either 16 or 24 weeks and CBT administered for 16 weeks, leading to a total of five contrasts. At 16 weeks, CBT and combination therapy were superior to medication alone in reducing binge eating and purging. At 32 weeks, patients receiving CBT alone and CBT in combination with medication (continued for 24 weeks) had better outcomes than those given medication for 16 weeks, suggesting that the addition of CBT acts to prevent relapse. This pattern was maintained at 1-year follow-up (Agras et al., 1994a).

Leitenberg et al. (1994) assigned patients to three conditions—CBT alone, desipramine alone, and CBT and desipramine in combination. Although the original design planned for 12 patients in each condition, as the trial progressed, it became evident that patients receiving desipramine alone were responding poorly and dropping out. This led the investigators to discontinue the trial early, when only seven patients had been assigned to each condition.

CBT alone was biweekly for 2 weeks, and weekly for a further 18 sessions, and followed Fairburn's (1985) model, with the addition of exposure to feared foods. Patients receiving desipramine alone met once a week for medication management; therapists were scrupulous in avoiding offering any discussion or advice regarding bulimic symptoms. Four of the seven patients dropped out of the desipramine-alone condition, contrasted to one in the CBT and two in the combined conditions. The reasons given for dropout usually related to side effects or the patient's expressed wish for a broader treatment approach. On a range of measures, CBT appeared to show benefit at both posttreatment and 6-month follow-up; the combined treatment appeared to confer no greater gains than CBT alone, and the high rate of dropout from the desipramine condition made data analysis meaningless.

Goldbloom et al. (1997) compared fluoxetine alone, CBT alone, and their combination in 76 patients. After 16 weeks of treatment, patients evinced clinical improvement in all three conditions. Though, on some measures, combination treatment showed a significant advantage over medication alone, it was no more effective than CBT alone. However, there was substantial attrition across all arms of the trial.

Jacobi et al. (2002) allocated 53 patients to 20 weeks of group-based

CBT alone, fluoxetine alone, or a combination of the two, reporting results both at posttherapy and at 1 year. Though all three treatments led to significant reduction in frequency of bingeing and purging, there was no evidence that adding medication to CBT enhanced its efficacy. Interpretation of results from this study are limited both by high refusal rates after initial randomization and high attrition rates (particularly and unusually from the CBT arm of the trial).

These trials (which suggest that there is no additional treatment benefit from the addition of medication to CBT) contrast outcomes from Walsh et al. (1997), who adopted a two-stage approach to medication (desipramine followed by flouxetine, if there was no appropriate treatment response). One hundred twenty patients were randomized to five treatment arms—active medication alone, or medication in combination with psychodynamically oriented psychotherapy or with CBT; within each of the psychological therapy arms, half the patients received active medication, and half, placebo. Remission rates for binge eating and vomiting favored CBT over supportive therapy. The addition of medication to CBT enhanced outcomes relative both to medication alone and to CBT in combination with placebo; in contrast, medication did not enhance outcomes with supportive therapy.

Tuschen-Caffier et al. (2001) reported an open trial of manualized CBT for 73 women presenting for treatment in a standard outpatient program, setting out to benchmark outcomes against research. Though marred by minor changes in assessment procedures over the period of the study and low rates of follow-up, there were indications that outcomes in this unselected sample were equivalent to those in studies reported earlier.

COGNITIVE-BEHAVIORAL THERAPY VERSUS SUPPORTIVE THERAPY

Two trials have contrasted CBT against supportive psychotherapy combined with self-monitoring (though, as noted earlier, self-monitoring may in itself be helpful, reducing any likely between-treatment variance). Kirley et al. (1985), employing group therapy, found CBT to be superior in its effect at posttreatment, though at 4-month follow-up there were no between-treatment differences. Agras et al. (1989) found that CBT offered individually was more effective than supportive psychotherapy at both posttreatment and at 6-month follow-up.

Freeman et al. (1988) contrasted CBT, behavior therapy, group psychotherapy, and a wait-list control, finding that all treatments were equally effective, and all were superior to control patients. Fairburn et al. (1986) found that CBT and a brief focal psychotherapy (focused not on eating problems but on understanding triggers for maladaptive eating) were equally effective in managing binge eating and purging, though CBT appeared to be somewhat more effective in reducing other symptoms, such as depression.

COGNITIVE-BEHAVIORAL THERAPY VERSUS NUTRITIONAL ADVICE/THERAPY

Hsu et al. (2001) randomized 100 participants to 14 weeks of CBT alone, to nutritional therapy alone, to CBT and nutritional therapy combined, or to a self-help support group. In this trial, CBT alone was offered without nutritional advice in order to highlight any contrast with nutritional counseling, making it somewhat distinct from CBT treatments described elsewhere in this section, and akin to a dismantling study. Overall, efficacy was greatest with the addition of the cognitive component, whether alone or in combination. Contrasted to the support group, only combined treatment showed significantly higher abstinence rates for vomiting and purging in the week preceding posttherapy (52 and 24%, respectively), suggesting the benefit of each element of the treatment.

COGNITIVE-BEHAVIORAL THERAPY VERSUS INTERPERSONAL PSYCHOTHERAPY

Fairburn et al. (1991) contrasted CBT, behavior therapy, and interpersonal psychotherapy (IPT) in 75 patients. Posttherapy, IPT performed more poorly than either behavior therapy or CBT. However, follow-up at 4, 8, and 12 months indicated that behavior therapy patients showed a significantly higher rate of relapse than the other treatment conditions, most usually within the first 4 months of follow-up. In contrast, those receiving IPT continued to improve. At 12 months, the proportion of patients meeting a strict criterion of recovery and no relapse were 44% for IPT, 35% for CBT, and 20% for behavior therapy. In addition, 48% of patients treated with behavior therapy dropped out during the trial or were withdrawn because of their worsening condition (Fairburn et al., 1993).

These trends appear to be maintained over the longer term. Ninety-one patients (from studies reported in Fairburn et al., 1986, 1991) were followed up at a mean of 5.8 years (Fairburn et al., 1995). "Remission" (defined as the absence of any DSM-IV-TR eating disorder) was significantly more frequent in patients who had received either CBT or IPT/focal therapy (63 and 72%, respectively) than those who had received behavior therapy (14%). Much of this difference is accounted for by the high proportion of behavior therapy patients who received a follow-up diagnosis of EDNOS; the proportion of patients diagnosed with bulimia nervosa or anorexia nervosa at follow-up was approximately equal across treatments.

A larger, multisite study (Agras et al., 2000b) aimed to replicate the CBT and IPT contrasts of the Fairburn trial, randomizing 220 patients to 19 sessions of these treatments, and following up patients over 1 year. Broadly, a similar pattern of results was obtained. Patients were classified as recovered if, over the previous 28 days, they had not binged or purged, and as remitted if they binged or purged less than twice a week in this period. On this basis, at posttherapy, CBT patients were more likely to have recovered than those receiving IPT (29 vs. 6%), or to have remitted (48 vs. 28%). At 4-month and 1-year follow-up, there was evidence of a slight decline in the proportion of CBT-treated patients remaining well, and a slight improvement in those treated with IPT, such that by 1 year, there was no statistical difference between the two groups. This pattern of outcomes does suggests a faster response to CBT, and the (untested) possibility that IPT achieves its impact less through direct modification of eating behavior than through amelioration of depressive symptoms and interpersonal factors that maintain problem eating.

Wilfley et al. (1993) examined the efficacy of group CBT and group IPT in nonpurging bulimics. Fifty-six patients were assigned to wait-list control or to treatment, which comprised 16 weekly sessions. Posttherapy, both treatment groups showed significant and equivalent improvement in binge eating contrasted to controls; these gains were sustained at 6-month and at 1-year follow-up.

COGNITIVE-BEHAVIORAL THERAPY VERSUS PSYCHODYNAMIC THERAPY

Garner et al. (1993) contrasted CBT with psychodynamic therapy (supportive–expressive psychotherapy; Luborsky, 1984) in 50 patients with bulimia. Both treatments were effective in reducing binge eating, though CBT was more effective in improving purging, and had more impact on attitudes toward eating and on measures of psychological distress. Follow-up data have not been reported, though Fairburn et al.'s (1993) data suggest that this may be critical to any conclusions about differential therapeutic efficacy. Bachar et al. (1999) allocated 33 patients to nutritional counseling alone or to nutritional therapy combined with psychodynamic therapy (based on Kohut's self psychology) or "cognitive orientation" therapy (COT, which focuses on beliefs but has important differences from CBT, as described in other studies); both active therapies were offered over 1 year. Though there appeared to be significant advantage on some measures to psychodynamic therapy over nutritional counseling alone, COT had no additional benefit. However, interpretation of this result is complicated by the inclusion of eight participants with anorexia; attempts to separate results by each condition render the sample size inappropriately small.

The trials reviewed here offer some, though limited, evidence for mode-specific effects for CBT over other therapies. Thus, studies show evidence of a reduction in dietary restraint (Fairburn et al., 1991; Garner et al., 1993; Wilson et al., 1991), more food eaten between bulimic episodes (Rossiter et al., 1988), and better attitudes toward body size and shape (Fairburn et al., 1993; Garner et al., 1993; Wilson et al., 1991). However, studies by Fairburn et al. (1993), Wilfley et al. (1993), and Agras et al. (2000a, 2000b), though based on slightly different patient populations, suggest that IPT may be equally effective despite an apparently broader focus.

Dialectical Behavior Therapy

DBT assumes that eating patterns reflect attempts to control emotional dysregulation; to date, only one small trial has examined its efficacy (Safer et al., 2001). Thirty-one participants were randomized to 20 weeks of DBT or to wait list, resulting in a significant reduction in bingeing and purging.

Overall Recovery and Relapse

Relapse after treatment is relatively common. In a broader review of long-term outcomes for bulimia, Keel and Mitchell (1997) identified 18 studies in which patients were followed up after treatment for between 6 months and 9 years (though the most usual period was between 6 and 12 months). Across these studies, there is a rather wide range of outcomes, with remission rates varying from 5 to 83%, and the number of fully symptomatic patients between 5 and 79%, with a mean percentage of 28%. Fairburn et al. (1993) found that although 44% of patients achieved abstinence from bingeing and purging at posttherapy, 27% had relapsed at 1 year, with level of self-esteem and cognitions relating to ideas about weight and shape predicting outcome. Halmi et al. (2002) identified 57 patients who achieved abstinence from bingeing and purging after treatment with 16 weeks of CBT (described in Agras et al., 2000b), but had relapsed at 4-month follow-up (representing a 44% relapse rate). These patients had higher levels of preoccupation with eating and were less likely to have achieved a period of continuous abstinence during treatment (possibly suggesting the utility of monitoring progress and adjusting treatment duration accordingly—an approach adopted by Eldredge et al., 1997, discussed below).

Stepped Care and Self-Help

There have been a number of studies of the efficacy of self-help manuals (most of which adopt a CBT model), sometimes against wait-list control and other times contrasted to varying levels of therapist input (e.g., J. C. Carter et al., 2003; Cooper et al., 1994, 1996; Ghaderi & Scott, 2003; Mitchell et al., 2001; Palmer et al., 2002; Thiels et al., 1998; Treasure et al., 1994, 1996). Ostensibly, these studies suggest that therapist contact does not necessarily enhance outcomes, though this conclusion is tempered by methodological problems (Wilson et al., 2000). Overall, the efficacy of self-help seems greatest when combined with at least some level of therapist input, in part because this ensures greater fidelity to the treatment program. As an example, Carter and Fairburn (1998) allocated 72 women to pure self-help or to guided self-help (which comprised six to eight brief sessions in which clients reviewed the book with a facilitator); a subgroup was allocated to wait list and subsequently to one of the two active treatments. Contrasted to wait list, there were significant and equivalent reductions in binge-eating episodes in both active interventions, though at 3 and 6 months, there was advantage to guided self-help. Subanalyses indicated that only 6% of pure self-help participants completed the program, contrasted to 68% of those receiving guided help, and 89% sought additional therapies during the treatment or follow-up (compared to 32% of the guided self-help group). Both findings represent a threat to the internal validity of the study and are suggestive both of the importance of therapist contact and the possibility that one impact of pure self-help was an enhanced motivation for treatment. Palmer et al. (2002) randomized 120 patients to wait-list, to pure self-help, to self-help with telephone guidance or self-help with face-to-face guidance—each condition representing incremental additions in therapist contact. Four sessions of therapist contact were provided over 4 months; at the end of this period, only patients receiving face-to-face guidance showed significant advantage to wait list, though the data were suggestive of the benefits of providing guidance for patients.

The use of a stepped-care approach to bulimia has been discussed by a number of authors (e.g., Wilson et al., 2000), in part based on evidence that psychoeducational approaches can help at least some patients. Rather few trials are available to assess the appropriateness of this approach. J. C. Carter et al. (2003) allocated 85 women on a wait list for treatment to one of two self-help manuals or to a wait-list control over 8 weeks. One manual gave advice on the management of bulimia, while the other acted as a nonspecific, though plausible, control (discussing self-assertion in women). There was only limited impact on eating disorder pathology, and no statistical differences on measures of eating disorder pathology across treatment conditions. However, there were indications on a range of measures that those in receipt of both self-help manuals showed greater improvement than the wait list, raising some questions about the specificity of action of manual-based interventions.

Treasure et al. (1996) randomized 110 patients to a sequential treatment group (comprising 8 weeks using a self-help manual followed [if still symptomatic] by 8 weeks of CBT), or to 16 weeks of CBT. At posttherapy and 18-month follow-up, both groups showed equal gains; at this latter point, the proportion of patients in remission was about 40% in both groups. Sixteen patients assigned to sequential treatment made significant improvement with self-help and did not require further intervention from a therapist. Interpretation of outcomes for sequential treatment is difficult, because 16% of nonimprovers in sequential treatment refused further intervention after the midpoint, and the remainder received a median of only 2.8 sessions of CBT. Troop et al. (1996) showed that there was a strong association between compliance with the manual and outcome—5% of noncompliers contrasted to 40% of compliers were in remission at 8 weeks. This same research group implemented a broadly similar research design in Germany (Thiels et al., 1998), though self-care was modified, with both therapist and patient working through the manual together (hence termed "guided self-care" and making this less obviously a stepped-care approach). Sixty-two patients were randomized to treatment, and though rate of abstinence from binge eating and vomiting at posttherapy was significantly lower in the guided self-care group (13 vs. 55%), by follow-up (at a mean of 43 weeks), outcomes were equivalent (61 and 71%, respectively).

Davis et al. (1997) used a quasi-experimental design to allocate two cohorts of patients (n = 81) either to five sessions of group psychoeducation alone or to psychoeducation followed by an additional seven sessions of group therapy (which appeared to contain some elements of CBT). Both groups evidenced equivalent levels of change, and there appeared to be no advantage to extending treatment. A later trial (Davis et al., 1999) randomized 56 patients to group psychoeducation, followed by either 16 sessions of individual CBT or no further treatment. Those receiving CBT evidenced a significant reduction in bingeing and purging, and higher levels of remission over 16-week follow-up—at this point, rates of remission from bingeing and purging were 38 and 16%, respectively. One issue raised by these studies is the difficulty of predicting which patients will benefit from minimal input alone, which patients will respond to additional therapy, and which will be unresponsive to the intervention package as a whole. Davis et al. note that a combination of low self-esteem, higher bingeing frequency after psychoeducation, and greater negatively reinforcing properties of the bingeing system predicted poorer response to CBT. Further work is required to clarify this issue.

Stepped-care approaches need to pay as much attention to the frequent problem of treatment resistance as they do to the possibility that some patients will make appropriate gains with minimal input. However, little research explicitly explores the former issue. Mitchell et al. (2002) reported a secondary phase from the multicenter trial reported by Agras et al. (2000b), in which 194 patients were initially treated with CBT; 62 participants identified as nonresponders were randomized to receive IPT or fluoxetine. Attrition from this stage was high (at 40%), and remission rates in completer patients was low—16% for IPT and 10% for medication, implying that the additive benefits of this intervention were low. In contrast, Eldredge et al. (1997) found evidence for the benefits of identifying nonresponders to a 12-week, group-based CBT program for binge eaters, and treating them in a further

12-week program. On the basis of such limited evidence, the benefits of stepped-care for treatment nonresponders with bulimia or binge-eating disorder are unclear. However, these studies raise questions about the most appropriate duration of treatment, and whether failure to respond to one therapy is best managed by extending treatment with the same therapy or by switching to another approach.

Prediction of Response to Treatment

Bulik et al. (1999) identified 19 individuals from a larger sample of 106 who showed a rapid and sustained response to "treatment" (defined as abstinence from bingeing and purging by 8 weeks of therapy). Regression analysis indicated that lower levels of bingeing at intake was predictive of rapid response, along with higher levels of self-directedness. This link between initial symptom severity and later outcome has been found in a number of studies (e.g., Mussell et al., 2000; Wilson et al., 1999), though some studies report an association only for bingeing (e.g., Garner et al., 1990) or purging (e.g., Davis et al., 1992). Comorbid substance abuse may (Wilson et al., 1999) or may not (Mitchell et al., 1990) be associated with poorer outcomes. Agras et al. (2000b) collated data from 194 participants who received 16 weeks of manual-based CBT. Treatment response was defined as no bingeing or purging in the previous 4 weeks (a criterion met by 58 patients), and a signal detection analysis used to determine pretreatment factors predictive of good outcome. Attrition was associated with higher levels of bulimic cognitions, a greater concern about body shape, and greater impulsivity. A poorer response to treatment was associated with comorbid depression and a low body mass index (BMI), but the best predictor variable was poor social adjustment. A dose–response relationship was also evident: Examining initial response to treatment and later outcome, those who reduced purging by more than 70% by session six were more likely to be treatment responders. Wilfley et al. (2000) found that the presence of a cluster B personality disorder did not impact on the efficacy of treatment but did predict higher symptom levels at pretreatment and a poorer outcome at 1-year follow-up. Variations in predictor variables across studies may relate to sample size, differences in treatment, or differences in outcome criteria; more precise conclusions regarding which patients are most likely to benefit from treatment requires further research.

TREATMENTS FOR BINGE-EATING DISORDER

Though a common feature in other eating disorders, binge-eating disorder involves persistent and frequent episodes of uncontrollable binge eating in the absence of purging. There is evidence suggesting the diagnostic utility of this classification (e.g., Castonguay et al., 1995), but also suggestions that there may be further subtypes to this presentation, one reflecting dietary preoccupation, the other associated with mood disorder (Grilo et al., 2001; Stice et al., 2001). This distinction may have implications for treatment outcome that have not been systematically explored. In most trials individuals will present with obesity as well as binge-eating.

A number of studies suggest that CBT has utility. Telch et al. (1990) randomized 44 women to 10 weeks of CBT or to a wait list; 79% reported abstinence from binge eating at posttherapy contrasted to 9% of the wait list, though at 10-week follow-up, the CBT group's abstinence rates had declined to 46%. Agras et al. (1994b) contrasted four conditions—9 months of behavioral treatment focused on weight loss or 3 months CBT followed by 6 months of the behavioral treatment; both programs were also conducted with or without desipramine. One hundred eight individuals participated. At 3 months, CBT showed gains over behavioral treatment (67% abstinence contrasted to 44%). Though by 9 months this had declined to 41%, this contrasts a rate of 19% in those receiving behavioral therapy.

Three studies explore the possibility that outcomes could be improved by supplementing a basic CBT package. Agras et al. (1995) allocated 50 individuals either to wait list or to 12 sessions of CBT. At this point, 55% of participants were classified as responders and were further assigned to 12 weeks of behavioral weight-loss treatment. Nonresponders were treated with 12 weeks of group IPT; no further gains were made. Following a similar research design, Eldredge et al. (1997) allocated 46 participants to 12 weeks of CBT or to wait list. About 50% of those receiving CBT responded. Nonresponders were offered a further 12 sessions of CBT; among these, 42% achieved abstinence. Whether these two trials indicate a specificity of action for CBT is unclear; at the point of reallocation, sample sizes were small, and given the positive outcomes for IPT reviewed immediately below, it would be prudent to base any conclusions on a larger trial. Pendleton et al. (2002) randomized 84 women to a basic package of CBT over 4 months, CBT supplemented by exercise, CBT with an extended period of maintenance treatment (12 fortnightly meetings over 6 months), or CBT with exercise and with maintenance. Adding exercise yielded gains over CBT, and adding maintenance resulted in yet further gain. At 16 months, abstinence rates for CBT alone or for CBT with maintenance were 18 and 39%, respectively. In conditions where exercise was added, abstinence rates were 65% for CBT and exercise, and 58% for the most intensive program (CBT with both exercise and maintenance). Perhaps most relevant is an association between exercising and weight loss.

Agras et al. (1997) reported aggregated data on 1-year follow-up from 75 obese participants in three CBT trials (Agras et al., 1994b, 1995; Eldredge et al., 1997), and found that about half of those who had achieved abstinence at posttherapy ($n = 31$) remained abstinent at 1 year. Of the 44 not abstinent at posttherapy, 11 were abstinent at 1 year. Reductions in frequency of binge eating were associated with weight loss.

Within-study contrasts of IPT and CBT suggest some equivalence of outcome. Wilfley et al. (1993) contrasted group IPT to group CBT and wait list in 44 individuals. After 16 weeks of treatment, abstinence rates were 44 and 28%, respectively (contrasted to 10% for wait-list patients). At 1 year, abstinence rates were 50 and 55%, respectively. A more recent and larger trial (Wilfley et al., 2002) allocated 162 patients to 20 sessions of group IPT or group CBT. Abstinence rates at posttherapy and at 1-year follow-up for IPT were 73 and 62%, respectively, and for CBT 79 and 59%, respectively.

Telch et al. (2001) report on the impact of DBT aimed at managing emotional dysregulation rather than eating behaviors. Forty-four women were assigned to 20 weeks of DBT or to wait list and then to DBT. Data are only given for the completer sample. At 6-month follow-up, 56% of those treated immediately were abstinent; of those initially assigned to wait list, 67% were abstinent.

A small number of trials examine the impact of self-help manuals. Carter and Fairburn (1998) allocated 72 women to self-help, guided (therapist-assisted) self-help, or to wait list. While rates of abstinence with both forms of self-help were equivalent and significantly better than wait list, there were substantial differences between them: Compliance was markedly higher with guided self-help (68 vs. 6%), and significantly fewer sought further help over follow-up (89 vs. 32%). Loeb et al. (2000) found significant advantage to guided over pure self-help in relation to abstinence and other measures of eating pathology. Peterson et al. (1998) contrasted guided self-help offered in a group format with self-help (again in a group format) and wait list. No significant differences were found between guided self-help or self-help either at posttherapy or at 1-year follow-up (Peterson et al., 2001). Taken together, these studies suggest that self-help approaches may be useful as part of a stepped-care approach, though researchers do note that self-help under research conditions involves at least some degree of monitoring, a factor pertinent to compliance in ordinary service settings (e.g., Loeb et al., 2000).

SUMMARY AND CLINICAL IMPLICATIONS
Anorexia Nervosa

Despite the potential health consequences of this condition, there are rather few studies of psychological treatments for anorexia nervosa. The overwhelming majority of participants are young females in adolescence or young adulthood; sample sizes tend to be small and attrition rates tend to be fairly high. Because researched treatments are almost invariably offered through specialist centers, patients usually represent the more severe end of the spectrum of presentation. Because of the paucity of research, the conclusions that can be drawn in relation both to efficacy and to generalization are necessarily tentative.

Psychological treatments invariably include dietary advice. In relation to specific approaches, inpatient contingency management treatments of anorexia nervosa appear to be effective in ensuring immediate weight gain. There is some evidence that family therapy, focal psychodynamic therapy, and CAT show benefit over standard care or no treatment. For cognitive therapy, evidence is somewhat inconclusive in relation to younger people with anorexia, though there is some indication of efficacy for its use in relapse prevention with older women. For younger people with anorexia (under the age of 18), there is some evidence of advantage to family over individual therapy. However, against robust criteria, recovery rates are rather low.

Inpatient treatment for severely anorectic individuals might be considered justified when there is anxiety about their physical health. However, though evidence on the benefit of treatment location is limited, the one available RCT tends to indicate equivalent outcomes from in- and outpatient treatments. While this challenges assumptions about the need for routine admission, it seems reasonable that clinical judgment should guide decisions about the appropriate milieu for treatment, particularly where very low body weight indicates a need for active medical intervention.

Though there are few indicators of prognosis, there does seem to be an association between very low weight (as defined by BMI) at referral and poorer response to treatment. More positively, better, longer term outcomes are linked to the speed with which weight is gained, as well as the capacity of the patient to maintain a target weight. These indicators make sense in relation to the clinical picture, since issues of motivation are especially important when referral—especially in adolescents—is often driven by the concern of those around the patient rather than the patient themselves. Although the use of motivational techniques has been subject to some exploration, results are inconclusive; developing techniques for the engagement of patients in their own treatment is an important challenge in this area.

Bulimia Nervosa

The majority of studies for eating disorders focus on bulimia, though many are small scale and the number of RCTs is somewhat limited. As for anorexia, this tempers any conclusions that can be drawn.

Most trials employ CBT, with rather few contrasts between CBT and alternative active therapies. Meta-analyses indicate relatively large posttherapy effect sizes for CBT, though these appear to decline substantially with follow-up, and a significant number of patients will continue to exhibit disturbed eating patterns at posttherapy. Contrast of CBT alone to antidepressant medication alone is hampered by high attrition rates from the latter condition, and though there appears to be some benefit to combination of medication and CBT, this also appears to increase dropout rates. Therapies often contain both behavioral and cognitive components, but it is difficult to discern the relative benefits of these techniques, partly because different studies place different levels of emphasis on each approach. However, the limited evidence offers little support for the benefit of exposure and response prevention alone, and suggests that this does not appear to add to the efficacy of CBT (and may even reduce its impact).

Contrast of CBT to IPT suggests that, whereas CBT shows significant benefit at posttherapy, over follow-up, patients who received CBT show some decline in functioning, while those in receipt of IPT continue to show improvement. This is a curious result, and because longer term follow-up is uncontrolled, some caution in interpretation would be advisable. Nonetheless, there is some indication of an "incubation" effect, perhaps attributable to the different focus of each approach—with CBT tending to attempt modification of eating behaviors, and IPT concentrating on depressive symptoms and interpersonal behaviors that may maintain the eating disorder. This pattern of outcome is, at the least, intriguing and invites speculation about the potential advantage of developing a treatment model that integrates these two approaches.

There is some limited evidence from one trial for the benefit of supportive–expressive therapy, which appeared to be of equal short-term efficacy to CBT, but interpretation is limited by the absence of follow-up data.

Stepped-care approaches have been used with reasonable success, and in this context, there is some value to self-help, though most obviously when it is combined with therapist input. There is only limited evidence of benefit to extending treatment for those initially unresponsive to treatment, though this appears most successful when the model adopted is consistent throughout as opposed to switching patients from one therapy to another.

While it seems clear that unstructured treatments are ineffective, even the best approaches show only moderate levels of efficacy. Initial treatment response appears to be poorer for patients with greater initial symptom severity, greater preoccupation with body shape, and more bulimic concerns. There are some indications that a more rapid response to treatment is indicative of later success. Rates of relapse after treatment are relatively high, with indications that levels of self-esteem, greater preoccupation with eating, and concerns about body shape are associated with longer term outcome.

Binge-Eating Disorder

Binge-eating disorder has attracted an increasing amount if research in recent years. A number of studies have suggested that CBT is an effective approach; in contrast, trials of DBT have not demonstrated evidence for efficacy. Though pure self-help approaches are of limited effectiveness, guided self-help offered as part of stepped care, and with therapeutic contact, appears more effective.

Generalizing research findings to standard settings may require consideration of a number of issues. Because recruitment usually takes place in specialist settings, treated patients represent the more severe end of the spectrum of eating disorders. Given that greater severity is associated with poorer outcomes, it may be that the outlook for patients seen in clinical settings will be more positive than research indicates. Equally, researchers usually exclude individuals with significant comorbidities; since these are common in eating disorders, many clinicians will treat individuals whose eating disorder presents in the context of other significant psychiatric conditions. However, there is as yet little evidence on the degree to which treatment approaches will remain effective with differing permutations of disorder.

Most research focuses on the DSM categories of anorexia and bulimia, despite the fact that evidence indicates a relatively higher community prevalence of EDNOS, and it is this form of presentation with which clinicians will be most familiar. Although this research bias can be justified (those meeting diagnostic criteria will be severely impacted by their disorder), it does mean that knowledge of treatment outcomes is restricted to a diagnostic grouping that is in some ways unrepresentative of eating disorders in the community. Although it would be very reasonable to apply treatment strategies employed for anorexia and bulimia to those with EDNOS, it should be acknowledged that there is no evidential basis for doing this, and hence no guidance as to likely outcomes. There is a risk that this could lead clinicians erroneously to interpret EDNOS status as a "subthreshold" condition as a justification for withholding treatment. This would be inappropriate, partly because individuals with this diagnosis exhibit a significant level of pathological behavior in relation to eating. More critically, the fluidity of eating disorder diagnoses across time makes restrictions on intervention based on current diagnosis inappropriate; for a significant number of patients, their diagnosis at any one point in time seems to represent the developmental progression of their eating pathology, and intervention at any stage in this process could well have preventive value. Finally, many more male presentations of eating disorders are classified as EDNOS rather than anorexia or bulimia, and when this diagnosis is considered, the overrepresentation of females within eating disorders is much less striking. Because there is so little research on EDNOS, the literature is essentially silent in relation to the likely treatment outcomes of boys and men, or the degree to which treatment strategies might need to be adapted to manage their needs.

CHAPTER 10

SCHIZOPHRENIA

DEFINITION

DSM-IV-TR describes a range of symptoms of schizophrenia. Diagnosis is based on a complex pattern that usually involves disturbance in several of the following areas: content and form of thought, perception, affect, sense of self, volition, relation to the external world, and psychomotor behavior. No single feature is invariably present, or seen only in schizophrenia. The disorder is usually associated (at some point in its course) with severe impairment in social and work functioning and difficulties in self-care. Supervision may be required to ensure that the person's basic needs are met and that he/she is protected from the consequences of actions deriving from the disorder. Between episodes, the extent of disability may range from none to disability so severe that institutional care is required.

A distinction is often made clinically between acute (or positive) symptoms, such as delusions or hallucinations, and residual (or negative) symptoms, such as social withdrawal and marked impairment in social role functioning.

PREVALENCE AND NATURAL HISTORY

Prevalence

On the basis of a systematic review of relevant studies, Goldner et al. (2002) estimate annual incidence at 11 per 100,000, and lifetime prevalence at 340 per 100,000.

Natural History

The course of this disorder is usually chronic, though recovery occurs in some patients after one or two brief, acute psychotic episodes. However, a more chronic course is found in patients who have recurrent episodes of longer duration; in these individuals, a "defect" state can develop, marked by lack of motivation, apathy, and social withdrawal (R. E. Kendall, 1993). Florid symptoms may or may not persist between acute episodes, and depressive symptoms are frequent.

PSYCHOLOGICAL INTERVENTIONS

While neuroleptic medication is widely recognized as the treatment of choice for schizophrenia, a substantial proportion of patients will remain troubled by symptoms. There is evidence that despite appropriate levels of medication, many patients continue to experience residual psychotic symptoms that, though often less severe than those occurring in acute episodes, are unresponsive to further medication. Full remission of symptoms occurs in less than two-thirds of patients (Shepherd et al., 1989). Curson et al. (1985), in a 7-year community follow-up study, reported that 23% of patients continue to experience florid symptoms; in a hospital setting, nearly half did so (Curson et al., 1988). About 40% of patients continue to experience some psychotic symptoms, (Kane, 1996), and though for some "treatment-resistant" individuals the newer "atypical" antipsychotics are of benefit, their potential gains should not be overstated. A significant proportion of such patients show only slight improvements when placed on these medications (Chakos et al., 2001), and it is not clear that their general efficacy is greater than traditional antipsychotics in treating initial presentations (Geddes et al., 2000). The need for psychological interventions also arises from patients' difficulty in maintaining themselves on long-term medication, and the fact that high relapse rates are evident even in patients who continue with this regimen.

Before the introduction of effective antipsychotic medication, there were reports of individual case studies examining the usefulness of psychodynamic treatments for schizophrenia. Because these studies antedate the development of reliable diagnostic criteria for the disorder, they are not reviewed here. In recent years, there have been important developments in three areas: (1) family intervention programs aimed at modification of the support network of the schizophrenic person, (2) cognitive-behavioral treatment (CBT) of acute symptoms, and (3) cognitive remediation, which addresses itself directly to amelioration of cognitive deficits. A fourth area of research—social skills training—represents a more traditional area of intervention.

FAMILY INTERVENTIONS

Family and Patient Psychoeducation

Lam (1991) reviewed the impact of educational packages, delivered either with or without the patient and to a single family or multifamily groups (Abramowitz & Coursey, 1989; Barrowclough et al., 1987; Berkowitz et al., 1984; Cozolino et al., 1988; McGill et al., 1983; Smith & Birchwood, 1987). Packages were usually fairly brief, in four studies consisting of two sessions; the longest (Abramowitz & Coursey, 1989) comprised six 2-hour sessions every 2 weeks. Studies have used different educational content, different measures, and differing lengths of follow-up (ranging from 2 to 9 months); some of these follow-up measures are contaminated by intervening treatments. However, with one exception, all studies demonstrated an increase in family knowledge regarding the condition at follow-up, contrasted with controls. In the exceptional case, this may relate to the fact that only one 3-hour education session was offered. There was no difference between families high or low in expressed emotion (EE), though there was a trend indicating that relatives of recent-onset patients gained more knowledge from the intervention. There was only limited and inconsistent evidence of change in family belief systems; those receiving education showed some greater optimism about the patient's future and less self-blame, though this effect was not stable over follow-up. There was no evidence that relapse rates—perhaps the most clinically rigorous test of these interventions—differed between experimental and control groups.

A more recent narrative review (Merinder, 2000) reached conclusions similar to those of Lam (1991), though there is no overlap in the studies each review considers. Merinder identified seven randomized studies—four naturalistic studies and eight trials that included mixed populations of psychiatric patients. Though most included family education, there was little consistency in the educational packages used, which ranged from basic information about medication to more complex interventions encompassing relapse prevention and problem solving. In addition, some programs were delivered to individuals and some to groups, and they varied in intensity and duration. Although patients showed a consistent benefit in relation to knowledge about their condition and compliance, this was not mirrored by a reduction in the key index of relapse rates. Perhaps surprisingly, in view of its overlap in coverage and authorship, a Cochrane review (Pekkala & Merinder, 2002) concluded that psychoeducation significantly reduces relapse or readmission rates, citing a number needed to treat (NNT) of 9 (confidence interval = 6–22). However, this result is based on pooled data, which does not reflect the wide variation in outcomes across individual studies.

Clearly, patients are entitled to careful education about their condition, but the risk is that the benefit will be pedagogic rather than mutative. Tarrier et al.'s (1988) study directly contrasted psychoeducation alone or in combination with a family intervention; contrasted to routine treatment, education made no impact on relapse rates. Educational packages alone may not be effective, in part because they do not address the gap between knowledge and attitudes. For example, Cunningham et al. (2001) offered a simple didactic education package to 61 patients, and found no differences in outcome relative to 53 patients receiving standard care. Overall, psychoeducation appears to show best results when combined with techniques recognizable as psychological interventions, with little therapeutic gain from psychoeducation alone.

Family Intervention Programs

The development of psychosocial intervention programs was prompted by both evidence of relatively high relapse rates for schizophrenia (Johnson, 1976; Leff & Wing, 1971) and the success of measures of EE in predicting relapse (Bebbington & Kuipers, 1994; Brown et al., 1972; Butzlaff & Hooley, 1998; Leff & Vaughn, 1985; Vaughn & Leff, 1976). In brief, these early studies indicated that relapse is more likely if patients live with, or have extensive contact with, relatives who are excessively critical and/or overinvolved. Two factors appear to be protective and additive in their effect: regular maintenance therapy with neuroleptic medication, and the establishment of a social distance between the patient and relative. Some studies (Halford et al., 1999) have criticized the measurement of EE for reliance only on negative interactions (and therefore failing to recognize the importance of positive support from caregivers), and for difficulties in its measurement. Families were assessed shortly after admission using a 10-minute videotaped interaction. On the basis of a cumulative measure of positive and negative responses made by both the patients and their relatives, families were defined as affect regulated or unregulated. At 6 months, patients from affect-regulated families had significantly lower relapse rates than those from unregulated families (15 vs. 50%).

Intervention programs have as an aim the prevention of relapse and improvement in functioning rather than direct amelioration or "cure" of the condition. All assume that it is useful to regard schizophrenia as an illness. Importantly, none regard the family as the cause of schizophrenia but take as their focus the family burden imposed in attempting to care for their relative. Finally, treatments are offered in conjunction with routine medical management. There are usually two components to intervention programs: (1) education regarding the illness, and (2) education and treatment aiming at influencing family functioning. With one exception (Glick et al., 1993), all trials discussed below were carried out on an outpatient basis. Though this gives some broad consistency to the form of intervention, there are some important variations in implementation. In particular intervention periods vary widely—from eight sessions over a short time period to fortnightly over 2 years, with additional monthly sessions over a further 2 years.

The use of relapse as an outcome criterion for these interventions is appropriate; it is a rigorous marker of successful intervention, and relapse not only impacts severely on patients and their families but also incurs direct costs to health care systems and indirect costs to society. However, the term "relapse event" might be a better one (as noted by Pharoah et al., 2002), since definitions of relapse vary across trials. In some, it denotes clinical change (such as recurrence of symptoms in patients who had previously obtained full remission, or deterioration from baseline), while in others, it reflects an index event such as hospitalization (meaning that factors other than symptomatic change could account for apparent relapse). A different concern is that indicators such as shifts in symptom levels or levels of functioning would be a more sensitive indicator than relapse rates, since it is likely that individuals who manage not to relapse will vary widely in their presentations.

Meta-Analyses

Meta-analytic reviews of family interventions have been carried out by Mari and Streiner (1994), Pharoah et al. (2002) and Pilling et al. (2002b). A meta-analysis by Mojtabai et al. (1998) is not considered further here; although a useful review of the impact of psychosocial treatments, it does not separate family interventions for relapse from other therapies. Pitschel-Walz et al.'s (2001) review of family interventions is also somewhat problematic. Although it includes two German-language papers, it also includes a number of studies in which psychoeducation alone was offered, some studies that antedate the development of family intervention programs, and some trials in which patients received diagnoses other than schizophrenia, placing at least some of its analyses outside the scope of the definition noted earlier.

Mari and Streiner (1994) examined data from six early trials, which included 169 patients in receipt of family intervention, with 181 patients acting as controls. The former showed a significantly lower relapse rate than controls (at 9 months, a mean relapse rate of 15.6% vs. 47.2%); as follow-up progressed, the relapse rate in the two groups of patients increased, though more so among controls (at 2 years, mean relapse rates were 24 and 65%, respectively). The pooled odds ratio was 0.3 at 6 months, 0.22 at 9 months, and 0.17 at 2 years, indicating a significant reduction in relapse rates. A more conservative intention-to-treat analysis (ITT) (which treated dropouts as though they had relapsed rather than using end point data) suggested a more marginal level of efficacy (odds ratios were 0.65 at 6 months, 0.59 at 9 months, and 0.80 at 2 years). Secondary analyses indicated that treated patients showed a significant increase in compliance with medication, and that their families showed a marginally significant reduction in EE.

Coverage of Pharoah et al.'s (2002) review extended to 1999, and included 13 trials at centers in North America, Europe, Asia, and Australia. Family interventions significantly reduced the rate of relapse events at both 12 and 24 months (odds ratio = 0.57 and 0.52, respectively), with longer term follow-up based on too few studies to make analysis reliable. Significant heterogeneity in the data was resolved by removal of one trial (Buchkremer et al., 1995), which employed family groups rather than seeing each family individually, resulting in improved odds ratios (0.45 and 0.31, respectively). On the basis of these figures, the NNT was 6.5. Admission rates at 1 year appear to be reduced by family interventions, though the robustness of this finding depends on the data set chosen for analysis—using the "homogenized" sample, the odds ratio is 0.53; for the completer sample, the odds ratio is 0.4. Less clear is the degree to which compliance with medication was influenced by this intervention; an odds ratio of 0.63 was not significant.

Pilling et al. (2002b) identified 23 trials with 1,467 participants. Relapse rates were reported for 765 patients; of the 381 who received a family intervention, the overall relapse rate at up to 4 years was 37.8%, and for the 384 who received "other treatments," it was 53.6%. Contrasted to standard care, at 12 months the NNT was 8, with a 12.8% absolute reduction in risk of relapse. Contrasted to other active interventions, there was no advantage to family interventions. The impact of family interventions was reduced with longer follow-up time; where studies report data at between 1 and 2 years posttherapy, relapse rates were not significantly lower than for controls. Using readmission as an index of improvement, there were very significant advantage to family interventions, with an NNT of 3 and a 48.8% absolute difference in the risk of readmission at 1 year. At 2 years, this benefit was maintained, with an NNT of 11 and a 9.7% absolute difference in risk of readmission. Evidence from five trials suggests that compliance with medication was enhanced by both formats of treatment delivery (odds ratio = 0.63).

Over recent years, some centers have implemented family interventions through multiple-family groups rather than treating single-family units; Pilling et al.'s (2002b) review includes four examples of this mode of delivery, though Pharoah et al. (2002) only included one. Pilling et al. (2002b) analyzed these group interventions separately, finding that this mode of delivery had no more impact than standard care (and that multiple-family groups were an inappropriate mode of delivery). This conclusion is inappropriate given that some of the four trials offered psychoeducation alone (which is known to be of dubious value), conflating mode of delivery with treatment type. Pilling et al. suggested that the lower impact of multiple-family groups would be an explanation for Pharoaoh et al.'s (2002) observation that ordering trials by year of publication yielded a decreasing effect size, since reports of multiple-family groups tended to be more recently published. However, it is also the case that more recent investigators are also moving away from using standard care as a comparator treatment, and employing an alternative active intervention, diminishing the degree to which differences in outcome will be expected.

Qualitative Reviews

Qualitative reviews by Barrowclough and Tarrier (1984), Strachan (1986), and Kuipers and Bebbington (1988) considered early trials; those by Lam (1991) and Barbato and D'Avanzo (2000) broadened coverage to include a more representative sample of studies. Lam (1991) identified five family intervention programs carried out with patients with a diagnosis of schizophrenia based on standard research tools such as the Present State Examination (PSE; Wing et al., 1974) or research diagnostic criteria (RDC, Spitzer et al., 1978), which randomly allocate patients to control or experimental groups, and in which some attempt was made to control for the impact of medication (Falloon et al., 1982, 1985, 1987; Hogarty et al., 1986, 1987; Kottgen et al. 1984; Leff et al., 1982, 1985, 1988, 1990; Tarrier et al., 1988, 1989). Four of these studies offered very similar treatments. Despite differences of detail, all focused on positive (rather than negative) areas of family functioning, acknowledging family burden and increasing family structure and stability (e.g., through problem solving, behavioral goal setting, cognitive restructuring, or techniques derived from family therapy). In contrast, Kottgen et al. (1984) adopted a psychodynamic approach.

Effects of family intervention appear to be marked. With the exception of the Kottgen study (1984), significant reductions in relapse rates were evident. At 9 months to 1 year, rates in patients from treated families ranged from 6 to 23%, contrasted with 40 to 53% in patients from control families. Levels of EE within families were usually reduced in these programs, and measures of household, social, and work functioning indicated that patients from treated families had improved relative to control patients.

At 2 years, less dramatic differences were observed; contrasting patients in high EE families (who have the most elevated risk of relapse), rates were 17–44% in patients from treated groups and 59–83% in controls. Although this suggests that intervention delays rather than prevents relapse, in most studies, there was only minimal contact between therapists and patients during the follow-up phase. Falloon's group maintained contact once every 6 months over the 2-year follow-up, obtaining a 17% relapse rate. There may be some indication, therefore, that better outcomes would be obtained by use of a maintenance model of treatment.

Barbato and D'Avanzo (2000) reviewed 25 studies of family intervention; there is considerable overlap with the previous meta-analyses, but they include in their review some trials of psychoeducation and two studies that employed nonbehavioral models—Levene et al. (1989), who employed a psychodynamic approach, and De Giacomo et al. (1997) who used a systemic paradoxical model. Overall, at 1 year, the median relapse rates for patients receiving a family intervention was 18%, and for controls, 44%; at 2 years, the equivalent figures were 33% and 64%. However, the range of outcomes across studies was quite broad; at 1 year, relapse rates among "treated" patients ranged from 6 to 52%, and for controls, from 15 to 67%. There may be a number of reasons for this variation in outcome, of which differences in therapeutic methods may be only one; methodological differences may also be relevant. For example, as noted earlier, differences between family intervention and an alternative treatment are greatest where the comparator is standard care, and usually least where an alternative active intervention is offered. Sampling frames are also important, with some studies focusing on more refractory cases (as was certainly the case in earlier trials), while others (e.g., Linszen et al., 1996) included an unselected group of younger patients in whom there was a very low overall relapse rate (and no differences between the different active interventions offered).

Individual Studies

Glick et al. (1993) reported outcomes following a relatively brief family intervention program offered on an inpatient basis. The study included 169 patients with a range of diagnoses, of whom 92 had a diagnosis of schizophrenia. All patients received standard hospital care, but half received additional family treatment (a mean of 8.6 sessions over a mean hospital stay of 51 days). This comprised an educational package, an examination of family interaction patterns that might exacerbate stress, and training in identifying potential sources of stress. Patients were followed up for 18 months after discharge, with no control on subsequent treatment, though results were reported only for patients who had six or more therapy sessions. Using Jacobson et al.'s (1984) criteria for establishing clinical significance, at discharge, 86% of patients receiving family therapy showed significant improvement, contrasted with 63% of controls. As follow-up progressed, differential treatment effects diminished such that at 18 months 54 and 50%, respectively, of the family therapy and control groups showed significant improvement.

Although the success of interventions in this group of studies could be attributable to better adherence to drug regimens and to the nonspecific effects of greater therapeutic input, this seems unlikely. Evidence from Tarrier et al. (1989) suggests that amount of contact with the clinical team and degree of drug compliance were equivalent across treatment and control groups.

Few trials use a non-CBT approach to family intervention. Kottgen et al. (1984) failed to demonstrate a benefit for their psychodynamic intervention in a nonrandomized study. Levene et al. (1989) conducted a small pilot study in which 10 patients received psychodynamic family treatment or problem solving. Though there was some evidence of differential gains in favor of the experimental treatment, the sample size was too low to support any firm conclusions. De Giacomo et al. (1997) assigned 38 participants either to 10 sessions of a paradoxical model of systemic therapy, with medication prescribed by the therapy team, or to pharmacological treatment; it is unclear whether allocation was random. At 1 year, those receiving family therapy had lower symptom scores than those receiving medication alone. While no patients required rehospitalization (an unusual finding for a sample such as this), this may reflect practices in the Italian health system, which emphasizes community care. Medication was not standardized in either condition, and post hoc analysis suggested wide variations in prescribing practice both within and between groups. On this basis, outcomes are difficult to interpret.

Buchkremer et al. (1997) attempted to identify the differential or additive efficacy of psychoeducation, relative support, and CBT. One hundred ninety-one patients were allocated to one of four active treatments or to a control treatment in which occupational activities were offered on an organized basis. All active treatments offered medication psychoeducation to patients in combination with (1) the control treatment, (2) the control treatment and counseling for relatives, (3) problem-solving skills training, (4) problem solving and counseling for relatives. At 2-year follow-up, there were no statistical differences in rates of rehospitalization across groups or between treatment groups and control, though rates for patients in receipt of the most intensive intervention (group 4) were lowest—24%, contrasted to 50% in the control group. While this hints at the benefits of more intensive intervention, the effect is not robust and could be attributable to intensity of input rather than the impact of specific techniques.

Schooler et al. (1997) attempted a rather complex study with 313 patients, manipulating both level of medication and the type of psychosocial intervention. Recruitment followed acute admission; after medication stabilization, patients were assigned to different medication protocols—a continuous standard dose, continuous low dose, or targeted medication given only in response to prodromal signs. Within this framework, all patients were further randomized; all received monthly, multifamily group psychoeducation or group psychoeducation plus individual family problem solving weekly for 13 weeks, biweekly for a further 13 weeks, and then monthly until the end of the first year. Follow-up over 2 years indicated no differential impact for psychosocial intervention in terms of relapse within each medication condition. Delivery of medication showed a clear impact on outcomes, with significantly higher relapse rates for those receiving a targeted dose. The overall relapse rate for standard and low-dose patients was lower than usually reported (at about 25%), though whether the family interventions contributed to this is unclear.

One cautionary note is struck by Linszen et al. (1996), most of whose sample were in their first admission, and were younger than other samples (with an average age of 20.5 years). All patients received standard care and individual therapy, which contained problem-solving and supportive elements. The authors examined the impact of adding a family intervention to this package, finding no differential benefit (though the overall relapse rate was low, at 16% over 1 year). However, though sample sizes are too small to be reliable, among low EE families, relapse rates were higher for family intervention (13%) than for individual therapy (0%). Linszen et al. (1998) noted that low-EE families tended to interpret a focus on communication skills as implying a deficiency in such skills, which increased rather than decreased family stresses. Nonetheless, while at 5-year follow-up (Lenior et al., 2001) there continued to be no differences between treatment groups in terms of clinical course, those in receipt of family interventions had a shorter duration of inpatient stays consequent on relapse.

MULTIFAMILY GROUPS

McFarlane et al. (1995b) argued that multifamily groups may be more effective than single-family treatments on the basis that the "social networking" afforded by this approach would enhance treatment effects. In the first of two trials reported by this group, patients were assigned to 2 years of fortnightly family psychoeducation and intervention based on a problem-solving approach, delivered in two formats—either to single families or as part of a multiple (five family) group. The original research design included a third condition offering multifamily therapy that contained no psychoeducational component, avoided direct discussion of schizophrenia as an illness, and focused on family dynamics and communication. High relapse rates in this condition relative to the others led to removal of this condition from the protocol. The treated sample comprised patients from 16 families treated in multifamily groups and 18 as single families. Over a 4-year follow-up, relapse rates in single-family treatments and multifamily groups were 77.8 and 50%, respectively.

In a larger, multisite study McFarlane et al. (1995a) allocated 172 patients to single- or multifamily (six family) treatment, again over 2 years. Recruitment took place after an acute admission, and family treatments were adjunctive to standard care. Though benefit was found for both approaches, there was a significant advantage to multifamily over single-family approaches, with relapse rates at over 2 years of 28 and 42%, respectively, in the total sample. The multifamily approach showed more obvious advantage in patients who had higher levels of positive symptoms at index discharge. Again comparing relapse rates in single- and multifamily groups, these were essentially equivalent for the 96 patients discharged with no or few positive symptoms. However, for the 76 patients discharged in partial remission, 19% relapsed with multifamily groups, contrasted to 51% for single-family groups, and it is this difference that largely accounts for the overall finding of differential relapse. This finding is clinically relevant, the more so because it was consistent on five of the six study sites, suggesting that it is robust across settings and therapists.

Buchkremer et al. (1995) adopted a rather different approach, excluding patients, and contrasting two forms of relatives-only groups against a control (which appears to have been standard treatment plus some form of group contact). Both active treatments started with 6 months of therapist-led psychoeducation and problem solving; over the subsequent 6 months, one group continued to be led by therapists, while the other ran as a self-help group. Relatives of 99 patients were allocated to interventions. After 1 year, and contrasted to a control, relapse rates were higher in the patients whose relatives attended either form of active treatment group (52 vs. 42%), though much of this difference is accounted for by the fact that by nine months, 60% of patients whose relatives were allocated to self-help had relapsed. The speed with which this pattern of differential relapse established itself makes it possible that it was underpinned by factors other than the treatment condition. However, the authors note that though the groups that shifted to a self-help format were prepared, group members found the prospect and the transition disorienting. Clearly, this trial offers no support for this form of intervention.

Dropout

Despite these promising findings, it is important to note that in all the above trials, a number of families refused to enter treatment, and there is a moderate level of attrition from treatment. Tarrier (1991a) discusses this issue, noting that across studies, the rate of families refusing treatment is between 7 and 21% (median = 13%), the rate of withdrawal from treatment is 7–14% (median = 9.5%), and the rate of noncompliance is between 8 and 35% (median = 16%). This is a significant problem in that there is evidence that patients from families that refuse or drop out of treatment have a higher relapse rate than those who follow the intervention program (Hogarty et al., 1986).

Tarrier (1991a) suggests a number of features that may be associated with adherence. There is some—though little—evidence that families high in EE may be more likely to drop out (Tarrier et al., 1989). Other characteristics (e.g., age of relatives, degree of chronicity in the index patient, or level of family burden) remain unclear; further research in this area would be helpful.

Implementation in Routine Settings

As is usual in research trials, most data on the efficacy of family interventions have been culled in the context of high levels of therapeutic expertise and supervision. However, some trials have been conducted closer to everyday practice. Brooker et al. (1992) reported a pilot study in which psychiatric nurses were trained to deliver intervention packages composed of education and family stress management. In a naturalistic design, 54 families were recruited either to experimental or control conditions and followed up for 12 months; control families received treatment as usual (TAU) from nursing staff. For families receiving the intervention package, significant gains were found in social and personal functioning, and in relatives' General Health Questionnaire scores. However, no differences in relapse rates were found.

In a subsequent trial (Brooker et al., 1994), a similar intervention package was employed with families receiving either treatment immediately or after a 6-month delay, thus forming a wait-list control group. Broadly similar gains in functioning to those found in the earlier trial were achieved, together with a marked reduction in the length of inpatient admissions.

Randolph et al. (1994) reported on the impact of behavioral family interventions (as described by Falloon et al., 1984) in a standard clinical setting. Forty-one patients were allocated either to a mean of 21 family sessions over 1 year or to routine care, which comprised monthly sessions of medical management. At the end of this treatment period, 15% of the treatment group had an exacerbation of their condition, contrasted to 55% of those receiving routine care. However, there was no difference between the groups in the number of days spent as inpatients.

Leff et al. (2001) reported on family interventions conducted by community psychiatric nurses (CPNs); though training was by a CPN involved in some of the original trials of this approach, the intervention took place in a routine clinical setting. All families scored high on EE at the start of the trial; 16 families were allocated to standard care plus family psychoeducation and intervention, and 14 to standard care plus family psychoeducation alone. Difficulties in recruitment led to sequential as well as random allocation. At 1-year follow-up, relapse rates in the family intervention and control groups were statistically equivalent at 25 and 36%, respectively. The relapse rate for controls is rather lower than that in other studies, though only 11 patients were available for analysis (one patient died and two were hospitalized for the duration of the follow-up), and the power of this study to detect differences is questionable. Though in this respect outcomes are open to interpretation, evidence that CPNs were able to learn the skills required to conduct therapy is afforded by the significantly greater reduction in EE with the family treatment (with seven of the family intervention and two of the control families moving from high to low EE status).

Barrowclough et al. (1999) report a needs-based CBT family intervention. A notable feature of this study was that it recruited on the basis of a geographical sampling frame, with potential subjects identified through hospital admission records. The aim was to achieve a sample that was representative of service users, and inclusion criteria specified that patients should have been ill for longer than 2 years, and have had at least one relapse in the previous 2 years. Given that prolonged contact with high-EE relatives is a known risk factor for relapse, participants also needed to be in contact with a carer for at least 10 hours a week. Overall, participants in the study had a mean duration of illness of 13 years.

All participants received standard care, which included assessment and psychosocial support, and some contact with a family support worker. Seventy nine participants were randomized to standard care alone or to standard care supplemented with a CBT family intervention based on systematic assessment of carer needs. The family intervention was delivered by a clinical psychologist experienced in this technique, usually in conjunction with the patient's key worker. Treatment was delivered over 6 months in between 10 and 12 sessions. Six-month follow-up (Sellwood et al., 2001) suggested a marked benefit to the family intervention; in contrast to the control, relapse rates were reduced (37 and 72%, respectively), as were the number of relapses not requiring admission (16 and 49%, respectively), though the number of admission was equivalent (29% and 38%, respectively).

This trial is appropriately described by its authors as an effectiveness study, but though its success is clear, it is worth bearing in mind that clinical services were operating with the input of a well-known research group, and while family intervention was offered by key workers, they worked with an experienced clinician. This caveat is important, because a number of commentators have commented on the difficulty of organizing and integrating family interventions in the context of routine care (e.g., Baguley et al., 2000; Fadden, 1997).

The first issue is that recruitment may prove a challenge. Although conducting a randomized trial, Wiedemann et al. (1994) recruited from a standard clinical population and noted that from a sample of 441 patients, though 60% were eligible for a family treatment, only 34% agreed to participate, and a further 40% dropped out of treatment. In the Barrowclough et al. trial (1999) reported earlier, 671 casenotes were examined. From these, 146 (22%) patient-carers were deemed eligible to participate; 35% of patients and 27% of carers refused, and of the 38 patient-carers randomized to treatment, 28 (73%) completed more than 10 sessions.

Certainly, there is evidence that rather few families receive these interventions. Dixon et al. (1999) examined the services received in 1991 by 20,818 persons with schizophrenia, using administrative claims data from Medicare and Medicaid; more detailed information was provided by a randomly selected field sample of 719 individuals with schizophrenia in two states of the United States. Of those receiving Medicare and Medicaid, 0.7% and 7.1%, respectively had a received a family intervention. In the field sample, 82% were in contact with family members, and of these, 30% reported at least some minimal family psychoeducation or support. Staff training seemed to influence this pattern; though didactic education made no difference to implementation, intensive training was associated with higher levels of provision. Both this and other studies (e.g., Amenson & Liberman, 2001; Baguley et al., 2000; Dixon et al., 2001; Hughes et al., 1996; McFarlane et al., 2001) suggest that without support from and integration into the clinical system, training individual practitioners in family intervention methods will not be sufficient to ensure their adoption.

A further trial of multifamily groups offered a broad set of interventions to individuals with first-episode psychosis (Nordentoft et al., 2002). Three hundred forty-one patients were randomized to standard care or to an integrated treatment package that comprised intensive community support, education about medication, multifamily groups (meeting over 18 months) and social skills training (for those who appeared to lack the skills for independent living). Initial reports of outcomes 1-year posttherapy suggested that integrated treatment was associated with reduced hospital stay and relapse. Although a good result clinically, the design of the trial makes it impossible to attribute outcomes to any specific feature of the treatment package.

Family Interventions and Service Costs

It is evident that family intervention programs can reduce relapse rates. Given the high cost of inpatient care and attendant interventions, it seems likely that such programs would be cost-effective. This issue has been investigated in detail by Tarrier (1991b). Eighty-three patients and their families were entered for a treatment trial, receiving either a full family intervention program, an educational program, or routine treatment. All contacts with mental health services were monitored and costed. Low-EE families in the control group made no more demands on services than high-EE families in the intervention group. However, comparison between high-EE families in the control and intervention groups revealed significantly greater costs accrued as a result of admission and professional contact time. Although there is a significant cost involved in offering family interventions, high-EE patients in receipt of the program had an estimated mean cost per patient of £1,171 ($1,760), contrasted with £1,603 ($2,400) for high-EE controls and £822 ($1,230) for low-EE controls. Cardin et al. (1986) reported that, over 12 months, the costs of family management were 19% lower than individually managed care, attributable to reduced rates of admission and crisis management. Some caution may be required in considering these figures, in that the studies reviewed here suggest that over longer time frames, increased relapse would be observed even in treated patients.

SOCIAL SKILLS TRAINING

Many people with schizophrenia have deficiencies in their social functioning, an observation that is used as the rationale for offering social skills training. There are two meta-analyses of the impact of this approach (Benton & Scroeder, 1990; Pilling et al., 2002a), and a number of qualitative reviews (e.g., Donahoe & Driesenga, 1989; Halford & Haynes, 1991; Heinssen et al., 2000; Huxley et al., 2000; Smith et al., 1996). Unfortunately, some (usually earlier) studies included nonschizophrenic patients or failed to ensure that diagnostic inclusion criteria were met. Overall, the wide variation in the form and length of interventions makes it difficult to draw firm conclusions about efficacy. A basic concern is that even if social skills training leads to improvements within the context in which training takes place, there is evidence that these fail to generalize over a longer time span and to community settings (e.g., Emmelkamp, 1994; Wallace et al., 1980). Though not always explicitly acknowledged by reviewers, an appropriate distinction would be between trials of "traditional" behavioral social skills training and broader programs, either augmented to include an explicit focus on generalization (e.g., Glynn et al., 2002), or focused on a narrower band of social skills considered pertinent to life functioning (e.g., Tsang, 2001).

Benton and Schroeder (1990) present a meta-analytic review of 23 studies in which at least 75% of subjects had a diagnosis of schizophrenia and had been inpatients for more than 6 months. Social skills training was characterized as containing elements of modeling, rehearsal, and homework assignments; studies not adhering to this specification were excluded. Overall, mean effect sizes based on naturalistic measures of outcome were rather lower than those closely related to treatment process, such as role-play-based measures (0.68 and 0.83, respectively). Self-rated assertiveness yielded an effect size of 0.69. Effect sizes based on measures of general functioning, self-rated symptomatology, and discharge and relapse rates were small and nonsignificant. In concordance with qualitative reviews, there appears to be some rather limited evidence of positive impacts using this technique, though only a modest degree of generalization of skills.

A more recent meta-analysis (Pilling et al., 2002a) considered outcomes only for individuals with a diagnosis of schizophrenia. On this basis, nine trials with 471 patients were identified. There was little consistency in domains of outcome or measures used across studies, which restricted the comprehensiveness of the review. Only in two cases was the contrast to standard care; in the remainder, the contrast to an alternative psychosocial intervention would tend to reduce the expected effect size. Overall, there were no indications that social skills training reduced relapse rates, nor was there any benefit in relation to measures of global adjustment. Given that gains in social functioning would be a pertinent outcome measure, it is surprising that only two studies provided appropriate measures, only one of which found a significant gain for social skills.

Huxley et al. (2000) concurred with the conclusions of earlier reviews that traditional social skills training has very modest impact, but also separately considered programs that explicitly facilitate generalization of skills to community settings. Four controlled trials of the UCLA Social and Independent Living approach were identified. (It should be noted that only a part of this modular program addressed itself to social skills; additional psychoeducational input on medication and symptom management made it harder to attribute gains to specific components). There were some—again, modest—gains over control treatments. Overall, it is unclear that social skills training offered alone—either in traditional or augmented form—has substantive benefit.

COGNITIVE-BEHAVIORAL THERAPY

A range of behavioral and cognitive-behavioral techniques have been employed in an attempt to alleviate psychotic symptoms (Haddock et al., 1998b). Early trials examined the efficacy of more behavioral techniques (such as operant methods, exposure, and distraction), but advances in models of cognitive functioning in schizophrenia have led to a rapid growth of interest in cognitive-behavioral strategies (Garety & Freeman, 1999). Although these vary in their emphasis and, to some degree, rationale, interventions have the primary aim of modification of hallucinations and delusional beliefs. One set of trials focus on individuals with chronic or treatment-resistant presentations, another on patients with a recent onset of symptoms. Whereas younger and more acute patients are prone to cycles of relapse and recovery, this is less the case for chronic patients; in this group, measures of mental state and global functioning will be a more sensitive and appropriate indicator of efficacy than relapse.

Meta-Analyses and Qualitative Reviews

Studies of CBT applied to the management of schizophrenic symptoms are not homogenous in their aims or their techniques. Broadly, one set of studies focus on the modification of delusional beliefs, with some variation in the repertoire of psychosocial techniques that they employ. Others aim to achieve better compliance with medication or other aspects of treatment.

Both approaches examine key beliefs and coping strategies, and both empha-size engaging clients and working with and through the way they understand their symptoms. However, there is an important difference in the level of beliefs they address, and in important ways, their aims are distinct. Some reviews subsume both approaches under the label of CBT, risking conflation of two different interventions and obscuring rather than illuminating issues of efficacy. A further issue is that reviews do not distinguish trials in relation to the chronicity of patient presentations, though—as noted earlier—this is likely to impact on the type of outcomes that can be expected.

This problem is inherent in two of the four meta-analyses of this area (Cormac et al., 2002; Gould et al., 2001; Pilling et al., 2002b; Rector & Beck, 2001). Rector and Beck's review focused only on CBT for delusions and covered seven trials, five of which are included in Gould et al. (2001), six in Pilling et al. (2002b) and six in Cormac et al. (2002). Cormac et al. (2002) identified 13 trials of CBT, two of which focused on compliance issues (Kemp et al., 1998; Lecompte & Pelc, 1996), one on psychoeducation (Buchkremer et al., 1997), one on social skills training (Daniels, 1998), and one on a small-scale trial of group therapy (Levine et al., 1998), leaving a pool of eight examining the direct modification of beliefs. Pilling et al. (2002b) examined eight trials, of which one focused on compliance. Of the 11 trials in Cormac et al. (2002), six were also included by Pilling et al. (2002b), while two trials reviewed by this latter group were not included in Cormac et al.

Rector and Beck's review (2001) identified six studies that included three arms—CBT, varying forms of psychosocial interventions, and routine care. Against routine care, pre- to posttherapy measures of positive symptoms yielded an effect size of 1.3 in favor of CBT and 0.6 in favor of psychosocial interventions; on measures of negative symptoms, the equivalent effect sizes were 1.1 and 0.5. Taking the primary outcome measure from each trial and contrasting the relative impacts of CBT and psychosocial interventions against routine care yielded an effect-size of 0.91 in favor of CBT. Gould et al. (2001) derived similar conclusions to this review.

Pilling et al. (2002b) examined relapse rates using data from six trials, though, as discussed earlier (in relation to family interventions), studies defined this either as an event (such as readmission) or as symptomatic deteri-oration. There were also variations in the contrast treatment, usually to an alternative psychosocial intervention (which itself varied in the degree to which this was a formal intervention); only in three studies was the compara-tor standard care. CBT did not appear to reduce the likelihood of relapse or readmission but did confer significant improvement in mental state—though defined in different ways across studies. Patients receiving CBT had a 22% greater chance of meeting criteria for improved mental state than those in receipt of treatments. Evidence of benefit at follow-up was less clear. Cormac et al. (2002) concurred with Pilling et al.'s (2002b) conclusions, finding that CBT does not reduce relapse rates when contrasted to standard care. Measures of mental state showed a significant improvement for CBT over routine care at between 13 and 26 weeks (NNT = 4), but this was no longer apparent at 1 year.

A narrative review by Dickerson (2000) noted the heterogeneity in aim and focus of CBT studies, identifying 20 trials with a focus on modification and challenge of delusional beliefs, on redirecting attention away from auditory hallucinations, on normalization of psychotic experiences and reduction of anxiety associated with them, on enhancing coping strategies, and trials focused on early intervention. Overall, trials showed benefit in relation to the problems they most directly targeted—principally reducing the conviction with which delusions are held, and the distress that they engender, with little benefit for negative symptoms or social functioning.

Individual Studies

Haddock et al. (1998a) contrasted the efficacy of two approaches to hallucinations, randomizing 33 patients with chronic hallucinations to distraction (n = 14), to focusing combined with anxiety-management techniques (n = 11), or to a control (n = 8). Experimental treatments were delivered in 18–20 weekly sessions. At posttherapy and 2-year follow-up, both groups showed equivalent gains in relation to measures of time spent hallucinating, though the effect was not robust over follow-up. Interpretation of this trial is hampered by the small sample size and wide variability in the response of individual patients.

Tarrier et al. (1993a) allocated 27 patients to two forms of CBT aimed at alleviating residual delusions and hallucinations: coping strategy enhancement (CSE) or problem solving. CSE is a method that identifies potential stressors and triggers to psychotic phenomena, and aims to develop patients' skills in controlling both these cues and their reactions to them. Problem solving was selected as a control treatment because, though not directly addressing psychotic processes, it is commonly used in family management trials. Treatment was delivered in 10 sessions over 5 weeks, with no maintenance sessions after this time. Baseline measures of functioning were obtained by monitoring patients over a 6-week period prior to initiating treatment.

Contrasted to baseline, both treatments resulted in significant, though specific, improvements in functioning. Delusions (but not hallucinations) improved, as did levels of anxiety, but depression, wider areas of functioning, and negative symptoms were not affected. Gains were maintained at 6-month follow-up, though there was evidence of some relapse at this point. There was some, though limited, evidence for the greater efficacy of CSE over problem solving, raising some questions about the mode of action of these techniques (Tarrier et al., 1993b).

A further trial by this group (Tarrier et al., 1998) surveyed a geographical cohort of patients in receipt of National Health Service (NHS) services, identifying 87 eligible patients meeting entry criteria (symptoms present for a minimum of 6 months). Participants were allocated to CBT plus routine care, to supportive counseling plus routine care, or to routine care alone. CBT included specific strategies aimed at coping with symptoms and reducing risk of relapse. Both CBT and counseling were delivered in 20 twice-weekly sessions over 10 weeks. Attrition from all arms of the trial was minimal. Overall, patients receiving CBT improved to the greatest extent; an index of 50% improvement was met by 33% of those in the CBT group, 15% of the supportive counseling group, and 11% of those allocated to routine care. This advantage was still apparent at 12-month follow-up (Tarrier et al., 1999c). Though differences between the active treatments diminished at 2-year follow-up (Tarrier et al., 2000), both continued to show significant benefit over routine care.

Garety et al. (1994) reported a small controlled trial that recruited patients who suffered persistent, drug-resistant psychotic symptoms that had been present for at least 6 months. The first 13 patients to be recruited formed the experimental group, with seven subsequently referred patients forming a wait-list control. Therapy was weekly or biweekly over 6 months, with an average of 16 sessions (range 11–22), and comprised a manualized intervention (Fowler et al., 1995) using cognitive-behavioral coping strategies, modification of delusional beliefs, psychoeducation, and techniques aimed at remoralization. Significant reductions were found in the conviction with which delusional beliefs were held, together with reductions in measures of distress and preoccupation with delusions. However, there were no differences between treatment and control groups on measures of functioning.

A larger controlled trial conducted by this group (across two sites in London and East Anglia) allocated 60 patients either to CBT plus standard care or to standard care alone (Kuipers et al., 1997). CBT was delivered individually, initially weekly and later fortnightly, for up to 9 months using the same manualized treatment as in Garety et al. (1994). Clinically significant change was indicated by a 5- or 10-point change in the Brief Psychiatric Rating Scale, signaling, respectively, a reliable or a large degree of improvement. On these criteria, 21% of the CBT group achieved large improvements, and a further 29% reliable improvement. In the control group, 3% showed a large improvement, 28% reliable improvement, and a further 9% a significant worsening. Improvement in the CBT group was associated with measures of cognitive flexibility in relation to persistent delusions, suggesting some degree of specificity in the link between treatment and outcome (Garety et al., 1997). At 18-month follow-up (Kuipers et al., 1998), those in the CBT group showed continuing and significant improvement, while controls showed no gain over their initial level of functioning. In addition, the CBT group required fewer inpatient episodes and made less use of day services, suggesting some cost–offset against the original treatment phase.

Hogarty et al. (1997a, 1997b) reported two trials of "personal therapy," usually classified by reviewers as a CBT planned on a modular, individualized basis. This means that not all patients receive all elements of the intervention, which includes strategies aimed at improving coping, increasing self-awareness, and managing stress (especially in relation to indicators of relapse), as well as planning for social and vocational rehabilitation.

About 25% (151 patients) of patients admitted to a specialist unit were recruited (with the remainder excluded on the basis of comorbid substance abuse and uncertainty regarding diagnosis). Both trials started after discharge and continued over 3 years; patients were also offered routine care, which included medication. In the first trial, 97 patients living with family were assigned to one of four treatments: (1) personal therapy alone, (2) family psychoeducation and management alone, (3) personal and family therapy combined, or (4) supportive therapy. In the second trial, 54 patients living alone or with nonrelatives were assigned to either personal therapy or supportive therapy. Patients in the two trials differed on a number of indices: Those living alone were older, had more previous hospitalizations, and were more likely to have been separated or divorced; in addition, this group contained significantly more African Americans. Because treatment intensity was matched to clinical need, it varied across patients, and patients in receipt of personal therapy received significantly more sessions than those in either family therapy or supportive therapy.

Overall relapse rates were lower than those usually observed in clinical trials, at around 30%. For patients living with their families, rates of psychotic relapse were lowest in those receiving personal therapy alone. However, patients living alone and receiving supportive therapy had significantly lower rates of relapse than those receiving personal therapy. Survival analysis over the 3 years of the study (which takes into account both the speed and the number of relapses) suggests that for patients living with their families, there was a trend for personal therapy to delay relapse, though this did not reach significance.

Interpreting this trial is difficult. The generally low rate of relapse across all conditions may be an reflection of the intensive support offered to patients across all treatment conditions; whether this effect is general or relates to specific elements of the treatment package is confused by the fact that the therapies contained many elements and were delivered both in "partial" and "full" versions. The adverse impact of personal therapy for patients living alone deserves to be more fully explored, since it may indicate that more intensive therapies will be poorly tolerated in more vulnerable individuals.

Sensky et al. (2000) allocated 90 patients to 19 individual sessions of manualized CBT or to a control "befriending" condition (in which discussion of difficulties was restricted to supportive comments). All interventions were delivered by two nurse–therapists under supervision. At posttherapy, both groups had improved equally. However, at 9-month follow-up, there were significant differences attributable to continued gains in the CBT condition and loss of benefits in the befriending group. "Incubation" effects such as this are hard to interpret given that posttherapy changes are no longer subject to the controls conferred by randomization. Nonetheless, results from this study, taken with others discussed previously, suggest that supportive interventions have some benefit, but that the immediate and longer term efficacy of targeted interventions is not attributable simply to the impact of general relationship factors.

Rector et al. (2003) randomized 42 patients to either "enriched" standard care (which optimized medication and care management, and included psychoeducation) or CBT plus enriched standard care; CBT comprised 20 sessions over 6 months. Both interventions resulted in equivalent and significant gains on posttherapy measures of symptom severity, though at 6-month follow-up, there was differential impact in relation to negative symptoms: Some 67% of patients receiving CBT met criteria for treatment response, contrasted to 31% of controls. Benchmarked against outcomes from other trials, there is some evidence that optimization of standard care led to better than usual outcomes across the whole cohort, though most particularly in relation to positive symptoms.

CBT in Routine Settings

There is relatively little evidence regarding the effectiveness of CBT interventions in routine practice, beyond the expertise of the research groups developing these techniques. Jenner et al. (1998) reported an open trial of 40 patients, with follow-up at 2–4 years (Wiersma et al., 2001). Though there appeared to be positive outcomes, results are difficult to interpret because a number of treatment strategies were employed, and assessments were based on retrospective recall of initial difficulties. Jakes et al. (1999) used a single-case, multiple-baseline design to assess the sequential impact of an initial phase of problem-solving therapy, followed by CBT. Although the two therapists were experienced in CBT technique, they and the patients were part of a standard NHS service. Of 18 participants, six showed significant and sustained changes in conviction of delusional belief during cognitive therapy but not during the control treatment, five showed positive but unstable response, and seven showed no response. Though this rate of mean improvement may be somewhat lower than that found in studies discussed earlier, conclusions drawn from analysis of individual cases may be somewhat more rigorous than analysis based on meaned data. Consistent with Garety et al. (1994; discussed earlier), the patients who improved showed some variability in the strength of their delusional conviction during the baseline period, which implies that not all patients can be expected to derive equal benefit from this intervention. Given the implications of this post hoc finding, this suggestion would benefit from further research.

Turkington et al. (2002) conducted a multicenter trial in which CPNs received 10 days' training in a manualized form of CBT. Four hundred twenty-two patients seen in routine settings were assigned to either standard care or CBT plus standard care. The addition of CBT led to significant posttherapy improvements in overall symptom levels, insight, and level of depression, but there was no evidence that specific symptoms of schizophrenia were impacted by the intervention. Durham et al. (2003b) contrasted CBT delivered by nurse-specialists with supportive therapy (broadly psychodynamic in orientation and also largely delivered by nurses) and treatment as usual (TAU). Sixty-six patients were randomized to approximately 9 months of treatment and followed up at 3 months. Both the CBT and supportive therapy conditions resulted in significantly greater reduction in severity of delusions than TAU. The proportions of patients receiving CBT, supportive therapy, and TAU who evidenced clinically significant change in delusions were 33%, 16%, and 12%, respectively, though these differences are not statistically significant; no differential impact was noted for hallucinations. Although these studies suggest that there may be some utility to offering these interventions in routine practice, overall, outcomes are more modest than those obtained in specialist contexts.

Group Treatment

Three studies explored the impact of group-based CBT for delusions (Chadwick et al., 2000; Gledhill et al., 1998; Wykes et al., 1999). All were open trials in naturalistic clinical settings, and all found some gains for group members in a number of specific measures of symptomatic distress, suggesting that there may be some utility to more systematic exploration of this mode of treatment delivery.

Trials with Patients with Acute Onset

In contrast to the previous studies, a small number of trials focused on the impact of CBT in younger individuals in a more acute stage of the disorder, and on those with subthreshold symptoms (with the aim of preventing progression). Drury et al. (1996a, 1996b) combined cognitive therapy for positive symptoms with a stress management package. Of 117 patients with acute nonaffective psychosis, 69 satisfied inclusion criteria and 40 were allocated to one of two groups on the basis of demographic and psychiatric variables. The first was a cognitive therapy program (CT) that comprised four elements in addition to routine supervision and monitoring: (1) individual CT designed to challenge and modify delusional beliefs; (2) group CT designed to enhance the work undertaken in individual therapy and to develop more general coping skills; (3) family psychoeducation and support, which was offered either in the hospital or in the family home, intended to facilitate patients' attempts to manage their symptoms—particularly their delusional beliefs; and (4) a "meaningful activity program" away from the ward, aimed at reducing negative symptoms. The control group comprised element (4) of the CT program, and was designed to raise patients' activity level and provide informal support. All patients received neuroleptic medication; poststudy checks indicated that the two groups were prescribed this at equivalent levels.

Overall, patients in the CT group showed marked improvement in symptom status, functioning, and speed of recovery, contrasted to the control group. Their stay in the hospital was significantly shorter (a mean of 54 days compared to 119 days), and the mean length of time to full resolution of positive symptoms was also reduced (108 days and 151 days, respectively). Patients in the CT program showed a significantly faster decline in positive symptoms and a significant reduction in the conviction with which they held, and were preoccupied by, core delusional beliefs. These group differences were maintained at 9-month follow-up, with 95% of the CT group, contrasted to 44% of the control group, displaying no or minor positive symptoms. In addition, the rates at which delusional beliefs were reported, and held with conviction, were significantly lower in the CT group. At 4-year follow-up (Drury et al., 2000), relapse rates in both groups were almost identical, though patients in the CT group showed greater perceived control over their illness than those in the control group. While this suggests that the initial benefits are lost over time in the overall sample, in the subgroup of patients who had either no or at most one relapse, the CT group showed significantly fewer positive symptoms and lower delusional conviction than controls. Although an interesting study, it should be noted that its design provides only partial control for the impact of cognitive interventions per se, since family interventions are themselves are known to be of demonstrable benefit to patients.

A small pilot trial (Haddock et al., 1999) allocated 9 patients to approximately 10 sessions of CBT and 11 to approximately nine sessions of supportive psychotherapy combined with psychoeducation; all participants had a recent onset of schizophrenia and were treated during a 5-week inpatient admission. No between-groups differences were found, though all patients showed significant improvement in mental state, and there was no differential acceleration of time to discharge. Although 2-year follow-up suggested a reduced rate of relapse in those receiving CBT, the time to readmission was shorter. The duration of CBT and supportive therapy in this trial was relatively brief (at 8 and 5 hours, respectively), and interpretation is also hampered by the low sample size.

This approach was examined as part of a large, multicenter trial (Lewis et al., 2002) exploring the impact of CBT on time to remission in 315 patients in the acute phase of their first or second episode of schizophrenia. Participants were randomized to "cognitive reality alignment therapy," to manual-based supportive counseling, or to routine care. CBT comprised 15–20 sessions over 5 weeks, with four booster sessions over 3 months, and focused on management of positive symptoms. Though there were no differences in length of hospital admission between groups, and no consistent differences overall in rate of improvement in symptom measures, there were indications that patients with auditory hallucinations responded better to CBT than to supportive counseling or routine care. At 18-month follow-up (Tarrier et al., 2004), both experimental treatments led to gains on measures of symptomatic improvement contrasted to routine care, though no differences in relapse rates (which were approximately 50% across all conditions). As in the acute phase, there was a trend for CBT to show advantage on measures of auditory hallucinations.

While this result suggests the benefit of psychosocial interventions, it offers only weak support for a structured compared to an unstructured approach. This equivalence of outcome is an interesting and to some degree challenging finding. The brevity of treatments and their restriction to the acute phase of illness may be pertinent, and it is also relevant that supportive therapy was manualized (and hence structured). Given that this and the Drury et al. (2000) studies represent the only large-scale studies with this acute population, more research is needed before definitive conclusions can be drawn.

Two further studies have a preventive focus, exploring the impact of CBT on individuals with subthreshold symptoms who may be at risk of progression to schizophrenia. McGorry et al. (2002) randomized 59 patients either to psychoeducation and supportive therapy or to this package combined with antipsychotic medication and CBT (which appeared to have a broad focus on stress management strategies). It should be noted that patients in the control condition did not receive antipsychotic medication, and although the experimental intervention resulted in a greater latency to a first episode of psychosis, it is not clear whether this is attributable to pharmacotherapy or to CBT. A further trial of a CBT intervention is in progress, targeting individuals at high risk of transition to psychosis (Morrison et al., 2002), but outcome data are not yet available.

"COMPLIANCE" AND RELAPSE PREVENTION THERAPIES

Compliance therapy (Kemp et al., 1996) includes discussion of pa___ ___ beliefs regarding their condition and their attitudes to treatment, and aims to identify and manage factors that mitigate against medication maintenance over 4–6 twice-weekly sessions. Kemp et al. (1998) assigned 39 patients to receive this intervention, in contrast to 35 patients who received an equivalent period of supportive counseling. At 18-month follow-up, there was evidence that the intervention led to better medication compliance and that the length of time to readmission was increased (though it should be noted that there was a high level of attrition from the study over the follow-up period). Lecompte and Pelc (1996) randomized 64 noncompliant patients to either CBT (tailored to address compliance with medication and other aspects of treatment) or to an "unstructured discussion" with the therapist, resulting in some gains in a number of areas of management (such as recognition of prodromal signs and attendance at outpatient clinics), but with unclear outcomes in relation to indices such as relapse.

Herz et al. (2000) describe a relapse-prevention program aimed at managing prodromal signs more effectively. Eighty-two patients were randomized to either this program (which comprised individual and group multifamily psychoeducation, group coping-skills therapy and active monitoring of, and intervention in relation to, prodromal signs) or TAU (which included supportive group therapy and medication management). Over 18 months, there were significant advantages to the active intervention both in relation to rates of relapse (17 vs. 34%) and rehospitalization (22 vs. 39%). However, while this may reflect changes in patient and family behaviors, the program also resulted in better recognition and management of prodromal states by clinicians, making it difficult to attribute gains to a specific cause.

Gumley et al. (2003) identified a group of 144 patients from community mental health teams who were considered at risk of relapse (on the basis of indicators such as a relapse in the previous 2 years, social isolation, failure to adhere to medication or a planned reduction in neuroleptics). Patients were randomized to receive TAU, or five sessions of CBT over 12 weeks (aimed at engagement), followed by intensive therapy (two to three sessions a week) if indicators of relapse became evident; 28 individuals in the active treatment group were targeted for this intensive treatment. At the end of the 12-month study period, relapse, as indicated by worsening of symptoms, was lower for CBT than for TAU (18 vs. 35%), though hospital admission rates were equivalent (15 vs. 26%).

Though these are promising (rather than conclusive) studies, greater clinical attention to the development of prodromal states is an important but nonspecific aspect of these programs. Contrast to TAU does not control for this; further research would be necessary before concluding that the form of therapy, rather than the systemic changes associated with its introduction, was mutative.

COGNITIVE REMEDIATION

People with schizophrenia often complain of difficulties in cognitive functioning—for example, in attention, concentration, and memory. Research suggests that they demonstrate deficits in "executive functioning" (the capacity for planning and decision making based on accurate processing of information), and that this may be linked to some of their functional difficulties (e.g., Green et al., 2000). On this basis, cognitive remediation seeks directly to train individuals in these areas. Although the 1990s saw considerable growth in the number of studies of this approach (Wykes & van der Gaag, 2001), meta-analyses by Hayes and McGrath (2000) and Pilling et al. (2002a) identified only three and five well-controlled studies, respectively (all those in Hayes and McGrath are included in Pilling et al.). The targets of remediation within these trials varied widely (with a focus on memory, attention, planning, and problem solving), as did the intensity of interventions. Both reviews concluded that there was no evidence that remediation improved specific areas of cognitive functioning. For example, Pilling et al. extracted separate effect sizes for attention, verbal and visual memory, executive functioning, and mental state, finding no significant differences between experimental and control patients.

Some studies published subsequent to the review period of these meta-analyses have more positive findings. Though these trials tend to demonstrate the feasibility of improving cognitive functioning, the broader benefits for other areas of functioning are not clear (e.g., Bark et al., 2003; Bell et al., 2001; Bellack et al., 2001), and on the whole studies are underpowered. Wykes et al. (1999b, 2003) allocated 33 patients already participating in a day program to receive cognitive remediation or occupational therapy, with therapies delivered for 1 hour a day over 40 days. Although, at posttherapy, there were no between-group differences on symptom measures, there was a gain in self-esteem. Patients who passed a threshold of improvement in cognitive flexibility also showed some improvement in social functioning. However, at 1 year, effects of remediation were apparent only on cognitive measures. In exceptions to this pattern, Hadas-Lidor et al. (2001) randomized 58 patients in receipt of standard care to either remediation or occupational therapy; after 1 year, there appeared to be some gains in measures of cognitive functioning, but more importantly, some evidence of gains in social and work functioning. Bellucci et al. (2002) allocated 34 patients (half with schizophrenia and half with schizoaffective disorder) to 8 weeks of remediation or to a wait-list control, with subsequent gains on cognitive measures and some reduction in measures of negative symptoms (affective flattening, anhedonia, and attentional impairment).

With few good-quality studies available, firm conclusions regarding the benefits of remediation may be premature, especially in the absence of strong evidence of generalization from the intervention itself into broader areas of social and clinical functioning.

INDIVIDUAL PSYCHODYNAMIC THERAPY

There are few methodologically rigorous trials of psychodynamic psychotherapy, with the result that usual inclusion criteria for reviews result in high exclusion rates. Two recent meta-analyses reflect this problem. Malmberg and Fenton (2001) and Gottdiener and Haslam (2002) included 3 and 27 trials, respectively, a difference largely accounted for by the fact that the latter included nonrandomized trials, as well as identifying studies dating from a much earlier period.

On the basis of the three available trials (Gunderson et al., 1984; 1976; O'Brien et al., 1972), all included in Gottdiener and Haslam (2002), Malmberg and Fenton (2001) concluded that psychodynamic therapy confers no additional benefit when combined with medication, and is less effective than medication when contrast is between those receiving therapy alone or medication alone. Gottdiener and Haslam (2002) identified 37 trials of individual therapy for schizophrenia; of these, 27 focused on psychodynamic therapy, 5 on CBT, and 5 on supportive therapy. Publication dates for reviewed studies ranged from 1951 to 1998. Though within-group pre- to posttherapy effect sizes are moderate (0.58), the average effect size for between-group contrasts (available only for seven comparisons) was small at 0.10. Contrast of psychodynamic therapy, CBT, and supportive therapy (based on within-group effect sizes) yielded effect sizes of 0.33, 0.35, and 0.23, respectively. Perhaps surprisingly, equivalent effect sizes were determined for the efficacy of individual therapy, with and without conjoint medication, and for acute contrasted to chronic presentations. Some caution needs to be attached to this review which, while helpful in identifying the extent of available research, includes many studies whose methodological quality falls short of current standards. For example, criteria used to establish outcomes vary widely, as do those for establishing diagnoses (17 trials antedate the more rigorous diagnostic criteria introduced by DSM-III in 1980, and only four trials of psychodynamic therapy adopted DSM or RDC criteria). Reliance on within-group effect sizes is also problematic, though this reflects the lack of available between-treatment contrasts.

On the whole, research into the efficacy of expressive, insight-oriented psychotherapy tends to be largely negative (Goldstein, 1991); indeed, there is some evidence that the emotional intensity of psychodynamic treatments may be harmful for at least some patients (Drake & Sedere, 1986; Mueser & Berenbaum, 1990). Illustrating this, Gunderson et al. (1984) contrasted psychodynamic–expressive therapy with supportive therapy oriented toward coping with problems of daily living. Therapies were carried out over 2 years, and patients were maintained on medication. Supportive therapy appeared to be significantly more helpful, particularly on measures such as relapse and the number of days in employment. This study also indicated, however, that the 31% of patients who remained in their assigned therapy over 2 years had the best outcomes, a finding similar to that of Alanen et al. (1985). However, it is not clear whether better outcomes can be attributed to therapy or to self-selection of patients who were able to maintain extended therapeutic contact and who therefore (by definition) had better levels of functioning. Although these studies indicate that therapy—particularly of a more supportive nature—may be useful to some patients, the very high drop-out rate from both studies (over 50% by 6 months) suggests that it may have limited application in practice.

Although formal psychotherapy may not be judged appropriate, there is some suggestion that the development of a good therapeutic alliance between clinician and patient promotes better compliance with medication (Frank & Gunderson, 1990) and may be a helpful adjunct to treatment (e.g., Liberman, 1994; Weiden & Havens, 1994).

SUMMARY AND CLINICAL IMPLICATIONS

Though pharmacotherapy is often effective in the management of schizo-phrenic symptoms, not all individuals benefit, and relapse rates are significant even in those maintained on medication. For this reason, there is increasing interest in the efficacy of psychosocial interventions, almost always offered adjunctively to pharmacotherapy.

Although social skills training has shown efficacy when examined in treatment-based assessments, its value in enhancing social performance in everyday contexts is less clear, and there is little evidence that it improves overall functioning. Some programs have focused on enhancing skills directly pertinent to community living (e.g., performance in job interviews), but because these have been investigated as part of multicomponent interventions, it is difficult to attribute any gains to specific treatment strategies.

Studies of individual psychotherapy indicate that, on the whole, this is not helpful. Psychodynamic therapy has not been demonstrated to be effective with this group of patients. Though there are indications that when patients value this contact (and are therefore retained in therapy) it can be helpful, its overall efficacy is low.

Recent years have seen developments in three areas of active research: (1) psychoeducation and family intervention programs aimed at modifying the support network of the person with schizophrenia; (2) cognitive-behavioral treatments of acute symptoms; and (3) cognitive remediation, which addresses itself to the amelioration of cognitive deficits.

Psychoeducation should be distinguished from family intervention; the aim of the former is to impart knowledge about schizophrenia, and that of the latter to reduce expressed emotion, and enhance family structure and positive social interaction. Psychoeducation appears to show best results when combined with techniques recognizable as psychological intervention, with little therapeutic gain from psychoeducation alone apart from increases in knowledge and short-term increases in compliance. Trials of family interventions have important variations in implementation, particularly in terms of their frequency and duration, and also in methods for their evaluation. Some studies define outcome using index events, such as hospitalization, while others examine the extent of clinical change. Each of these approaches has merit, but each reflects differing concerns. Hospitalization in particular can be an ambiguous proxy for change; while it often indicates relapse, admissions take place as much for social reasons as clinical (e.g., reflecting variations in family tolerance of difficult behavior, for good or for ill).

Meta-analytic reviews vary in coverage but concur in their conclusion that in comparison to standard care, those receiving family intervention are at significantly reduced risk of relapse. The impact of family intervention reduces with follow-up over 1–2 years, raising an obvious but as yet unresearched question about the potential utility of offering maintenance or booster sessions. There is little evidence for the efficacy of family work other than that based on variants of CBT. In relation to form of delivery, there has been interest in offering multifamily group therapy, partly on grounds of efficiency, but also because it affords relatives greater social support and opportunities for networking. However, only one study has directly contrasted single- and multifamily groups, showing benefit to the latter when patients were discharged in partial remission. However, in other trials, multifamily approaches have failed to demonstrate an advantage over standard care, and more research may be needed to clarify this issue.

The majority of trials examining the implementation of family interventions in routine settings have positive outcomes. However, despite their potential to reduce the cost of care for individuals with schizophrenia, they appear to be difficult to implement. There is some evidence that this is more likely to happen when appropriate training is offered in the context of a service framework that supports this approach. While it remains a moot point as to whether these interventions are—or could be—offered as part of a routine service, their potential utility suggests that even if offered by specialist services, they should be routinely available to those for whom there are indications of benefit. In this respect, it is worth noting that there may be disbenefits to family work, particularly when there are a few indications of family tension or conflict. There is a risk that, in clinical settings, the criteria for offering family work relate more to traditional criteria of psychotherapeutic suitability (e.g., evidence of verbal skills and receptivity to psychological ideas) than to the indicators by which the intervention has shown efficacy (reducing relapse in individuals living in a stressful family environment).

Two broad approaches have been taken in the exploration of CBT with schizophrenia. One focuses on the amelioration of symptoms, while the other aims to achieve better adherence to medication or other aspects of treatment. Both examine key beliefs and coping strategies and working with and through the way in which clients understand their symptoms. Because some reviews conflate these approaches, which actually differ quite markedly in their aims and the type of beliefs that they address, some meta-analyses are difficult to interpret.

Studies of CBT that focus on reducing symptoms are aimed at two populations—on the one hand, chronic patients, and on the other, patients who are acutely ill and often in their first episode of schizophrenia. Within this framework, approaches vary in focus, approach, and length of input. In more chronic patients, CBT does not reduce the likelihood of relapse or readmission but does confer significant improvement in mental state, more so on delusions than hallucinations. This population is less prone to cycles of relapse, and gains in functioning in chronically ill individuals are a significant contribution to quality of life. In more acute populations, there is mixed evidence regarding the capacity of CBT to shorten initial episodes or to ameliorate specific symptoms, and no indication that it reduces relapse rates. Overall, it seems reasonable to conclude that though expectations of improvement should be modest, CBT can make an important contribution to patients' quality of life and mental state. Its long-term effects are unclear from meta-analyses, though some individual studies suggest an incubation effect. It needs to be noted that some forms of CBT—largely, as delivered in individual format—appear to have adverse impacts, particularly for more vulnerable individuals. It is also relevant that CBT is almost invariably implemented in the context of optimized clinical services, and this may well affect its impact. On this basis, offering CBT in isolation may be ill-advised. Finally, it should be noted that in some studies, unstructured supportive interventions, used as a control for CBT, show efficacy—in some cases, equivalent efficacy to CBT. This needs to be considered carefully: Whether it implies that claims for the specificity of action of CBT are inappropriate (e.g., Paley & Shapiro, 2002) or whether this reflects the relatively immature state of research in this area (Tarrier et al., 2002) is yet to be decided.

Outcomes from compliance therapies are somewhat mixed; overall, there appears to be benefit in the form of reduced relapse rates, but the degree to which this relates to specific elements of the therapy is not clear, particularly when there are indications that research protocols increase staff attentiveness to prodromal signs.

Research on cognitive deficits in schizophrenia has recently been reflected in treatment programs aimed at cognitive remediation, adopting a rehabilitative model to train individuals in areas of attention, concentration, memory, and executive functioning. Notwithstanding some variability in the focus and intensity of the intervention, meta-analytic review yields little evidence that remediation therapy improves specific areas of cognitive functioning. Though some studies show more positive results, the breadth of measures used to detect outcome are limited, and more work needs to be done to show the pertinence of any changes in the patient's everyday functioning. Although the current status of cognitive remediation is disappointing, its potential is great, if the analogy with rehabilitation in traumatic brain damage is appropriate. It may be that many of the interventions employed have failed to consider performance differences associated with different states of arousal. Since cognitive deficits become more marked when the information to be processed is emotionally significant, the value of cognitive remediation may be improved by taking emotional salience more fully into account.

The trend in psychotherapy research concerning schizophrenia is toward study of an increasingly narrow range of orientations, and more decisive reviews of the lack of efficacy of psychodynamic therapy make it more rather than less likely that this trend will continue. With an increasing focus on specific forms of intervention, mostly based on variants of CBT, there is some risk that variable evidence for the efficacy of generic psychosocial interventions will be overlooked in favor of reasonably consistent evidence for the value of structured techniques. This observation may be most pertinent for individuals in acute stages of the disorder, when the corrosive impact of psychotic illness on usual developmental trajectories is particularly obvious and—at least, potentially—subject to some amelioration. The emergence of studies focusing on this issue is therefore to be welcomed.

As promising as psychotherapeutic approaches might seem, some caution is appropriate. Both in clinical trials and in routine settings, rates of refusal and dropout are relatively high. In some respects this is unsurprising—a significant proportion of this client group finds it difficult to engage with services. However, it does indicate an obvious limitation to generalization of trial effects. It is possible that further studies with improved techniques will indicate ways of increasing acceptability, but refusal rates should also focus attention on the skills and supervision that may be required to implement these techniques. Evidence from family interventions suggests that systemic change is required in order to allow these techniques to be implemented.

Because CBT can be offered on a one-on-one basis, it may be more readily transportable, but there are enough indications from the literature to suggest that care should be taken in its adoption into routine settings. Most practitioners would recognize that working directly to modify psychotic symptoms is a highly skilled process that requires both adequate training and supervision, the more so because of evidence of iatrogenic effects. The current state of research is not so compelling as to justify assumptions of effectiveness in routine settings, implying that monitoring of outcomes should be a critical part of implementation.

CHAPTER 11

PERSONALITY DISORDERS

DEFINITIONS

Problems in the Definition of Personality Disorders

Defining and describing personality disorders is controversial. Although clinical and research instruments make it possible to make reasonably reliable diagnoses, there is debate about whether the descriptions on which these diagnoses are based have clinical utility or meaning. An additional problem is that DSM-IV-TR describes the traits associated with these disorders as stable and enduring, logically—and unhelpfully—rendering the notion of treatment an oxymoron. As with other areas covered in this review, much of the literature on treatment effectiveness is organized according to Axis II diagnoses. While we do not necessarily regard this to be the most appropriate for designing treatment interventions or for assessing effectiveness, it is undoubtedly the most commonly used heuristic device for organizing treatment outcome in this area.

Axis II of DSM-IV-TR identifies 10 personality disorders. These are grouped into three "clusters," which better reflects the fact that individuals rarely belong to just one category of personality disorder. Patients with presentations in cluster B command most clinical and research attention, based on the challenge to services posed by a combination of poor impulse control, self-harm, and aggression and tendency to present in crisis.

Cluster A: "Odd–Eccentric"

Paranoid Personality Disorder

The essential feature of this disorder is a pervasive tendency to interpret the actions of others as deliberately demeaning or threatening. People with this disorder are usually argumentative and exaggerate difficulties, "making mountains out of molehills."

Schizoid Personality Disorder

This disorder is characterized by a pervasive pattern of indifference to social relationships. There is little enjoyment of or desire for close relationships, and people with this disorder tend to be loners, having no (or only one) close friends or confidants. They appear cold and aloof, and display a restricted range of affect.

Schizotypal Personality Disorder

In this disorder, there is a pervasive pattern of peculiarities of ideation, appearance, and behavior that is not severe enough to meet the criteria for schizophrenia. Disturbances of thought content may include paranoid ideas, ideas of reference, and magical thinking. There may be disturbances of perception or peculiarities of speech content (such as vagueness or impoverishment, but not a loosening of associations). People with this disorder often appear odd and eccentric in their behavior; there may be inappropriate or constricted affect, and social relationships are few and often restricted to first-degree relatives.

Cluster B: "Dramatic–Erratic"

Antisocial Personality Disorder

People with this disorder have a pattern of antisocial and irresponsible behavior beginning in childhood and continuing into adulthood. In adulthood, there is a pattern of behavior that often renders the person liable to arrest, such as harassing others, stealing, destroying property, or failing to honor financial obligations. These individuals tend to be irritable or aggressive, often getting into fights or assaulting others. There is rarely expression of remorse for the effects of their behavior on others.

Borderline Personality Disorder

The essential feature of this disorder is a pervasive pattern of instability of self-image, interpersonal relationships, and mood. The person's sense of identity is profoundly uncertain. Interpersonal relationships are unstable and intense, fluctuating between the extremes of idealization and devaluation. There is often a terror of being alone, with great efforts being made to avoid real or imagined abandonment. Affect is extremely unstable, with marked shifts from baseline mood to depression or anxiety usually lasting a few hours. Inappropriate anger and impulsive behavior are common, and often this behavior is self-harming. Suicidal threats and self-mutilation are common in more severe forms of this disorder.

Histrionic Personality Disorder

This disorder is characterized by a pervasive pattern of excessive emotionality and attention seeking. People with this disorder often seek reassurance, approval, or praise from others, and often display rapidly shifting and shallow expression of emotions.

Narcissistic Personality Disorder

People with this disorder often display a pervasive pattern of grandiosity, either in fantasy or in behavior, together with hypersensitivity to the evaluation of others. There is an exaggerated sense of self-importance that often alternates with a sense of special unworthiness. Self-esteem is very fragile.

Cluster C: "Anxious–Fearful"

Avoidant Personality Disorder

The essential feature of this disorder is a pervasive pattern of social discomfort and timidity, together with a fear of negative evaluation. There is a reluctance to enter into social relationships, unless there is a guarantee of uncritical acceptance; consequently, people with this disorder rarely have close friends or confidants. Although there is strong desire for affection, social situations are avoided.

Dependent Personality Disorder

People with this disorder have a pervasive pattern of dependent and submissive behavior, characterized by an inability to make decisions without reassurance from others. There is a sense of helplessness when alone, and there is often great anxiety about abandonment when in close relationships.

Obsessive–Compulsive Personality Disorder

This disorder is characterized by a pervasive pattern of perfectionism and inflexibility. There is an adherence to unusually strict and often unattainable standards, which often results in interference with the completion of projects. In addition, there is a preoccupation with rules and trivial detail. People with this disorder are always mindful of their status relative to others, often resisting the authority of others and stubbornly insisting that others conform to their own way of doing things. These individuals frequently have difficulty expressing affect, and they are often perceived as stilted or "stiff."

PREVALENCE, COMORBIDITY, AND NATURAL HISTORY

Prevalence

Weissman (1993) reviewed epidemiological surveys conducted using a range of standardized interview schedules. Overall, around 10–13% of personality disorders were diagnosed in community samples or in samples made up of relatives of patients with psychiatric problems. Two more recent surveys based on community samples confirm these rates (Samuels et al., 2002; Torgersen et al., 2001).

Cluster A

Lifetime prevalence rates vary between 0.4 and 1.8% for paranoid personality disorder, between 0.4 and 0.9% for schizoid personality disorder, and between 0.7 and 5.6% for schizotypal personality disorder, with more usual figures in the range from 3 to 5.6%.

Cluster B

Prevalence rates for histrionic personality disorder range between 1.3 and 3.0%; for narcissistic personality disorder, rates vary between 0.0 and 0.4%, and for borderline personality disorder, between 1.1 and 4.6%. Rates for antisocial personality disorder vary between 1.5 and 3.2%.

Cluster C

Rates for avoidant personality disorder vary between 1.1 and 1.4%, for dependent personality disorder, between 1.5 and 1.7%, and for obsessive–compulsive personality disorder, between 1.7 and 2.2%. Rates for passive–aggressive personality disorder vary between 0.0 and 1.8%.

Although these percentages suggest that relatively few individuals suffer from personality disorders, the acute nature of their symptoms and the chronicity of their condition lead to their being overrepresented in psychotherapeutic caseloads (Berelowitz & Tarnopolsky, 1993).

Comorbidity

Comorbidity within Personality Disorders

Zimmerman and Coryell (1990) reported that paranoid, avoidant, and borderline personality disorders were almost always comorbid; 23% of subjects with borderline personality disorder also met criteria for schizotypal personality disorder. Antisocial personality disorder was frequently diagnosed in people with borderline or schizotypal personality disorder. Half of those diagnosed with avoidant personality disorder also met criteria for schizotypal personality disorder.

Comorbidity with Axis I Disorders

Swartz et al. (1990) reported very high rates of comorbid Axis I disorders in patients with borderline personality disorder. In the year prior to the survey, 56.4%, had generalized anxiety disorder; 41.1%, specific phobia disorder; 40.7%, major depression disorder; 36.9%, agoraphobia; 34.6%, social phobia; 21.9%, alcohol abuse; and 6.1%, obsessive–compulsive disorder.

Natural History

The course of borderline personality disorder has been more extensively researched than other diagnoses. Although follow-up over 5 years suggests that symptomatic patterns change little (Carpenter et al., 1977; Pope et al., 1983; Werble, 1970), follow-up over 15 years suggests that by middle age, many borderline patients no longer meet relevant diagnostic criteria, though this does not indicate that recovery is complete (McGlashan, 1986; Paris et al., 1987; Stone, 1993). At this point, approximately 10% of patients will have committed suicide. Zanarini et al. (2003) conducted a prospective follow-up study of 290 individuals originally admitted as inpatients. After 6 years, 74% no longer met diagnostic criteria for borderline personality disorder. Though symptoms associated with impulsiveness (such as self-harm and substance abuse) declined, most participants continued to suffer from affective disorders, along with chronic feelings of anger and emptiness. In this sense, borderline personality disorder appears to be a chronic disorder with some moderation in its severity over time.

Treatment utilization by individuals with personality disorders is extensive. Bender et al. (2001) contrasted service use by 664 patients, 97 with depression and 567 with personality disorders, finding that the presence of personality disorder was associated with a significant increase in the probability of receiving multiple psychosocial and psychiatric interventions, especially hospitalization (odds ratio = 4.9).

IMPACT OF PERSONALITY DISORDERS ON OUTCOME IN TREATMENT OF AXIS I DISORDERS

The impact of personality disorders on the treatment of Axis I conditions is reviewed in the relevant chapters of this book, and interested readers should refer to these sections (though it should be noted that appropriate evidence is not available across all conditions, and for some, diagnoses are based on a limited number of trials). Briefly, while many studies of depressive disorder find that the presence of a personality disorder reduces efficacy, this broad conclusion needs to be tempered by evidence of some inconsistency across studies, and by concerns about the impact of methodological quality. In relation to the anxiety disorders, individuals with social phobia and comorbid avoidant personality disorder present as more symptomatic and have poorer outcomes than those without this comorbidity. Dependent or avoidant personality disorder reduces the probability of remission in generalized anxiety disorder. Many trials find that personality disorders reduce treatment efficacy for panic disorder, but this is not a consistent finding. For obsessive–compulsive disorder, there is consistent evidence that schizotypal personality disorder has a negative impact on outcome. In eating disorders, there are indications that the presence of a cluster B personality disorder predicts higher symptom levels at pretreatment and a poorer outcome at follow-up.

Overall, research implies that the presence of a personality disorder will be associated with more complex and severe initial presentation, and that while improvements will be evident, outcomes will be more modest than when comorbidity is not present (e.g., Tyrer et al., 1993, 1994). However, the strength of evidence for this assertion is variable across diagnoses, and in some cases, findings are inconsistent. On this basis, it seems reasonable to suggest that clinicians carefully assess patients with comorbid personality disorders in relation to the ways in which their presentation may or may not imply a challenge to treatment, rather than to assume that comorbidity will necessarily prejudice therapy.

TREATMENT APPROACHES

General Considerations in the Evaluation of Treatments for Personality Disorder

In earlier sections, we have observed that the outcome of treatment for Axis I disorders is likely to be varied by the presence of a comorbid personality disorder. Equally, evaluation of treatments for personality disorders is made problematic when, as is frequently the case, Axis I disorders are present. Woody et al. (1985) have demonstrated this influence for antisocial personality disorder (discussed further below). Shea (1993) suggested that research could control for this by excluding patients with Axis I disorders from clinical trials but also notes that some disorders, such as borderline personality disorder, are almost always associated with significant Axis I psychopathology. An ideal strategy, but one that no current trial has attempted, might be to assign patients to treatment groups on the basis of matched Axis I disorders.

A further difficulty for evaluation studies is that such comorbidity can be difficult to assess. For example, in studies by Soloff et al. (1986) and Kelly et al. (1992), two cohorts of inpatients with borderline personality disorder were assessed on admission. Though apparent rates of major depressive disorder were between 64 and 75%, depression resolved in a significant proportion of these patients after 2 weeks, and this without any active treatment (intervention being limited to observation without medication). Similar findings under the same "observational" regimen have been reported by Siever et al. (1985); depression resolved in 17 of 22 (90%) patients. Such observations raise questions about whether these patients are presenting with comorbid depression or with characterological symptomatology reflective of the borderline syndrome, such as chronically low self-esteem. The extent to which resolution of such problems should constitute a marker for treatment efficacy is therefore a matter for debate.

Psychopharmacological Studies

A review of pharmacological treatments for patients with personality disorders is beyond the scope of this chapter. Usually, medication aims to manage specific symptomatic manifestations of personality disorders, and though there is evidence for the efficacy of this approach, there is no drug treatment of choice for personality disorders. This is unsurprising, since patients vary markedly in the domains in which impairment is presented and, hence, the extent to which medication is indicated. A wide range of medications are used in clinical practice, including neuroleptics, antidepressants, and mood stabilizers.

Reviews (Roy & Tyrer, 2001; Sanislow & McGlashan, 1998; Soloff, 1994) indicate that there is relatively little research evidence on which to base treatment recommendations. Trials of neuroleptics in patients with borderline or schizotypal personality disorder (Brinkley et al., 1979; Cowdrey & Gardener, 1988; Goldberg et al., 1986; Leone, 1982; Soloff et al., 1986, 1989) suggest that patients with moderately severe schizotypal symptoms appear to benefit most from neuroleptic medication. In addition, neuroleptics have some efficacy relative to depression (Soloff et al., 1986) and impulsive behavior (Soloff et al., 1989). Neuroleptics administered tend to be low-dose and contribute to global improvement primarily through addressing psychotic-like symptoms, depression, anxiety, and impulse control.

The efficacy of tricyclic antidepressants tends to be modest (Perry, 1985; Soloff et al., 1986, 1989). Indeed, in some patients, the response to tricyclics can be one of increasing anger and poorer impulse control (Soloff et al., 1986). Even the effect on depressive symptomatology is not reliably demonstrated (Links et al., 1990). Monoamine oxidase inhibitors (MAOIs) may be more effective than tricyclics in treating symptoms of depression in patients with borderline personality disorder (Parsons et al., 1989) and are certainly superior to placebo in terms of improving mood (Cowdrey & Gardener, 1988). Two trials (Coccaro & Kavoussi, 1997; Salzman et al., 1995) suggest that fluoxetine may be helpful in reducing impulsiveness and anger. There is some (limited) evidence for the benefits of mood stabilizers for impulsive and aggressive behaviors (e.g., Cowdrey & Gardener, 1988; Hollander et al., 2001; Stein et al., 1995).

Waldinger and Frank (1989) surveyed 40 American clinicians in private practice with experience of psychotherapy with patients with borderline personality disorder; 90% of these clinicians prescribed medication; 87% of the therapists reported problems of patients abusing their prescribed medication at some time. Anecdotal reviews of clinical experience indicate that specific problems may arise when psychotherapy is combined with pharmacological treatment, because many of these individuals have specific problems with dependency on drugs and on individuals, and have a potential for abusing both (see Elkin et al., 1988a, 1988b; Perry, 1990). Trials of long-term maintenance therapy have shown little additional benefit beyond the acute phase (e.g., Cornelius et al., 1993). Nonetheless, short-term adjunctive use of medication may be important in the management of these patients (Soloff, 1994).

Psychological Therapies

Meta-Analyses

Perry et al. (1999) reviewed 15 studies published between 1981 and 1999, of which six were randomized, covering several subtypes of personality disorder treated using a range of therapies (cognitive-behavioral therapy [CBT], psychodynamic therapy, supportive therapy, and interpersonal psychotherapy [IPT]), with a wide range in the length of therapy (from 10 days to 2 years). Some were trials in which the primary aim was not the direct management of personality disorder but of associated problems (such as eating disorder or depression). The mean pretreatment to follow-up effect size was 1.1 and 1.3 for self-reported and observer-rated measures respectively, indicating a significant impact of psychological therapy. Three studies that contrasted active to control treatment yielded an effect size of 0.75, though in no case were controls active therapy (being a wait list in two cases, and treatment as usual [TAU] in the other).

Four studies reported the percentage of cases no longer meeting criteria for personality disorder. In these trials, 53% of patients had borderline personality disorder; all had cluster B or C diagnoses. At follow-up (mean = 67 weeks), 52% met recovery criterion. Treatment length was associated with recovery; Perry et al. (1999) calculated that while the recovery rate in natural history studies is 3.7% per year, recovery rates in these four trials were about seven times faster, at 25.8%.

Leichsenring and Leibing's (2003) review is somewhat more focused, considering only trials that employed psychodynamic therapy or CBT, and attempting some disaggregation of personality disorder subtypes. They identified 22 studies (of which 11 were randomized), published between 1974 and 2001. This review includes all relevant studies from Perry et al. (1999), with most (but not all) additional studies explained by its later publication date. Because of the relative paucity of randomized trials, effect sizes were (as in Perry et al.) calculated on the basis of pre- to posttherapy change. For borderline personality disorder, the effect size for psychodynamic therapy was 1.31 ($n = 8$), and for CBT, 0.95 ($n = 4$). Combining data for all personality disorders, the effect size for psychodynamic therapy was 1.46 ($n = 15$ contrasts) and for CBT, 1.0 ($n = 10$ contrasts). Six exclusively psychodynamic studies employed measures oriented to the core pathology of personality disorders, yielding an effect size of 1.56. Treatment length showed a positive but nonsignificant correlation with outcome in psychodynamic studies ($r = .41$); the smaller number of CBT trials precluded an equivalent analysis. Overall, this review suggests that both therapies are of equal efficacy.

Although these are promising results, the relative paucity of trials—and especially of good quality trials—restricts the conclusions that can be drawn for meta-analysis. Rather few studies are randomized, there are few direct contrasts of therapies, and in only a limited number is the primary aim to treat Axis II disorders. Even when this is the case, the range of personality disorder subtypes is restricted, with borderline presentations being best represented. On this basis, it could be argued that these meta-analyses, while welcome, are somewhat premature.

The remaining sections of this chapter review outcomes in relation to subtype of personality disorder.

TREATMENTS FOR BORDERLINE PERSONALITY DISORDER

Psychodynamic Therapy

Uncontrolled Trials

The Menninger study (overviewed in Wallerstein, 1989) treated 42 patients with intensive psychodynamic psychotherapy. The trial was carried out in the 1950s, and follow-up has continued since that date. Although it antedates the development of diagnostic systems, clinical descriptions suggest that the majority of patients would merit a diagnosis of borderline personality disorder. Patients were treated with psychoanalysis, expressive psychotherapy, or supportive psychotherapy. Reports from therapists indicated that rarely was analysis carried out in a pure form, and that (presumably pragmatically) therapy was characterized by a significant degree of supportive (ego-building) elements. Of 27 patients for whom full follow-up data were available, good outcomes were obtained in 11, and a partial resolution in a further 7. Better outcomes were obtained in patients with higher levels of ego strength. Those with high levels of ego strength and better quality of interpersonal relationships seemed to respond better to psychoanalytic or expressive therapy than to supportive therapy. In contrast, those with low ego strength responded better to supportive psychotherapy combined, where necessary, with hospitalization.

Waldinger and Gunderson (1984) reported a survey of analysts who, between them, had treated 78 moderately impaired patients with borderline personality disorder. Treatments were either psychoanalysis or psychoanalytic psychotherapy, and were intensive; patients averaged three sessions per week over 4.5 years. Therapist reports indicated significant improvements in all areas, with some relationship between the duration of therapy and better outcomes.

Antikainen et al. (1995) reported a cohort study of 69 patients who spent at least 3 weeks on an inpatient therapeutic community unit (range, 3–42 weeks). Although most were reported as meeting psychodynamic criteria for borderline personality disorder, a formal diagnosis was assigned in around half the sample. While there were some gains on measures of depressive symptoms at posttherapy and 3-year follow-up, there was an increase in suicidal thoughts at follow-up. Nearly all patients were referred for further treatment after admission, and about a half had further inpatient treatment, making it difficult to attribute any changes to the initial admission.

Wilberg et al. (1998) conducted a naturalistic study in a specialist day treatment unit run as a therapeutic community. Outcomes in 31 patients who received day treatment alone were contrasted with 12 patients who were given an additional 1 year of outpatient group therapy after leaving the unit. Although outcomes were better for those who received outpatient treatment, there are several reasons for caution. In particular, the study was carried out over many years, and most patients receiving the day program alone were seen early in the life of the unit (when staff were less experienced), and when treatment duration was shorter. Finally, allocation to outpatient treatment was elective, further reducing the likelihood that the two treatment groups are comparable.

Stevenson and Meares (1992) and Meares et al. (1999) reported an open trial for 48 borderline patients receiving twice-weekly outpatient therapy over 12 months using an interpersonal/psychodynamic therapy. Outcomes in the cohort of 30 patients who completed 1-year of planned treatment were contrasted with patients placed onto a 12-month wait list. Allocation to treatment or wait list was based on therapist availability, and the somewhat lower

levels of severity in the wait-list group may have reflected selective reallocation to other sources of help based on clinical need. Ratings of DSM diagnostic status suggested that 30% of patients no longer met DSM-III-R criteria
for borderline personality, with little indication of change in the wait-list
group. A cost–benefit analysis (Stevenson & Meares, 1999) followed up the
30 completer patients and contrasted health service utilization in the years
preceding and following the intervention. The significant reduction in costs
was largely attributable to reduced inpatient stays.

Monsen et al. (1995) described outcomes for a diverse group of 25 individuals treated as outpatients for a mean of 2 years (range, 5 months to 3.5
years). At baseline, 7 participants were reported as meeting criteria for borderline personality disorder, 16 for various other personality disorders, 2 for
no personality disorder, and 4 for a psychotic diagnosis. Nineteen patients
stayed for more than 1 year, and mean follow-up was 5 years. Although at
termination there was an apparent reduction in the number meeting diagnostic criteria, the methods for establishing diagnoses were inconsistent and
hence unreliable. Pretreatment diagnoses were derived from information
supplied by therapists, whereas posttherapy diagnoses were closer to a formal
evaluation, based on independent interviews using a structured diagnostic
instrument.

Dolan et al. (1997) presented information on patients referred to a therapeutic community specializing in "severe personality disorder," all of whom
were asked to complete a questionnaire pack on referral; about 40% of these
patients were admitted. A second pack was sent 1 year after discharge for
patients entered into the program, and 1 year after referral for untreated individuals. Of an initial cohort of 598, 137 patients returned questionnaires at
both assessment points, evenly distributed between admitted and non-
admitted patients. Of these, around 80% met criteria for borderline personality disorder at referral. Scores on measures of borderline psychopathology
were equivalent at baseline, but there were significant gains for treated over
untreated patients, with 43 and 18%, respectively, showing clinically significant change. Length of stay was associated with improvement; contrasting
those who made clinically significant improvement with those who did not,
average length of admission was 35.7 and 21.1 weeks, respectively. The
untreated group did not constitute a formal comparison group, partly because
the reasons for their nonattendance varied (from refusal, to exclusion on clinical or financial grounds), and their "follow-up" questionnaires were solicited
1 year after referral, contrasted to an average of 19 months for treated
patients. Although this limits the inferences that can be drawn, this study was
able to demonstrate meaningful clinical improvements in a specialist but routine service.

Clarkin et al. (2001) described outcomes from a cohort study of 23
female patients after 1 year of treatment. At this point, a decrease in suicidal

behavior and inpatient stays was apparent. Chiesa and Fonagy (2000) contrasted two forms of hospital-based psychodynamic treatment. In the first, patients were admitted for 11–16 months, with no aftercare; the second comprised a shorter inpatient stay of 6 months followed by 12–18 months of outpatient therapy, along with community support. Allocation to each program was based on distance from the patient's home to the clinic (and hence availability for outpatient treatment). Of 90 patients who started treatment, approximately 75% met criteria for borderline personality disorder. In practice, length of hospital stay was almost equivalent between the two groups, but more rapid and greater improvement was apparent in patients whose treatment spanned both in- and outpatient contexts, and this differential was maintained at 36-month follow-up (Chiesa & Fonagy, 2003). The reasons for this differential outcome are not clear, though the more explicit structure of care in the postdischarge period may be relevant. Whatever the mechanisms underpinning outcome, this study suggests that long-term admission is neither necessary nor necessarily helpful for these patients.

Gabbard et al. (2000) presented data from a prospective, naturalistic study of outcomes from a cohort of patients treated in two inpatient programs using therapeutic community principles. Although program content was broadly consistent, treatment offered was on the basis of clinical judgment, and the length of stay varied widely (with a median of 58 days). Of 689 patients admitted, data were reported on (a possibly unrepresentative) 216 patients who completed treatment and were available for follow-up at 1 year. Although all patients were classified as having "serious" personality disorders, the precise composition of the group is unclear—around half had a diagnosis of personality disorder not otherwise specified (NOS), or of mixed personality disorder, and 35% had a diagnosis of borderline personality disorder. Significant improvements were noted on a range of measures, which were sustained at follow-up. For example, whereas at admission only 3.7% of patients had scores greater than 50 on the Global Assessment Scale, at discharge this rose to 55%, and 66% at 1 year. Although this result is broadly positive, the report is limited by a lack of information on the specific treatments received and the reporting of outcome data only for those cases available to follow-up.

Reviewing the results of follow-up and uncontrolled outcome studies, Higgitt and Fonagy (1993) concluded that (1) psychotherapy is more likely to be effective for less severely borderline patients; (2) in patients under age 30, the greatest risk comes from suicide, and the aim of treatment may legitimately be the reduction in this risk rather than cure; (3) patients with chronic depression, psychological mindedness, low impulsivity, and good social support appear to be most likely to benefit from expressive therapy; (4) patients with impulse control disorders associated with cluster B diagnoses appear to benefit from a limit-setting group; and (5) patients with substance abuse require their dependency problems to be specifically and separately addressed before psychotherapy is likely to be effective.

Controlled Trials

Bateman and Fonagy (1999) assigned 38 patients to either an 18-month program of intensive, structured psychodynamically informed day treatment ("partial hospitalization") or routine care. Though both treatments were offered in
the context of standard NHS services, the day unit specialized in work with
borderline patients. Over 18 months, patients receiving partial hospitalization
showed significant gains over controls on measures of suicidality, self-harm, and
inpatient stay, and also on measures of symptoms and functioning. These gains
became apparent only after 6 months of treatment and became more robust
over time, suggesting that shorter periods of therapy may not be effective.
Follow-up at 18 months (Bateman & Fonagy, 2001), which included an intent-
to-treat analysis, suggested that patients who completed the program maintained gains, and that further improvements in symptomatic and interpersonal
functioning were evident. A cost–benefit analysis (Bateman & Fonagy, 2003)
suggested that the additional costs of the program were offset by reductions in
inpatient and emergency-room care, as well as reduced medication.

Cognitive-Behavioral Therapy

Uncontrolled Trials

Turkat and Maisto (1985) reported results from a case series of 35 patients
with a range of personality disorders. Treatment was based on the derivation
of detailed formulations for each patient's problems, and cognitive-behavioral
interventions were employed. Of 16 cases with outcome data, only four
showed a good outcome.

   Davidson and Tyrer (1996) reported a case series of seven patients,
though detailed clinical data were presented only for three clients, who
attended between 14 and 17 sessions of treated schema-focused CBT.
Although outcomes were positive, interpretation is limited by the small sample size and lack of information on the remaining patients in the trial. Blum
et al. (2002) reported on the development of Systems Training for Emotional
Predictability and Problem Solving (STEPPS), a 20-week manualized program that deploys psychoeducation, behavioral management, and a focus on
maladaptive schemas in a systemic context (which includes both professional
and family carers). Data from a cohort of 52 patients entering the program
suggest some reduction in impulsive and suicidal behavior and some improvement on measures of depression, but no follow-up data are available to
indicate the durability of this effect.

Controlled Trials

Evans et al. (1999) recruited 34 patients who had been referred after an episode of self-harm within the previous 12 months and had a personality disor-

der within cluster B. Patients were randomized to a manualized CBT treatment (which contained elements of dialectical behavior therapy [DBT], and
whose intensity varied from bibliotherapy to six sessions of CBT) or to TAU.
Though CBT led to a significant reduction in depressive symptomatology,
the rate of suicidal acts was not significantly different in the two groups.
Tyrer et al. (2003) reported outcomes from a large multicenter trial of this
approach, in which 480 individuals who presented to emergency services
after self-harm were randomized to either brief manualized CBT (five sessions over 3 months) or TAU. Though approximately 40% of individuals in
this study had a personality disorder, their actions, rather than their diagnosis,
formed the basis for trial entry, and the relevance of these results for personality disorder per se is unclear. There were no differences in the rate of self-
harm or rates of suicide over 12-months follow-up. Though there were some
indications of greater cost-effectiveness for active treatment (related largely to
the costs of hospital, social and criminal justice services), these were significant only at up to 6-month follow-up (Byford et al., 2003a).

Dialectical Behavior Therapy

Uncontrolled Trials

Bohus et al. (2000) implemented DBT in two phases, the first as part of a 3-
month inpatient treatment, followed by outpatient treatment. Twenty four
women who had at least two parasuicidal acts in the 2 years prior to admission entered the trial; assessment 1 month after the inpatient phase suggested
a decrease in impulsive acts and some improvement in symptom levels. Low
et al. (2001) implemented DBT in a high-security hospital. Ten patients
entered the trial; at 6-month follow-up, there was evidence of reduced rates
of self-harm, and lower levels of depression and dissociative experiences. Barley et al. (1993) tracked the impact of introducing DBT into an inpatient unit
for borderline personality disorder, with the milieu shifting from a primarily
psychodynamic approach to one in which, while psychodynamically informed, closely followed DBT principles. One hundred thirty patients were
monitored, and the shift to a DBT program was considered as three phases
(the 19 months prior to its introduction, the 10 months while it was introduced, and the subsequent 14 months). Introduction of the program was
associated with reduced levels of parasuicidal behavior.

Controlled Trials

Linehan et al. (1991) contrasted DBT with TAU. DBT is a manualized therapy (Linehan, 1993) that contains elements of behavioral, cognitive, and supportive psychotherapies. Therapy was conducted weekly, and treatment was

offered both individually and in groups over 1 year. By definition, interventions received by patients receiving TAU were not controlled.

Patients were admitted to the trial if they met DSM-III-R criteria and had at least two incidents of parasuicide in the 5 years preceding the trial (with one in the immediately preceding 8 weeks); 22 female patients were assigned to DBT and 22 to the control condition. Assessment was carried out during and at the end of therapy, and again after 1-year follow-up (Linehan et al., 1993). Control patients, as contrasted with those receiving DBT, were significantly more likely to make suicide attempts (the mean number of attempts in control and DBT patients, respectively, was 33.5 and 6.8) and spent significantly more time as inpatients over the year of treatment (mean = 38.8 and 8.5 days, respectively). In addition, they were also significantly more likely to drop out of the therapies they were assigned to as part of TAU. Attrition from DBT was 16.7% contrasted with 50% for other therapies.

Follow-up was naturalistic, based on the proposition that the morbidity of this group precluded termination of therapy at the end of the experimental period. At 6-month follow-up, DBT patients continued to have less parasuicidal behavior than controls receiving TAU, though at 1 year, there were no between-group differences. While at 1 year DBT patients had fewer days as inpatients, at the 6-month assessment, there were no between-group differences. Although on some measures (employment performance and anxious ruminations) there were no between-group differences, most assessments of adjustment favored the patients receiving DBT.

In a small-scale trial, Koons et al. (2001) randomized 20 women to a shortened (6-month) version of DBT or to TAU, and found that DBT resulted in a significant reduction in suicidal behavior, hopelessness, and depression at posttherapy. Verheul et al. (2003) assigned 58 female patients to 12 months of DBT or to TAU (which usually comprised contact with metal health services). DBT did not reduce the rate of suicidal behavior, but it did show a greater reduction in high-risk behaviors (such as self-mutilation), and greater retention of patients in treatment. Stratification of the patient sample by severity of presentation suggested a greater impact for more disordered individuals, though this was statistically significant only for self-mutilation. As in Linehan's studies, while there is evidence that DBT is helpful in the management of impulsive behaviors associated with borderline personality disorder, there is little evidence that it impacts on other symptomatic or functional features of the disorder, and neither trial presents follow-up data.

Bohus et al. (2004) reported a contrast of 40 female patients assigned to a 3-month inpatient DBT program against 20 female patients placed on a wait-list control. On assessment, 1 month after the end of the treatment program, those receiving DBT showed significant improvement over wait-list members on indices of self-injurious behavior and on a number of symptom measures. Approximately 40% of patients receiving active treatment met criteria for reliable and clinically significant change on the Symptom Checklist 90 (SCL-90). Some constraints on interpretation of this trial are pertinent. Patients were allocated to treatment or wait list on a consecutive rather than random basis, analysis is available only for treatment completers, and no follow-up data are available.

A small number of trials have examined the efficacy of DBT for patients with comorbid substance abuse and borderline personality disorder. Linehan et al. (1999) contrasted DBT and TAU in 28 substance-abusing female patients (showing dependence on both prescription and nonprescription drugs). DBT resulted in greater treatment retention, and at posttherapy and 16-month follow-up, there was a significant reduction in substance abuse. Linehan et al. (2002) randomized 23 heroin-dependent women to DBT or to a combination of the 12-step program and "comprehensive validation therapy" (a nondirective approach developed as a contrast therapy for this trial, which includes the validation component of DBT). Both interventions showed equivalent efficacy in reducing opiate use and levels of psychopathology, and, indeed, DBT had poorer retention rates. However, it did result in better maintenance of reduction in drug use over treatment and follow-up.

Inpatient and Therapeutic Community Programs

Tucker et al. (1987) reported data on 40 of 62 inpatients treated for between 6 months and 1 year in a specialized unit for borderline personality disorders. Treatment included individual and group therapies in a milieu that seemed to correspond to a therapeutic community setting. Moderate improvements were found at 2-year follow-up, particularly in a reduced rate of suicidal behavior, together with some improvement in social functioning.

All studies with borderline patients emphasize the importance of extremely long follow-up, because the benefits of therapy may not be apparent upon discharge. Of course, longer term follow-ups are very hard to interpret because of intervening variables, and none of these studies can be considered much more than studies of prognosis. A 5-year follow-up of treatment offered at the Cassel Hospital in London showed that patients who, on admission, showed borderline pathology tended to be those who showed a poor response to the inpatient psychotherapeutic program and did no better than at a standard psychiatric institution (Rosser et al., 1987). Stone's (1993) report of the follow-up of 550 patients at the New York State Psychiatric Institute indicates that, regardless of mental state at discharge, many patients appear to have utilized long-term hospitalization and inpatient therapy as a springboard toward normal functioning, autonomy, and independence. At up to 20-year follow-up, 66% of patients were functioning well. Individuals successfully treated with psychotherapy probably fall into a higher order, less dysfunctional group.

Cognitive Analytic Therapy

Ryle and Golynkina (2000) described outcomes from a case series of 27 patients with borderline personality disorder treated with 24 sessions of cognitive analytic therapy (CAT). At 6-month follow-up, 52% of the sample no longer met diagnostic criteria for personality disorder and were classified as improved. Wildgoose et al. (2001) described a case series of five patients treated with 16 sessions of CAT; clinical improvements were seen in three participants. Though these reports are clinically interesting, more definitive statements regarding the efficacy of CAT await results from a randomized trial of CAT in progress (Ryle & Golynkina, 2000).

TREATMENTS FOR AVOIDANT PERSONALITY DISORDER

Many studies of social phobia include individuals with avoidant personality disorder, and as discussed elsewhere in this book, there is controversy over the distinction between generalized social phobia and avoidant personality disorder. Perhaps reflecting this, there are few trials that explicitly focus on this disorder per se. Alden (1989), Cappe and Alden (1986), and Marzillier et al. (1976) have employed behavioral methods in the treatment of social difficulties encountered by these patients. These studies are reviewed in more detail in the section of this book detailing treatments for social phobia. Briefly, patients were treated using behavioral methods including exposure, social skills training, and systematic desensitization, with resulting improvements relative to wait-list controls. Though intervention programs are often designated as social skills training, they invariably include exposure procedures and are better described as a behavioral intervention package.

Argyle et al. (1974) found a trend toward improvement for both social skills and psychodynamic treatment in a trial in which patients acted as their own controls in a waiting period. Stravynski et al. (1982) assigned 22 patients to 14 sessions of social skills alone or with the addition of cognitive techniques aimed at challenging maladaptive beliefs. Equal and significant gains were found for both treatment groups. Stravynski et al. (1994) contrasted outcomes in 28 patients assigned to social skills training conducted either in a clinic or in a mix of clinic and real-life settings. The two treatments were equally effective, though only 3-month follow-up data are available. In addition, attrition from the real-life condition was markedly higher than when treatment was conducted in the clinic (58 vs. 21%); patients indicated that they found this form of therapy delivery stressful.

Though improvements can be found following treatment using social skills alone or in combination with cognitive techniques, many patients in these studies do not achieve normal levels of functioning, and there was limited generalization of improvements to broader social environments than those tested within studies. Alden and Capreol (1993) suggested that patients with avoidant personality disorder can be distinguished into two groups: those in whom distrustful and angry behavior is prominent, and those who are underassertive. In a trial of 76 patients, those with the former characteristics benefited more from exposure but not from skills training, while the latter benefited from both procedures. This result, though preliminary, suggests that greater targeting of therapeutic strategies may be associated with better outcomes.

Barber et al. (1997) reported an open trial of outcomes after 1 year of supportive–expressive therapy in 38 individuals, 24 of whom had avoidant personality disorder, and 14 with obsessive–compulsive personality disorder. Attrition was high in those with avoidant personality disorder (about 50% left therapy prematurely), and of those remaining in treatment, 40% retained their diagnosis. In contrast, patients with obsessive–compulsive personality disorder had much higher retention rates and superior outcomes.

TREATMENTS FOR ANTISOCIAL PERSONALITY DISORDER

There appear to be very few trials for antisocial personality disorder. This is a common comorbid diagnosis in substance abusers (e.g., Brooner et al., 1997), and a small number of trials contrast persons with antisocial personality disorder alone, and those with an additional comorbidity of depression. Studies are consistent in finding that outcomes with antisocial personality disorder alone are poorer than when it is associated with depression. This result was obtained in Woody et al. (1985), employing psychodynamic therapy for opiate-dependent men; Alterman et al. (1996), offering drug counseling for opiate-dependent individuals; and V. L. King et al. (2001), in a large study that contrasted outcomes from 513 participants in a methadone maintenance program (which included counseling).

Davidson and Tyrer (1996) reported detailed clinical data on two of five patients treated with between 9 and 18 sessions of schema-focused CBT. As for patients with borderline personality disorder also seen in this pilot study (discussed earlier), outcomes were broadly positive, but interpretation is limited by the small sample size and lack of information on the remaining patients in the trial.

A small number of studies (though few controlled trials) examined the impact of treatment on individuals within the penal system. Though it is likely that at least some of patients in these trials meet criteria for antisocial personality disorder, this cannot be assumed. Most studies select for commonalities in offending behavior (e.g., sexual offenses), or for people presenting with problematic behavior (e.g., violence). Alternatively, studies focus on individuals who are "psychopathic," a concept that, while well-defined in relation to measurement techniques, is not coterminous with DSM definitions of antisocial personality disorder (e.g., Hare et al., 1991). A detailed discussion of this area can be found in Warren et al. (2003), who reviewed treatments for "severe personality disorder" for the U.K. Home Office. There are a small number of observational studies of individuals detained in high-security settings using group CBT (Quayle & Moore, 1998), individual and group CBT in the context of a therapeutic milieu (Hughes et al., 1997) or psychodynamic therapy (Reiss et al., 1996). While improvements in functioning are noted, all share a number of methodological problems. Saunders (1996) contrasted CBT and psychodynamic therapy delivered in a group format in men who had assaulted their female partners; 40% of 136 participants met criteria for antisocial personality disorder. There were no differences in recidivism rates between groups, an outcome that is hard to benchmark in the absence of a no-treatment control group. Taylor (2000) describes outcomes from a 7-year follow-up of 700 individuals treated in a therapeutic community unit within Grendon Prison, contrasting their outcomes with those of 142 individuals allocated to a wait list but not admitted to the unit, and 1,400 inmates from the general prison population. Although there were some indications of reduced rates of reoffending, control for prior criminal histories reduces the apparent impact of this result. However, there did seem to be a link between length of stay on the unit and better outcome, with individuals who stayed less than 1 year showing no treatment effect. Thornton et al. (1996) evaluated progress in a dedicated unit for sex offenders within Grendon, finding better outcomes than for inmates with similar forensic histories treated within the general therapeutic program. Of interest is the fact that this benefit was restricted to those with at least two previous sexual convictions.

TREATMENTS FOR MIXED PERSONALITY DISORDERS

Liberman and Eckman (1981) reported the results of a brief, intensive treatment for inpatients with a range of personality disorders, though the selection criterion of a history of repeated suicide attempts suggests that many would have a diagnosis of borderline personality disorder. Treatment contrasted behavior therapy (which largely comprised social skills training) and insight-oriented therapy; outcome measures at 6- and 9-month follow-up suggested a reduction in suicidal ideation for the behavioral group but no between-treatment differences in the number of suicide attempts.

Winston et al. (1991) treated 32 patients with a range of personality disorders (predominantly in DSM-III-R cluster C), using two forms of brief psychodynamic therapy (short-term dynamic psychotherapy or brief adaptational therapy), contrasting both with a wait-list control. Because of ethical constraints, wait-list subjects began treatment after 15 weeks. Although both therapies used psychodynamic techniques, brief adaptational therapy employed more cognitive strategies. Patients with borderline, schizotypal, and narcissistic personality disorder were excluded from the trial, which comprised weekly sessions over 40 weeks. Contrasted to wait-list controls, treated patients showed moderate improvements in symptoms and target complaints at posttherapy. Though there were few between-treatment differences, there was more variance in outcome for the patients treated with short-term dynamic therapy, suggesting that for some patients the technique was unhelpful. Gains appeared to be maintained at 18-month follow-up. A larger trial of these therapies by the same authors (Winston et al., 1994) was conducted with 81 patients (of an original sample of 93). Again, the patient sample predominantly constituted those with cluster C disorders, with approximately one-fifth having cluster B disorders (primarily hysterical personality disorder). As in the earlier trial, significant and equivalent gains were found with both treatments.

Karterud et al. (2003) reported outcomes for a large sample of 1,244 consecutive admissions to eight day hospitals in Norway between 1992 and 2000. All clinics used similar programs, with therapists trained in group analytic methods but employing a nonmanualized approach that included both psychodynamic and cognitive-behavioral methods. Patients were usually offered 18 weeks of therapy, with treatment intensity varying from 8 to 16 hours per week; following discharge, patients were offered weekly therapy for up to 3.5 years. Approximately 80% of patients had personality disorders; of these borderline (22%), avoidant (20%) and paranoid (12%) personality disorder were the most frequent. Overall, outcomes at 1-year follow-up were positive. Although the absence of a contrast group limits interpretation, response rates were equivalent to those found in randomized trials reported earlier (Bateman & Fonagy, 1999; Wilberg et al., 1998), suggesting the utility of this approach in routine settings. Of particular note is comparative outcome across personality disorder diagnoses. Patients with borderline personality disorder without comorbid cluster A diagnoses had markedly better outcomes than those with borderline/paranoid or paranoid presentations, suggesting that this treatment format may not be appropriate for the latter presentations.

SUMMARY AND CLINICAL IMPLICATIONS

There are rather few controlled trials of treatments for personality disorders. The paucity of evidence from controlled trials may reflect the fact that, with the exception of cluster B disorders, many individuals with personality disorders present to services for help with Axis I disorders. In this context, their treatment is less for their "personality disorder" than for the symptomatic state for which they are presenting. In contrast, many of the features of individuals with borderline or antisocial personality disorder create such distress for the person, or for others around them, that clinicians need directly to attend to the intra- and interpersonal consequences of the personality disorder, and will usually privilege these over symptomatic states when setting goals for treatment. While this makes it more likely that studies focused on these personality disorders will be attempted, the challenge of running a randomized trial should not be underestimated. This group of individuals is difficult to retain in treatment and tends to be reluctant to accept randomization, to challenge the administration of manualized interventions, and to be difficult to follow-up.

While there is some evidence that personality disorders will usually impact negatively on treatments for Axis I presentations, the strength and specificity of evidence for this proposition varies across Axis I diagnoses and also across personality disorders. While clinicians should consider the possibility that a person with comorbid personality disorder may be less responsive to symptom-oriented treatment for an Axis I problem, treatment planning should not assume this to be so.

Medication (both prescribed and nonprescribed) is frequently used to manage particular symptoms, and no single form of pharmacological intervention seems to be recommended for treating any one category of disorder. This aspect of treatment is often poorly controlled in trials and has not been subjected to systematic evaluation.

The main research into treatments for antisocial personality disorder has been centered on patients seeking help for substance abuse, or individuals seen within the penal system. There is no clear evidence of treatment efficacy, with conclusions limited not only by the small number of trials but also by the methodological limitations of these studies. The recent growth in the evidence base for borderline personality disorder indicates the feasibility of coherent research programs, with a patient group usually seen as presenting problems of engagement. The practical problems of mounting trials should not be underestimated, but it seems reasonable to emphasize the need for further research in this area given the social impact of this disorder.

Avoidant personality disorder has received a modest amount of research attention. There are indications that this may be addressed using social skills training or cognitive techniques, but the generalization of improvements to other social contexts is not well demonstrated.

Most extensively researched are interventions for people with borderline personality disorder, where there is evidence from randomized trials that structured treatments employing DBT or a psychodynamic approach have efficacy over routine care. Unfortunately, the majority of studies present data from open trials or case series, which means that while a number of approaches have been exposed to empirical scrutiny, at this point, only two approaches can be considered "evidence-based."

Although the available randomized trials of DBT and psychodynamic treatment are methodologically sound, they can be criticized on the grounds that they are limited by relatively small sample sizes and were conducted in the context of clear leadership from the principal investigators. More pertinent is the fact that because contrast is to routine care, it is difficult to ascertain whether outcomes are attributable to the structured nature of the programs or the therapeutic orientation and models which they employ. To a degree, this represents a conundrum: Since clinicians working in this area are clear about the importance of offering structure for these patients, disaggregation of structure from orientation is clearly not an option. More realistically, studies need to contrast one orientation against another in the context of high levels of structure, and also against routine care. Unfortunately, this will require a much larger sample size than has been mustered by any extant trial, and, as noted earlier, there are practical problems in achieving this (e.g., Bateman & Fonagy, 2004). Finally, rather few trials conduct follow-up over an appropriate period—for example, a minimum of 18 months to 2 years—or include a contrast or control group over follow-up. This is needed to capture the tendency for many individuals to show periods of complete remission followed by episodes of great severity, and it is the impact of treatment on this often chronic and cyclic course that should form a critical index of efficacy.

While there is good evidence for the immediate impact of DBT, its focus is largely on the management of behavioral problems of impulsivity and suicidality. A concern for these areas is shared by psychodynamic approaches, but these have a more conscious aim of changing the way the person thinks, and there is some evidence that this results in a greater impact on mood states and interpersonal functioning. Inevitably, this emphasis on engaging the patient in cognitive change results in greater length of therapy, with some indication of not only slower rates of change but also more sustained gains over follow-up. While shorter interventions are likely to have lower immediate costs, longer ones would be justified were they to demonstrate greater cost-effectiveness. This being so, there needs to be further exploration of issues of dosage, as well as focus and intensity, in order to have greater clarity about the most appropriate service model.

Perhaps more than in many areas, debate about particular forms of therapy should not preclude concern for the clinical observation that attention to nonspecific factors is integral in treating individuals with cluster B personality disorders. Successful approaches usually emphasize the importance of structure, a coherent theoretical base, a higher intensity of treatment than for many Axis I disorders, and, especially, attention to the unique set of problems presented by the individual, with a psychological formulation guiding treatment. This means that decisions about choice of treatment might be best made with regard to pragmatic considerations rather than argument about which particular approach is "best." This means that the competence and training of senior clinicians who can offer supervision will be especially important, as will the skills mix of staff and the resources (including staffing level) available to the service. These "nonspecific" issues may be especially pertinent when considering the performance of evidence-based treatments in routine practice. Since systemic factors related to the context into which a treatment is introduced may be as relevant to success as the type of treatment, pragmatic trials would be especially useful in indicating the conditions required to implement evidence-based therapies in routine services.

CHAPTER 12

SUBSTANCE ABUSE

Alcohol, Cocaine, and Opiate Dependence and Abuse

Though a wide range of prescription and nonprescription drugs have the potential for abusive use, this chapter restricts its scope to interventions for alcohol, cocaine, and opiates, largely for reasons of space.

The majority of trials we review describe the efficacy of interventions in research populations selected for one primary drug of abuse, but it is worth bearing in mind that patients seen in community settings often abuse more than one substance. While studying polydrug abusers would enhance external validity (e.g., Rounsaville et al., 2003), reducing internal validity at this stage of treatment development may make it difficult to be clear about the efficacy of interventions in relation to particular drugs (e.g., O'Brien & Lynch, 2003). This review suggests that there can be variation in outcome from similar treatments applied in relation to different substances, and this suggests that even if a somewhat artificial strategy in relation to clinical presentation, it is helpful to consider specific substances of abuse independently.

DEFINITIONS

Within DSM–IV–TR substance dependence is characterized by a maladaptive pattern of substance use leading to clinically significant impairment or distress, as indicated by three or more of the following features occurring in the same 12-month period: (1) tolerance, marked by a need for increasing amounts of the substance, or a decreased effect from taking the same quantity of the substance; (2) withdrawal, as manifested by the characteristic withdrawal syndrome for the substance; (3) the substance is taken in larger amounts and over longer periods than the person intended; (4) a persistent desire, or one or more unsuccessful efforts to cut down or control substance use; (5) a great deal of time spent in activities necessary in getting the substance, taking the substance, or recovering from its effects; (6) important activities given up because of substance use; and (7) continued substance use despite knowledge of personal problems caused by its use.

DSM-IV-TR distinguishes substance abuse from substance dependence; abuse is indicated by evidence of a maladaptive pattern of substance use leading to clinically significant impairment or distress, manifested by the occurrence of one or more of the following within the same 12-month period, but in the absence of criteria for substance dependence: (1) recurrent substance abuse resulting in a failure to fulfill major role expectations (e.g., leading to absenteeism or neglect of household or children); (2) recurrent use in physically hazardous situations (e.g., driving when impaired by substance use); (3) recurrent substance-related legal problems (e.g., arrests for substance-related disorderly conduct); (4) continued substance use despite social problems caused or exacerbated by the effects of the drug (e.g., fights).

PREVALENCE AND COMORBIDITY

Prevalence

Data from the Epidemiologic Catchment Area (ECA) survey estimated lifetime prevalence of alcohol dependence at between 10.7 and 15.9% across study sites (Helzer et al., 1991), with 6-month prevalence rates between 4.5 and 6.1%. Significantly higher rates were found in men than women (9 vs. 1.5%), and greater prevalence in younger age groups (Warheit & Auth, 1993).

Although data from the National Comorbidity Survey indicate a lifetime prevalence for drug dependence of 7.5% (Kessler et al., 1994), it is difficult to derive accurate prevalence rates for illicit drugs such as opiates and cocaine. Kraus et al. (2003) estimated national prevalence rates for drug use in the European Union and Norway by applying weighted multipliers to data on rates of treatment for drug abuse, drug-related mortality, HIV rates, and police reports. On this basis, estimated rates of opiate use per 1,000 individuals between ages 15 and 64 vary in different countries—from 2.6 in the Netherlands to 6.3 in the United Kingdom and 7.1 in Italy. Estimates of prevalence rates for cocaine are restricted to France, where it is estimated at between 3.9 and 4.7. Inevitably, different computational systems produces different estimates, and it needs to be recognized that figures for prevalence can only be approximations. Inner-city prevalence rates will be higher than national rates. Thus, Hickman et al. (1999) derived estimates of prevalence rates for opiate use in three areas of inner-London at between 1.3 and 3.6%, for people ages 18–49 years.

Comorbidity

Comorbidity rates between alcohol dependence and DSM Axis I disorders vary according to the population sample under study, though both in community and treatment-seeking samples there is a higher rate of comorbidity with depression and dysthymic disorder than would be expected by chance (Lynskey, 1998). Kessler et al. (1994) reported an odds ratio (OR) of 2.0 for the association between major depression and alcohol dependence. Ross (1995) found that 28.1% of individuals with alcohol dependence had a comorbid affective disorder, contrasted to 8.6% who were not alcohol dependent. Regier et al. (1992) reviewed 17 studies of patients presenting for treatment of alcohol abuse, estimating lifetime prevalence rates for panic and phobic disorders at 2–60%, though most studies yielded rates under 15% for panic and generalized anxiety, with a median rate of about 20% for phobic disorders. Antisocial personality disorder was relatively common, with rates in two studies of 41% and 44%, respectively. Within community samples, comorbidity rates are lower. Regier et al. (1992) noted that the presence of a comorbid Axis I disorder increases the likelihood of attendance for specialist care by a factor of 3 or 4. This suggests that there may be significant differences in the psychiatric profile of clinic attenders and people with drinking problems within the community. Among individuals with substance abuse other than alcohol, there are indications of even higher rates of comorbidity. Merikangas et al. (1998) reported data from six international studies, finding consistent evidence that individuals with drug dependence have elevated rates for mood disorders (OR = 2.9–5.3), anxiety disorders (OR = 3.3–5.2) and antisocial personality disorder (OR = 9.8–15.2).

Unsurprisingly, substance dependence is often not restricted to one class of drug. Comorbidity between alcohol and other drugs is estimated at 22% (Regier et al., 1990). Burns and Teesson (2002) reported an odds ratio for the association between the co-occurrence of alcohol and opiate abuse at 7.2, and for alcohol abuse and any another substance abuse, 10.1. Among a sample of injecting heroin users, 75% met criteria for alcohol abuse, and 25% for benzodiazepine dependence (Dinwiddie et al., 1996); within this sample, there was a mean of 3.3 dependence/abuse diagnoses. Darke and Ross (1997), also surveying injecting heroin users, reported a linear relationship between the number of drug dependencies and the number of comorbid psychiatric diagnoses, indicating that persons with the highest levels of distress will also be those with the greatest likelihood of presenting with polydrug abuse.

Although comorbidity is clearly common, the structure of this chapter—and most trials—do not reflect this. Clinics frequently encounter individuals with a pattern of abuse and need not easily classified into discrete categories, a disparity between research and practice that needs to be recognized when considering the implications of material presented here.

TREATMENTS FOR ALCOHOL DEPENDENCE AND ABUSE

The focus of treatment for alcohol problems has shifted over the years. As awareness of the risks of excessive drinking has grown, treatment has shifted from provision of services for "alcoholics" toward treatment of patients with a broader range of difficulties with drinking, of which the classical alcoholic picture is one extreme (Thom et al., 1992). On this basis, treatment has moved away from intensive residential treatment and rehabilitation toward brief interventions (Bien et al., 1993), now widely employed for early intervention with both problem drinkers (Heather & Robertson, 1989) and heavy drinkers (Wallace et al., 1988). Although specific treatment approaches can be identified, classification can be difficult. Miller and Wilbourne (2002), whose Mesa Grande project reviews outcomes across all domains of treatment, note that because treatments often include a range of procedures (only some of which constitute distinctive therapies), classification of treatments for review purposes can be difficult. Although most studies use one leading model, there can be wide variation in the detail of implementation. Some of the major approaches in this area include the following:

1. *Twelve-step approaches.* Developed from that employed by self-help groups such as Alcoholics Anonymous, this approach adopts an illness model that views substance abuse as the consequence of an innate vulnerability, and acceptance of a lack of control over addiction is a key therapeutic target. On this basis, abstinence is seen the only acceptable goal of treatment.

2. *Motivational interviewing/motivational enhancement.* This directive but collaborative counseling style focuses on the readiness of patients to deal with their drinking and to examine ambivalence and resistance to and about change.

3. *Behavioral and cognitive-behavioral approaches.* This heading subsumes a wide range of approaches that assume substance abuse is a learned, maladaptive behavior, maintained partly because of beliefs about the addictive power of abused substances, and also by the use of drugs as a means of managing stress. Therapies have varying aims but often focus on developing more adaptive coping skills and challenging beliefs, and most approaches include a functional analysis of drinking behavior. Specifically, behavioral techniques include cue exposure and retraining, which involves relearning responses to

addictive substances (on the basis that these can be a trigger to relapse). Contingency management is based on the reinforcement of abstinence through (for example) voucher systems. Aversion therapy (counterconditioning) has also been used by some investigators. Coping skills training is a cognitive-behavioral approach that aims to enhance and extend the individual's repertoire of coping responses; because of this focus, it overlaps somewhat with response prevention approaches.

4. *Community reinforcement approaches.* This behavioral approach is based on the belief that substance abuse is strongly influenced by environmental contingencies, and hence uses a variety of techniques to shift the balance of social, familial, recreational, and vocational reinforcers in a way that makes sobriety more rewarding than substance use.

5. *Relapse prevention.* Many treatment approaches include "relapse prevention," and in this sense, relapse prevention is more a procedure than a therapy. Nonetheless, it can be provided as a distinct program with a focus on identification of triggers and indicators for relapse, and facilitation of coping strategies to maintain abstinence or control.

6. *Other approaches.* The involvement of partners and families through marital and family therapy recognizes the social context of substance abuse, both as a source of stress that triggers abuse and as a source of potential support for abstinence. Other common therapies include counseling, psychodynamic therapy, other insight-oriented therapies, solution-focused therapy, group therapy, and milieu approaches.

General Methodological Considerations

External Validity

The possibility that exclusion criteria impact adversely on the external validity of studies is a general concern across the field of psychotherapy outcome research. However, this may impact especially significantly in the field of substance abuse, particularly because the social and economic consequences of severe dependence are likely to impact adversely on patient motivation. Humphreys and Wiesner (2000) applied eight exclusion criteria found by an earlier meta-analysis (Monahan & Finney, 1996) to be commonly applied in trials. These include the presence of serious psychiatric disturbance, lack of motivation, comorbid medical problems, polydrug use, unsuccessful prior treatment, and social and family instability. When applied to 593 patients treated in public and private settings, these criteria resulted in disproportionate exclusion of African Americans, those on low income, and those with more severe psychiatric and substance abuse histories. This resulted in research samples with lower levels of vulnerability than are likely to be seen in clinical settings, making it plausible to suggest that the effectiveness of treatments will be lower than that observed in research trials. There is very limited evidence on this point. Westerberg et al. (2000) contrasted demographic and clinical characteristics and outcomes for 348 individuals who accepted or refused randomization into a clinical trial, finding that though the refusers had somewhat greater problem severity, outcomes were broadly equivalent.

Measurement of Outcome in Alcohol Treatment

The treatment goals of studies and of treatment centers vary. For some, complete abstinence is the aim, while for others, harm reduction (and controlled drinking) is seen as a viable option. Though it is usual—and reasonable—for most studies to employ measures that reflect both abstinence and measures of drinking behavior in those who do return to drinking, this does imply that the interpretation placed on outcomes by practitioners is likely to vary in relation to their orientation, since, for some services, the notion of controlled drinking is inimical to their philosophy.

Reviews of Treatments

Meta-Analyses

Most quantitative reviews focus on the efficacy of brief treatments. Bien et al. (1993) identified 13 randomized controlled trials (RCTs) and 32 controlled studies of brief interventions, covering approximately 6,000 patients. These authors did not distinguish between the target drinking populations, with the result that there is some potential for a confound between outcomes and client characteristics (in particular, motivation and levels of dependence). Meta-analyses of 19 studies contrasting brief interventions against control (no or very minimal intervention) yield an effect size of 0.38. Of note is the finding that there is no evidence of differential impact when brief interventions are contrasted against extended therapies—13 studies yielded an effect size of 0.06. Wilk et al. (1997) reviewed 12 trials of brief interventions in heavy drinkers, in which sample sizes were greater than 30, and in which brief interventions lasted less than 1 hour and included motivational interviewing techniques. Contrasted to no intervention, the odds ratio for the proportion of individuals drinking moderately 6 to 12 months after intervention was 1.91. Poikolainen (1999) identified seven trials of brief interventions in a primary care context that randomly allocated patients to treatment and included a follow-up at 6–12 months, distinguishing between very brief interventions (e.g., a few minutes of advice on drinking reduction from a health professional) and more extended, though still brief, interventions. Studies that included individuals with severe alcohol dependence were excluded. Though effect size estimates for both forms of intervention indicated a significant reduction in alcohol consumption, the lack of statistical homogeneity for these estimates suggests important differences in the content of the methods used in trials.

Heather (1995) helpfully distinguished studies of non-treatment-seeking individuals (e.g., those whose problematic alcohol consumption is identified in the context of their seeking treatment for an unrelated problem) from those in which individuals specifically seek help. Moyer et al. (2002) reviewed brief interventions lasting less than four sessions, separating studies along these lines. Thirty-four trials contrasted brief intervention against control in non-treatment-seeking patients; on an aggregate measure of all drinking-related outcomes, effect size at 3-month follow-up was 0.3, reducing to 0.13 at 1 year; on all measures, the largest effect sizes were apparent proximal to treatment. When individuals with more severe alcohol problems were excluded from the analysis, effect sizes were greater. Twenty studies contrasted brief treatments against extended interventions in treatment-seeking individuals. At most assessment points, effect sizes were not significantly different from zero (though, at 3 months, extended treatments showed greater benefit [effect size = 0.42]). Moyer et al. suggest that this latter finding should be interpreted carefully, since their narrative review indicates that brief treatments were intensive and often accompanied by additional formal and informal treatment. Though, in this sense, they argue that the term "brief" may be misleading, it remains the case that the trials in their analysis offer a contrast between interventions of different duration and intensity.

Although these analyses converge in finding little evidence for extended-over brief treatments, Monahan and Finney (1996) reached a different conclusion. These authors restricted their review to controlled and uncontrolled studies that cited abstinence rates and disaggregated data into different forms of intervention rather than utilizing paired comparison. On this basis, they found that higher intensity—and especially inpatient—treatment resulted in higher abstinence rates. This result was reasonably robust; for example, it survived control for private versus public treatment (on the basis that the former would be more likely to select patient intakes). However, the inclusion of uncontrolled studies means that the observed associations may still relate to patients with better or worse prognoses being attracted to different treatment locations.

Qualitative Reviews

William Miller's research group has produced a number of iterations of a qualitative review of outcomes and cost-effectiveness that aggregate cumulative evidence for outcomes in relation to therapeutic method. This is based on a continuously updated database of studies; in their most recent publication, this comprises 381 trials (Miller & Wilbourne, 2002; Miller et al., 2003).

Inclusion criteria restrict review to comparative trials of reasonable methodological adequacy, and the relative efficacy of approaches is tabulated by producing a box score that reflects the sum of positive and negative outcomes
across trials, as well as the methodological quality of the studies. On this basis,
treatments are rank-ordered for efficacy. The authors note that this approach
can be criticized, because it does not weight relative efficacy in relation to the
number of trials or individuals within trials, and interventions with a large
number of trials but with mixed results will incur lower ranking than those
with fewer but consistently positive contrasts. Because of this, the specific
rank ordering of treatments may be misleading.

Examining the orderings for psychological treatments, the highest
ranked are brief interventions and motivational enhancement, with the
reviewers separating "brief therapies" from interventions explicitly based on
motivational interviewing. Community reinforcement and bibliotherapy follow (though the latter is usually examined in populations of lesser severity).
Next come behavioral self-control training and behavior contracting, both
forms of behavioral self-management that aim to assist individuals to adopt
strategies for regulating their alcohol intake. Social skills training follows,
though it should be noted that this approach is usually offered with the intention of enhancing coping skills that maintain sobriety, as well as improving
relationships—a similar aim to the next therapy listed, behavioral marital
therapy. Aversion therapy is the last treatment with scores that suggest efficacy. Treatments ranked in positions that indicate little or no evidence for
efficacy include counseling, problem solving, nonbehavioral marital therapy,
hypnosis, 12-step programs and Alcoholics Anonymous, confrontational
approaches, and psychotherapy, with those placed later having the least evidence for efficacy. The positioning of Alcoholics Anonymous and the 12-
step approach may, however, be somewhat misleading. In relation to the former, studies reviewed were of individuals coerced into treatment. Trials of
the 12-step approach contrasted it to well-defined treatments, meaning that
the box-score method is likely to underestimate its efficacy.

The approach to classification of efficacy employed by this group has
been criticized, and attempts have been made to refine the method. For
example, Finney and Monahan (1996) refined an earlier review (Holder et
al., 1991) by estimating the probability of studies producing at least one statistically significant effect, based on the number of tests for treatment effects.
They also attempted to control for the fact that contrast of a therapy against a
"weak" intervention will artificially boost apparent efficacy (noting that most
therapies had been contrasted to relatively weak competition). On this basis,
they computed an adjusted measure of efficacy. Though, on the whole, this
confirmed the rankings of most interventions identified as having good evidence for effectiveness, this was not true for all therapies. Clearly, there is
scope for debate about the most appropriate method for tallying studies using
a box-score approach, and the degree to which the specific rankings of thera-

pies in Miller et al. (2003) would shift if exposed to the same reanalysis is unclear.

An important question is the rate of improvement that can be expected. Miller et al. (2001) estimated that in the year following a treatment episode, about 1 in 4 clients remained continuously abstinent, and 1 in 10 drank moderately and without problems. Of those who drank in the year following treatment, there was evidence of improvement, with abstention on 3 out of 4 days; overall alcohol consumption was reduced by 87% on average, with a 60% reduction in alcohol-related problems. Though not based on a literature review, Ritsher et al. (2002) examined outcomes from a cohort of 2,805 male patients treated in Veterans Affairs substance abuse programs, 28% of whom were abstinent 2 years after treatment. Better outcome was not predicted by the type of treatment, but was predicted by the initial severity of substance abuse and presence of comorbid psychiatric problems. There was also evidence that participants with more contact with outpatient follow-up services or with self-help groups had higher levels of remission, with some suggestion that it was the duration rather than the number of contacts that was significant. Whether this association reflects patient compliance or a treatment effect is not clear and requires further research, but it may suggest the importance of maintenance therapy.

Evidence for the Efficacy of Individual Treatment Approaches

Medication

DISULFIRAM (ANTABUSE)

Disulfiram has been widely used in the treatment of problem drinking, both as an implant and as an oral medication. Though earlier studies claimed to demonstrate the superiority of Antabuse contrasted to control, they are characterized by poor methodological quality and short follow-up (e.g., Gerrein et al., 1973; Reinert, 1958; Wallerstein et al., 1957). Later studies provide evidence of a strong placebo effect. Fuller and Roth (1979) allocated 128 patients to an active dose of disulfiram, an inactive dose, or no medication. At 1 year, there was a higher abstinence rate among both the active and inactive medication groups (23%) than among those given no pill (12%). A similar effect has been found for disulfiram implants. Wilson et al. (1978) gave either a disulfiram implant or sham surgery. At 2-year follow-up, the implant group showed some advantage over the sham surgery, but there was a clear and substantial placebo effect. The implant and sham surgery groups had a mean of 367 and 307 days of abstinence, respectively, contrasted with 27 abstinent days for an unoperated control group.

In line with these findings, Mattick and Jarvis (1993) meta-analyzed results from five controlled studies, finding no difference between the impact of oral disulfiram and placebo (effect size = −0.14), though there was a small difference between the impact of disulfiram and no medication (effect size = 0.33). However, there was a moderate effect size when contrasting placebo and no medication (0.47), confirming the placebo effect noted earlier. Meta-analysis of studies of disulfiram implants (four studies) again confirms this pattern. Given that patient compliance is relatively low (e.g., Fuller et al., 1986; Meyer, 1989), evidence in support of the use of for disulfiram is not strong.

OPIATE AGONISTS (NALTREXONE)

Three recent meta-analyses (Kranzler & Van Kirk, 2001; Srisurapanont & Jarusuraisin, 2002; Streeton & Whelan, 2001) suggest that there is good evidence for the short-term efficacy of naltrexone. When contrasted to placebo, there is a reduction in rates of both relapse and alcohol consumption, with medication appearing to confer some protection against resumption of heavy drinking when patients drink after a period of abstinence. However, these reviewers note that there are few trials of medium to longer term efficacy, and caution against the use of naltrexone in the absence of psychosocial treatments. A small number of trials examined the efficacy of this combination. Volpicelli et al. (O'Brien, 1992) conducted a 12-week, double-blind placebo-controlled trial with 70 male alcoholics as an adjunct to outpatient rehabilitation (comprising 1 month of day treatment counseling and psychoeducation, followed by twice-weekly group psychotherapy). Over 12 weeks, 23% of those receiving naltrexone relapsed, contrasted with 54% of those receiving placebo. A particularly marked effect was seen in patients who took alcohol at any point in their treatment; 95% of such patients who had received placebo relapsed, contrasted with 50% of those receiving active medication.

O'Malley et al. (1992) randomized 97 patients to receive either naltrexone or placebo, combined either with coping skills/relapse prevention therapy or a nondirective supportive psychotherapy that encouraged abstinence, but did not offer any strategies for achieving this. Coping skills taught were those that assisted self-management in situations associated with relapse and incorporated self-monitoring, social skills training, and a range of cognitive-behavioral therapy (CBT) methods. Survival analyses were conducted for each treatment group at 12 weeks and at 6 months (O'Malley et al., 1996). At 12 weeks, patients treated with naltrexone were significantly more likely than those receiving placebo to remain abstinent, to show lower relapse rates, and to have fewer drinking-related problems, but this difference was only sustained through the first month of the follow-up period. The trajectory of patients who received therapy was somewhat complex. For patients who received naltrexone, there was no difference between the therapies at any assessment point. However, for those given placebo, there was a significant benefit to coping skills therapy, which (contrasted to supportive therapy) evidenced a significant reduction in rates of relapse and heavy drinking. Consistent with the findings of Volpicelli et al. (1992), for patients who had at least one drink over the study period, subsequent abstinence was lowest for those receiving naltrexone and coping skills therapy.

Anton et al. (1999) allocated 131 patients with moderate alcohol dependence to receive naltrexone or placebo; all received 12 weeks of CBT. At the end of this period, those receiving naltrexone showed a significantly greater time to relapse (a mean of 60 vs. 48 days), and if they relapsed, showed lower levels of drinking. Krystal et al. (2001) randomized 627 veterans with chronic and severe alcohol dependence to receive short- or long-term therapy with naltrexone (3 or 12 months, respectively), or to receive placebo over the same period. Patients were seen in the context of standard public treatment centers; all received individual 12-step counseling and were encouraged to attend Alcoholics Anonymous (AA) meetings. At 3- and 12-month assessment, naltrexone did not show any benefit over placebo. This study is somewhat unusual in that patients had higher levels of dependence than in many trials, and were seen in routine clinical settings, and it is unclear whether either or both factors may have led to a decrease in the apparent efficacy of naltrexone.

OTHER MEDICATIONS

The efficacy of acamprosate has been investigated in a number of trials and appears to be equivalent to that of naltrexone (Kranzler & Van Kirk, 2001). Peachey et al. (1989) have conducted the only RCT examining the efficacy of citrated calcium carbimide with 128 patients. A crossover design was employed, with subjects receiving either placebo or active medication for 56 days, followed by the alternative for the succeeding 56 days. Active medication reduced levels of alcohol consumption to the same extent as placebo, suggesting no specific impact for this medication. Trials of metronidazole suggest that it has no greater impact than placebo (e.g., Gallant et al., 1968; Merry & Whitehead, 1968).

PSYCHOTROPIC MEDICATION

Though commonly used in the acute withdrawal phase from alcohol, there appears to be no evidence for the benefits of chlordiazepoxide in sustaining abstinence (e.g., Rosenberg, 1974). Evidence for the benefits of antidepressants is equivocal, though there may be some impact on mood. Kissin and Gross (1968) administered chlordiazepoxide and imipramine in combination, each drug alone, or placebo, finding reduced drinking rates of 28%, 19%, 0%, and 13%, respectively, at 6-month follow-up. Miller and Hester (1986) reviewed the limited number of available studies, noting poor methodology, a failure to control for levels of depression, and inadequate follow-up periods. Investigations of the benefits of lithium carbonate have produced a similarly equivocal picture (e.g., Dorus et al., 1989).

Behavioral and Cognitive-Behavioral Approaches

AVERSION THERAPIES

Aversion therapies attempt to countercondition alcohol consumption with an aversive stimulus. Apnea, chemical aversion (emetics), electrical aversion, or covert sensitization have been employed. Laverty (1966) and Vanderhoof and Campbell (1967) induced apnea with succinylcholine, showing some success and no impact, respectively, for this intervention. The combination of these contradictory results and the dangers of the technique make it difficult to recommend its use.

A number of studies have examined the impact of pairing various emetics and alcohol in open trials (e.g., Boland et al., 1978; Smith & Fawley, 1990) or in RCTs (e.g., Cannon & Baker, 1981; Cannon et al., 1981). A further seven RCTs have employed electrical aversion (Mattick & Jarvis, 1993). Although results are not consistent across trials, there appears to be only a short-term impact with both variants of this technique. There has been little research on this approach in recent years; in an exception to this trend Smith et al. (1997) matched 249 patients treated as inpatients in a multimodal treatment program (which included chemical or electrical aversion) with an equivalent number of controls from a separate outcome program (an inpatient treatment that largely employed counseling). Although at 6 months, those who had received aversion therapy showed higher rates of abstinence, this benefit was not sustained at 1 year. In addition, the matching procedure makes it difficult to attribute any differential outcomes to the delivery of aversion therapy. Overall, there is little support for aversion techniques, and it is hard to recommend its use in standard service settings, given that there is (unsurprisingly) a high rate of attrition from such therapies.

Covert sensitization involves the imaginal pairing of drinking behavior with nausea–inducing scenes. Six RCTs have been conducted (Mattick & Jarvis, 1993); in five of these, covert sensitization is associated with lower drinking at 6 months compared to control groups. The average effect size for all studies is 0.85. Though there is some evidential support for this approach, good outcomes rest on its successful implementation (Elkins, 1980; Elkins & Murdoch, 1977), and there is little evidence of its greater efficacy over alternative interventions (e.g., Fleiger & Zingle, 1973; Piorkowsky & Mann, 1975).

SOCIAL SKILLS TRAINING

Consistent gains have been demonstrated for the addition of social skills training to treatment programs. On the basis of 12 studies comparing social skills training to a range of alternative treatments (usually standard treatment and group discussion), Mattick and Jarvis (1993) calculated an effect size of 0.78 at

12-month follow-up. The benefits of this intervention appear to be robust regardless of whether patients are screened for social skills deficits (Mattick & Jarvis, 1993), and particularly when the focus of this intervention lies in increasing assertiveness (e.g., Chaney et al., 1978; Ferrell & Galassi, 1981; Freedberg & Johnson, 1978).

Oei and Jackson (1982) contrasted social skills training alone, social skills with the addition of cognitive restructuring (aimed at modifying beliefs that inhibited assertion), and a group discussion control condition. Both social skills interventions were more successful than control, but at 12 months, those who had received additional cognitive restructuring showed the greatest gains. Oei and Jackson (1980) compared the delivery of a combined package of social skills and cognitive restructuring in individual and group formats, finding that alcohol consumption at 12 months was significantly lower for those treated in groups.

RELAPSE PREVENTION

More frequently than not, relapse prevention (RP) techniques are offered as part of other interventions, with the result that the number of trials with a relapse prevention component is greater than those that declare this as the major intervention method (Dimeff & Marlatt, 1998). There are a small number of reviews focusing on the efficacy of relapse prevention as an explicit method. These examine efficacy across the whole field of substance abuse, and some disaggregation is needed to determine the efficacy of RP for alcohol abuse. Carroll's (1996) review identified 24 studies of relapse prevention, concluding that efficacy was equivalent across all classes of substance use, and that while RP was more effective than no treatment, it was equivalent to alternative active interventions. Irvin et al.'s (1999) meta-analysis identified 10 trials of RP for alcohol, yielding a pre- to posttherapy effect size of 0.37. Congruent with Carroll's (1996) review, effect sizes were modest when contrasting RP to an alternative active intervention, though RP appeared more effective in the management of alcohol abuse than for other classes of substance abuse. The efficacy of RP was significantly greater when it was combined with the adjunctive use of medication (effect size = 0.09 and 0.48, respectively). Few studies provided follow-up data, and where this was available, it suggested that effects decease over time.

CUE EXPOSURE

This intervention is intended to strengthen resilience in the face of drinking-related cues, and while it can be implemented through exposure to alcohol cues alone, it is often combined with exposure to social cues (introducing some overlap between this and a coping skills approach). This rationale for this approach assumes that conditioning models can account for drinking behavior, an assertion for which there is mixed evidence (Conklin & Tiffany, 2002; Kadden, 2001). While early work (e.g., Rankin et al., 1983) confirmed that *in vivo* exposure is more effective than imaginal exposure, the form of exposure varies, in that few trials expose clients to a priming dose of alcohol (partly because many studies set abstinence as a goal, while others set moderate drinking as an acceptable outcome).

Drummond and Glautier (1994) randomized 35 inpatients receiving a standard program to receive additionally either cue exposure or relaxation training. Though the time to initial lapse from abstinence was equivalent, over 6-month follow-up, there was significant benefit to cue exposure in terms of latency to relapse to heavy drinking and the amount of alcohol consumed. Monti et al. (1993) contrasted standard inpatient treatment with inpatient treatment augmented by cue exposure combined with coping skills training in 40 male participants. Though at 3 months there were no differences between groups, at 6 months there appeared to be a benefit to cue exposure, with a greater proportion of patients maintaining abstinence and showing reduced levels of drinking if they did relapse, whereas the control group worsened. A later trial from this research group (Rohsenow et al., 2001) randomized 100 inpatients to receive combinations of individual and group treatments—either individual cue exposure or relaxation, and either group coping skills training or group psychoeducation (trying to control in each case for contact time). This yielded four possible programs: cue-exposure combined with coping skills training, cue exposure combined with psychoeducation, relaxation training combined with coping skills training, and relaxation training combined with psychoeducation. Though at 6 months and 1 year overall rates of drinking were lower for cue exposure or skills training, this effect was more marked among those individuals who returned to drinking, suggesting that treatment may have assisted more moderate drinking in those who relapsed. Whether these results can be attributed to cue extinction or coping skills is unclear, since, in this study, cue exposure included teaching of coping skills, making it difficult to distinguish their relative impacts. It is also noteworthy that almost half the patients approached refused randomization to cue exposure, suggesting that this approach may be unacceptable to many patients.

The use of cue exposure with the goal of moderation (rather than abstinence) has been explored in a small number of studies. Sithartan et al. (1997) randomized 52 "problem drinkers" (defined as those without high levels of dependence) to six sessions of cue exposure or CBT. While at 6-months both interventions showed evidence of reduced drinking frequency and lower consumption per drinking occasion, there was significant advantage to cue exposure on both these measures. A further trial by this group (Dawe et al., 2002) was less selective in its recruitment, requiring only that patients had a goal of moderation rather than abstinence. Again, cue exposure was contrasted to CBT, though in this sample ($n = 100$) both interventions were of equal efficacy. Interestingly, the degree to which moderation was achieved did not appear to be related to initial levels of dependency. Similar results were reported by Heather et al. (2000), who allocated 91 clients to cue exposure or to behavioral self-control training, and found each treatment to be equally effective; again, initial severity did not predict the achievement of moderation. These studies suggest no strong advantage to cue exposure over other forms of behavioral intervention, but they do indicate that drinking severity does not preclude offering clients a goal of moderation.

The impact of cue exposure in combination with medication has rarely been studied; Monti et al. (1999) combined naltrexone and cue exposure, finding that though 24% of patients reported urge to drink with this combination, among those who continued to experience urge to drink, the magnitude of urges was not reduced.

CONTINGENCY MANAGEMENT

This approach reinforces abstinence through the use of reinforcement, most usually in the form of vouchers exchangeable for retail goods. There are few studies of this approach for the management of alcohol problems (Higgins & Petry, 1999), though as described below, it has been widely researched in relation to cocaine and opiate abuse. Petry et al. (2000) assigned 42 males to either a standard (but intensive) 8-week outpatient program, or this program augmented by contingency management (CM). The addition of CM resulted in significantly greater retention rates over the complete program (84 vs. 22%) and significantly higher levels of abstinence; 26% of the CM group had relapsed to heavy drinking by the end of treatment, contrasted to 61% of the standard treatment group. One challenge to the application of CM for alcohol abuse is that it is hard to verify abstinence; whereas opiate and cocaine use is easily detected through urinalysis, techniques for detecting alcohol use (such as Breathalyzers) yield information about alcohol use proximal to testing.

COMMUNITY REINFORCEMENT APPROACHES

There is good research evidence for the efficacy of community reinforcement approaches (CRAs), which usually combine a broad spectrum of interventions (including social skills, problem solving, behavior contracting, stress management, and behavioral marital therapy). Meta-analysis of six controlled studies (Mattick & Jarvis, 1993) suggests that while there is evidence for its short-term efficacy (with an effect size of 0.87 at 6-month follow-up), its longer-term efficacy may be limited; at 1-year follow-up, effect sizes diminish almost to zero.

Hunt and Azrin (1973) included problem solving, behavioral family therapy, social counseling, and (for unemployed clients) job-finding training. This package was added to an inpatient program and contrasted with patients receiving the standard milieu therapy. At 6 months, patients receiving the treatment package were drinking on 14% of days, contrasted with 79% in control patients. Broader gains in social adjustment were also evident. All marriages in the experimental group remained intact, contrasted with a 25% rate of separation or divorce in controls. In addition, there were 12 times the number of unemployed days in the control group than in the experimental group.

Azrin (1976) added disulfiram, a behavioral program aimed at increasing disulfiram compliance, a "buddy" system, and daily self-monitoring of mood, contrasting the addition of this program to inpatient treatment to treatment as usual (TAU). Again, significant gains were obtained in the experimental group, which were maintained at 2-year follow-up. Azrin et al. (1982) contrasted the full package from their 1976 trial with disulfiram alone (though combined with the behavioral compliance program), both contrasted with routine outpatient treatment. Drinking in the outpatient group was almost double that in the disulfiram–alone group, but both treatments were significantly inferior to the community reinforcement package. Although Azrin et al. (1982) found that married clients benefited more from treatments than unmarried ones, this differential effect was not found by Miller et al. (1990, cited in Mattick & Jarvis, 1993).

Smith et al. (1998) examined outcomes in 106 (mainly male) homeless individuals, all of whom were housed for 3 months (conditional on abstinence) and randomly assigned to CRA or to "standard" care (which comprised access to a day shelter and to AA-oriented individual and case management for those with a dual diagnoses). CRA involved an extensive program that included skills training groups, disulfiram compliance for a subgroup taking this medication, social support groups, couple therapy (where appropriate), and a job club. There was no evidence of benefit for disulfiram. Both groups showed improvement. Significantly better outcomes for CRA were evident at up to 9-month follow-up, through by 1 year, rates of drinking had increased, leading to statistical equivalence between groups.

A variant of CRA—community reinforcement and family training (CRAFT)—attempts to change the family environment through unilateral work with the partners of drinkers. Miller et al. (1999) randomized 130 (largely female) "significant others" of otherwise unmotivated drinkers to CRAFT, to counseling aimed at encouraging attendance at a 12-step program, or to a Johnson Institute intervention (in which the family works toward involving the identified patient in a family confrontation meeting). The CRAFT approach led to significantly more drinkers attending for treatment (64 vs. 13 and 30%, respectively). Broadly similar rates of attendance were observed in an open trial of this approach (Meyers et al., 1999).

COGNITIVE THERAPY VERSUS ALTERNATIVE ACTIVE TREATMENT

Longabaugh and Morgenstern (1999) reported on 26 trials of CBT interventions conducted up to 1998. In 11 of these, CBT was delivered as a stand-alone treatment, in 10 of which it was found to be as effective as alternative approaches; in one case (Project MATCH, reviewed below), it was found to be less effective than a 12-step approach or motivational interviewing. However, the addition of CBT to a broader treatment package conferred an advantage in 15 of 21 studies, suggesting that while its benefit over other treatments is doubtful, it has a significant role as an adjunctive component of therapy. Morgenstern and Longabaugh (2000) noted that while contrast to non-bona fide therapies indicates greater efficacy for CBT, contrast to bona fide interventions results in equivalent outcomes.

Three large-scale trials contrasted the efficacy of CBT with a 12-step approach—a contrast of major interest, since both are widely used in clinical settings but have very different rationales. Though Project MATCH (described more fully below) was primarily interested in the relation of process factors to outcome, it compared CBT, a 12-step approach, and motivational enhancement in both in- and outpatient contexts, finding no substantive differences in outcome across treatments (Project MATCH Research Group, 1997a). Ouimette et al. (1997) contrasted CBT, a 12-step approach, and a combined CBT and 12-step program in a multisite study of 3,018 patients recruited while undergoing inpatient detoxification in Veterans Affairs centers. All programs were effective at both posttherapy and 1-year follow-up. Though there was a greater probability of abstinence at 1 year for 12-step participants, all interventions showed equal outcomes for rates of substance use and a range of measures of symptomatic and functional status. Morgenstern et al. (2001) also found little evidence for the benefit of short-term CBT (delivered in either a "high-quality" manualized form or in a form that allowed therapists to implement CBT as they wished) as contrasted to drug counseling (which contained many elements of the 12-step approach). Two separate arms of the study examined the efficacy of these approaches either as stand-alone treatments ($n = 103$), or as an adjunct to an intensive outpatient program ($n = 149$); just under half the sample had a primary problem with alcohol abuse (the majority of remaining clients had a primary problem of cocaine abuse). While gains were made for all interventions in all conditions, there was no incremental benefit for the addition of CBT to standard treatment for alcohol users.

Although CBT emphasizes the development of coping skills, there are few studies that make it clear whether this is the mechanism through which it exerts its action. Morgenstern and Longabaugh (2000) identified 10 trials in which CBT was contrasted to an alternative intervention. Though the main criterion for this contrast was that the alternative treatment did not place explicit emphasis on coping skills, only three of these contrasts were against a bona fide treatment. While, overall, there was evidence that an increase in coping skills was associated with better outcome, only one trial suggested a mediating role for coping skills; in the remainder, there was either an increase in coping skills but no concomitant decrease in substance abuse, or there was no evidence that CBT increased coping skills to a greater extent than the contrast treatment. Congruent with this outcome, Litt et al. (2003) studied the development of coping skills in 128 patients randomized to group treatment that emphasized either coping skills or interactional issues. Both approaches resulted in equivalent drinking outcomes, and both produced similar improvements in coping skills. Though treatment type did not impact on outcome, improvement in coping skills was associated with better rates of abstinence, reduced substance abuse, and longer time to relapse—the latter being a consistent finding from other studies (Chung et al., 2001; Morgenstern & Longabaugh, 2000).

Psychotherapy and Counseling

Evidence for the efficacy of psychotherapy and counseling is limited. Levinson and Sereny (1969) assigned inpatients either to insight–oriented therapy (which included individual and group therapy, as well as educational sessions) or to TAU, which comprised occupational and recreational therapy. At 1-year follow-up, no differences in drinking behavior were found between groups. In this study, somewhat greater improvements were found in control patients; a similar pattern of results has been found by other studies (Bjornvoll, 1972, cited in Miller & Hester, 1986; Pattison et al., 1967; Tomsovic, 1970).

Psychodynamic Therapy

Though the contrast of dynamic psychotherapy to no treatment yields positive results (e.g., Brandsma et al., 1980; Kissin et al., 1970), its contrast to minimal intervention strategies indicates that there is little extra benefit to the addition of therapy (e.g., Crumbach & Carr, 1979; Zimberg, 1974). Early studies contrasting psychodynamic therapy and counseling (Ends & Page, 1957) or psychodynamic therapy and behavior therapy (Pomerleau et al., 1978) suggest few differences between therapies or between therapies and controls, and studies that do indicate such differences appear to have been characterized by poor methodology (Miller & Hester, 1986). A more recent, small trial by Sandahl et al. (1998) contrasted group psychodynamic and group CBT in 49 patients who had completed a prior period of inpatient treatment. Posttherapy and at 15-month follow-up, both groups showed improvement. Though there were no statistically significant differences between treatments, there was a trend toward greater maintenance of gains among patients in the psychodynamic group.

Marital and Family Therapy

In most trials of marital therapy, it is usually the male partner who has an identified drinking problems. Mattick and Jarvis (1993) reviewed eight trials of marital and family therapy, concluding that whereas their impact is better than no treatment at all, there is little evidence for their long-term impact (contrasts of such therapies with control treatments at between 6- and 11-month follow-up yield an effect size of 0.06). This conclusion contrasts that of Miller and Hester (1986), who suggest some gains, at least in the short term, for this intervention. Discrepancies between these reviews are difficult to account for and may reflect differing interpretations of a rather inconsistent literature.

MARITAL THERAPY VERSUS NO/MINIMAL INTERVENTION

There are few contrasts of marital therapy and minimal intervention. Corder et al. (1972) added a marital therapy workshop to inpatient milieu therapy, and found that at 6 months, 42% of this group had relapsed, contrasted with 85% of a previous cohort receiving the milieu therapy alone. Cadogan (1973) assigned 40 inpatients to either an additional outpatient marital therapy group or a wait-list control group. At 6 months, 45% of the marital therapy group and 10% of the controls were abstinent. However, Zweben et al. (1988) found no advantage to eight sessions of marital therapy over one 90-minute session with the drinker and his/her spouse, though this study incorporated a large number of follow-ups that, in effect, may have increased the level of intervention.

MARITAL THERAPY COMBINED WITH OTHER THERAPIES

McCrady et al. (1999) assigned 90 couples to receive behavioral couple therapy alone, in combination with attendance at AA meetings, or with relapse prevention. All three conditions showed equal gains, suggesting no benefit to the additional treatment elements. O'Farrell et al. (1993, 1998) assigned 59 couples to receive 5 months of behavioral marital therapy, after which half were randomized to no additional treatment, and half to 15 sessions of a couple-based relapse prevention program over the next year. For the whole sample, results at posththerapy and at 6-month follow-up favored the addition of relapse prevention; for patients with more severe marital and alcohol problems, the superiority of the combined package continued to be evident at 30-month follow-up.

MARITAL THERAPY VERSUS INDIVIDUAL COUNSELING

There are few relevant trials of this important contrast, but outcomes are reasonably consistent. McCrady et al. (1979) compared a control group receiving individual counseling with two treatments: In the first, subjects received
outpatient marital therapy; in the second, both patient and spouse were
admitted to an inpatient unit. Though significant reductions in drinking were
reported for the two treatment groups, effect size analyses by Mattick and
Jarvis (1993) suggested that there were no between-group differences in the
quantity and frequency of drinking. However, at 4-year follow-up (McCrady
et al., 1982), those treated as inpatients evidenced more abstinence and a
greater reduction in drinking than either outpatient or individually counseled
patients, presumably reflecting the benefit of the greater spousal involvement
under this treatment condition. A further study (McCrady et al., 1986) examined the impact of three levels of spousal involvement. In the first, the spouse
was merely present while the patient received individual cognitive training
(acting as a control group). In the second, the patient received the same training, while the spouse was trained in behaviors aimed at reinforcing abstinence. A third group received both these interventions, together with behavioral marital therapy. Some advantage to marital therapy was evident. In a
small trial, Bowers and Al-Redha (1990) assigned 16 couples to either individual treatment or group couple therapy. Though at posttreatment both
interventions were of equal efficacy, there was evidence of reduced drinking
at 6 months and 1 year for those who had received couple therapy. O'Farrell
et al. (1985) randomized male patients receiving individual counseling to
receive either marital therapy or no additional treatment. Though initially
there were greater gains for conjoint treatment, these had disappeared at 2-
year follow-up (O'Farrell et al., 1992).

Motivational Interviewing

Accurately defining the practice of motivational interviewing has proved
complex, because its spirit relies on therapists maintaining a nonjudgmental
and nonconfrontational position (Rollnick & Miller, 1995). This issue is
reflected in Dunn et al.'s (2001) comprehensive meta-analysis, in which
uncertainty about the precision with which motivational interviewing was
implemented led to the exclusion of many trials—an initial sample of 107
reduced to 29 (of which 10 focused on alcohol abuse). Across the sample of
29, the length of treatment sessions varied from 5 to 360 minutes, suggesting
further variation in implementation of this method. Because of this heterogeneity, a common effect size was not reported, though effect sizes for individual studies are usually positive, ranging from 0.3 to 0.83. Though there was

evidence across studies for the maintenance of gains, within studies there is some inconsistency in longer term outcome. However, evidence for motivational interviewing was strongest when it was added in a planned fashion to a more extended treatment rather than as a stand-alone brief intervention. Illustrating this mode of application, Connors et al. (2002) contrasted both attrition rates and outcomes from standard outpatient therapy, or this therapy preceded by one session of role induction or motivational interviewing. The addition of motivational interviewing led to significantly better retention in therapy and more abstinence in the first 3 months of follow-up.

Whatever its mode of action, there is some preliminary evidence that the more structured elements of this approach may be relevant to its efficacy. Sellman et al. (2001) provided 6-month follow-up data for 122 mild to moderate drinkers randomized to receive one session of psychoeducation alone, or psychoeducation followed by either four sessions of motivational enhancement therapy or nondirective counseling. Motivational enhancement—but not nondirective counseling—led to significantly greater reductions in drinking behavior than psychoeducation alone.

Matching Clients to Treatments

Project MATCH, a very large and ambitious trial (Project MATCH Research Group, 1997a), aimed to determine whether outcomes from three different treatments would have differential impacts in relation to a range of client characteristics. There were two parallel arms: outpatients (n = 952), and those treated following inpatient or intensive day hospital treatment (n = 774). Three therapies were contrasted—cognitive-behavioral coping skills therapy (CBT), motivational enhancement (ME), and twelve-step facilitation (TSF)—all delivered over 12 weeks, though CBT and TSF comprised 12 weekly sessions, and ME comprised four sessions spaced over the study period. The primary measures of outcome were percentage of days abstinent from drinking (PDA) and drinks per drinking day (DDD). All treatments resulted in significant reductions in PDA and DDA at posttherapy and at 1- and 3-year (Project MATCH Research Group, 1998a) follow-up.

Although aftercare patients had more severe levels of pathology, abstinence rates among this group were lower than for outpatients. Among aftercare patients, 35% were abstinent for 1 year, and 60% never had more than 3 days of heavy drinking; for outpatients, the equivalent figures are 20 and 50%. The reasons for this difference are unclear. While it may reflect selective recruitment (in order to enter the trial, aftercare patients had to complete an intensive day or inpatient program and demonstrate a period of abstinence), it may also indicate the benefit of a combined residential and aftercare program.

Only one significant difference between treatments was apparent: Outpatients receiving TSF were more likely to remain abstinent over the first year of follow-up (24%) than those receiving CBT (14%) or ME (15%). Forty-one percent of CBT and TSF clients were abstinent or drinking moderately, contrasted to 28% of ME clients. Wherever differences were observed between treatments, they favored TSF. However, the lack of between-treatment differences is unlikely to represent a Type II error, and this study suggests that a very brief intervention (ME) is as effective as longer therapies across all levels of severity.

While the primary purpose of the trial was to identify client × treatment matches, few emerged. Clients with fewer psychological problems had greater rates of abstinence than those receiving CBT over the first follow-up year. Those outpatients high in anger had better outcomes with ME than with CBT, and aftercare patients with high levels of alcohol dependence did better with TSF than with CBT (Project MATCH Research Group, 1997b). Overall, patients had poorer outcomes if their social networks supported drinking. Longabaugh et al. (1998) also found that such patients had better outcomes with TSF, though this effect was only evident at 3-year follow-up, and was partially (though not wholly) attributable to greater involvement in AA.

It has been suggested that clients low in coping skills would be expected to show greater gains with CBT (since their deficits lie within the treatment focus of this approach). However, few studies support this proposition. Though Kadden et al. (1992) found that patients who performed poorly in role-play tests of drinking-related scenarios did better with CBT, most of the few trials that explore this issue suggest that those lowest in coping skills did no better (Kadden et al., 2001) or worse with CBT contrasted to supportive or more socially oriented treatments (Project MATCH Research Group, 1997b; Rohsenow et al., 1991). Jaffe et al. (1996) assigned 97 patients to receive naltrexone or placebo in combination with either relapse prevention or supportive therapy. This study examined impact of verbal learning ability, as a proxy for cognitive capacity and the capacity to learn new coping skills. While outcomes from supportive therapy were equivalent on this variable, patients with poorer verbal learning had worse outcomes from relapse prevention, and those with higher levels of verbal learning had better outcomes. A similar pattern of outcomes was observed by Kadden et al. (1989), who contrasted outcomes from coping skills or interactional therapy. A later study by this group (Kadden et al., 2001) set out to determine the impact of prospective matching to these two therapies. Two hundred fifty participants were either matched to treatment or randomly allocated; contrary to prediction, randomized clients had better outcomes, and there was no evidence of benefit from pretreatment matching. Though prior research tentatively suggested that the task demands of treatments may be a factor to take into account when planning individual treatment, this later study casts doubt on the robustness of this effect.

Noting the practical problems associated with treatment matching in clinical settings, McLellan et al. (1997) matched clients to services rather than to specific treatments. In this trial 94 patients referred to one of four treatment centers were prospectively assessed for indications of employment, family or psychiatric problems. They then either received the standard package of treatment, or this treatment supplemented by assignment to targeted services matching problem areas. Significant gains were made by both groups, though matched patients stayed in treatment longer, and showed greater gains on some (but not all) measures.

A large multicenter trial in progress, the U.K. Alcohol Treatment Trial (UKATT Research Team, 2001) is designed to build on Project MATCH and should contribute to the debate on treatment matching. This project contrasts ME with social behavior and network therapy (SBNT). SBNT was developed for the trial on the basis of good evidence for the importance of social factors in managing substance abuse, and contains aspects of marital and family therapy, community reinforcement, relapse prevention, and social skills training.

Length and Setting of Treatment

There is little evidence that longer treatments are more successful than briefer interventions, or that inpatient therapy shows greater efficacy than outpatient treatment. Miller and Hester (1986) reviewed 12 controlled studies of contrasts between in- and outpatient treatment, none of which favored inpatient treatment, and some of which showed greater gains for outpatients. Similarly, five studies of the length of treatment showed no gain for longer treatment and some advantage for shorter interventions. Contrasts of seven RCTs of in- and outpatient treatments by Miller and Jarvis (1993) yield an effect size close to zero, suggesting no advantage to inpatient regimens.

This picture is complicated by the likelihood of an interaction between inpatient treatment and the use of outpatient aftercare. Pittman and Tate (1972) found that success following inpatient treatment was correlated with subsequent use of outpatient services. Robson et al. (1965) and Smart and Gray (1978) both contrasted high users of outpatient services with patients who attended for only short periods, finding that high users tended to have lower rates of drinking problems. However, these results are based on naturalistic studies using post hoc analysis, and there is the possibility of a confound between motivation and attendance.

Though these general reviews usually find that there is no advantage to inpatient compared to outpatient treatment, Rychtarik et al. (2000) hypothesized that inpatient stay would be of particular benefit for clients with greater levels of dependence, and for those whose social networks were supportive of drinking. One hundred ninety-two participants were randomized to 1-

month programs of inpatient treatment, intensive outpatient therapy (identical to the inpatient program except for the milieu component), or standard outpatient treatment (which contained similar therapies to the first two conditions, but delivered at lower intensity). Although there was no overall difference in outcomes across treatments, individuals with higher levels of dependence had significantly better outcomes from inpatient care, while those with lower levels benefited more from outpatient treatment; there was no association between treatment type and network support for drinking.

Brief Interventions for Problem Drinkers and for Alcohol-Dependent Individuals

As noted earlier, there have been many studies of brief therapy, with most reviews indicating no advantage for extended over brief intervention. Whether this observation holds true over different populations of drinkers is an important question. Mattick and Jarvis (1993) distinguished between patients who are alcohol-dependent, "problem drinkers" (who have difficulties limiting their alcohol intake but are not alcohol-dependent), and those who are excessive drinkers but not necessarily alcohol-dependent.

Brief versus Extended Treatment for Alochol-Dependent Individuals

Edwards et al. (1977) contrasted one 3-hour session of advice with several months of in- or outpatient treatment in 100 married male alcoholics. No differences in outcome were found between these conditions at posttreatment. Although yielding an apparently clear-cut result, this study is open to criticism; subjects were not comorbid and were relatively well-adjusted, and there was some blurring in treatment intensity (only one-third of patients randomized to the more intensively treated condition actually continued in treatment). Additionally, there is some evidence from 2-year follow-up data (Orford et al., 1976) that more severely dependent individuals benefited from more extensive interventions.

Chick et al. (1988) and Chapman and Huygens (1988) replicated the Edwards et al. (1976) trial using essentially similar research designs. Though Chick et al. (1988) suggested some advantage to extended treatment, Chapman and Huygens (1988) found no differences in outcome between conditions. However, both studies are flawed by the fact that the minimal intervention condition was, for many patients, relatively extensive. In Chick et al.'s (1988) trial, this was because additional treatment was offered to, and accepted by, many patients randomized to minimal intervention. Chapman and Huygen's (1988) study was conducted in the context of a 2-week inpatient detoxification program, and more accurately examines the adjunctive impacts of treatments to this program.

Brief Interventions for Problem Drinkers

Although individuals who drink excessively have the potential to develop more serious dependence, this is not an inevitable trajectory, and it is reasonable to question whether this group should be targeted for active intervention. However, both earlier and more recent trials of minimal intervention support the proposition that brief interventions in a range of settings can lead to significant reductions in alcohol consumption when contrasted to TAU (e.g., Chick et al., 1985; Elvy et al., 1988; Heather et al., 1987a, 1987b; Kristenson et al., 1983; Wallace et al., 1988).

Fleming et al. (2002) identified 2,450 patients with moderate levels of alcohol intake from 17,695 individuals who attended one of 64 primary care physicians' offices for routine medical care. Of these, 774 met exclusion criteria and agreed to be randomized to receive standard care or a brief intervention that comprised two 15-minute meetings with their physician 1 month apart, and two follow-up phone calls 2 weeks after these meetings from office nurses. All patients received a booklet focused on a number of health promotion issues. At 4-year follow-up, the intervention group had significantly lower rates of alcohol use and binge drinking. Though at 2-year follow-up the intervention led to lower rates of heavy drinking, at 4 years this advantage had eroded. Ockene et al. (1999) screened 9,772 patients in primary care settings. Five hundred thirty heavy drinkers were randomized to TAU or to a program based on a brief, structured, 5–10 minute intervention (which included motivational interviewing and psychoeducation). Although problems in randomization meant that the intervention group had higher initial rates of drinking, brief intervention resulted in a significant reduction in drinking. In this trial, both male and female patients showed equivalent responses; in contrast an earlier multisite international trial (World Health Organization [WHO] Brief Intervention Study Group, 1996) allocated 1,559 patients with moderate drinking but no history of alcohol dependence to assessment only, to receive 5 minutes of advice, or to receive 15 or 60 minutes of brief counseling. At 9-month follow-up, male patients responded equally to both advice and counseling, though women in all conditions (including assessment alone) reduced their alcohol intake. To some degree this echoes Kahan et al.'s (1995) review of physician-based interventions that identified 11 relevant trials, four of which met appropriate quality criteria, and indicated that interventions led to consistent reduction in drinking for men but inconsistent outcomes for women. A 10-year follow-up of the Australian cohort of the WHO study (Wutzke et al., 2001) reported data on an initial cohort of 554 individuals, 370 of whom were reinterviewed at 10 years. While 9-month outcomes followed the same pattern as the main trial, at 10 years, there were no differences between treatment groups. Though this suggests that, over the very long term, the impact of these interventions will dissipate, the fact of their brevity and the magnitude of initial effects makes this an unsurprising finding. Overall research suggests that brief interventions in primary care contexts may be useful, though their cost-effectiveness needs to be considered; the likely prevalence of problem drinking means that, in most settings, the amount of screening needed to identify appropriate patients may be burdensome in terms of both time and money (e.g., Yarnall et al., 2003).

Shakeshaft et al. (2002) contrasted the impact of brief intervention and CBT in 295 problem drinkers seeking help from a community drug and alcohol service. All clients received a prior assessment and a self-help manual. Brief interventions lasted no more than 90 minutes (though they could take place over more than one session), and comprised psychoeducation and counseling tailored to individual need (as indicated by the assessment). CBT was delivered in six weekly sessions, with a maximum time of 270 minutes. Despite these differences in the extent and complexity of treatment, at 6-month follow-up, both groups showed equivalent outcomes.

Hall and Heather (1991) examined contrasts of minimal and intensive interventions for problem drinkers (those who are not dependent on alcohol). Though many studies suggest that the two interventions are of equal efficacy, this is not a consistent finding. They suggest that inconsistencies across studies may reflect variations in subject motivation, attributable to the better prognosis (hence, treatment responsiveness) associated with self-referred as contrasted to referred patients, which in turn reduce the likelihood of finding a benefit to additional therapist input.

Successful interventions are more than simple advice. Consistent common elements (as identified by Miller & Sanchez, 1993) are feedback regarding personal risk, emphasis on personal responsibility for change, clear advice to change, offering a range of options to achieve change, therapeutic empathy, enhancement of client self-efficacy, and optimism. Indeed, Miller and Sanchez (1993) monitored the interventions employed by counselors in a study of brief treatment, finding a close association between the number of confrontational responses from counselors and the amount being drunk by the client at 1-year follow-up.

In summary, there is good evidence that brief interventions will help a significant proportion of patients, though it is important to note that such an approach may not be suitable for all patients, and particularly not for those who are more disabled (Thom et al., 1994). Nonetheless, it may be appropriate for services to ensure that such a service is offered to clients, since there is evidence that allocating patients to a wait list until therapists become available may result in significant levels of attrition. Leigh et al. (1984), Rees and Farmer (1985), and Thom et al. (1992) have demonstrated an association between greater waiting time and a reduced probability of patients attending for their first appointment, reinforcing arguments for the utility of relatively rapid and brief interventions.

TREATMENTS FOR COCAINE DEPENDENCE AND ABUSE

Though not analyzed in relation to treatment type, Simpson et al.'s (1999) naturalistic study of the impacts of community treatments (offered as part of the national Drug Abuse Treatment Outcome Studies program) offered a helpful orientation to expected outcomes for cocaine abuse. One thousand six hundred five sequential admissions to 55 community treatment programs were identified, and their treatments classified as long-term residential (LTR; a primarily therapeutic community), short-term inpatient (STI), or outpatient drug-free (ODF) programs. The study also examined the impact of retaining patients in treatment for an optimal period. On the basis of prior research, this was set as 90 days for LTR and ODF, and 21 days for STI. Across the sample, 23% of patients relapsed, with the probability of relapse related both to initial severity and the length of time patients were retained in treatment. Patients with the lowest levels of dependence had the lowest rates of subsequent relapse (between 15 and 20% across the treatment settings), and appeared to benefit from all treatment types, implying that shorter outpatient intervention would be cost-effective for this group. For individuals with medium levels of severity, better outcomes were obtained if they stayed in treatment for the optimal period; these patients had half the rates of relapse of those who had shorter durations of therapy. Overall, patients with the most severe problems were treated in LTR settings, and these also did best if retained for the optimal period in longer term programs. Relapse rates for LTR, STI, and ODF were 15, 38, and 29%, respectively. These percentages may be underestimates, because one in four patients reported a return to treatment over 1-year follow-up. Because of evidence of underreporting of cocaine use, Simpson et al. suggested a figure between 10 and 20% higher than those cited here. However, while actual rates of outcome may be hard to determine, relative rates appear robust and emphasize the importance of treatment exposure to longer term outcome. Five-year follow-up of 708 individuals (Simpson et al., 2002) confirms an overall pattern of reasonably stable rates of cocaine use (at this point, 25% of the sample reported weekly cocaine use), but with significantly poorer outcomes for individuals with more severe drug and psychosocial problems who had not engaged with treatment.

Relapse Prevention

Carroll et al. (1991) contrasted 12 weekly sessions of CBT relapse prevention (RP) and interpersonal psychotherapy (IPT) in 42 patients; though more individuals in CBT were abstinent for more than 3 weeks during the treatment period (57 and 33%, respectively), this difference was not statistically significant. Stratification by level of severity suggested that high-dependence users were significantly more likely to show abstinence after RP than with IPT (54 and 9%, respectively); participants with low dependence had equivalent outcomes from both treatments.

Carroll et al. (1994a) randomized 139 participants to four conditions (all of which took place over 12 weeks): RP combined with desipramine or with placebo, and clinical management combined with desipramine or placebo. All groups showed some improvement, but there was no difference between conditions. However, at 1-year follow-up, there was some indication that patients who received RP had better outcomes (Carroll et al., 1994b). Post hoc analysis suggested that patients with higher levels of dependence attended more RP sessions than those with lower levels. It also seemed that level of dependence was associated with a differential response to treatment; those with higher levels of dependence had greater levels of abstinence from RP than clinical management, whereas low-severity patients had better outcomes from clinical management than from RP.

Contrast of CBT-RP to 12-step approaches yields inconsistent findings. Wells et al. (1994) compared RP and a 12-step approach in 110 participants, and also found no differences between treatments (though the informative value of this trial is weakened by the fact that almost one-fourth of trial entrants had been abstinent in the month prior to study entry). Maude-Griffin et al. (1998) assigned 128 individuals to a 12-week program of CBT-RP or to a 12 step approach and found that, overall, CBT was more effective than the 12 steps. The percentages of patients achieving 4 weeks of continuous abstinence were 44 and 32%, respectively, with this advantage maintained over 26-week follow-up. Of interest are several post hoc analyses of matching effects, which suggested that RP is particularly suited to depressed patients (a finding also noted by Carroll et al., 1994a), and to those high in abstract reasoning. McKay et al. (1997) contrasted 12-step counseling and RP, finding that counseling led to higher rates of abstinence, but RP was more effective in limiting cocaine use in those who relapsed. The pattern suggests that coping skills training may help reduce cocaine use once relapse occurs.

In an approach that overlaps with CBT-RP, Monti et al. (1997) compared cocaine-specific coping skills training and attention control in 108 participants who were also receiving inpatient care. Though relapse rates were equivalent, as in McKay et al. (1997), coping skills training resulted in lower rates of cocaine use over the first 6 months of follow-up (though at 12 months its impact had dissipated; Rohsenow et al., 2000).

Community Reinforcement Approach and Contingency Management

Higgins et al. (1993) compared CRA with drug counseling. Treatment was intensive—biweekly for 12 weeks, and weekly for a further 12 weeks. Sixty-

eight percent of patients receiving CRA were abstinent for 8 weeks, dropping to 42% over 16 weeks; for drug counseling, the equivalent figures were
11 and 5%. Variations of the CRA approach aim to enhance attendance of
individuals through "concerned significant others" (CSOs). Kirby et al.
(1999) assigned 32 CSOs either to CRA or to a 12-step program. About half
the identified patients were abusing cocaine, about one-fourth heroin, and
the remainder, other drugs. Attendance of CSOs and identified patients was
significantly greater in CRA: 86% of CSOs and 64% of users attended CRA,
contrasted to 39 and 17%, respectively for the 12-step program. Meyers et al.
(2002) identified 90 CSOs with treatment-refusing family members with a
range of substance abuse problems. CSOs were randomized to a 12-step program or to CRAFT, offered either as a 12-session program or with the addition of optional aftercare groups over 6 months. CRAFT alone engaged 57%
of identified patients; CRAFT with aftercare, 77%, and the 12-step program,
29%, suggesting a clear benefit to this approach.

    Higgins et al. (1994) examined the efficacy of adding contingency man-
agement to CRA. In exchange for a cocaine-negative urine sample, participants were given vouchers that could be exchanged for retail goods. The
addition of this component resulted in higher levels of retention (75 vs. 40%
attended 24 weeks of treatment), and higher levels of abstinence (in the first
12 weeks, 50 and 20%, respectively, with and without vouchers). This
advantage was maintained at 1-year follow-up (Higgins et al., 1995). Higgins
et al. (2000) randomized 70 participants to receive vouchers either contingent
or noncontingent on negative urinalysis, in order to establish whether better
outcomes reflected greater contact time rather than reinforcement. Although
both groups were retained in the trial at approximately the same rate, levels
of abstinence were greater when vouchers were issued contingently, giving
support to the theoretical rationale for this approach. Analysis of data from
several trials conducted by this group (Higgins et al., 2000) suggests that the
probability of continuous abstinence during follow-up is predicted by the
amount of abstinence during treatment rather than the type of treatment
received. However, the use of contingent vouchers appears to promote abstinence more effectively than other approaches to which it has been compared
(on the basis of urinalysis and across all assessment points, abstinence rates
were 21%, contrasted to 12% for control treatments).

    Rawson et al. (2002) identified 120 cocaine-abusing individuals main-
tained on methadone in order to manage their opiate abuse. Participants were
randomized to receive one of four treatments over 16 weeks—CM alone,
CBT-RP, CM combined with CBT, or methadone maintenance only. Urinalysis indicated that CM resulted in greater gains during treatment; at 17
weeks, rates of cocaine-free samples were (for CBT, CM, CBT + CM, and
methadone, respectively) 40, 60, 47, and 23%. Results were maintained over
1-year follow-up, though participants receiving CBT continued to make

gains, and at this point rates for cocaine-free samples were 60, 53, 40, and 27%, respectively. In this trial, there were no indications of an additive effect of CM and CBT. Epstein et al. (2003) examined outcomes for 193 methadone-maintained participants assigned to 12 weeks of group CBT or control therapy combined with contingent or noncontingent vouchers. Although at posttreatment the addition of CBT appeared to reduce the impact of CM, at 3-month and 1-year follow-up there was evidence of significant additive benefit. Other trials have also showed promising outcomes for this population (Petry & Martin, 2002; Preston et al., 2001).

Focusing on homeless cocaine users, Milby et al. (1996) contrasted usual care (which comprised individual and group counseling) to day treatment and contingency management (which allowed access to housing and to work therapy) in 131 individuals. The combination of day treatment and contingency management led to significantly higher retention, to higher levels of abstinence, though by 12 months, loss of gains was evident. A further trial (Milby et al., 2000) attempted to separate the contribution of day treatment from contingency management. One hundred ten homeless cocaine users with a coexisting nonpsychotic DSM disorder were allocated either to an intensive day treatment program, or to this program accompanied by CM (which allowed access to housing and employment advice and opportunity). The addition of CM significantly improved the percentage of negative urine samples; at week 8, the proportion of negative samples were 71% and 31%, respectively, and while this difference declined over time (to 39 and 19%, respectively, at week 24), group differences remained. However, at 12-month follow-up (Milby et al., 2003), maintenance of gains had declined, resulting in equivalent outcomes for each group. It is not clear whether the immediate treatment effect in this difficult-to-treat group is attributable to CM alone or to its combination with day treatment.

The cost of running a CM program in standard clinical settings may be an important issue. Conventionally, the voucher system increases the amount of reward for each successive negative urine sample, with a loss of incentives for positive samples. In studies conducted by Higgins's research group participants could earn approximately $1,000, and on average received $600. Though increasing reward could have benefit, it would threaten the cost-effectiveness of programs. K. Silverman et al. (1999) found that patients who had previously been unresponsive to CM were more likely to achieve abstinence as the amount they could earn increased—ultimately to $3,500, an unrealistic figure for most clinical settings. Petry and Martin (2002) evaluated a low-cost CM program in which participants drew vouchers that could range from $1 to $100. About half the vouchers were nonwinning slips, but there were also a small number of large prizes. Forty-two cocaine- and opiate-abusing patients maintained on methadone were randomly assigned to standard methadone treatment or to standard treatment with CM. At posttreatment and 6-

month follow-up, there was an advantage to CM, with average earnings of $137. Although this study examined outcomes for polydrug abusers, it suggests that programs may be able to set reward systems at lower levels than are seen in some research trials. Some caution is warranted, however. Kirby et al. (1998) contrasted CBT and problem-solving sessions, with or without the addition of CM, in 90 patients. The voucher system was of low value and depended on the results of weekly (rather than the usual daily) urinalysis, and did not enhance retention or abstinence rates. A second trial adapted CM by increasing the potential reward and also (in effect) making the voucher system more contingent on consistent negative urine samples. Contrast of this new schedule to the original (in a small sample of 23 patients) resulted in significantly improved rates of abstinence. This suggests that some care might be needed to ensure that the precise form of voucher delivery conforms to that identified as effective in research trials.

Preston et al. (2001) reported a variation on CM in which vouchers were initially given for successive reductions in cocaine levels at urinalysis, in an attempt to shape behavior on the principle of successive approximation. Ninety-five methadone-maintained patients were randomized to an 8-week program that contrasted standard CM and 3 weeks of successive approximation, followed by 5 weeks of standard CM. In the initial 3 weeks, outcomes were identical, but once both groups were receiving standard CM those receiving successive approximation showed an advantage, suggesting that this method better prepared participants for CM.

Other Psychotherapies

Kang et al. (1991) contrasted family therapy, supportive–expressive psychotherapy (SE; a form of psychodynamic therapy), and group therapy (led by paraprofessionals) in 122 individuals, 72% of whom were smoking crack cocaine. Attrition was very high; only 50% attended more than one session, and 22%, more than six sessions. Only 25% were abstinent during treatment, and 19% of those who attended more than three sessions reported abstinence at 6-month follow-up.

A major trial—the National Institute on Drug Abuse Collaborative Cocaine Study (Crits-Christoph et al., 1997)—randomized 487 patients to one of four treatments. All treatments included group drug counseling, which followed a 12-step model, encouraged participation in 12-step programs, and included social support. This was either offered alone or combined with one of three individual therapies: individual drug counseling (which focused on achieving abstinence and followed a 12-step model); CBT; or individual SE psychotherapy. These were all offered over 6 months (with a maximum of 36 individual combined with 24 group sessions), biweekly for the first 3 months, and weekly for the final 3 months; after this time, three further sessions were held at monthly intervals. Overall, attrition rates were high; by month 3, about half of study participants had left treatment and only 28% completed treatment, though attrition was significantly lower for CBT and SE therapy. Though all interventions led to reduction in drug use, this was greatest for individual combined with group counseling. The proportion of patients (based on the intention-to-treat sample) who achieved 3 months of consecutive abstinence was 38% for this approach, contrasted to 23, 18, and 27% for CBT, SE, and group counseling, respectively (Crits-Christoph et al., 1999). This study raises important issues, not least of which is the suggestion that the most effective therapy was one that required the shortest professional training—an explicit research question posed in the planning stage of the trial (Crits-Christoph et al., 1997). While it may be relevant that the aim and focus of drug counseling is coterminous with the primary outcome measure of this trial, there were no differences across treatments on a wide range of outcome measures (Crits-Christoph et al., 2001). It is of interest to note that this trial failed to replicate earlier patterns of outcome from a trial for opiate abusers (Woody et al., 1987, discussed below, and on which many features of this trial design were based; Woody et al., 1983), in which psychotherapeutic models appeared to have benefit over the delivery of a "disease" model by paraprofessional therapists.

Though this study was conducted to very high levels of methodological adequacy, it is relevant to note that all trial entrants were required to undergo a 2-week assessment phase prior to randomization. This resulted in the loss of 383 of the initial 870 participants, many of whom had higher levels of dependence and lower levels of educational achievement than those who started treatment (Siqueland et al., 1998). This has led some commentators to suggest that the high levels of attrition could relate to overtreatment (Carroll, 1999). Unfortunately, it also led to difficulties in testing a secondary hypothesis: that the addition of formal psychotherapies to counseling would be especially beneficial to individuals with dual diagnoses and antisocial personality disorder. No evidence was found to support this contention (Crits-Christoph et al., 1999), a finding that could reflect the lack of variance in psychopathology across the sample.

Outcomes from this study contrast somewhat with other trials, which find either no differences between psychological therapies or greater efficacy for CBT. Gottheil et al. (1998) randomized 447 patients to receive one of three treatments over 12 weeks—weekly individual counseling, weekly individual counseling combined with weekly group meetings, or an intensive group program 3 days a week. All three interventions led to improvements, and all therapies showed equal efficacy. Most patients were unmarried and unemployed, and most were African American; while this may limit generalization, it may also reflect the demographics of inner-city, publicly funded services.

The impact of behavioral couple therapy (BCT) has been investigated in two trials by the same research group. Fals-Stewart et al. (1996) randomized 80 male substance abusers to 24 weeks of individual and group CBT alone, or to these therapies combined with BCT. The primary drug of abuse was cocaine in 50% of the sample, and opiates in 32%. During the treatment phase, there were equal reductions in substance use, though over 12-month follow-up, those receiving BCT had a significantly higher percentage of days abstinent (at 12 months, 76 and 69%, respectively). BCT also showed a significantly slower rate of relapse over the first 90 days of follow-up. A reanalysis of this trial (Fals-Stewart et al., 2000) computed rates of clinically significant change. In relation to rates of abstinence, the percentage of individuals who improved or were unchanged with BCT were 83 and 17%, respectively; for individual therapy, the equivalent figures were 60 and 40%. Winters et al. (2002) assigned 75 substance-abusing women (of whom 60 and 40%, respectively, met criteria for cocaine or opiate abuse) to the same pattern of treatments. Again, there were equal reductions in substance use during the treatment phase and some advantage to BCT over follow-up. Relapse rates were slower for BCT than for individual therapy, and in the 9 months after treatment, percentage of days abstinent was significantly higher for BCT than for individual therapy (81 and 72%, respectively). However, this difference was not sustained at 12-month follow-up.

TREATMENTS FOR OPIATE DEPENDENCE AND ABUSE
Meta-Analyses

Brewer et al. (1998) identified 69 trials, published between 1943 an 1996, that examined the impact of treatments for opiate addiction in order to identify patient characteristics that predict continued opiate use posttreatment. Meta-analysis revealed rather few predictors of continued use, though poorer outcomes were associated with higher levels of pretreatment abuse, prior treatment, a social network supportive of continuing abuse, poorer psychiatric and social adjustment, short length of treatment, and leaving treatment prior to completion. A similar conclusion was drawn by Prendergast et al. (2002), who identified 78 studies of pharmacological and psychological treatments, published between 1965 and 1996, and conducted in the U.S. or Canada, the majority of which focused on opiate addiction, with a smaller number examining outcomes for cocaine or polydrug abuse. Although they determined an overall effect size of 0.3, there were few clear links among client characteristics or program specifications and outcome. Nonetheless, greater success appeared to be related to treatment integrity, reflected in higher levels of staff training, monitoring of and adherence to protocols, and lower attrition rates. However, this finding contrasts the fact that programs with less explicit theoretical rationales had larger effect sizes, an association that is puzzling and difficult to explain. Furthermore, no treatment type emerged as specifically beneficial.

Stanton and Shadish (1997) identified 15 studies that contrasted family therapy and individual therapy, peer group therapy and family psychoeducation, and that treated adults and adolescents. Although the analysis excluded studies in which alcohol was the primary drug of abuse, across studies, there is some variation in the specific drugs abused by individuals. Most participants were being treated primarily for opiate abuse, less frequently cocaine, and in some studies other drugs (such as cannabis). Contrasting family interventions with nonfamily interventions yielded an effect size of 0.48 on measures of drug use, with no difference in effect sizes for studies of adults or adolescents. Attrition rates were significantly higher for nonfamily than for family interventions. Given evidence of an association between attrition rates and higher levels of substance abuse (Stark, 1992), this raises the possibility that differential retention will reduce the impact of family interventions, hence, underestimating their relative impact.

Cue Exposure

While a number of studies have examined the responsiveness of opiate-dependent individuals to drug-related cues (e.g., Powell et al., 1993), rather fewer examine the impact of cue exposure as a treatment technique. These offer little support for the efficacy of this approach. McLellan et al. (1986) contrasted CBT, with and without cue exposure, to drug counseling alone; while CBT showed an advantage over drug counseling, there was no evidence of added benefit to cue exposure. Dawe et al. (1993) allocated 186 individuals to a specialist unit or a general psychiatric ward; in each setting, patients were further randomized to receive either 6 weeks of cue exposure or a control condition. At 6-week and 6-month follow-up, there were no differences between groups. Other trials from this same research group reached similar conclusions (Kasvikis et al., 1991).

Community Reinforcement Approaches and Contingency Management

A meta-analytic review of CM, based on 30 studies, yielded an effect size of 0.25 (Griffith et al., 2000). As discussed below, there are a number of variations in the delivery of CM. Examining these, Griffiths et al. noted that the largest effect sizes were obtained from studies in which contingencies allowed for an increase in methadone or for take-home methadone, where reinforcement was offered on an immediate rather than a delayed schedule, and where urine samples were collected more frequently (more than twice weekly).

Bickel et al. (1997) combined CM and CRA with a 26-week outpatient detoxification program using buprenorphine, contrasting this with bu-prenorphine alone. Thirty-nine individuals were allocated to treatments; contingent on both negative urine samples and attendance at the CRA pro-gram, participants received vouchers exchangeable for goods and services. Completion rates were significantly higher with CM-CRA than for control (53 and 20%, respectively). The percentage of patients achieving 8 weeks of abstinence were 47 and 15%, and 16 weeks' abstinence, 11 and 0%, respec-tively.

Iguchi et al. (1997) also employed a voucher system in a 12-week trial, but contingencies were based either on urinalysis or on the successful com-pletion of therapeutic activity (such as vocational training). Their design was based on two propositions. First, because some individuals do not submit negative urine samples, they are never reinforced by the CM approach. Sec-ond, making reinforcement contingent on undertaking therapeutic activities allows for individual shaping of the required outcomes, making this a poten-tially more powerful intervention. One hundred three patients were random-ized to one of the two CM conditions, or to standard outpatient treatment; outcomes were significantly better for those with contingencies reinforcing therapeutic activities. The failure of the urinalysis condition contrasts with positive outcomes in other studies and may reflect the fact that the amount earned for each voucher was lower than that in most trials.

Gruber et al. (2000) reported a trial of contingency management for opi-ate abusers who did not wish to use methadone, modeled on the work of Milby et al. (1996; reported earlier). Fifty-two heroin users who contacted a rapid inpatient detoxification unit were assigned to standard outpatient after-care (which assigned patients to outpatient treatment centers), or to receive a 1 month of abstinence-contingent CRA, along with 3 months of non-contingent counseling. At the end of the 1 month, CM-phase, postdetox-ification retention levels were significantly greater (61 vs. 17%), as were levels of abstinence (50 vs. 21%); however, at 3 months, the groups showed equiva-lent levels of heroin use. An open trial by this same group (Katz et al., 2001) extended the CM program to 3 months with a similar population of 37 indi-viduals, demonstrating better outcomes for those retained in the full program.

Although it has a number of advantages over methadone, naltrexone is less commonly used as part of detoxification programs, largely because attri-tion and noncompliance rates are high. Carroll et al. (2001) contrasted out-comes in 127 individuals for CM, CM enhanced with family therapy involv-ing a significant other, and standard treatment. Both CM conditions showed significant advantage over standard treatment, though, overall, there was no extra benefit to the addition of family work. Preston et al. (1999) assigned 58 clients to contingent or noncontingent vouchers, or to standard treatment, finding significantly improved retention and abstinence rates for the addition of vouchers. Roozen et al. (2003) found significant gains for individuals offered naltrexone combined with CRA treatment over patients assigned to standard methadone maintenance. Rothenberg et al. (2002) attempted to improve compliance by using a significant other to monitor medication, as part of an open trial that combined this with individual therapy and CRA. However, attrition rates were high, especially for patients who had been previously maintained on methadone (though slightly better for those who were heroin-dependent). Fals-Stewart and O'Farrell (2003) also examined the impact of family involvement on compliance, assigning 124 men maintained on naltrexone to one of two 24-week treatments—individual coping skills therapy or individual therapy combined with behavioral family therapy. In the family therapy condition, the patient took a daily dose of naltrexone in the presence of a family member. Family involvement led to higher levels of compliance with naltrexone in the year after treatment, and a higher percentage of days abstinent from opiates in this period (69 vs. 56%). Although this is a more promising result, the study population was derived from an initial sample of 459 individuals, of whom 318 refused to take naltrexone, and contrasted to these individuals, the study sample was younger, better educated, and had a shorter history of opiate abuse. Overall, these studies suggest that while the efficacy of naltrexone can be potentiated by its combination with behavioral therapies, medication compliance remains a challenge.

A small number of trials explored the use of CM in polydrug-abusing individuals with a history of continuing to take heroin or benzodiazepines while on methadone (the latter representing a group with a particularly poor prognosis; Condelli & Dunteman, 1993). Stitzer et al. (1992) allocated 53 individuals to receive take-home methadone either on the basis of contingent drug-free urinalysis, or noncontingently. A significant advantage to contingent scheduling was demonstrated, and a subgroup of those originally allocated to noncontingent privileges showed gains when subsequently switched to contingent scheduling. Chutuape et al. (1999a) demonstrated the efficacy of this approach in a small sample of individuals ($n = 14$) who had been detoxified in a short residential program, had a history of using heroin or cocaine during methadone treatment, and also abused benzodiazepines. Chatuape et al. (1999b) constructed a pattern of CM that recognized that some polydrug-abusing patients might never receive reinforcement for abstinence. On this basis, 34 patients were assigned to either a daily or a weekly contingency protocol, or were not given take-home privileges; for all patients, urine needed to be clear of heroin or cocaine, but not of benzodiazepines. Similar outcomes were observed for both contingency conditions, but while the proportion of drug-free samples were lower for this group, they were not significantly different from control. Nonetheless, five of 21 patients showed marked reductions in positive urine samples, an effect absent in control patients. Though this outcome is statistically modest, the clinical challenge posed by these patients suggests that this approach may be worth pursuing.

Psychological Therapies Other Than Behavioral and Cognitive Therapies

Woody et al. (1983) randomized 110 methadone-maintained individuals to 24 weeks of drug counseling alone, counseling and SE therapy, or CBT (a sample derived from participants who attended an intake screening and a further three sessions). The number of sessions attended varied across interventions (an average 17 sessions for drug counseling alone, 12 for SE therapy and 9.5 for CBT). Although at 7 months there were improvements in all three groups, there were greater gains for the clients who received both counseling and psychotherapy, with gains maintained at 12-month follow-up (Woody et al., 1987). Patients with higher levels of psychiatric symptomatology had better outcomes with the addition of psychotherapy; such clients showed little improvement with drug counseling alone (Woody et al., 1984).

Woody et al. (1995) conducted a partial replication of this study, locating it in a community setting (rather than a university research facility), and addressing the fact that, in the original study, clients in the psychotherapy conditions had access both to a counselor and a therapist. Forty-one clients were randomized to drug counseling alone, and 82 to counseling and SE therapy; those receiving drug counseling alone had access to two counselors. Both groups evidenced significant and equivalent gains at 1-month follow-up (suggesting a benefit to adding an additional counselor), but at 6 months, counseling clients showed a decline, while those receiving psychotherapy maintained their gains.

Rounsaville et al. (1983) randomized 72 patients in a methadone maintenance program to either a low contact group (a 20-minute monthly visit with a psychiatrist) or weekly IPT delivered over 6 months. Gains were made in both conditions, but there was no advantage to the addition of IPT. Interpretation of this trial is limited by a number of factors. Attrition levels were very high, and only 38% of IPT and 54% of low-contact clients completed treatment. Perhaps more critically, the methadone program required all clients to attend weekly group therapy along with daily contact for urinalysis and counseling as requested, reducing the potential for demonstrating any benefit for additional therapeutic input. Furthermore, the authors noted that (unlike other studies in this section) delivery of IPT was not integrated with the methadone program, perhaps contributing to higher attrition rates. Whether these methodological and procedural problems account for the lack of impact for IPT is, however, unclear.

Fals-Stewart et al. (2001) examined the impact of adding weekly BCT (which focuses on the maintenance of sobriety, as well as on relationship issues) to weekly individual drug counseling. Thirty-six married or cohabiting men maintained on methadone were randomized to 12 weeks of individual counseling alone or to counseling plus BCT. Contrasting the two treatments, at 4 months, those receiving BCT had significantly lower opiate use and reported better quality of family and social relationships. Curiously, the benefit of the intervention was specific only to opiates; use of cocaine was equivalent in both groups.

An important question is whether outcomes can be enhanced by adding psychosocial interventions to methadone. McLellan et al. (1993) assigned 92 male participants to 24 weeks of methadone alone with minimal contact, to standard methadone maintenance with access to counselors (initially required, and subsequently contingent on negative urine tests), or to an enhanced program that added psychiatric treatment, employment counseling, and family work. Randomization failed, because 69% of clients in the methadone-alone condition had to be "protectively transferred"; urinalysis showed continued use of opiates (contrasted to 41% of standard care and 19% of enhanced care clients). Though there appeared to be a relationship between the amount of service contact and improvement, the range of ancillary services offered makes it difficult to attribute this to any specific intervention. In an attempt to reexamine this apparent dose–response relationship, Avants et al. (1999) randomized 291 individuals to a 12-week program contrasting standard day treatment (which offered weekly group CBT therapy, psychoeducation, and vocational support) with an enhanced, 5 day per week program. Outcomes for both approaches were significant and equivalent. This concurs with a cost-effectiveness analysis of the McLellan trial (Kraft et al., 1997), which suggests that the most cost-effective intervention was methadone plus counseling, and indicating that there may be no advantage to enhanced programs.

Treatment Setting

Although many individuals are treated in specialist settings, there are reasonable questions about whether this improves outcomes over equivalent treatment in general psychiatric settings. Strang et al. (1997) randomized 186 participants to receive care in specialist or general wards within the same hospital. While all patients randomized to specialist treatment accepted their randomization, 77% of those allocated to general wards refused, and the proportions of patients actually admitted were 60 and 42%, respectively. Significantly more patients completed detoxification in the specialist unit, and at (approximately) 6-month follow-up, abstinence rates were significantly lower (the proportion of opiate-free patients in the preceding month were 79 and

31%, respectively). Although this suggests benefit to specialist treatment, there were differences in treatment delivery in each setting. Gossop et al. (1986) allocated patients to inpatient or outpatient detoxification, with assignment based either on randomization or on patient preference. Cost–benefit analysis of this study and Strang et al. (1997) suggests that the costs of specialist treatment are higher, but that this is at least partially offset by better outcomes (Gossop & Strang, 2000). Clearly, the relative costs (both financial and organizational) of in- and outpatient services differ, as do those for specialized and generic services. Because these studies indicate that their cost-efficiency may vary, it is a matter of concern that there appears to be so little relevant research on which to judge an issue that has clear implications for service organization and delivery.

Gossop et al. (2003) present long-term follow-up data from a large-scale survey of outcomes from about 20% of routine services in the United Kingdom (the National Treatment Outcome Research Study). Four types of service were identified—inpatient drug-dependence units (DDUs), residential rehabilitation units, methadone maintenance clinics, and methadone reduction programs. Psychological therapies were more usual in DDUs and residential rehabilitation, though their precise nature varied by location and type of service. Typically, they included 12-step and therapeutic community programs, as well as psychosocial and supportive interventions. An initial sample of 1,077 patients attending 54 programs were followed up, with complete 5-year data available for 418 patients. For both methadone and residential patients, opiate use in the first year of treatment was reduced by approximately 50%, with this reduction maintained over 5 years. Patterns of abuse of other drugs—particularly cocaine—varied across settings at intake, making interpretation of subsequent outcomes more difficult. Nonetheless, at 5 years, 26% of methadone and 38% of residential patients were abstinent from illicit drugs (defined as opiates, cocaine, tranquilizers, and amphetamines). Though this study gives a useful estimate of likely outcomes from standard settings, its design means that it cannot contribute to knowledge of any differential impact from specific psychological treatments or different service settings.

SUMMARY AND CLINICAL IMPLICATIONS

Although this chapter and these summaries distinguish among alcohol, cocaine, and opiate abuse, substance abuse tends not to be restricted to one class of drug, and some authorities suggest that polydrug abuse is almost normative in many clinical settings. Alongside this, frequent comorbidity with other Axis I and II disorders adds to the challenge of mapping broad conclusions to the context of individual clinical presentations.

Alcohol Abuse and Dependence

A wide variety of techniques have been employed to manage alcohol abuse. These approaches are usually well defined, though they are often implemented in different contexts and combinations, and this as much as the approach itself may be pertinent to efficacy. This caution needs to be borne in mind when considering the summary that follows; since it is usual for the intervention under study to be embedded in broader programs of care, support for that approach does not indicate that it necessarily can be offered in isolation.

The external validity of trials may be reduced by the fact that exclusion criteria tend to bias samples toward those with lower levels of comorbid psychiatric and substance abuse histories, and higher levels of social stability and motivation for treatment. This may result in a treatment sample that is more treatment-responsive. An additional, but inadvertent, consequence is that these exclusion criteria also appear to skew the demographics of research samples and reduce the number of nonwhite participants. A final point is that the goal of research treatments varies across studies: In some, the aim is abstinence; in others, moderate, controlled drinking is seen as legitimate and feasible. This may or may not be congruent with the approach of individual service providers.

Many studies consider the efficacy of "brief interventions," though the definition of this term is broad and can include interventions of high intensity offered in the context of formal and informal treatment. While many reviews find that brief and more extended treatments are of equal efficacy, some indicate that higher intensity treatment and inpatient stay result in higher abstinence rates. Estimates of the likely efficacy of interventions vary, but better outcomes are associated with lower initial severity of alcohol abuse and an absence of comorbid psychiatric problems.

In relation to medication, there is only equivocal evidence for the efficacy of disulfiram (Antabuse). Naltrexone in combination with psychosocial treatment shows some benefit in reducing relapse, particularly when patients have failed to maintain complete abstinence from drinking. Acamprosate appears equivalent in efficacy to naltrexone.

Considering psychological therapies and approaches, there is only limited evidence for the short-term benefit of aversion therapy, and this technique is associated with high attrition rates. A number of interventions, often offered adjunctively and in various combinations as part of a broader package of treatment, show benefit—including social skills training, RP, cue exposure, coping skills training, CM, and motivational interviewing. CRAs usually combine a range of approaches and show evidence of efficacy, most obviously in the shorter term. These approaches may be especially relevant to homeless individuals, and their extension to include family members may be useful for improving attendance. For problem drinkers, often seen in nonspecialist contexts, very brief interventions appear to be helpful, particularly in the shorter term.

Formal psychological therapies do not appear to be especially helpful when offered as stand-alone treatments. This observation applies both to CBT (though there may be more value when this is offered as part of a broader program) and to psychodynamic therapy. There is rather mixed evidence of the benefit of marital therapy. Direct contrasts of 12-steps programs and drug counseling against CBT suggest an equivalence of outcome.

On the whole, the most successful interventions appear to be those that directly target drinking behavior, and it is striking that user-based interventions such as 12-step programs sometimes appear to be as, if not more, effective as "professional" programs.

Attempts to match treatment to patient characteristics have been largely unsuccessful, although this area has seen some of the most methodologically robust attempts to detect such effects. Only in one area has some indication of matching emerged, with some suggestion that those with more sever dependence may have better outcomes from inpatient or day hospital treatment.

Cocaine Abuse and Dependence

As for alcohol abuse, better outcomes are likely with individuals who have lower levels of cocaine use and fewer psychosocial problems. For lower levels of dependence, briefer treatments seem appropriate (and are of equal efficacy to longer interventions). For individuals with moderate and greater levels of dependence, a capacity to stay in treatment appears important, and there is also some indication that longer (usually residential) treatment is beneficial.

There is good evidence for the benefit of CBT-based relapse prevention and 12-steps programs. A large trial of SE psychotherapy did not find evidence for its efficacy (contrasting somewhat with outcomes in opiate users). Contrast of individual CBT and behavioral marital therapy suggests that they are equivalent at posttherapy, though there may be some advantage to marital therapy in reducing relapse rates over follow-up.

CM and CRAs seem to be efficacious. It is notable that these approaches show benefit for homeless individuals with severe drug dependence, who might be expected to be difficult to treat. Although studies have included a range of adjunctive techniques, with somewhat mixed results in relation to specific combinations of treatments, the general value of this approach, and particularly of CM, appears clear. This is an important, though potentially challenging finding. By bringing together systems of health and social care, CRAs and CM offer a structure that is—for this chaotic group—probably vital. Unfortunately, the immediate cost of establishing these programs, together with the level of organization and rigor required to manage them, may act to restrict their transfer from research to clinical settings.

As in treatment of alcohol abuse, there often appears to be only marginal gain from adding additional elements to programs; in this sense, there appears to be little relationship between the dose or extent of therapy and the likely response. What seems most effective is when psychological techniques are focused directly onto the problem of drug use. While there are sometimes indications that there is longer term benefit to adding adjunctive methods, in terms of achieving abstinence, this strategy seems to add little and can indeed decrease the efficacy of treatment. It may be that when patients present with many problems and comorbid conditions, it is possible to lose sight of a primary focus of managing drug abuse, and hence to create more complexity than patients can manage—in a sense, overtreatment.

Opiate Abuse

Psychological treatments for opiate abuse have been rather less well researched than those for alcohol or cocaine abuse. At a general level, it seems hard to predict who will respond to treatment, though higher levels of abuse are associated with poorer outcome, as is poor compliance with treatment and the maintenance of a social network supportive of drug use.

Treatments are usually researched in the context of a program that includes methadone maintenance. As in other areas of drug abuse, there is robust evidence for the effectiveness of CM and CRAs. While SE therapy shows efficacy, this is not the case for IPT or cue exposure. There are indications that adding counseling to methadone treatment enhances its effectiveness over methadone alone. There is some evidence of additional benefit for family contrasted to individual treatments, especially in relation to treatment retention and compliance. Finally, although evidence is sparse, there are also indications that better outcomes will be obtained from treatment in specialist settings.

Considering the field of substance abuse as a whole, outcomes from programs are often rather disappointing and relapse rates are relatively high, particularly among individuals with more severe histories of drug abuse. There are indications that initial treatment response and willingness to engage in treatment act as a marker for outcome, and this is congruent with the general finding that briefer treatments are often as effective as longer ones, and that adding adjunctive elements does not usually result in significant gains in efficacy. On the other hand, longer treatments offered in more intensive and residential contexts may be helpful for individuals with more severe problems, especially when there is planned contact after discharge. At present, evidence is rather equivocal about benefit, though rather more decisive about the advantage of specialist units for the management of opiate abuse (where arguments about their greater cost-effectiveness may be more persuasive than for other areas).

The pattern of results in this area seems somewhat different than that reported in other chapters; essentially, the best outcomes seem to be achieved when the focus of intervention is on direct modification of drug-related behavior, and when high levels of social support are offered. Because many individuals with drug problems also have fairly obvious psychological difficulties, there is high face validity to offering formal psychological therapies adjunctively or as a primary treatment. Studies are not persuasive about the advantage of this approach, and on this basis, it would be difficult to recommend their use routinely. However, an as yet unresearched possibility is that the value of psychological interventions may lie at a later stage of treatment, when dependency issues are less acute and patients are more able to focus on broader psychological issues.

CHAPTER 13

SEXUAL DYSFUNCTIONS

DEFINITIONS

As defined in DSM-IV-TR, the essential feature of these disorders is an inhibition in the appetitive or psychophysiological changes that characterize the complete sexual cycle. A diagnosis can only be made if the problem is judged clinically significant and causes marked distress or interpersonal difficulty, and in cases where the dysfunction cannot be attributed to organic factors or to another Axis I disorder. Four classes of disorder are distinguished: sexual desire disorders, sexual arousal disorders, orgasmic disorders, and sexual pain disorders.

Sexual Desire Disorders

- *Hypoactive sexual desire disorder:* persistently or recurrently absent sexual fantasies and desire for sexual activity.
- *Sexual aversion disorder:* persistent or recurrent aversion to, and avoidance of, all or almost all genital sexual contact with a sexual partner.

Sexual Arousal Disorders

- *Female sexual arousal disorder:* persistent or recurrent partial or complete failure to maintain until completion of the sexual activity an adequate lubrication–swelling response of sexual excitement.
- *Male erectile disorder:* persistent or recurrent partial or complete failure to maintain an erection until completion of the sexual activity.

Within DSM-IV-TR these diagnoses can only be given when there is a difficulty with physiological arousal.

Orgasmic Disorders

• *Female orgasmic disorder:* persistent or recurrent delay in achieving orgasm following a period of normal sexual excitement. DSM-IV-TR notes that diagnosis will depend on a clinical judgment that the woman's orgasmic capacity is less than would be expected given her age, sexual experience, and the adequacy of sexual stimulation she receives.
• *Male orgasmic disorder:* persistent or recurrent delay in, or absence of, orgasm following a phase of normal sexual excitement.
• *Premature ejaculation:* persistent or recurrent ejaculation with minimal sexual stimulation before or shortly after penetration, and before the person wishes it.

Sexual Pain Disorders

• *Dyspareunia:* recurrent or persistent pain in either a male or female during, before, or after intercourse, which is not caused by lack of lubrication or by vaginismus.
• *Vaginismus:* recurrent or persistent involuntary spasm of the muscula-ture of the outer third of the vagina that interferes with coitus.

Relevance of Subtypes of Dysfunction to Expected Outcome

All disorders are subclassified in terms of the onset of the dysfunction and the context in which it appears. Individuals who have always suffered from the disorder are distinguished from those in whom the dysfunction develops after a period of normal functioning (primary or lifelong vs. secondary or acquired type). A second subtype differentiates between individuals in whom the dis-order is present only in the presence of certain types of stimulation, situations, or partner as opposed to those in whom it is always present (situational vs. generalized type). Since it is probable that these subtypes reflect different degrees of associated psychopathology (Kaplan, 1974; Masters & Johnson, 1970), it follows that expected outcomes for these patients are likely to vary in relation to the particular form of patient presentation.

Problems in Defining Sexual Dysfunctions

While DSM provides a clear framework for classifying sexual problems, deci-sions about the presence or absence of a dysfunction may at times reflect the values and standards of both clinicians and patients, which in turn are also likely to reflect shifting cultural opinions regarding sexual functioning. The definition and understanding of sexual dysfunctions is complex and at times controversial, especially when dysfunctions imply reference to a normative level of activity or interest.

In addition, the identification of sexual dysfunctions as a separate class of disorder within the DSM could lead to a misleading impression of homogeneity. Almost certainly, there are several etiological routes to each of the dysfunctions; reflecting this, sexual difficulties are often found as part of the clinical picture in both Axis I and Axis II disorders. While diagnosis of a sexual dysfunction is only made when this is considered to be the primary Axis I disorder, there remains the difficulty of ascertaining the role of comorbidity in varying outcomes, both within research and clinical practice.

PREVALENCE, COMORBIDITY, AND ASSOCIATED DIFFICULTIES
Prevalence

In recent years, there has been a marked increase in epidemiological research into the sexual dysfunctions. Spector and Carey (1990) noted 23 relevant studies; a later paper (Simons & Carey, 2001) identified a further 52 studies published in the intervening period. Though the studies were based on a large number of surveys, Simons and Carey noted that lack of methodological rigor limits the confidence that can be placed in these figures. Rather few surveys employed DSM criteria, introducing potential problems of interpretation, and most attempted to assess the presence of symptomatic difficulties rather than the DSM disorder. Current prevalence in community samples is estimated at 0–3% for male orgasmic disorder, 0–5% for erectile disorder, 0–3% for male hypoactive sexual desire disorder, and 4–5% for premature ejaculation. Considering female dysfunctions, prevalence is 4–7% for female orgasmic disorder, 6–8% for female arousal disorder, 5–16% for hypoactive sexual desire disorder, 3–18% for dyspareunia, and 0.5–1.0% for vaginismus (though this latter range is based on a very small number of surveys).

Comorbidity and Associated Difficulties

Sexual problems do not arise in isolation from other psychological difficulties, nor are their effects limited to the sexual arena. However, when comorbidity is present, distinguishing cause from effect can be difficult. Thus, while there is evidence that sexual dysfunctions do not necessarily lead to relationship problems, it appears to be the case that sexual difficulties are associated with higher rates of marital separation (Hawton, 1985). There is also evidence to suggest that many individuals with sexual dysfunction are likely to experience distress, reduced self-esteem, and symptoms of anxiety and depression;

although studies are not always consistent, a relatively high proportion of patients exhibit psychiatric symptoms and suffer from psychiatric disorders (Hawton, 1985). In some cases, psychiatric problems are reactive to sexual problems; in others, sexual problems reflect coexisting psychopathology. Although distinguishing these patterns may not always be easy, it is obvious that the choice of treatment strategies will be influenced by judgments regarding the relative primacy of the presenting problems.

TREATMENT APPROACHES

The treatment of sexual dysfunctions has undergone two revolutions. Whereas in the 1960s and 1970s, Masters and Johnson pioneered the development of psychological interventions, in the 1990s, attention shifted to pharmacological approaches as treatments for erectile dysfunction established a high public profile both for the disorder and for its therapy (and to some degree shifted the focus for treatment of sexual dysfunctions from specialist units into primary care). Though most pharmacological research has focused on just one disorder, any review of psychological approaches needs to consider the impact of this medical advance, partly in relation to issues of efficacy and also in relation to its potential to shift perceptions regarding the most appropriate approaches to the management of sexual dysfunctions.

Masters and Johnson's (1966) descriptions of the physiology of normal sexual response laid the groundwork for their exposition of a range of essentially behavioral strategies that are central to most approaches to sex therapy (Masters & Johnson, 1970). These methods include information and education about sex, encouraging communication between partners, and using specific techniques such as sensate focus exercises. Patients treated by Masters and Johnson were usually seen with their partners by a dual-sex, male-and-female therapy team, and were treated intensively, receiving daily sessions over a 2-week period. This form of delivery is unusual in most settings, and it would be rare for patients to be seen so intensively—weekly sessions being more normative. In addition, resource constraints, perhaps more than research evidence (discussed below), make it more likely that couples will be seen by a single therapist. Finally, sex therapists frequently make explicit use of a variety of alternative behavioral techniques (such as systematic desensitization), and many have adopted an explicitly integrationist approach. When considered relevant to the presenting problem, therapists may explore conscious and unconscious thoughts and feelings about sex, and engage in marital/relationship therapy (e.g., Hartman & Fithian, 1972; Kaplan, 1974).

This deliberate mixing of methods introduces uncertainty into studies of therapeutic outcome, since it is not always easy to identify the form of therapy implemented. While this reflects clinical reality, it is important to note that the few studies that "dismantle" the various components of therapy or contrast standard sex therapy with alternative techniques (reviewed below) suggest that some sex therapy approaches may be less specific in their impact than has been supposed.

Limitations of the Research Literature on Treatments for Sexual Dysfunctions

There is only a small outcome literature relevant to the treatment of sexual dysfunctions, and for some dysfunctions, there is no research at all. O'Donohue et al. (1997, 1999), in comprehensive reviews of treatments of male and female dysfunctions, suggest that the pervasiveness of methodological problems in this area is sufficient to make treatment recommendations inappropriate. Much of the evidence in this chapter is based on studies performed in the 1970s and 1980s, subsequent to which there appears to have been little research and innovation into psychological (as contrasted to pharmacological) approaches in this area (Heiman, 2002; Schover & Leiblum, 1994). Unfortunately, this means that few studies achieve the level of required rigor currently expected of outcome trials, seriously limiting the conclusions that can be drawn. Rather than critically review each individual study, it is more efficient to make the following observations:

1. Most studies are relatively small scale, few contrast treatment approaches, and when they do, small sample sizes invariably result in studies of very low statistical power (Bancroft et al., 1986). Larger studies are usually open trials reporting results from sexual dysfunction clinics. As noted in Chapter 2, in theory, very large open trials could overcome the major problems associated with this design—principally, that the patient sample is representative only of those patients treated. Unfortunately, available, larger scale reports tend to be problematic either because outcome data are based on rather crude assessments (e.g., Bancroft & Coles, 1976; Warner, Bancroft, & Members of the Edinburgh Human Sexuality Group, 1987), or because their patient samples are demonstrably unrepresentative of the usual clinical population (e.g., Masters & Johnson, 1970).

2. Even when trials are based on usual clinical populations, differential attrition both before and during therapy appears particularly high during sex therapy. Some of this can be attributed to the fact that not all patients presenting with sexual dysfunctions will be appropriately treated using sex therapy; treatment of a dysfunction is unlikely to succeed when it is secondary to other mental health problems or reflects general relationship difficulties (Hawton, 1995). Catalan et al. (1990) reported on the fate of 200 consecutive referrals to a sex therapy clinic. Only 55% of members of this sample were considered suitable for therapy, of whom 30% did not enter treatment. Yet

more bias is introduced by the high rates of attrition from sex therapy commonly reported in specialist centers (e.g., Bancroft & Coles, 1976; Warner et al., 1987), a problem compounded by the fact that very few studies cite outcomes for "intent-to-treat" samples.

3. Few trials clearly specify the treatments used or procedures for monitoring treatment fidelity.

4. Over time, diagnostic precision has increased, but many studies predate this development. Interpretation is further limited by the use of mixed diagnostic samples in many earlier trials, especially when there is no disaggregation of outcomes in relation to individual dysfunctions. These trials can make little contribution to considerations of efficacy, since (as discussed below) specific dysfunctions appear to be differentially responsive to treatment.

5. Not all dysfunctions are equally well researched; the bulk of studies focus on erectile dysfunction.

Results from Masters and Johnson (1970)

Masters and Johnson (1970) provided information on outcome for patients seen at their research center. Because these data were based on a large sample and appeared to indicate very high rates of improvement for almost all dysfunctions, their work was influential in popularizing sex therapy with both professionals and, particularly in the United States, the public.

More recent trials of sex therapy tend to report less impressive results, at least for some dysfunctions. The manner in which Masters and Johnson's treatment programs were implemented may go some way in explaining this difference. The therapy programs, as originally devised, were offered on a daily basis over 2 weeks. Since only 10% of the patients lived near the research unit, most patients were required to spend this time in local hotels—to some extent ensuring that only patients committed to the program actually entered into treatment. Though the early part of the research program treatment was offered free, most patients were middle-class, an unusually high proportion had received higher education (73%), and nearly 20% were physicians or mental health professionals. Taken together, this combination of characteristics undoubtedly favors better outcomes, in part because of demographic factors, and also because the effort made physically to attend the unit in itself acted as an inclusion factor for patients of higher motivation.

Approximately 800 individuals were assessed over the 11 years of the research program; almost all were seen with their partners. Information about outcomes was collected immediately after treatment and at 5-year follow-up. However, there are a number of problems of analysis and presentation. Masters and Johnson chose to provide details of treatment failure, rather than treatment success, on the grounds that this produces data less prone to subjective bias—the suggestion being that failure is easier to discern unequivocally. Unfortunately, this argument is less than persuasive, particularly since details of assessment procedures were not given, and without them, there are no obvious criteria for defining success or failure. The potential for bias in reporting of results is clear. For example, if only those patients showing a complete absence of improvement were classified as failures, this would inflate the apparent success rate; patients showing a partial response to treatment would have been classified as successes. In summary, significant problems of sample bias and problematic reporting of data necessitate caution in generalizing Masters and Johnson's figures.

Data for outcome are presented at two points—immediately after the 2-week treatment period and at 5-year follow-up. This is reproduced using DSM categories rather than Masters and Johnson's terminology (see Table 13.1).

Data for inhibited female orgasm (Table 13.2) are separately coded by Masters and Johnson, distinguishing women who are orgasmic only during masturbation, those who are anorgasmic during coitus, and a third category described as "random orgasmic inadequacy," which refers to women who are orgasmic but only rarely, and who "usually are aware of little or no physical need for sexual expression" (Masters & Johnson, 1970, p. 240). It should be noted that within the DSM, these women would probably be seen as suffering from sexual arousal disorder.

Taken as a whole, these data suggest a very high rate of immediate symptom relief for both male and female sexual dysfunctions, together with a

TABLE 13.1. Masters and Johnson's (1970) Outcome Data following Treatment for Sexual Dysfunctions

Complaint	n	Immediate failure (n)	Immediate failure rate (%)	Relapse (n)	Overall failure rate (%)
Primary erectile disorder	32	13	40.6	0	40.6
Secondary erectile disorder	213	56	26.2	10	30.9
Premature ejaculation	186	4	2.2	1	2.7
Inhibited male orgasm	17	3	17.6	0	17.6
Primary inhibited female orgasm	193	32	16.6	2	17.6
Secondary inhibited female orgasm	149	34	22.8	3	24.8
Vaginismus	193	32	16.6	—[a]	—[a]

[a] Masters and Johnson do not report follow-up data for vaginismus.

TABLE 13.2. Masters and Johnson's (1970) Outcome Data following Treatment for Inhibited Female Orgasm

Complaint	n	Failure (n)	Failure rate (%)
Orgasmic only when masturbating	11	1	9.1
Anorgasmic during coitus	106	21	19.8
"Random orgasmic inadequacy"	32	12	37.5

low rate of relapse at follow-up. Indeed, for conditions such as premature ejaculation, almost complete success is reported. On publication, these figures generated considerable optimism about results likely to be obtained in routine clinical practice. However, results from more recent studies often suggest poorer outcomes, perhaps lending weight to the caution we expressed earlier about both the representativeness of Masters and Johnson's patient samples and their reporting methods.

Treatments for Male Erectile Disorder

This disorder is the most frequent problem in men presenting to sexual dysfunction clinics (Bhugra & Cordle, 1988; Catalan et al., 1990; Warner et al., 1987). Though relatively prevalent, it is important to note that spontaneous remission will be observed in between 14 and 30% of men with psychogenic impotence (Segraves et al., 1982). The development of pharmacological treatment for erectile dysfunction has resulted in a marked increase in awareness of and presentations for this disorder. While sildenafil (Viagra) was the first to market, a number of second-generation medications are available or in development (Brock & Bochinski, 2001). The strength of evidence for the efficacy of sildenafil (e.g., Burls et al., 2001; Fink et al., 2002) raises obvious and reasonable questions about the status of psychological treatments within current provision. Models of adjunctive practice have been proposed (e.g., Rosen, 2000), based on the clinical observation, that in some patients, interpersonal issues continue to be pertinent to successful treatment with sildenafil and similar compounds, though there is as yet no research on this.

Understanding the relative role of physiological or psychological factors in the development of erectile dysfunction is an important and basic issue. Though Masters and Johnson (1970) asserted that 95% of erectile failure was psychogenic in origin, more recent studies suggest that approximately 50% of patients presenting with erectile failure have some vascular, neurological, or hormonal involvement. Melman et al. (1988) found that of 406 cases of erectile dysfunction, approximately 30% were purely organic in origin, 40% were psychogenic, and 25% were combined organic and psychogenic.

Most usually, the presence of nocturnal erections is used to differentiate between organic and psychological causes for this dysfunction. Though not always a reliable indicator (Mohr & Beutler, 1990), it appears to be as effective as the complex and expensive investigations sometimes employed to make this distinction (Segraves et al., 1987). However, although etiology is clearly important to treatment planning, it may be a less helpful distinction than at first appears; organic and psychogenic factors may be present to varying degrees and interact with each other to produce the dysfunction. For this reason, LoPiccolo and Stock (1986) have suggested that the relationship between these elements is best conceptualized as orthogonal rather than unidimensional.

A number of physical intervention methods have been developed for the treatment of erectile dysfunction. These include penile implants, revascularization for patients with vasculogenic erectile dysfunction, administration of exogenous testosterone, use of intracavernosal papaverine injections, and use of vacuum constriction devices (Gregoire, 1992). Full discussion of the efficacy of these treatments is beyond the scope of this review, though the short-term efficacy of many of these interventions appears to be good (Mohr & Beutler, 1990). However, there are indications that the rate of attrition from somatic therapies—particularly from autoinjection—can be very high. Althof et al. (1991), in a 1-year study of 42 self-injectors, found a dropout rate of 57%, often associated with physical complications. In addition, there is evidence that patients with psychogenic erectile dysfunction will respond poorly to such interventions (Hartmann & Langer, 1993). Current treatment algorithms (Rosen, 1999) suggest that these more invasive procedures represent second- or third-line therapies, with oral therapies and sex therapy being the preferred options for initial presentations.

The major factors considered to underlie psychogenic impotence are performance anxiety or performance demands, distraction, misinformation or inhibition about sex, and relationship problems, such as poor communication or hostility (Kinder & Curtiss, 1988). Given this range of issues, it is unsurprising that most psychological treatments are multimodal and employ anxiety reduction techniques in tandem with a focus on communication or relationship issues. These intervention formats are the most frequently studied and have been comprehensively reviewed by Mohr and Beutler (1990). On the basis of 23 studies, they suggest that "approximately two-thirds of men suffering from erectile failure will be satisfied with their improvement at follow-up ranging from 6 weeks to 6 years" (p. 134). These figures are comparable to those obtained by Masters and Johnson (1970). Trials of reasonable sample size and rigor report similar proportions of improved cases, both immediately posttherapy and at long-term follow-up (e.g., De Amicis et al., 1985; Hawton & Catalan, 1986; Hawton et al., 1992). However, there are exceptions to this picture; Heiman and LoPiccolo (1983) reported only modest decreases in the frequency of erectile problems, though their data analysis makes it difficult to ascertain the proportion of men in whom improvement was seen.

Though this conclusion appears broadly favorable, it is not clear what components of the therapy are effective. There are only a small number of studies that focus on deconstructing techniques or contrasting different approaches to treatment. Of these, statistical power is almost invariably low, either because of small total sample sizes or small numbers of patients within treatment cells. As a result, their conclusions, while of interest, are in no sense definitive.

A number of studies have contrasted systematic desensitization (either imaginal or *in vivo*) with the sensate focus techniques employed by Masters and Johnson. Everaerd and Dekker (1985) compared these approaches in 24 couples, finding an equivalent improvement in sexual functioning. Mathews et al. (1976) contrasted the relative efficacy of systematic imaginal desensitization and an intervention based on Master and Johnson's method. After assessment, both these procedures involved weekly therapeutic contact. To gauge the impact of this aspect of treatment, a third condition offered assessment followed by written instruction in Masters and Johnson's method, offered in the form of materials mailed to participants. Thirty-six couples with mixed sexual dysfunctions participated in the study; of these, the majority of men (13 of 18) had a presenting complaint of erectile dysfunction. At 4-month follow-up, there were no significant differences between treatment methods, with each showing some benefit. However, the low statistical power of this study makes it important to note a trend in which Masters and Johnson's technique, conducted in conjunction with therapist contact, showed the greatest efficacy. Unfortunately, there was no matched assignment of couples to treatment groups on the basis of dysfunctions, nor were dysfunctions distinguished in the data analysis. Consequently, it is not possible to be certain whether results for erectile dysfunctions followed this overall pattern. A further drawback of this study is the use of imaginal rather than *in vivo* desensitization, a weaker form of intervention. Since *in vivo* desensitization could be seen as approximating the sensate focus techniques employed by Masters and Johnson, there would be more value in a direct contrast of these techniques.

Cognitive approaches to treatment—almost exclusively rational–emotive therapy (RET)—have also been contrasted to sensate focus. Everaerd and Dekker (1985) examined the relative impact of these techniques in 32 couples. While the two methods produced equivalent improvements in sexual functioning, there was a very high rate of attrition from RET, which makes interpretation of this study more difficult. Munjack et al. (1984) assigned 16 men to either 6 weeks of biweekly RET or a 6-week wait-list control group. Though immediately after therapy, treated patients demonstrated some gains relative to controls, at 9 months they reported only 25% of attempts at intercourse to have been successful. Contrasted to the overall improvement rates derived by Mohr and Beutler (1990), this is a poor result.

A number of authors (e.g., Mohr & Beutler, 1990; Reynolds et al., 1981; Stravynski, 1986) have suggested that social or communication skills training may be helpful in treating erectile dysfunction, on the basis that social and sexual anxiety are likely to be linked. Kilmann et al. (1987) assigned 20 couples to three treatment groups—communication training, sexual technique training, or a combination of the two. In addition there were two control groups—attention–placebo or no treatment. The three treatments produced equivalent gains, though the small sample sizes make it unlikely that any differences would have been detectable. Using post hoc analyses, Hawton and Catalan (1986) found that good long-term outcome was associated with better communication between couples, marked by an ability to discuss difficulties as they arose and to implement appropriate strategies for managing them. However, while suggesting the possible utility of communication training, this result may reflect as much preexisting characteristics of the couples as any benefits from therapy (Hawton et al., 1992).

Treatment of Men without Partners

In the studies reviewed earlier, treatment strategies are largely predicated on the availability and cooperation of the patient's partner. However, some patients present for treatment by themselves. Others may be temporarily single because their sexual dysfunction has inhibited the development of relationships, or their partners may be unwilling to undergo therapy. Still others may have more fundamental difficulties, and there are suggestions that individuals presenting in this way may display significant comorbidity with other mental health problems (Cole, 1986).

A number of treatment strategies have been developed to overcome this problem. Masters and Johnson (1970) employed surrogate partners and reported satisfactory results, as have other workers (e.g., Apfelbaum, 1984; Dauw, 1988). However, the use of surrogate partners remains controversial and (except in specialized settings) difficult to arrange. Other workers have used structured men's group treatment comprising sex education, group discussion, and homework exercises, usually with a focus on social skills training. Reviewing six studies of such groups, Reynolds (1991) reported improvement rates in open trials varying between 40 and 70%, though across studies, there are indications of relatively high relapse rates. Auerbach and Kilmann (1977) contrasted systematic desensitization offered in combination with relaxation with relaxation alone. Sixteen men were treated over 15 sessions, with an improvement rate of 40% for those receiving systematic desensitization, as contrasted to 3% for those receiving only relaxation. Reynolds (1991) reported three further studies in which patients were treated on an individual basis. Two (Csillag, 1976; Reynolds, 1982) employed biofeedback. Poor results were obtained, perhaps predictably, given that this technique is likely to focus attention on performance and hence increase performance anxiety. The third (Kuruvilla, 1984) treated 13 men using sex education, guided imagery, and directed masturbation. At 2-year follow-up, 7 of 11 men (64%) reported continued improvement.

There are three relevant randomized trials. Price et al. (1981) assigned 21 men to sex therapy or a wait-list control, and found no significant difference in rates of successful intercourse between groups. Reynolds et al. (1981) assigned 11 men to either sex therapy or sex therapy augmented by social skills training (on the basis that participants might be deficient in "courtship" skills); at posttherapy (but not at 6-month follow-up), the augmented therapy showed significant advantage on indices of sexual performance. A larger scale trial (Stravynski et al., 1997) randomized 69 men to sex therapy, a focused form of social skills training, or a combination of the two. Nineteen patients were initially allocated to a wait list for 15 weeks prior to randomization. Patients in all conditions showed significant improvements that were sustained at 1-year follow-up; wait-list patients showed no gains prior to treatment. However, there was evidence that the combined condition showed the most rapid results, confirming the importance of attending to both interpersonal and sexual difficulties.

As noted earlier, men who have never had sexual partners may have comorbid interpersonal problems. Where studies provide separate analyses for men with and without partners, the relevance of this factor to outcome is clear. Everaerd et al. (1982) treated 21 men with erectile or ejaculatory problems in groups, using a mix of RET, sensate focus exercises, masturbation exercises, and social skills training. Thirteen of the 21 men remained dysfunctional; improvements tended to be found only in men who already had partners prior to treatment (Dekker et al., 1985). For partnerless men, social dysfunction may be a more primary problem than sexual difficulties and may account for the rather poor outcomes in many studies (Stravynski & Greenberg, 1990).

Relapse

Relapse rates following treatment appear to be quite high (Mohr & Beutler, 1990), though outcome in erectile dysfunction is better than that for most other forms of sexual difficulty (Hawton & Catalan, 1986). These authors reported a naturalistic study of outcomes in a sex therapy clinic and contrasted rates of improvement in 18 (of an original 31) couples treated using a modified Masters and Johnson procedure, and for whom follow-up data at between 1 and 6 years were available. Immediately after treatment, 14 of 18 couples (78%) reported the problem wholly or partially resolved. At follow-up, 11 of 18 couples (61%) reported this level of outcome. These figures are similar to those of De Amicis et al. (1985), who reported ratings of "improved" functioning in 12 of 18 men posttherapy (66%) and 10 of 17 men (59%) at 3-year follow-up.

Treatments for Premature Ejaculation

Clinical observation that selective serotonin reuptake inhibitors (SSRIs) were associated with difficulty in achieving orgasm has led to increasing research into their efficacy in the treatment of premature ejaculation. Though outside the scope of this review, a number of controlled trials suggest that SSRIs are effective in increasing ejaculatory latency (McMahon & Samali, 1999).

Good short-term success rates have been reported for the stop–start and squeeze techniques developed by Masters and Johnson (e.g., 1970; Yulis, 1976), with some early research claiming success rates as high as 90 and 98% (Kilmann & Auerbach, 1979). St. Lawrence and Madakasira (1992) suggested a clustering in initial improvement rates between 43 and 65%, with a range of 43 to 100%. However, this conclusion is based on a limited range of studies (Cooper, 1969; Meyer et al., 1983; Shapiro, 1943; Watson & Brockman, 1982), some of which antedate current sex therapy techniques.

Even if the evidence of posttherapy gains were taken at face value, there is some suggestion that gains are poorly maintained. Three studies contain data relevant to this issue. In a trial with 21 men, Heiman and LoPiccolo (1983) reported significant average increases in the duration of intercourse immediately after therapy (from 1 to 2 minutes to 5 to 8 minutes), with some loss of gains at 3 months (with duration of intercourse reducing to 3–6 minutes). Longer term follow-up suggests poorer results. In De Amicis et al.'s (1985) study, 15 of 20 men reported their dysfunction to have improved immediately following therapy, with a significant increase in mean duration of both intercourse and foreplay. However, this declined by 3 months, and at 3 years had returned to pretherapy levels. Similarly, Hawton and Catalan (1986) found that at 1- to 6-year follow-up, only two of eight men reported some degree of problem resolution, with the remainder reporting the problem to be unresolved or worse.

Treatments for Inhibited Female Orgasm

Heiman and LoPiccolo (1983) treated women with primary and secondary orgasmic dysfunction (n = 25 and 16, respectively). Posttherapy, women with primary dysfunction showed a significant increase in orgasm during masturbation (from an average rate of 0 to 60%), during manual stimulation (from 0 to 40%), and during coitus (from 0 to 25%), with good maintenance of gains at 3-month follow-up. Women with secondary dysfunction showed little gain in orgasmic frequency during masturbation or manual stimulation, and only a moderate (nonsignificant) increase in the average rate of coital orgasm (from 12 to 30% posttherapy).

De Amicis et al. (1985) followed up 22 women with a mix of primary, secondary, and situational orgasmic dysfunction over 3 years, all treated using procedures described by Masters and Johnson (1970). Across all subtypes, there were posttherapy gains in sexual satisfaction, though there was less evidence of behavioral change. Women with primary dysfunctions showed an increase in orgasmic frequency during masturbation and "genital caress." This improvement was not evident for women with situational dysfunction, and across subtypes, there was no improvement in orgasmic functioning during coitus.

Similar results are reported by Libman et al. (1984), who treated 23 couples whose main complaint was secondary orgasmic dysfunction, using either "standard" couple therapy (as described by Masters & Johnson, 1970), group therapy (in which women were treated in groups on a weekly basis, and their partners once a month), or minimal-contact bibliotherapy. A wide variety of measures of sexual functioning were employed, and where there were differences between treatment conditions, these favored the standard treatment over other treatment options. However, though gains in orgasmic frequency were statistically significant, their clinical significance is less clear. Posttherapy, women were more likely to achieve orgasm during masturbation (77% were orgasmic at follow-up, contrasted with 55% at intake), though a significant proportion remained anorgasmic in interpersonal contexts. Thus, at 3-month follow-up, and dependent on the type of sexual activity engaged in, between 6 and 27% of women were orgasmic. Further analysis of data from this study (Fichten et al., 1986) suggests that though enjoyment and satisfaction did increase as a consequence of treatment, there was little behavioral change. In addition, daily recording of sexual activity suggested even poorer therapeutic response than when patients were asked to make retrospective judgments of their sexual responsiveness.

Kilmann et al. (1986) reported outcomes in 55 couples for whom secondary orgasmic dysfunction was the presenting complaint. Patients were assigned to four treatment groups—communication training, sexual technique training, or two variants of the combination of the two (communication training followed by sexual technique training, or vice versa). In addition, there were two control groups—attention–placebo or no-treatment. There was no evidence that treatment formats exerted differential effects. Overall, contrasts between couples receiving therapy and those in control conditions suggest some moderate gains. Improvement was defined in terms of reaching orgasm during coitus more than 50% of the time. Pretherapy, no women met this criterion. Posttherapy, it was achieved by 9 of 35 treated women (26%), with a slight increase in this rate at 6-month follow-up (11 out of 30 women; 37%). In contrast, no patient from the control groups (n = 20) met this criterion at posttherapy, and only 1 of 10 did at follow-up. Longer term follow-up of these patients at between 2 and 6 years (Milan et al., 1988) suggests that coital orgasmic frequency was reasonably stable over follow-up, though there was a decline in the frequency of intercourse. However, approximately one-fourth of the sample sought additional help during this time. Overall, it appears that greater gains can be expected for orgasm during masturbation and manual stimulation—particularly for women with primary dysfunction—than is the case for orgasm during coitus, where most studies suggest only moderate improvements.

Treatments for Vaginismus

Treatment approaches include systematic desensitization in combination with the use of graded dilators. A Cochrane review by McGuire and Hawton (2003) identified 16 case series, 6 open trials and 12 RCTs, but considered only 3 RCTs to meet methodological criteria, of which only one contained analyzable data. Most RCTs were unanalyzable because of the inclusion of mixed dysfunctions or a failure to ensure that vaginismus was accurately diagnosed. The one remaining trial (Schnyder et al., 1998) randomized 44 patients to receive *in vivo* or *in vitro* desensitization (effectively, therapist or self-administered dilatation). After an average of 6.3 sessions, 43 of these patients reported that they were able to have sexual intercourse, with no differences reported between the two methods of desensitization. Of 36 patients followed up at a mean of 10 months, half remained in remission, and in half symptoms had improved. Although the impact of therapy was large, this trial is limited by the fact that it contrasted two variants of the same therapy in a relatively small sample.

A number of case series and open trials suggest reasonable outcomes from treatment. Bancroft and Coles (1976) and Warner et al. (1987) report outcomes from a sexual dysfunction clinic, though the reliability of results is limited by reliance on therapist-based ratings of outcome. In Bancroft and Coles (1976), six of eight women treated were reported to have had a successful outcome; of 52 women treated by Warner et al. (1987), 52% had a "good" outcome, and 65% a response rated as moderate or better.

Hawton and Catalan (1990) examined treatment outcomes in 30 couples; patients were consecutively referred to a sexual dysfunction clinic and were selected on the basis that the main sexual problem was vaginismus. The mean duration of the problem was 5 years. Therapy was based on Masters and Johnson's (1970) procedures and was conducted over an average of 18 sessions. Immediately after treatment, 43% of patients reported the problem resolved, with a further 37% reporting it largely resolved. At 3-month follow-up, more gains were evident, with 61% of patients reporting that the problem was resolved, and a further 26% that it was largely resolved.

Similar results were obtained in an earlier trial by the same authors (Hawton & Catalan, 1986). Twenty women with vaginismus were followed up at 1–6 years. Posttherapy, 10 women reported that the problem was resolved, and a further seven that it was largely resolved. At follow-up, 11 women reported the problem resolved, and seven reported that it was largely resolved, suggesting some stability in therapeutic gain.

Outcomes for women with vaginismus appear to be better than those for other sexual dysfunctions. This may relate to patient characteristics. Hawton and Catalan (1990) contrasted women referred with vaginismus with those referred for other sexual dysfunctions. Though patients with vaginismus tended to be younger and less sexually experienced, they also appeared to be more motivated and more interested in sex, to display less sexual aversion, and to enjoy greater arousal and pleasure from sexual activity prior to treatment.

Treatments for Sexual Desire Disorders

In the largest survey of outcomes for desire-phase disorders, Schover and Lo Piccolo (1982) retrospectively reanalyzed data from 152 couples who had attended their clinic between 1974 and 1981. However, nearly all these couples had been diagnosed using systems that antedated the recognition of desire disorders. A post hoc classification system was employed to identify such cases on the basis of questionnaire data from the couples' intake interviews, raising some questions about the reliability of diagnoses.

The sample included 58 men and 67 women with a diagnosis of inhibited sexual desire, and 27 women with an "aversion to sex." Treatments were broadly based, with "the usual sex therapy format" supplemented by behavioral, cognitive-behavioral, psychodynamic, and Gestalt techniques. Results for women with an aversion to sex were poor. For patients with inhibited sexual desire, there was a modest improvement in ratings of sexual satisfaction and a significant gain in the frequency of intercourse (from a mean of approximately once every 2–4 weeks to once or twice a week). This declined significantly over 3-month follow-up, to around once every 1–2 weeks. However, whereas men appeared to maintain this increase, the pattern for women was improvement followed by a decline. Relatedly, though there was an initial increase in the frequency with which the partner with low desire would initiate sex, this declined at follow-up, again, a trend more clearly seen in women than in men. These data suggest that overall treatment outcomes were modest, with men responding more to treatment than women.

Hawton and Catalan (1986) reported data for 32 couples in which the female partner's presenting problem was "impaired sexual interest." Though, posttherapy, 68% of patients reported that the problem was fully or partially resolved, at 1- to 6-year follow-up, this proportion had dropped to 34%.

De Amicis et al. (1985) presented data on a sample of six men and three women with desire dysfunction. Both posttherapy and at 3-year follow-up, there was little improvement in sexual functioning, with some suggestion that the frequency of intercourse decreased over the period of follow-up.

Whitehead et al. (1987) contrasted two treatment approaches for women presenting with a lack of sexual interest or enjoyment. In the first, women were treated with their partners. This conventional treatment, based on Masters and Johnson's (1970) procedures, was contrasted with a "woman-focused" treatment consisting of a graded series of educative elements and exercises designed to encourage sexual self-exploration. Both treatments resulted in significant posttherapy improvement on measures of quality of the sexual relationship. Though follow-up data appear to indicate good mainte-nance of gains, there is some evidence that couples who did worse tended not to return for evaluation.

Hurlbert (1993) assigned 39 women with hypoactive sexual desire disor-der either to small-group, couple-based treatment using marital and sexual therapy, or to this intervention combined with a training package focused on increasing orgasmic consistency. Although both groups showed significant improvement at 3- and 6-month follow-up, gains were greater in measures of sexual arousal for the combination approach. Hurlbert et al. (1993) contrasted the benefits of the training package in women-only or couple-based groups; 57 women and their partners were allocated to either an active treatment or a wait-list control. At 6-month follow-up, those treated as couples showed sig-nificantly greater benefit than those in women-only groups, with both groups showing significant gains over control patients.

Marital Therapy and Sex Therapy

Empirical studies suggest a link between marital and sexual difficulties (e.g., Frank & Kupfer, 1976; Schenk et al., 1983), and there are indications that couples showing higher levels of marital adjustment tend to have better clini-cal outcomes (Abramowitz & Sewell, 1980; Leiblum et al., 1976). However, it is not clear whether this implies that marital therapy is indicated prior to sex therapy for couples with significant relationship problems.

In an attempt to examine whether marital therapy enhanced the impact of sex therapy, Hartman and Daly (1983) carried out a small trial of 12 cou-ples with mixed sexual dysfunctions. Half the couples received standard sex therapy followed by behavioral marital therapy; for the other couples, the order of therapies was reversed. Therapy was conducted in small groups, with each form of therapy offered for 5 weeks. Examining outcomes at the point at which the form of therapy switched suggests that sex therapy had a greater impact on both sexual and marital satisfaction than did marital therapy, though this effect was not significant at the end of therapy. While results from this study broadly suggest that sexual problems can be managed without prior marital therapy, there was some suggestion that couples with major relationship problems did appear to benefit from receiving marital therapy before sex therapy.

Considerable caution is warranted in drawing conclusions from this study; the patient sample is very small, diagnostically heterogeneous, and uncontrolled for levels of marital distress within each condition. A larger scale examination of these issues was conducted by Zimmer (1987), who selected couples in which the female partner suffered from secondary sexual dysfunction; although this was a more homogeneous group than Hartman and Daly's (1983), the range of dysfunctions was again fairly diverse, including disorders of sexual desire, sexual arousal, and inhibited orgasm. In the majority of clients, at least one partner had considered separation. Couples were either placed on a wait list ($n = 9$) or received marital therapy followed by sex therapy ($n = 10$) or a "placebo" treatment (containing relaxation and general discussion of the partners' personal histories) followed by sex therapy ($n = 9$). Contrasted to couples on the wait list, patients receiving both active treatments showed comparable overall gains. However, on some measures, there was evidence of greater and more enduring gains for the couples who received the combination of marital and sex therapy. In addition, marital therapy appeared to have conferred some benefit on sexual satisfaction, whereas sex therapy did not improve marital satisfaction. Overall, the best results were obtained with those couples showing the best marital adjustment. In this regard, it is noteworthy that 16 couples allocated to treatment failed to complete therapy, in nearly all cases because the couples separated.

Apparent discrepancies between these two studies may reflect differences in their samples, since the degree of marital distress in Hartman and Daly's (1983) patients is not dear. Taken together, they provide some support for the clinical contention that marital therapy may be a useful and prior adjunctive treatment for couples presenting with sexual difficulties in the context of acute marital distress. However, this conclusion is weakened by the fact that the most severely maritally distressed couples tended to drop out of Zimmer's study, suggesting that such couples may be particularly hard to help.

Treatment Format

In developing sex therapy, Masters and Johnson employed dual-sex co-therapy teams, working usually, though not exclusively, with couples, and offering treatment daily. Available evidence suggests that more flexible formats are equally effective. Dual-therapist work has obvious resource implications; studies that have explored this issue suggest that outcome is equivalent whether dual-sex cotherapy teams or single therapists are used (Clement & Schmidt, 1983; Crowe et al., 1981; LoPiccolo et al., 1985). Though the gender of the therapist relative to the patient does not appear to influence outcome (Crowe et al., 1981; LoPiccolo et al., 1985), patient preference is likely to be important in clinical practice. Daily treatment does not appear to confer greater gains than delivering therapy either weekly (Heiman & LoPiccolo, 1983) or biweekly (Clement & Schmidt, 1983).

Beyond examining the structure of therapy, few studies deconstruct Masters and Johnson's techniques. In an exception to this rule, Takefman and Brender (1984) found that the ban on intercourse almost universally imposed at the start of treatment may not be as essential a component of therapy as is usually supposed. In their study, 16 couples in which the male partner presented with erectile dysfunction were assigned to two conditions. Though all patients were asked to focus on communication of sexual likes and dislikes during sexual activity, only in one condition were they asked to refrain from sexual intercourse. Equivalent outcomes were observed with and without the ban. The small sample size renders only tentative the implication that communication is a mutative factor in successful therapies.

Bibliotherapy

The efficacy of bibliotherapy was reviewed by van Lankveldt (1998), who identified 12 relevant studies. These almost exclusively focused on male and female orgasmic disorders, and employed directed practice techniques (rather than cognitive-behavioral approaches). Only three studies examined completely self-directed bibliotherapy, with the remainder offering varying degrees of therapist contact. A weighted within-groups effect size of 0.5 was evident at posttherapy, but this declined to 0.21 at follow-up. Few trials contrasted self-directed with varying levels of therapist contact, and results were somewhat mixed. Though some found therapist contact to be helpful (Libman et al., 1984; Mathews et al., 1976; Zeiss, 1978), others found greater benefit for minimal over intensive therapist contact (Morokoff & LoPiccolo, 1986).

SUMMARY AND CLINICAL IMPLICATIONS

Sexual dysfunctions are common and represent a potentially serious problem, particularly when they complicate preexisting disorders or lead to the development of psychological disorders, either directly or indirectly, through, for example, relationship difficulties. Perhaps more explicitly than is the case with psychological approaches to many other disorders, therapeutic approaches to sexual dysfunction often utilize a wide range of treatment procedures and can often be seen as multimodal therapies.

Much of our knowledge about treatment efficacy is derived from studies conducted prior to the 1990s. There have been few large-scale, controlled trials on the treatment of sexual disorders, and larger studies are often based on heterogeneous diagnoses of dysfunctions, and are usually open trials. Outcomes from uncontrolled studies should be viewed with caution in the light of relatively high rates of spontaneous remission for erectile dysfunction and the known situational specificity of other disorders. Reflecting the therapeutic eclecticism often seen in this area, some research reports are not always clear about the form of therapy administered, leaving open the possibility that variations in the effectiveness of treatment reflect differing combinations of procedures and emphases on technique. Finally, findings from studies are rendered ambiguous, because focusing on patient's sexual problems without comprehensive descriptions of their psychological functioning and comorbid status can make it difficult to interpret outcomes.

Outcomes for treatments of sexual dysfunction are highly variable, both across different classes and subtypes of dysfunction, and within disorders, presumably because of unmeasured aspects of comorbidity.

The proportion of *male erectile disorders* with underlying organic pathology has been underestimated by earlier researchers, and a substantial proportion of patients are likely to show a mix of organic and psychological pathology. While it is likely that psychological treatments may have some role in such patients, there is no direct evidence regarding this. Pharmacological treatments are increasingly available and have clear evidence of efficacy; although other physical treatments are available, some (such as autoinjection) may have limited acceptability. While there is evidence that patients with primarily psychological problems respond poorly to physical treatments, at this point, there is no evidence that this finding extends to pharmacological interventions. Despite the efficacy of pharmacological agents, the restoration of physical functioning may—in some cases—make it evident that interpersonal or relationship issues were pertinent in the development of sexual problems. Although data directly examining this issue are not available, adjunctive psychological treatment would be desirable in such cases.

Psychological treatment approaches aimed at reducing sexual anxiety and improving communication and the quality of relationships appear to be successful in approximately 60% of cases. In addition, there are suggestions that cognitive approaches and social/communication skills training may be helpful for some patients. Although there is little direct evidence, such approaches may be useful for patients deficient in these skills. The few trials that include longer term follow-up suggest that gains are maintained. Most of these success rates are only applicable to men who are already in relationships. Treatments for men without partners appear to be most successful for those who are temporarily outside a relationship rather those who have never had one.

Problems of *premature ejaculation* in men have been treated using specifically designed behavioral techniques. Reported success rates tends to vary considerably across studies; overall, although around half the patients tend to improve, available data suggest that these gains tend not to be maintained on follow-up.

Vaginismus appears to be an anxiety-related disorder that responds well to exposure-based behavioral techniques; up to 80% of patients show some or significant improvement, with good maintenance of gains.

Interventions for *inhibited female orgasm* tend to be principally psychoeducational. Findings suggest that women can be taught to achieve orgasm during masturbation, but this does not readily generalize to orgasm during intercourse. However, sex therapy does increase the enjoyment reported by these women.

Treatments for *sexual desire disorders* tend to be psychoeducational and behavioral; while there are indications of some modest initial improvement, outcome is poor in the longer term.

It would be helpful to signal several issues that would benefit from further research—all of them long-standing, but all remaining undeveloped in the absence of new research in this area. First, it is unclear whether marital therapy is always indicated before sex therapy in couples with problematic relationships, though clinical judgment might often suggest this to be an appropriate strategy. Second, there is very little research examining the relative importance of widely accepted elements of sex therapy. Such research as exists suggests that techniques such as the use of dual-sex therapy teams and the ban on intercourse during therapy may be less essential to success than has been supposed. Third, though advocates of sex therapy can make a strong argument for the virtues of a multimodal approach in an area where problems clearly have multiple etiologies, it remains true that sex therapy techniques are often poorly described; a systematic description of the "rules" for combining components of treatment has yet to be developed. More work needs to be done in this area before thorough evaluation of this treatment modality will be possible. Fourth, it may be important to be more specific about the role of emotional disorders—particularly anxiety—in sexual difficulties. The literature suggests that sexual difficulties in which anxiety appears to predominate (e.g., erectile dysfunction and vaginismus) are also better treated using behavioral techniques implicity or explicitly based on principles of exposure. When the etiological role of anxiety is less clear, psychoeducational approaches seem to be somewhat more valuable, but outcomes are also more limited. Given this, better techniques need to be developed, particularly in relation to premature ejaculation, inhibited female orgasm, and sexual aversion disorder. Finally, given the heterogeneous nature of patients who receive treatment for sexual problems, and the varied etiologies underlying their presentation, there is also a need for further information on the factors that determine the likelihood of successful outcomes in terms of a range of comorbid factors.

Researchers in the 1960s and 1970s established a climate that privileged psychological over organic factors in models of sexual dysfunctions, and this appeared to create—or to coexist with—a period of rapid development in psychological techniques for the management of sexual problems. Whether the absence of new research reflects changing attitudes in the management of sexual dysfunctions among clients, clinicians, researchers, or funding bodies is hard to discern. It may also be the case that the recent emergence of pharmacotherapy has created a climate in which the case for psychological treatment appears harder to defend—at least in relation to erectile dysfunction. Whatever the reasons, advances in psychological treatment require further well-designed, large, controlled trials investigating the efficacy of specified therapies in relation to specified dysfunctions. Without this, it may become more difficult to represent techniques in widespread use as "evidence-based," since this claim will rest on trials that increasingly fail to meet current methodological standards.

CHAPTER 14

THE PSYCHOLOGICAL TREATMENT OF CHILD AND ADOLESCENT PSYCHIATRIC DISORDERS

Mary Target and Peter Fonagy

In 2002, a companion volume considered the outcome evidence for treatment of child and adolescent disorders in considerable detail (Fonagy et al., 2002). This book gives readers requiring fuller details a more extensive discussion of the issues involved in studies of outcome with young people. This chapter is intended as a summary and update of this material, with statements of the current conclusions.

METHODOLOGICAL ISSUES

A number of methodological issues specific to the evaluation of child and adolescent interventions need to be borne in mind when reading this chapter.

1. Measures of symptomatology derived from parents, teachers, and children correlate poorly; thus, the overall outcome of an intervention is difficult to assess. Changes should be looked at in the context of potential dis-

crepancies among informants: teachers, parents, children, clinicians, and independent raters. Wherever possible, a mix of sources should be used.

2. Assessments of outcome must be made in the context of the natural history of disorders, in particular, changing symptom patterns over the course of development; otherwise, the usefulness of long-term treatments in particular may be misjudged. Impact of therapy should not be studied simply in terms of the child's symptomatology, but relative to impact of that symptomatology on normal developmental processes—psychological, social, and educational. Treatments should be evaluated in terms of their capacity to facilitate change, not just in target symptoms, but across a spectrum of aspects of psychological adaptation. This applies mainly to longer term therapies.

3. Certain treatments can only be offered to children whose life circumstances support them. Family therapy, for example, requires the child to have a family, and all therapies require the agreement and often the collaboration of the child's current caregivers. Some therapies also require cooperation from teachers. Some children need help partly because of environmental failure or stress, and the degree of support available and required must be considered realistically. In reviewing efficacy, it should be noted how many children were considered for treatment, how many were found suitable, and how many accepted it. These proportions set limits on the usefulness of the therapy in clinical settings.

4. Comorbidity affects the outcome of treatment in ways that are only now being clarified. Studies looking at children selected for lack of comorbidity (unrepresentative samples) should be treated with great caution, because the results are likely not to be applicable to the majority of clinic referrals.

5. It follows that a range of therapies need to be offered to fit different circumstances and combinations of disorders.

6. Measured outcome varies considerably depending on length of follow-up: Evidence from the adult literature suggests that "sleeper effects" may be particularly strong in more intensive forms of therapy aimed more at developing resilience than at reducing symptoms. All outcome studies should include follow-up for as long a period as is practicable, and with regard to natural history. For example, children treated for depression should be followed up for some years, because the disorder tends to remit spontaneously and then recur.

7. Serious ethical problems face randomized controlled trials (RCTs) that contrast long-term untreated outcome with a specific treatment condition, yet suitable control conditions for longer term treatments are hard to design and very expensive to implement; these need to be evaluated using a wider range of designs, such as open trials, with additional attention to linking outcome with processes of change.

SUMMARIES OF EVIDENCE IN RELATION
TO PARTICULAR DISORDERS
Autism

Definition

The definition of autism covers problems in three main areas of functioning, with onset in the first 3 years of life: (1) qualitative impairments in social interactions that may manifest as a failure to comprehend that others have feelings, a lack of interest in imitative or social play, and inability to seek friendships or comfort from others; (2) qualitative impairments in verbal and nonverbal communication; and (3) restriction of interests and a resistance to change, which may be expressed as an insistence on certain routines or a desire to take part in only a narrow range of interests or activities.

On the basis of 20 studies, the American Academy of Child and Adolescent Psychiatry (1999) suggested a prevalence rate of 4.8 cases per 10,000 (Fombonne, 1998a). However, Bryson (1997) reported a rate of 1 per 1,000. Autism is on a spectrum of severity and is highly disabling, especially in terms of social relationships. Though one of the least prevalent conditions seen in child services, the degree of disability and its implications for the family mean that this condition places considerable demand on resources. The outcome of autism is usually poor: there is deterioration in 50% of adolescents, some of which can be attributed to onset of seizures. However, 30% show some improvement in behavior and functioning. The outcome is best for children with later onset of autism (> 24 months), with higher general intelligence (IQ over 60) and intelligible speech by the age of 5 years.

Treatment Approaches

PLAY GROUPS

Play is often used to promote communication skills in children with autism (Cogher, 1999). Wolfberg and Schuler (1993, 1999) reported on the impact of integrated playgroups in a school setting on the play behavior of three children with autism. Treatment lasted for 7 months. Following the intervention, the amount of functional and/or symbolic play doubled and was accompanied by gains in language, with generalization to settings outside the playgroup. Similar results were obtained by Kohler et al. (1995), again in three autistic preschool children. Celiberti and Harris (1993) focused on modifying the play behavior of siblings or peers, who were trained to elicit play and play-related speech, to praise play behaviors, and to prompt the child with autism when he/she failed to respond. A study of this approach (Schleien et al., 1995) reported the inclusion of 15 autistic students, ages 4–11 years, in an integrated art program. However, although the nondisabled peers increased the frequency of social approaches during the intervention, this was not reciprocated by the autistic subjects.

More recently, Kok et al. (2002) examined the impact of two programs on communication and play of eight autistic children ages 4–5 years. In the first, teachers actively engaged the child in structured play; in the second, opportunities for play were taken as they emerged. Each approach showed benefit, but a different pattern of gains was evident. Structured play led to more appropriate communicative responses and appropriate play, whereas there were more appropriate initiations of communication and play in the contrast condition.

BEHAVIOR THERAPY

Howlin and Rutter (1987) described a detailed, long-term case–control study of the benefits of a home-based behavioral program on 16 high-functioning autistic boys with a mean age of 6 years at commencement of treatment. Their outcomes were contrasted to 14 short-term and 16 long-term controls. Treatment employed behavior modification to reduce inappropriate behaviors and encourage the development of language skills, and also offered psychological support for the family. Although intervention significantly improved social competence, use of language and behavior problems in the 6-month period of treatment, this was less evident at 18-month follow-up, and IQ was not affected.

Lovaas (1987) provided intensive behavioral treatment to an experimental group of 19 children under 4 years of age with autism. Treatment consisted of at least 40 hours per week of one-to-one behavioral treatment over 2 or more years, plus parent training. Discrete trial training (DTT) was used, in which skills were disaggregated into discrete components and practiced until each component was mastered. A control group of 19 children received 10 hours a week of one-to-one behavioral treatment in their home, in addition to a variety of other treatments, such as parent training or special education classes. When followed up at a mean age of 7 years, children in the experimental group had gained an average of 20 IQ points and had progressed in their education; nine were in normal classes and had an average IQ. Only one control subject reached normal levels of IQ and educational functioning. This sample was followed-up when experimental subjects were age 13, and controls were age 10 (McEachin et al., 1993). The proportion of children in regular classes was unchanged from the position at age 7—47% of the experimental subjects and none of the control group. On the Vineland tests assessing communication, daily living, and socialization, the mean scores in the treatment and control groups were 72 and 48, respectively (compared to 100 in the general population). In addition, the mean IQ of treated children was about 30 points higher than that of the control subjects.

Anderson et al. (1987) conducted an open study of 14 children under age 5. The intervention comprised (1) 15–25 hours of individual training to address individually assessed deficits, such as those of self-care, language, play, behavior, and socialization; and (2) parent training for 15–25 hours per week, in which the parent joined the therapist. Although there were statistically significant improvements in mental age and social maturity (as measured by the Vineland scales), these were less marked than in the Lovaas (1987) study, especially in relation to normalization of intelligence and the ability to be taught in a mainstream classroom.

There are a number of replications of the Lovaas findings. One of these (Birnbrauer & Leach, 1993) was based in the community. While apparently successful, the sample size was small (with only 9 children), and there was no statistical contrast of the treatment and control conditions. Eikeseth et al. (2002) contrasted intensive behavioral treatment with a placebo (eclectic therapy) in a school setting, matching the intensity of each intervention (at a mean of 39 hours a week). On standardized measures, there were significant gains for the experimental condition. On balance, there is good evidence for the benefit of behavioral interventions in the home and school setting.

All studies of behavioral interventions in autistic children have included a parent training approach. Several case reports (Celiberti & Harris, 1993) have also described the successful training of siblings of autistic probands, enabling them to elicit play and speech by prompting their autistic sibling when there was no initial response, and praising play behaviors.

SOCIAL SKILLS TRAINING

Lord and Rutter (1994) reviewed school programs that aim to encourage satisfactory vocational behaviors, such as task completion and self-management (e.g., Dunlap et al., 1987; Mesibov, 1986). They concluded that these individuals respond best to a well-structured environment in which the individual needs of each child are considered (Harris et al., 1990). By way of example, several case studies (Ingenmey & Van Houten, 1991; Matson et al., 1990, 1993) have reported that spontaneous verbalizations can be increased using either time-delay or visual cue prompting (Charlop-Christy et al., 2002). Adults mirroring or imitating their child in a playful way appears to have a positive impact on the child's social behavior with that adult (T. Field et al., 2001). In a test of this hypothesis, 20 autistic children were randomly assigned to a group in which an adult either imitated them or simply played with them. Imitation had the effect of increasing proximal social behaviors (e.g., touching). In a study of two 10-year-old boys with autism, Pierce and

Schreibman (1995) attempted to engage them in a variety of complex social behaviors by teaching peers to act as behavioral change agents. After the intervention, both children maintained prolonged interactions with the peer, initiated play and conversations, and increased engagement in language and joint attention behaviors. In addition, teachers reported positive changes in social behavior, with the largest increases in peer-preferred social behavior.

Despite the fact that a number of studies have examined variants of social skills training, there is little evidence that this approach significantly benefits autistic individuals beyond the environment in which training takes place (Campbell et al., 1996; Matson & Swiezy, 1994). Illustrating this, some recent studies have built on discoveries of deficits of social cognition to design appropriate programs. Ozonoff and Miller (1995) incorporated teaching theory of mind to 9 autistic male adolescents with IQs above 70. Five received weekly social skills sessions, and 4 acted as no-treatment controls. Although subjects were more likely to be more successful with false-belief tasks than were controls, social competence as observed by teachers and parents did not improve significantly.

Studies usually find little generalization beyond training conditions, and for this reason, more recent trials have tried to teach social understanding rather than social skills (Howlin et al., 1999). Most promising results are reported to follow using a social understanding task broken down into a sequence of small steps, beginning with simpler skills that are learned earlier in normal development. A series of studies (Hadwin et al., 1996, 1997) demonstrated that children with autism could be taught to understand emotions, belief, and pretense. This was maintained at 2-month follow-up but did not generalize to untaught domains or tasks with a different structure to the instruction task. Furthermore, no improvement in the use of mental-state terms was observed in the course of conversation. An RCT designed to explore the effects of a computer-based method of training emotion recognition and prediction established that autistic adolescents could improve on tasks calling for these abilities (Silver & Oakes, 2001). However, no evidence was provided that these gains generalized to real-life situations.

An innovative study looked at the value of behavioral training methods in teaching "joint attention," a social capacity thought to be both developmentally fundamental and completely lacking in autistic children (Whalen & Schreibman, 2003). Five young children with autism participated. All made gains in responding to joint attention, and this improvement generalized to unstructured assessments. There were substantial individual differences in the rate of acquisition of behaviors, but 4 of the 5 children showed improvement in joint attention initiations, and 3 showed improved supported joint attention. However, the study also reports significant loss of gains from post-treatment to follow-up, suggesting that parents were not able to maintain these behaviors, and that parent training programs might be a helpful addition. No observations were reported on generalization other than within the testing situation.

A conceptually linked study of parent training (Drew et al., 2002) focused on the development of joint attention skills and joint action routines in young children with autism (mean age, 23 months) randomly assigned to parent training or treatment as usual (TAU). Although, at 1-year follow-up, there were indications that language development was faster in the parent training group, this was based on parent report, which may have been biased. In addition, the two groups were poorly matched, and no attempt was made to monitor parental compliance with the protocol.

Summary

Behavioral treatments have been shown to reduce some of the secondary problems associated with autism, but social and communicative abnormalities have proved more resistant to intervention. In order to have an impact, interventions probably need to be intensive (e.g., offering a behavioral program both at home and at school) and involve both parents and teachers. In at least some studies, there is evidence of gains in IQ, improvements in daily living skills, communication and the ability to socialize, and a decrease in behavior problems.

Studies have tended to focus on children under the age of 4 years at the time of commencing treatment, but it is unclear whether early commencement is a necessary condition for successful treatment. Despite a variety of approaches, there is no good evidence that individual social skills training significantly benefits individuals with autism. A potentially promising line of studies is exploring interventions related to specific deficits of social cognition assumed to underpin many other behavioral dysfunctions, including difficulty in engaging in a teaching–learning process.

Conduct Problems

Definitions

Conduct problems include conduct disorder (CD) and oppositional defiant disorder (ODD). According to DSM-IV-TR, ODD must include a repetitive pattern of defiance and disobedience, and a negative and hostile attitude toward authority figures of at least 6 months' duration. Although ODD and CD overlap in definition, unlike ODD, CD entails violations of the basic rights of others or of age-appropriate societal norms or rules. CD with onset before puberty is generally considered more severe and more likely to entail neuropsychological deficits than adolescent-onset antisocial behavior, which may have peer influence as a major part of causation (Moffitt et al., 1996).

Psychosocial Treatment Interventions for Preadolescents

PARENT TRAINING

The parent training model is based on the assumption that ODD and CD reflect parental difficulty in adequately reinforcing socially appropriate forms of conduct, as well as a tendency to maintain inappropriate behavior through coercive interactions (Kazdin, 1995b; Miller & Prinz, 1990; Patterson, 1982). This 6- to 8-week intervention is conducted with the parents, with limited therapist–child contact. Parents are encouraged to refocus on prosocial behaviors rather than on the elimination of conduct problems. The training component of the program is based on behavioral management principles drawn from social learning theory. Although programs vary in terms of the exact syllabus and methods of delivery, in all programs, dyadic instruction is accompanied by other aids to learning, such as role playing, behavioral rehearsal, and structured homework exercises. Evidence that changing families' interaction patterns has the power to alter children's behavior is very strong (Ducharme et al., 2000; Forehand & Long, 1988; Long et al., 1994; Nixon et al., 2003; Nye et al., 1995; Patterson & Chamberlain, 1988; Schuhmann et al., 1998; Webster-Stratton & Hammond, 1997; Webster-Stratton & Reid, 2003). There is accumulating evidence that parent training programs generally may be applied in a wide range of conduct problems and effectively delivered in various settings, including clinical populations (Bradley et al., 1999; Cunningham et al., 1995; S. Scott et al., 2001).

The best evaluated program (Webster-Stratton, 1996a; Webster-Stratton & Reid, 2003) comprises three complementary training curricula, known as the Incredible Years Training Series, targeted at parents, teachers, and children ages 2–8 years. The program aims to promote parental competencies by increasing positive and decreasing negative parenting, improving problem-solving skills, increasing family support networks, and encouraging parents and teachers to work collaboratively. Although this program has been proposed as a pure videotape training program, therapist input appears to be a important component (Montgomery, 2003).

There have been six controlled trials with children with ODD and CD at the University of Washington (Webster-Stratton, 1981, 1982, 1984, 1990, 1994, 1998; Webster-Stratton & Hammond, 1997; Webster-Stratton et al., 1988, 1989) and two independent replications (Scott et al., 2001; Taylor et al., 1998). The teacher training curriculum has been separately assessed (Webster-Stratton & Reid, 2003), with evidence of benefit reported by both teachers and parents.

Among other approaches to the parent training approach, the Oregon Social Learning Center (e.g., Patterson, 1976; Patterson et al., 1975) is widely used, but there are few satisfactory evaluations of this approach. A promising, more intensive treatment is parent–child interaction therapy (Eyberg et al.,

1995), which has been subjected to some evaluation (e.g., Hembree-Kigin & McNeil, 1995; McNeil et al., 1991, 1999) with some evidence from follow-up studies (Funderburk et al., 1998). This program shows good evidence for generalization between changes observed in the home and those noted at school (Brestan et al., 1997), and maintenance of gains up to five years has been shown in two studies (Eyberg et al., 2001; Hood & Eyberg, 2003).

Parent training shows greater efficacy (fewer dropouts, greater gains, and better maintenance) when children are younger; the disturbance of conduct is less severe; there is less comorbidity; less socioeconomic disadvantage in the family (Holden et al., 1990; Kazdin et al., 1992; McMahon et al., 1981); the parents are together (Dumas & Albin, 1986; Farmer et al., 2002); parental discord and stress are low (Dadds et al., 1987; Dumas & Albin, 1986; Kazdin et al., 1992; McMahon et al., 1981; Webster-Stratton, 1996b); social support is high; and when there is no parental history of antisocial behavior. Failure to benefit from the program may be associated with parental disadvantage, lack of parental perception of a need for intervention, marital discord (Dadds et al., 1987; Nye et al., 1995), parental drug or alcohol problems (Nye et al., 1995), psychiatric difficulties (drug and alcohol problems, depression, personality difficulties), more severe and chronic antisocial behavior, and comorbidity in the child (Kazdin, 1995a; Ruma et al., 1996). However, inattention, impulsivity and hyperactivity problems increase the size of the response (Hartman et al., 2003). Maternal psychopathology, particularly depression and life events, has been found to reduce the effectiveness of parent training (Dumas & Albin, 1986; Kazdin et al., 1992; McMahon et al., 1981; Webster-Stratton, 1996b). There are also indications that single-parent status (Dumas & Albin, 1986), only one parent attending (Farmer et al., 2002), and maternal insecurity of attachment (Routh et al., 1995) may undermine progress, but these associations are not consistent across studies.

In the case of violent families, consequence procedures normally included in parent training packages can result in confrontation between the parent and the oppositional child that could provoke more serious aversive interactions in parents prone to child abuse (Lutzker, 1996). "Errorless" compliance training offers an alternative to the use of physical consequences for noncompliance (Ducharme et al., 2000). Parent training can have quite limited effects when parents themselves did not seek treatment (Barkley et al., 2000; Webster-Stratton & Hammond, 1997)

CHILD-ORIENTED INTERVENTIONS

Psychodynamic Therapy. Psychodynamic treatments have not been shown to be effective for children with conduct problems relative to an untreated or alternative treatment control group (Fonagy & Target, 1994).

Behavioral and Cognitive-Behavioral Approaches. Dush et al. (1989) identified 48 controlled studies of cognitive-behavioral therapy (CBT) that employed "self-statement modification." Trials were conducted in a variety of settings (inpatient, outpatient, school, etc.) and with a variety of disorders (anxiety, delinquency, hyperactivity, impulsivity). The effect size for measures of disruption and aggression was small (0.18), though this may reflect the comingling of disruptive and aggressive categories in the analysis, as well as the collapsing of data from school and clinical settings.

Mild conduct problems are ameliorated with the help of social skills and anger management coping skills training (see Quinn et al., 1999, for a review). In a school-based coping skills intervention (Lochman et al., 1993) children rated as aggressive and rejected benefited from this package in terms of reduced aggression (effect size = 0.85) and social acceptance (effect size = 0.89), but those who were aggressive but not socially rejected did not. Attrition was high, however, at 45%. There is no evidence for the use of social skills and anger management coping skills training approaches on their own with more chronic and severe cases (Fonagy et al., 2002).

Problem-solving skills training (PSST) is the most rigorously investigated singular approach to the cognitive-behavioral treatment of conduct problems. Its effectiveness in combination with parent training has been demonstrated by two independent studies (Kazdin & Wasser, 2000; Kazdin et al., 1992), and it seems to be the treatment of choice for conduct problems in school-age children (8–12). In a trial contrasting relationship therapy (RT) with (1) PSST, and (2) PSST and *in vivo* practice outside the treatment setting, PSST produced improvements with the outpatient, milder or moderate severity group, as well as the inpatient group. Children with more severe disturbance of conduct (either in terms of frequency or intensity) were more likely to drop out or to have negative outcomes (Kazdin et al., 1994), and there is some indication that ethnic/minority status may be associated with relatively poorer outcomes (Kazdin, 1996). Of 242 children ages 3–14 years referred to a specialist outpatient unit for treatment for oppositional, aggressive, and antisocial behavior, 39.9% dropped out (Kazdin et al., 1997). These individuals were more likely to be from minority groups or single-parent families, to be on public assistance, to have adverse child-rearing practices, to be of low socioeconomic status, and to have a child with a history of antisocial behavior. Families who dropped out had higher levels of stressors and obstacles that competed with treatment, including conflict with a significant other about coming to treatment, problems with other children, and seeing treatment as adding to other stressors. Those terminating early also perceived the treatment as less relevant to the child's problems and appeared to have poorer relationships with the therapist.

These conclusions were supported by an uncontrolled study of 250 children and families treated over 22 weeks with a combination of PSST and parent training (Kazdin & Wasser, 2000). The greater the severity of the child's dysfunction and the higher the perceived barriers, the smaller the observed changes. Helping parents deal with stress independently improves the outcome of already potent combinations of parent training and PSST (Kazdin & Nock, 2003).

INTERVENTIONS FOCUSED ON CLASSROOM BEHAVIOR

Although classroom contingency management methods are effective in controlling the behavior of children with conduct problems in that setting (e.g., Deitz, 1985; Walker et al., 1984), there is little evidence of generalization outside the classroom situation or beyond the termination of the programs (Barkley et al., 2000). Parent-administered reinforcements may enhance classroom contingency management in universal or selective prevention programs (Ayllon et al., 1975; Kahle & Kelley, 1994), and on this basis, their combination should be considered when children have behavior problems in school.

Treatment Interventions for Adolescents

FAMILY-BASED INTERVENTIONS

There are few studies of parent training specifically in relation to adolescents. Chamberlain and Rosicky (1995) identified seven studies of parent training conducted between 1988 and 1994. A more recent, somewhat broader, Cochrane review (Woolfenden et al., 2002, 2003) identified eight trials of parent training and multisystemic therapy (which includes parent training). Essentially, both concluded that family and parenting interventions for juvenile delinquents have beneficial effects in reducing time spent in institutions and the frequency of arrests.

The Oregon Model, designed for 6- to 10-year-olds, has been extended to adolescents by targeting risk behaviors for delinquency (e.g., class attendance, affiliation with antisocial peers, or drug use), enhancing parental monitoring, and replacing time-out procedures with more radical punishments (e.g., restriction of free time and restitution of stolen property). However, the effectiveness of this procedure appears limited (Bank et al., 1991; Forgatch & Patterson, 1989; Patterson & Forgatch, 1987). In addition, a controlled trial (Dishion & Andrews, 1995) found that instituting this approach in a group format was associated with particularly poor outcomes, possibly due to peer influence. Further studies show more positive benefit with children in foster care, where it appears to reduce behavior problems, as well as recidivism (Chamberlain & Reid, 1998; Chamberlain & Rozicky, 1995), perhaps because of a higher level of motivation in the foster parents.

Functional Family Therapy (a form of behavioral family therapy) has been shown to be effective in reducing recidivism in adolescents who have multiply offended. Nine studies carried out between 1973 and 1997 reported an improvement of 25–80% in recidivism, out-of-home placement, or future offending by siblings of the treated youths (Fonagy & Kurtz, 2002). Though a promising treatment, it has not yet been widely applied. There is less work on structural family therapy, mostly on Hispanic children, where it has been shown to be effective in youth with conduct problems (Coatsworth et al., 2001; Santiseban et al., 2003; Szapocznik et al., 1989).

MULTISYSTEMIC THERAPY

This home-based approach is offered by one therapist, who potentially offers a range of techniques, dependent on the clinical picture. These include marital and family therapies, parent training, behavioral and cognitive approaches, supportive therapy, and case management (which may involve liaison with outside agencies). A number of good-quality RCTs of this approach suggest that this is the most effective treatment for delinquent adolescents in reducing recidivism and improving individual and family pathology (Borduin, 1999; Henggeler et al., 1986, 1992, 1993, 1996a). It is substantially more effective than individual treatment even for quite troubled and disorganized families (Borduin et al., 1995). Multisystemic therapy (MST) shares a particular strength with other systemic family approaches in reducing attrition rates in this highly volatile group (Henggeler et al., 1996b). The success of this program is quite striking: at an average 4-year follow-up, recidivism in those who completed MST was significantly reduced (22.1%) relative to recipients of individual therapy (71.4%). The rate of arrest in the MST group was 26%, contrasted to 71% for those who received individual therapy; further, where they were arrested, their crimes were usually less serious (Borduin, 1999).

INDIVIDUAL APPROACHES

Social skills and social problem-solving approaches lead to desirable short-term changes, but do not generalize well across settings or engender lasting improvements (Feindler et al., 1984; Guerra & Slaby, 1990; Huey & Rank, 1984). Anger management is a promising treatment approach, but the evidence for its efficacy is quite limited (Feindler et al., 1984). School-based approaches have considerable potential, but studies to date have failed to demonstrate powerful effects on delinquency (Esbensen & Osgood, 1999; Gottfredson & Gottfredson, 1992). The evidence for communitywide implementation of psychosocial treatment programs is inadequate, and the results are mixed, although family preservation and systemic family therapy implementations appear most promising (Nugent et al., 1993).

Individual-treatment approaches appear to be less effective than family based approaches, but if individual approaches are implemented, these should focus on proximal causes for delinquent behavior rather than more distal underlying problems. The programs for these adolescents should be skills oriented, wherever possible identifying the skills deficits.

Summary

For young children with conduct problems, parent training is a highly effective intervention. Programs increasingly attempt to meet the challenge of comorbidity, severity, parental psychopathology, and social disadvantage, all of which threaten their efficacy. These interventions have evolved to become longer, and include children and teachers, which appears to improve generalization. Best outcomes are found with younger children with less comorbidity and severity, with lower levels of socioeconomic disadvantage, and with higher levels of parental stability. Failure to benefit is associated with parental psychiatric difficulties (e.g., substance abuse, depression, personality difficulties). There are indications that barriers such as parental stresses need to be managed in order for programs to show benefit. A particular clinical challenge is posed by parents who do not initiate treatment themselves, or who do not perceive the need for an intervention.

Psychodynamic treatments have not been shown to be effective for children with conduct problems relative to an untreated or alternative treatment control group. Mild—but not more chronic or severe—conduct problems benefit from social skills and anger management coping skills training.

Among cognitive-behavioral approaches, PSST is the most rigorously investigated and effective, perhaps because this helps children develop alternative strategies to resolve problems that cause disruptive behavior (rather than attempting to regulate it). It is particularly effective when offered in combination with parent training, and this is the treatment of choice for conduct problems in school-age children (8–12).

For adolescents, psychosocial interventions are less effective than for younger children. Though the strongest evidence of benefit is for multisystemic approaches, their complexity and intensity means that they are not yet widely available.

Attention-Deficit/Hyperactivity Disorder

The characteristics of attention-deficit/hyperactivity disorder (ADHD) are reduced levels of concentration or attention, impulsivity, and overactivity or restlessness. There is no clear demarcation between extremes of normality and truly abnormal degrees of these behaviors. Findings from several factor-analytic studies, such as the study by Lahey and Carlson (1992), suggest two separate dimensions in ADHD: the impulsive–hyperactive, and the inattentive–disorganized dimensions. DSM-IV-TR describes three types of ADHD:

predominantly inattentive, predominantly hyperactive, and combined (both sets of symptoms).

Medication

Systematic reviews of extended treatment studies underscore the value of stimulant medication (Farmer et al., 2002; Schachar et al., 2002). Seventy-five percent of children with ADHD show normalization of inattention, hyperactivity, and impulsivity when so treated. Attention and output during academic tasks improve by 70%, and efficiency and accuracy by approximately 50%, though there is little evidence for improved academic performance in the long term. Prosocial behaviors do not improve substantially, although there is evidence that these benefit from the additional use of clonidine (Hazell & Stuart, 2003). Despite improvement, behavior is not normalized with medication in all cases (MTA Cooperative Group, 1999).

Psychosocial Treatment Interventions

Although a number of behavioral or cognitive-behavioral treatments have been shown to be effective in ADHD when compared to wait-list controls (e.g., Anastopoulos et al., 1993; Hoath & Sanders, 2002; Sonuga-Barke et al., 2001), there is mixed evidence for their adjunctive benefit when the contrast is to medication. Some studies show little or no benefit from adding psychosocial interventions to well-administered medication treatments (Horn et al., 1991; Ialongo et al., 1993), while others suggest that the appropriate psychosocial intervention can help attain desired responses with lower doses of medication (Abikoff & Hechtman, 1996; Satterfield et al., 1981, 1987; Vitiello et al., 2001).

It is possible that greater benefit is found when there is comorbid anxiety (Jensen et al., 2001; MTA Cooperative Group, 1999) and high parental education (Pisterman et al., 1992; Rieppi et al., 2002) Overall, it seems reasonable to conclude that behavior therapy offered alone is less effective than stimulant medication. Nonetheless, it may improve task performance and reduce disruptive behavior, but there is little evidence of generalization beyond the treatment setting (Vitiello et al., 2001).

Most of these observations are derived from the Multimodal Treatment Study of ADHD (MTA), a 5-year study set up by the National Institute of Mental Health (Richters et al., 1995). Five hundred seventy-nine children with ADHD were randomly allocated to 14 months of treatment, with a control condition (standard care chosen by families obtained from community providers) contrasted to one of three experimental groups: (1) medication alone, (2) intensive behavioral management with the parents, child, and school (with therapist input reduced over time), or (3) the two "optimally" combined (MTA Cooperative Group, 1999).

In the 34% of the sample with comorbid anxiety, there was a trend toward a better response to the combined treatment than to medication alone, and behavioral intervention alone was better than the standard community care. The presence of comorbid anxiety reduced the relative advantage of medication over the other treatments, but it did not reduce the rate of response to medication (March et al., 2000). ADHD-only, and ADHD with comorbid CD or ODD subjects responded only to treatments that included medication. If comorbidity included anxiety as well as conduct syndromes, the combined treatment group fared best. Combined treatments were more effective for better educated families and yielded greater patient satisfaction (Rieppi et al., 2002). Treatments involving medication were more likely to ensure normalization in the absence of parental depression and less severe initial presentation (Owens et al., 2003). Beneficial effects of the behavioral treatment appeared to remain several months after the treatment had ceased, supporting the notion that combining treatments may allow earlier discontinuation of medication. Furthermore, parental disciplinary practices consistently predicted changes in child outcome at school (Hinshaw et al., 2000; Wells et al., 2000).

In cases of pure ADHD, there is no consistent evidence yet that any psychological approach increases the effectiveness of medication. CBT offered alone does not appear effective (e.g., Abikoff et al., 1988; Abikoff & Gittelman, 1985; Brown et al., 1986), and there is some indication that its effective component may be behavioral. For example Tutty et al. (2003) randomly assigned 100 children (ages 5–12, and newly diagnosed with ADHD) to receive either stimulant medication alone or medication combined with an 8-week behavioral and social skills (BSS) class. Compared to medication alone, the addition of BSS resulted in parental reports of significantly lower ratings of symptoms of ADHD, and significantly better and more consistent discipline practices. There is no evidence that social skills intervention leads to an improvement in relationships (Cousins & Weiss, 1993).

Parent training is effective in improving compliance with instructions (Pisterman et al., 1992, 1989) but not all families are able to persist with the approach. It is more likely to be effective with prepubertal children (Anastopoulos et al., 1996) and if participating mothers have low levels of ADHD symptoms (Rieppi et al., 2002; Sonuga-Barke et al., 2002) (indeed, parental ADHD may require treatment before parent training is likely to be effective). Attrition is higher among less-educated parents (Pisterman et al., 1992), suggesting that greater effort will be required to involve this group.

There is no evidence either for or against the effectiveness of systemic or psychodynamic therapy.

Summary

The benefit of psychosocial treatments relative to well-administered medication is unclear. While a number of studies show little benefit, others suggest that their addition can lead to equivalent outcomes with lower doses of medication. There are indications that the presence of comorbid anxiety and higher parental education is associated with greater benefit from intensive behavioral treatment.

Parent training improves compliance with instructions, but not all families are able to persist with the approach. There are a number of interventions with little supporting evidence for their use—multimodal treatments, CBT offered alone, social skills training, and systemic and psychodynamic therapy. A number of classroom-based programs have been evaluated; although these show efficacy, they tend not to generalize to other settings, and their impact is lost after the program is completed.

Tourette Syndrome

Tourette syndrome is a common childhood-onset disorder with unknown neurobiological etiology (Comings & Comings, 1985). It presents with motor and vocal tics. Motor tics vary from simple movements, such as blinking or shrugging, to more complex movements, such as facial expressions or gestures of the arms or legs (Leckman & Cohen, 1994).

Habit reversal (performing a movement that is opposite to the tic in question) and relaxation have been found successful in at least some children. Azrin and Peterson (1990) offered 10 months of habit reversal to 10 subjects. Children were randomized to immediate treatment or to a 3-month wait list, which acted as a control, and a 93% reduction in tics was found. Although this approach seems promising, further studies are required. Results from massed negative practice (in which the child performs the tic as quickly and forcefully as he/she can) have been uncertain (Azrin & Peterson, 1988). Leckman and Cohen (1994) found that families generally report only short-term benefits from these interventions. They also reported that while psychotherapy or supportive interventions may be useful in helping children and families cope with this syndrome, there have been no controlled studies of their use.

Deliberate Self-Harm

Definition and Prevalence

The definition of "deliberate self-harm" includes not only nonfatal or attempted suicide but also life-threatening behaviors, such as self-poisoning, in which the person does not necessarily intend to take his/her own life. Surveys of lifetime suicidality usually find higher suicide attempt rates among

U.S. teenagers compared to their European counterparts. For example, Smith and Crawford (1986) and Harkavy-Friedman et al. (1987) both reported lifetime suicide attempt rates of approximately 9% for U.S. high school students. Lifetime rates among 12- to 18-year-olds in Quebec were 3.5% (Pronovost et al., 1990), and 2.2% among Dutch students (ages 14–20 years) (Kienhorst et al., 1990). Larsson et al. (1991) reported that 4% of a sample of Swedish 13- to 18-year-olds had made a suicide attempt at some time in their lives, and 2% in the past year.

Treatment Interventions

Diekstra et al. (1995) and Hawton (1996) discussed approaches to the prevention of suicidal behavior in young people. These include school-based educational programs, the control and/or modification of methods used for committing suicide, efforts to reduce substance misuse, responsible media reporting of suicide, specialist services—often crisis intervention—for people seriously contemplating suicide, and aftercare programs for those who have deliberately harmed themselves. There is evidence that treatment effects on suicidality are divorced from treatment effects on depression (Miller & Glinski, 2000).

Aftercare programs for parasuicides treated in hospitals have increased substantially in most countries. Most studies lack both suitable controls and adequate follow-up, reflecting the fact that this is a difficult population to recruit in research or to engage in treatment. For example, among 129 young people admitted to Birmingham Children's Hospital following an overdose, only 33.3% agreed to participation (Dorer et al., 1999).

Crisis intervention centers typically provide a 24-hour hotline plus referral to other mental health or social work agencies. However, a meta-analysis by Dew et al. (1987) found no indication of impact on suicide rate in communities with such a center.

Allard et al. (1992) randomized 150 patients to an intensive intervention program or to TAU. The program included 18 therapy appointments over 1 year, links to other agencies, and various measures to improve attendance. Despite evidence that the program increased contact with professional services, the 2-year follow-up indicated that 35% of the experimental group and 30% of controls had carried out at least one parasuicidal act. Three of the experimental and one of the control patients completed suicides. A more recent study (Thompson et al., 2000) suggests better efficacy for a preventive school-based interventions focused on individuals showing signs related to suicide risk as opposed to programs with high-risk groups and entire school populations.

Harrington et al. (1998a) identified 162 consecutive cases of children under 17 years admitted with deliberate self-poisoning, allocating them either to routine care alone, or to routine care plus brief, home–based family intervention (which focused on family communication and problem solving). Although at 6-month follow-up there were no significant differences in measures of suicidality or hopelessness, compliance with family treatment was better than that for routine care, and parents in the intervention group were significantly more satisfied with treatment at 2-month assessment than were parents in the control group. The same group carried out the only RCT on the treatment of repeated deliberate self-harm in adolescence (Wood et al., 2001). They randomized 63 patients to routine care or to approximately 14 sessions of an eclectic group therapy, which incorporated techniques from CBT, dialectical behavior therapy (DBT), and psychodynamic therapy. Contrasted to the control, group treatment significantly reduced the risk of repeated self-harm (6 vs. 32%, equivalent to a number needed to treat [NNT] of 4). However, follow up of 7-months after baseline might be too brief to judge true treatment effects.

Cotgrove et al. (1995) examined outcomes in a group of 105 patients ages 12–17 years (85% of whom were female) admitted after deliberate self-harm. On discharge, 47 patients were assigned to standard care plus an emergency (green) card acting as a "passport" to readmission into the local pediatric ward; 58 controls received standard care. The percentage of repeaters at 12-month follow-up was 6.4% in the experimental group and 12.1% in the control group, not a statistically significant difference.

Lack of adherence to treatment regimens is a particular problem in adolescents who attempt suicide (Spirito et al., 1992). Zimmerman et al. (1995) found a psychoeducational module addressing issues of treatment adherence and adolescent suicidality to be ineffective. However, Rotheram-Borus et al. (1996) compared adherence to treatment among 140 female suicide attempters (ages 12–18 years) assigned to standard care or a specialized emergency room program (which included psychoeducation and individual and family therapy). The program reduced adolescents' self-reported depression and suicidality, and also showed benefit for their family functioning. In a more recent paper, Rotheram-Borus et al. (1999) reported a 6-month follow-up of 66 adolescents (ages 13–17 years) with significant suicidal thoughts, intent, or behaviors, hospitalized in an adolescent psychiatric unit. Compliance with medication (66.7%) and individual therapy (50.8%) were better than attendance at parent guidance/family therapy (33.3%). The poorest compliance for the latter approach was found with the most dysfunctional families, and those with the least involved/affectionate father–adolescent relationships. The same group applied a problem-solving intervention to increase adherence in 63 adolescents (Spirito et al., 2002). Three months postintervention, the compliance enhancement group attended significantly more (7.7 vs. 6.4 sessions), but the difference was not significant until adjusted for structural barriers to service use (e.g., length of wait list, insurance coverage).

Summary

Evidence for effective approaches to the prevention of further suicide attempts in young people is extremely limited, although there is suggestive value from programs that facilitate contact with professional services following admission. Round-the-clock "hotline" services have not been shown to reduce the incidence of suicide attempts among the populations served. There is some (though limited) evidence that brief eclectic group therapy with the families of adolescents following a suicide attempt can reduce adolescents' feelings of depression and suicidality, and improve family involvement (hence, further compliance with specialist programs).

Depression

Definition and Prevalence

In children and teenagers, a diagnosis of major depressive disorder (MDD) requires a minimum 2-week period of pervasive mood change toward sadness or irritability, and loss of interest or pleasure (American Psychiatric Association, 2000) that is not explicable by other illnesses, life events, and so on. Children and adolescents may show more anxiety and anger, fewer vegetative symptoms, and less verbalization of hopelessness than adults (American Academy of Child and Adolescent Psychiatry, 1998a). Dysthymic disorder is a chronic condition with depressed and/or irritable mood, with at least two other symptoms of MDD (American Psychiatric Association, 2000).

DD and dysthymic disorder both have point prevalence rates of about 2% among children and 2–5% for adolescents (Birmaher et al., 1996a; Lewinsohn & Clarke, 1999). Depression is equally common in girls and boys up to adolescence, but thereafter, girls outnumber boys by two to one (Lewinsohn et al., 1994; Weissman et al., 1997). The majority of clinically depressed children have other comorbid disorders, mostly anxiety and disruptive disorders (Beidel et al., 1999; Strauss & Last, 1993). There is a high rate of recovery from episodes of depression (mean length, 9 months), but a high rate of relapse (50% within 2 years). Childhood or adolescent depression is associated with raised rates of depression and other psychopathology in adult life (e.g., Harrington et al., 1990, 1991, 1994; Klein et al., 1997; Kovacs et al., 1997).

Treatment Interventions

The treatment of depression in children and adolescents has been reviewed by, among others, Harrington et al. (1998b), Birmaher et al. (1996b) the American Academy of Child and Adolescent Psychiatry (1998a), Lewinsohn and Clarke (1999), and Asarnow et al. (2001). Most treatment approaches are adaptations of techniques employed with adults, particularly medication and CBT.

COGNITIVE-BEHAVIORAL THERAPY

Reinecke and colleagues (1998) carried out a meta-analysis of six studies of CBT for adolescent depression, and found a robust effect size of 1.02 at termination and 0.61 at follow-up. Harrington and colleagues (1998c) also carried out a very useful systematic review of all methodologically sound CBT outcome studies ($n = 6$) for childhood depressive disorder. Their pooled odds ratio was 3.2, with children receiving CBT significantly more likely to be in remission by the end of treatment. This odds ratio fell to 2.2 if a (very conservative) intention-to-treat (ITT) analysis was applied (in which all dropouts from the control groups were counted as having remitted, and all those from the CBT groups as not having remitted).

CBT appears to be effective, whether provided individually or in a group (Brent et al., 1998; Clarke et al., 1999; Kroll et al., 1996; Lewinsohn et al., 1994, 1996; Wood et al., 1996). Providing longer courses of CBT (or booster sessions) in cases of nonresponse to a standard length of treatment improved recovery and reduced relapse (Clarke et al., 1999; Kroll et al., 1996).

Although these results are positive, it is worth noting that CBT has mainly been tested with mildly to moderately impaired adolescents, rather than with either severe cases or preadolescent children. Many early investigations focused on recruited children with mild symptoms of depression rather than referred patients with clinical levels of disturbance (e.g., Jaycox et al., 1994; King & Kirschenbaum, 1990; Liddle & Spence, 1990; Marcotte & Baron, 1993). They have produced mixed results on the efficacy of CBT approaches (see review by Asarnow et al., 2001). Recent studies have confirmed that referred, depressed adolescents are more difficult to treat successfully than recruited cases, even when severity is comparable (Birmaher et al., 2000; Brent et al., 1999). In a trial of CBT including 96 depressed adolescents (Lewinsohn et al., 1994, 1996), best results were found for those with less severe symptoms and better initial adaptation. The difference between CBT and other treatment tends to disappear at follow-up (Birmaher et al., 2000; Brent et al., 1999; Wood et al., 1996). Family factors such as maternal depression and family discord can reduce treatment response (e.g., Brent et al., 1998). Finally, and contrary to expectations based on the theory underpinning CBT, it is not more effective in cases where there are greater cognitive distortions, and its benefits are apparently not explained by a reduction in such cognitions (Brent et al., 1998; Lewinsohn et al., 1990).

Rohde and colleagues (2001) analyzed data from 151 adolescents from the combined Oregon cohorts (Clarke et al., 1999; Lewinsohn et al., 1990), to examine the influence of comorbidity on outcomes for CBT. Almost 40% of the sample had another lifetime diagnosis (in addition to the depressive disorder at intake). Contrary to expectations, although comorbidity was associated with greater impairment at intake, it did not predict poorer outcome (in fact, comorbidity with anxiety was a positive factor), nor did it predict slower recovery, with the exception of substance abuse, which did seem to delay improvement.

INTERPERSONAL PSYCHOTHERAPY

Interpersonal psychotherapy (IPT), adapted for adolescents (IPT-A; Moreau et al., 1991; Mufson et al., 1994), appears promising for treatment of adolescent depression. Two clinical RCTs have been reported (Mufson et al., 1999; Rosselló & Bernal, 1999). The Mufson et al. (1999) trial included 48 referred adolescents with MDD, of whom 32 completed the protocol. The majority of dropouts came from the control condition, which was "clinical monitoring." An ITT analysis showed that 75% of patients assigned to IPT-A recovered, as judged by Hamilton Rating Scale for Depression (HRSD) scores, in comparison with 46% of those in the control group.

Rosselló et al. (1999) studied 71 Puerto Rican adolescents meeting criteria for MDD, and showed that while both IPT and CBT reduced depressive symptoms (Child Depression Inventory [CDI] and Child Behavior Checklist [CBCL]), IPT was more effective in improving self-esteem (Piers–Harris Children's Self-Concept Scale) and social adaptation (Social Adjustment Scale for Children and Adolescents). This study was the first to compare IPT and CBT, but it needs to be replicated with other cultural groups, since the treatments were manualized to be specifically appropriate to Puerto Rican society.

Santor and Kusumakar (2001) reported a controlled study comparing 12 weeks of IPT with sertraline in the treatment of 49 moderately to severely impaired adolescents with MDD. The 25 IPT cases were compared with 24 who had previously been treated using sertraline in an open trial. Outcomes were compared on the Beck Depression Inventory (BDI), the Children's Global Assessment Scale (CGAS), and an index of clinical recovery. Both treatments led to significant improvement, but IPT was superior across all three measures.

FAMILY THERAPY

Although there is ample evidence of the importance of the family context and parental psychological problems in relation to child and adolescent depression (see Asarnow et al., 2001, for a clear description), there is little evidence of the effectiveness of family therapy for depression. Family therapy or parent work in parallel with individual treatment for the child has been included as a comparison condition in four RCTs (e.g., Brent et al., 1997), and has generally been found to be of less benefit than the experimental condition. However, Brent et al. (1997) employed systemic–behavioral family therapy as a control condition, and found that this form of family therapy was beneficial, especially in cases where the mother was perceived to be controlling. Recently, an RCT conducted by Diamond and colleagues (2002) evaluated the impact of "attachment-based family therapy" in comparison with wait list. Family therapy was associated with significantly greater reduction in depression scores on the BDI and HRSD, and with greater likelihood of remission by the end of treatment. This new model of therapy deserves further evaluation in comparison with active treatments.

SOCIAL SKILLS TRAINING AND INDIVIDUAL CHILD PSYCHOTHERAPY

To date, neither of these approaches has been shown to be an effective treatment. Matson (1989) reported on two cases of individualized social skills training, both of which improved substantially. Fine and colleagues (1991) compared two group therapies for depressed adolescents: 12-week therapy groups using either "therapeutic support" (27 patients) or social skills training (20 patients). Forty-one percent of the patients were receiving other treatment: psychotherapy, medication, or both. At posttreatment, adolescents in the therapeutic support group showed significantly greater improvement than those receiving social skills training, though these group differences were no longer significant at follow-up (more because sample size had dropped than because the difference had decreased).

A chart review study of 763 patients who had been in psychoanalytic therapy (Target & Fonagy, 1994b) included 65 children and adolescents with dysthymia and/or MDD who had been treated for an average of 2 years. By the end of therapy, over 75% showed reliable improvement in functioning and no depressive symptoms. However, the episodic course of depression means that these pre- to posttherapy findings with no control group or follow-up cannot be taken as evidence of efficacy. A clearer finding was that children and adolescents with depressive disorders appeared to benefit more from intensive (4–5 sessions per week) than from nonintensive (1–2 sessions per week) therapy, after controlling for length of treatment and level of impairment at referral. This is of some interest given that the depressed cases were mostly adolescents, who generally did not gain additional benefit from frequent sessions.

Summary

CBT appears to be effective, whether provided individually or in a group. However, it has mainly been tested with mildly to moderately impaired adolescents, rather than with either severe cases or preadolescent children. Family factors can reduce treatment response. Providing longer courses of CBT (or booster sessions) in cases of nonresponse to a standard length of treatment has been shown, at least in some studies, to hasten recovery.

IPT-A appears to be a promising treatment for adolescent depression. Family therapy, or parent work in parallel with individual treatment for the child, has rarely been the focus of evaluation. There is very limited evidence for the benefit of family therapies, though a recent attachment-based approach shows some promise. Social skills training and individual child psychotherapy have not yet been shown to be effective treatments.

As in studies for many other disorders, outcome of the treatment of depression has generally been defined in terms of change in symptoms and diagnostic status, leading to a neglect of other important indices of functioning, such as deficient social adaptation and academic performance. The inclusion of such adaptation variables, and of comorbidity and family history, promises to allow more fine-grained assessment of the efficacy of treatments for childhood depression in the coming years.

Anxiety Disorders

Definition and Prevalence

Anxiety disorders commonly present as part of a more complex picture, frequently including other disorders (e.g., Strauss & Last, 1993), and difficulties in adaptation such as shyness, academic underachievement, and unhappiness (e.g., Quay & LaGreca, 1986). Fears and worries are, of course, very common in normal development (e.g., Bell-Dolan et al., 1990; Muris et al., 1998), and only become diagnosable when a persistent and disabling pattern has become established. Nevertheless, for children starting school, it has been shown that anxiety symptoms that do not meet diagnostic criteria are associated with academic impairment over the following years (Ialongo et al., 1994, 1995). Here, we are concerned with treatments for symptoms that do meet the thresholds for at least one diagnosis.

Anxiety disorders in children and adolescents include the syndromes described for the adult population, so the following DSM-IV-TR categories can be applied to children: generalized anxiety disorder (GAD), obsessive–compulsive disorder (OCD), agoraphobia, panic disorder, specific phobia, social phobia, and anxiety states due to either medical disorder or substance use. In addition, separation anxiety disorder (SAD) can be diagnosed in children.

Anxiety disorders are very common, but most cases go untreated. Overall figures from epidemiological studies (e.g., see review by Bernstein & Borchardt, 1991) of children and adolescents spanning 4–20 years of age suggest that 8–12% of children in this age range suffer from one or more diagnosable anxiety disorders, making anxiety disorders the most common type of psychiatric disorder in children. Dadds et al. (1997) found that one in six schoolchildren in their study had an anxiety disorder or features of one. Anxiety disorders occur with equal frequency in boys and girls until adolescence, after which there is a predominance of girls (Cohen et al., 1993). These figures may seem surprisingly high, perhaps because children with emotional disorders are much less frequently referred for psychiatric attention than those with disruptive disorders (Beardslee et al., 1997; Beidel & Turner, 1997; Keller et al., 1992).

Different disorders have different prognoses, but moderate to severe cases are not likely to remit spontaneously, and when they do remit, it is quite common for other disorders to take their places (Flament et al., 1990; Kovacs & Devlin, 1998; Pollack et al., 1996). Anxiety disorders commonly evolve into other anxiety or depressive syndromes. Persistent anxiety disorders cause pervasive and lasting impairments. The high placebo response observed in child and adolescent patients makes demonstration of efficacy of all treatments problematic.

Treatment Interventions

BEHAVIORAL AND COGNITIVE-BEHAVIORAL TECHNIQUES

The methods and rationale of behavioral treatments for childhood anxiety are fully described by King and Ollendick (1997; Ollendick & King, 1998), who also give a clear and comprehensive overview of studies of the cognitive-behavioral treatment of childhood phobias. This form of treatment for anxiety disorders in general has been reviewed by P. C. Kendall (1993).

Behavioral techniques are often effective in the treatment of children with circumscribed phobias, especially younger children (King et al., 2001a; Ollendick & King, 1998). Exposure has been assumed to be a central aspect of the efficacy of CBT, but two well-designed studies of the treatment of school phobia found that therapeutic support without exposure was equally effective (Last et al., 1998; W. K. Silverman et al., 1999). Despite early evidence, from a nonrandomized controlled study, that "flooding" (rapid return to school) could be rapidly successful in managing school refusal (Blagg & Yule, 1984), RCTs for this condition have focused on more gradual exposure with added cognitive strategies. Where exposure treatment is used, it may well be more effective, as well as humane, to use a gradual rather than a flooding approach (King et al., 1998).

Thirty-two studies of cognitive-behavioral methods of treatment for OCD have been expertly reviewed by March (1995; March & Leonard, 1996; March & Mulle, 1995). March and coworkers (2001) have also described the rationale and effective elements of CBT for childhood OCD, together with issues of assessment and research. A more recent survey is provided in the practice parameters of the American Academy of Child and Adolescent Psychiatry (1998b). March's conclusion (1995) was that "although empirical support remains weak, CBT also may be the psychotherapeutic treatment of choice for children and adolescents with OCD [as for adults]" (p. 7). March and his colleagues (2001) repeated this view in a recent review paper; however, empirical support remains fairly weak. OCD can be improved in some cases, though generally not eliminated, by a CBT approach (March, 1995; March & Leonard, 1996; March & Mulle, 1995; March et al., 2001). This approach has so far mostly been evaluated with concurrent medication (e.g., Neziroglu et al., 2000), but there is some evidence that CBT makes a distinctive contribution (DeVeaugh-Geiss et al., 1992; March et al., 1994). The recent review paper by March and his colleagues (2001) stated that although there is some consensus that CBT is usually helpful for OCD, in practice, many patients will not comply with behavioral treatments, and parents claim that clinicians are inadequately trained in CBT procedures. This report from perhaps the foremost authority in this area reminds us of the importance of three things: maintaining more than one psychosocial treatment approach to provide options in cases where the child or family does not comply; making sure that treatment manuals and procedures are well-adapted to children, so that compliance is more likely; and, of course, the specific training for clinicians in the best-validated treatments.

Although generalized anxiety states in children are a frequent cause of referral for treatment (Last et al., 1987), treatments for this disorder were not evaluated using behavioral or cognitive methods until their value had begun to be demonstrated with more circumscribed problems. Certain CBT packages have been shown to be effective in the treatment of GAD and other anxiety disorders and, for those who improve, the gains can be maintained (Barrett et al., 1996; Beidel et al., 2000; Kendall et al., 1997; Toren et al., 2000; Tracey et al., 1999). In a small, open trial of parent–child group CBT for preadolescent children with anxiety disorders (Toren et al., 2000), the children whose mothers met criteria for an anxiety disorder (half the sample) did better than those whose mothers were not anxious, even though the anxious mothers' own anxiety levels were not reduced during treatment. This small study strongly justifies extension and clarification, because it involved a relatively brief and low-cost treatment that appears to have been helpful with a challenging group: clinically referred children, most with comorbid diagnoses, and half of whose mothers had similar symptoms.

There is accumulating evidence that CBT for childhood anxiety disorders can be delivered in a group as successfully as in an individual format (Flannery-Schroeder & Kendall, 2000; Manassis et al., 2002). Adding a family component to CBT may well be beneficial for younger children, or for families in which parental anxiety is also high (Barrett et al., 1996; Cobham et al., 1998; Howard & Kendall, 1996; Mendlowitz et al., 1999).

A study by Bernstein et al. (2000) deserves mention although it was intended as a test of a tricyclic drug (imipramine). In this double-blind RCT involving school-refusing adolescents with comorbid anxiety and depressive disorders, 63 subjects began the trial and 47 completed treatment. All adolescents were treated with individual CBT, while one group also received imipramine and the other received placebo, and the major outcome measure was school attendance. All the children received eight sessions of individual, manualized CBT that enlisted parental involvement, as well as working with the child, from therapists trained to mastery criteria and supervised by the developer of the therapy, who had previously tested its efficacy (see Last et al., 1998). Nonetheless, the children who received this therapy plus placebo showed a very poor rate of remission (16.7% return to school): Even with the additional drug treatment, remission was achieved for just over half the group, with poor results across both conditions at follow-up. One reason for this low success rate might be that treatments often perform more convincingly when they are the "active" treatment of interest. This highlights the importance of not judging treatments from their results as "control" conditions (in this case, a background constant across groups). It also cautions against assuming that the results achieved in an RCT will be repeated when that treatment is being offered as part of routine clinical care. This relates to important work being done currently exploring the reasons for treatments showing better results in the "lab" versus the clinic (Weersing & Weisz, 2002; Weisz & Weiss 1989; Weisz et al. 1995a, 1995b).

PSYCHODYNAMIC PSYCHOTHERAPY

Although psychodynamic psychotherapy is quite widely used in the treatment of anxious children (especially those with entrenched and complex problems), there have been few attempts to evaluate its effectiveness systematically. The attempts that have been made fall short of the methodological standards reached in evaluation of much briefer and more goal-directed therapies, because of the complexities of designing such studies, their much greater costs, and probably also due to greater resistance to research at that time among psychodynamic therapists.

There is preliminary evidence that psychodynamic psychotherapy may be effective in the treatment of anxiety disorders (Target & Fonagy, 1994a). Children with anxiety disorders (with or without comorbidity) showed greater improvements than those with other conditions, and greater improvements than would have been expected on the basis of studies of untreated outcome. Over 85% of 299 children with anxiety and depressive disorders no longer suffered any diagnosable emotional disorder after an average of 2 years' treatment. Looking in more detail at specific diagnostic groups, it was found that phobias ($n = 48$), SAD ($n = 58$), and overanxious disorder ($n = 145$) were resolved in around 86% of cases. OCD was more resistant, ceasing to meet diagnostic criteria in 70% of cases. There are serious limitations to a retrospective study, and there was no control group or follow-up; however, these rates of improvement appear to be above the level expected from longitudinal studies. A further finding was that children with severe or pervasive symptomatology, such as GAD or multiple comorbid disorders, required more frequent therapy sessions, whereas those with more circumscribed symptoms, such as phobias, even if quite severe, improved comparably with once or twice weekly sessions. Muratori et al. (2003) contrasted the efficacy of 11 weeks of psychodynamic therapy to TAU in 58 children with depression and anxiety. At 2-year follow-up, 34% of the treated group was in the clinical range on symptomatic measures, compared to 65% of the controls.

FAMILY THERAPY

No studies have so far examined the effectiveness of family therapy for childhood anxiety disorders, other than CBT delivered in a family format. One recent study compared "brief strategic family therapy" (BSFT) with a routine community treatment, in which the results for adolescents with CD were compared with those with anxiety disorders (Coatsworth et al., 2001). The study was mainly focused on outcome for the adolescents with CD, who did indeed fare better with BSFT. However, although families with anxious youngsters engaged well with treatment, results were quite poor, with few children making reliable improvements even if they stayed in treatment, either in the BSFT condition or in the community clinic setting (23% in both cases).

PREDICTORS OF OUTCOME

A number of studies have examined predictors of improvement in groups of treated children. Berman and colleagues (2000) studied 106 children, ages 6–17 years, with various anxiety disorders, who were given exposure-based treatment. Children did less well if they were also depressed, had trait anxiety, or had parents with more psychopathology (a factor that was most important in younger children). Southam-Gerow and colleagues (2001) evaluated predictors of response to individual CBT in a similar group of anxious children. Here, poor outcome was associated with more severe internalizing problems, more maternal depression, and the child being older. Kendall and colleagues (2001), examining the outcome of CBT in 173 children given 16–20 weeks of treatment, found that although comorbidity was associated with greater pre-treatment severity, but not with poorer outcome. This is consistent with a number of previous findings, including the Southam-Gerow study (2001). Layne and colleagues (2003) treated 41 adolescents, all of whom had diagnoses of both anxiety and depression, finding that poorer outcome was associated with worse school attendance at baseline, more SAD and avoidant disorder, and female gender.

Crawford and Manassis (2001) explored the importance of family factors on treatments for child anxiety using either individual or group CBT, with parallel parent training. Outcome was strongly mediated by family stress; specifically, clinician-rated child outcome was predicted by the child's rating (before treatment) of family dysfunction and of parental frustration. Greater dysfunction and frustration predicted worse treatment outcome.

Summary

Behavioral techniques are often effective in the treatment of children with circumscribed phobias, most especially with younger children. OCD can be improved by CBT in some cases, though generally not eliminated. Although this approach has usually been evaluated with concurrent medication, there is some evidence that CBT makes a distinctive contribution. Certain CBT packages have been shown to be effective in the treatment of GAD and other anxiety disorders, and for those who improve, the gains can be maintained. Exposure has been assumed to be a central aspect of the efficacy of CBT, but two recent, well-designed studies of the treatment of school phobia found that therapeutic support without exposure was equally effective. Where exposure treatment is used, it may well be more effective, as well as humane, to use a gradual rather than a "flooding" approach. There is accumulating evidence that CBT for childhood anxiety disorders can be delivered in a group as successfully as in an individual format. Adding a family component to CBT may be helpful for younger children or for families in which parental anxiety is also high. There is preliminary evidence that psychodynamic psychotherapy may be effective in the treatment of anxiety disorders. No studies have so far examined the effectiveness of family therapy for childhood anxiety disorders, other than CBT delivered in a family format.

Eating Disorders

Definition and Prevalence

DSM-IV-TR definitions of anorexia nervosa and bulimia nervosa can be found in Chapter 9. Bryant-Waugh and Lask (1995) noted that among referrals to a specialist eating disorders unit for children, 25% present disturbances of eating do not fit the existing DSM-IV-TR categories. Studies in children and adolescents have led to the suggestion that anorexia nervosa and bulimia nervosa may be different symptom patterns of one basic eating disorder, in which preoccupation with food and a disturbed body image are core symptoms (van der Ham et al., 1994). There are no reports of prepubertal bulimia nervosa and, until recently, very few cases with onset below the age of 14 have been noted (Schmidt et al., 1992).

Estimated prevalence rates for anorexia nervosa in young people vary quite widely—for example, 0 per 1,000 among Japanese schoolgirls (Suzuki et al., 1990), 1% in English private schools (Crisp et al., 1976; Szmukler, 1983), and 10.8% among Swedish girls below the age of 18 (Rastam & Gillberg, 1992). Both clinic and survey data show consistently higher rates for late-adolescent girls, with markedly lower rates for adolescent males (Barry & Lippman, 1990) (though a number of studies have reported that between 19 and 30% of cases among children are boys; Bryant-Waugh, 1993).

Steinhausen (1997) reviewed 31 outcome studies of patients with adolescent or preadolescent onset of eating disorder. Crude mortality rates ranged from 0 to 11%, with a mean of 2.2%; variations across studies were largely dependent upon the length of follow-up. Overall, about 52% of patients showed a full recovery, with some improvement in 29%, but 19% developed a chronic condition. At the end of treatment, a significant proportion continued to show evidence of psychiatric problems—for example, around 20% had affective disorders, 12% had OCD, 18% had personality disorders, and 19% had substance use disorders (see also Steinhausen et al., 2000).

There are rather few studies that focus specifically on interventions for children with eating disorders, and this section should be seen as complementary to the discussion of treatments for adults with eating disorders in Chapter 9.

Psychosocial Treatment Interventions

WEIGHT RESTORATION

Although the first goal of any treatment for children meeting DSM criteria for anorexia nervosa, beyond the evidence that early intervention and hospitalization might be a positive prognostic factor (especially among younger patients: see Bryant-Waugh et al., 1988), there are few data to assist selection of the type and setting of treatment intervention (Steinhausen & Glanville, 1983). As an alternative to full hospitalization, Danziger et al. (1988) treated 32 adolescents in a day treatment refeeding program that actively involved parents. At an average of 9 months after admission, 84% had reached and retained their ideal weight, 89% had resumed menstruation, 59% overcame body image distortions, and 88% stopped ritualistic exercise. Although the involvement of parents was regarded as very helpful, there were no formal measures of parental responses to the program. Operant conditioning programs have been shown to be effective in short-term weight gain, but there is no information about effects on the broader spectrum of pathology (Bemis, 1987).

Psychotherapeutic Approaches

The main approaches used with adolescent patients with anorexia are individual psychotherapy, behavior therapy, and family therapy. Steinhausen (1995) cautions that most experience comes from the treatment of adults, and also notes that individual psychotherapy requires the child to be motivated and to have the capacity to engage in therapy—factors that may not be present with very ill children.

BEHAVIORAL THERAPIES

Lacey (1983), Lee and Rush (1986), and Wolchik et al. (1986) found cognitive and behavior therapy techniques effective in reducing eating disorder symptoms when compared to wait-list controls. However, in a contrast of behavior modification and milieu therapy, Eckert et al. (1979) found no significant difference in weight gain between the two groups, nor was there any difference in long-term outcome. In a controlled outcome study, Channon et al. (1989) also failed to find significant differences between CBT, behavior therapy, and a no-treatment group of patients presenting with anorexia nervosa.

INDIVIDUAL AND FAMILY THERAPY

Russell et al. (1987) compared 1 year of family therapy or individual supportive therapy in 80 patients. Family therapy was found to be more effective than individual therapy in patients whose illness was not chronic and had begun before the age of 19 years. In older patients, individual supportive therapy tended to be more effective than family therapy in terms of weight gain, but the improvement fell short of recovery in most patients. Gowers et al. (1994) randomized 90 patients with anorexia to one inpatient and two outpatient groups, and one group offering an assessment interview only; thus, 20 patients received a package of outpatient individual and family psychotherapy. At 2-year follow-up, 12 of these 20 patients were classed as well, or very nearly well, according to operational defined criteria, with statistically significant improvements for weight and psychosocial adjustment (replicating an earlier finding of Hall & Crisp, 1983). Positive results were also obtained with conjoint family therapy and individual therapy in adolescents with recent-onset anorexia nervosa. At 5-year follow-up (Robin et al., 1995), improvement was most evident in patients with early onset and a short history. Results favored family therapy for patients with early onset and a short history of anorexia nervosa, and individual supportive therapy for patients with late-onset anorexia nervosa.

Robin and colleagues (1994, 1999) randomized 37 adolescent girls with anorexia either to behavioral family therapy or to ego-oriented individual therapy (EOIT). Each patient received 10–16 months of therapy, was assessed at posttherapy, and followed up at 1, 2.5, and 4 years. Both treatments were effective; two-thirds of the girls reached their target weights by the end of treatment, and at 1-year follow-up, 80% of those receiving family therapy and 69% of those treated individually had reached their target weights (a difference that was not statistically significant). Both therapies produced equally large improvements in attitudes toward eating and depressed affect and family functioning (Robin et al., 1995). Robin and colleagues concluded that parental involvement was essential to the success of their interventions for younger adolescents with anorexia nervosa, but that family dynamics could still be influenced without requiring the adolescent and her parents to be in the room together for all therapy sessions.

Dodge and colleagues (Dodge et al., 1995) reported an exploratory study of family therapy for bulimia nervosa in eight adolescents ages 14–17 years. Their approach to family therapy was based on the model developed by Eisler (1988) and Dare and Szmukler (1991). At 1-year follow-up, bulimic behaviors were significantly reduced, although patients continued to show symptoms. Schwartz and colleagues (1985) implemented a structural model of family therapy with 30 consecutive adolescent and adult bulimic referrals over a 9-month period; 66% of patients achieved abstinence from bulimic symptoms or had less than one episode per month.

Summary

Most psychosocial approaches to anorexia nervosa combine operant techniques for weight gain with other treatment techniques aiming to alter irrational beliefs, disturbance of body image, anxiety, poor interpersonal skills, and dysfunctional eating behavior; these have been shown to be effective in short-term weight gain. No particular benefit has been found for cognitive-behavioral treatments over other forms of brief psychotherapy. Although there is clinical consensus that multifaceted treatment programs are effective, there has been little evaluation of the effects of different components of treatment for different patients.

Family therapy appears to be somewhat more successful than individual therapy in patients with onset of anorexia before the age of 19 years and whose illness is not chronic. Family change may not be necessary to achieve individual change, and individual change appears to result in some family change. Individual psychodynamic therapy shows benefit in those with late-onset anorexia and may contribute to the prevention of relapses after discharge from hospital treatment. Evidence for the efficacy of family therapy in bulimia is equivocal. As yet, there is no evidence for the efficacy of cognitive-behavioral treatment of bulimia in children and adolescents.

Posttraumatic Stress Disorder

Definition

Trauma of various kinds is strongly associated with psychopathology, particularly emotional (e.g., Kliewer et al., 1998) and behavioral (e.g., Farrell & Bruce, 1997) problems, as well as developmental delay (e.g., Delaney-Black et al., 2002). Children who have subthreshold posttraumatic stress disorder (PTSD) have similar problems to those who meet full diagnostic criteria (Carrion et al., 2002). For example, follow-up studies of sexually abused children have identified both short- and long-term effects, including depression, anxiety, and eating disorders (Beitchman et al., 1991, 1992; Trowell et al., 1999). About 55% of children show substantial recovery from psychological symptoms over the 1 to 2 years after presenting, but 10–24% appear to become worse (Kendall-Tackett et al., 1993). The prevalence of posttraumatic reaction to some degree depends on the nature of the trauma. The large majority of children who are exposed to violence, either as witnesses or victims, experience some symptoms of PTSD, with a substantial minority meeting full diagnostic criteria (Berman et al., 1996; Cuffe et al., 1998; Horowitz et al., 1995).

Psychosocial Treatment Interventions

TREATMENTS FOR TRAUMA ASSOCIATED WITH A SINGLE-INCIDENT STRESSOR: NATURAL DISASTERS AND EXPOSURE TO VIOLENCE

With the exception of one small, poorly controlled investigation (Stallard & Law, 1993), there are no outcome studies of psychological debriefing with children. This should be a source of concern given the high prevalence of this type of intervention and evidence of its potential ill-effects in adult PTSD sufferers (see Chapter 8).

March et al. (1998) reported assessment outcomes from an 18-week group CBT program for youths with PSTD consequent to a single-incident stressor. Fourteen of 17 subjects completed treatment and, of these, 57% no longer met PTSD criteria after treatment and 86% no longer met criteria at 6-month follow-up. Benefit was also observed in the level of depression, anxiety, and anger. An exploratory study (Salloum et al., 2001) evaluated the effectiveness of time-limited group psychotherapy for 45 adolescents between ages 11 and 19 years who had a loved one die because of violence.

Posttherapy, participants reported a clinically significant decrease in traumatic symptoms, especially in the areas of reexperiencing and avoidance symptoms.

Goenjian et al. (1997) reported on the outcome of psychotherapeutically treated and untreated earthquake victims 1.5 years (pretreatment) and 3 years (posttreatment) after the earthquake. While the severity of PTSD symptoms significantly decreased among recipients of trauma/grief-focused brief psychotherapy, symptoms significantly worsened among untreated subjects.

Pynoos and colleagues developed a program for adolescents who experienced or witnessed violence (Layne et al., 2001a). The UCLA School-Based Trauma/Grief Intervention Program for children and adolescents includes a systematic method for screening students, a manualized 16- to 20-week group psychotherapy protocol, and adjunctive individual and family therapy, Saltzman et al. (2001) found that the screening procedure identified 58 (from 812) students with PTSD symptoms and functional impairment, of whom 26 agreed to participate. Participation was associated with improvements in trauma-related symptoms and in academic performance. The same group assessed a modification of this protocol for 55 war-traumatized Bosnian adolescents (Layne et al., 2001b; Soberman et al., 2002). There was an observed reduction in psychological distress and positive associations between distress reduction and improved psychosocial adaptation.

Chemtob et al. (2002b) evaluated the efficacy school-based screening and psychosocial treatment that identified 248 children with persistent trauma symptoms from 4,258 children in second through sixth grade who had been exposed to a hurricane. Children were randomly assigned to one of three consecutively treated cohorts, with those awaiting treatment serving as wait-list controls. Within each cohort, children were randomly assigned to four sessions of either individual ($n = 73$) or group treatment ($n = 176$). Though group and individual treatments did not differ in efficacy, treated children showed reductions in observed and self-reported trauma-related symptoms, which were maintained at the 1-year follow-up.

Chemtob, Nakashima, and Carlson (2002a) reported a controlled study of eye movement desensitization and reprocessing (EMDR) in children who had not responded to the brief intervention described earlier at 1-year follow-up. Three sessions of EMDR treatment were provided to 32 children, resulting in substantial reductions in PTSD scores (pre- to posteffect size = 1.55), with gains maintained at 6-month follow-up. A study of 29 adolescent boys drawn from a similar clinical population and treated with EMDR also showed large and significant reductions in memory-related distress (Soberman et al., 2002). studies In contrast, adding EMDR to routine treatment of 39 children in a child guidance center appeared to confer no additional benefit (Rubin et al., 2001).

TREATMENTS FOR POSTTRAUMATIC STRESS DISORDER FOLLOWING SEXUAL ABUSE

Maltreatment or sexual abuse rarely takes the form of a single overwhelming incident but usually involves prolonged exposure to highly stressful situations. Most research focuses on trauma related to sexual abuse.

Naturalistic studies offer mixed support for the value of psychosocial interventions in ameliorating the effects of childhood sexual abuse (CSA). At 5-year follow-up of 68 girls treated as victims of CSA, only 44% of those who were symptomatic at intake were improved at follow-up (Tebbutt et al., 1997). Furthermore, 41% of those who were asymptomatic at intake had deteriorated following treatment. In another naturalistic study of 64 children treated for an average of 9 months (Oates et al., 1994), 65% failed to change, and 48% remained in the dysfunctional range for behavior, and 35% for depression. There was no relationship between outcome and being in receipt of therapy, or the type or length of therapy.

A trial of CBT (Deblinger et al., 1996, 1999) assigned 100 school-age children with a history of CSA to one of four conditions: child-focused, mother-focused, mother and child combined, and standard community care control. The mother-only condition incorporated parent training and psychoeducation. All three active treatments were superior to standard care, with improvements maintained at 2-year follow-up (though treatment continued during the follow-up period, and attrition was high). Inclusion of parents resulted in greater improvement in the child's depression. A replication (Deblinger et al., 2001) explored the comparative effectiveness of supportive and cognitive-behavioral group therapy designed for young children (ages 2–8) with CSA and their nonoffending mothers. Mothers who participated in CBT groups reported greater reductions at posttest in their intrusive thoughts and negative parental emotional reactions regarding the sexual abuse.

These findings are consistent with those of Cohen and Mannarino (1996, 1997) who assigned 67 sexually abused preschool children and their parents either to 12 sessions of CBT adapted for sexually abused preschool children or to nondirective supportive therapy, acting as a control treatment. Those receiving CBT showed significantly greater symptomatic improvement on most outcome measures than controls. A further study (Cohen & Mannarino, 1998), assigned 49 recently sexually abused children (ages 7–14) and their nonoffending parent to 12 sessions of CBT or to a supportive therapy control. Children in the CBT group improved more on measures of depression and social competence.

Trowell et al. (2002) randomized 71 sexually abused girls to either 30 sessions of individual psychoanalytic psychotherapy or 18 sessions of group psychotherapy with psychoeducational components. Both treatments generated substantial improvements, but individual treatment had somewhat more powerful effects on PTSD symptoms.

Summary

The published literature of the treatment of PTSD in children is at an early phase. A number of studies suggest the efficacy of trauma-specific CBT in improving PTSD symptoms and associated depression, anxiety, and social functioning. Evidence regarding the status of EMDR is mixed. Although other psychotherapeutic approaches have been tested and show promise in both single-trauma and chronic or multiple-trauma-related conditions, evidence here is less strong, with no randomized controlled trial showing superiority to an active control group.

SUMMARY AND CLINICAL IMPLICATIONS

Epidemiological studies consistently report surprisingly high prevalence rates of diagnosable psychiatric disorders (at around 20%) in children and young people. Thus, for moderate and severe disorders, the frequent assumption that childhood problems are transient is clearly not justified. Another common belief is that what works for adults should also work for children. It is fairly easy to demonstrate that this belief is unjustified. For example, some drugs work in different (often opposite) ways in children and may have different side effects, and some psychosocial therapies (such as those relying on more mature cognitive capacities like abstract thinking) cannot be offered to children without extensive modification and testing. It is therefore vital to develop and evaluate therapies specifically for child and adolescent psychiatric disorders. However, it must be acknowledged that the current state of the research literature on the outcome of child treatments is sparse and somewhat less methodologically sophisticated than that available for adult disorders. It is worth highlighting some methodological and ethical issues specific to research with children that lie behind this relative dearth of evidence and that lead to problems in mounting well-designed studies as well as inherent difficulties in measuring outcomes. These difficulties include the following:

1. *Ethical issues.* There can be great difficulty in obtaining an ethical review board's agreement to conduct studies with children, reflecting the tension between methodological adequacy and clinical probity. This arises because children do not usually seek treatment themselves, and the consent of their parents may not fully safeguard their wishes and rights. This can mean that the design of a study, and hence its capacity to answer the research question, is compromised. For example, boards and researchers may be uneasy about leaving children untreated and commit to trials that compare two active treatments before either has convincingly been shown to be superior to an untreated control group (thus producing unclear evidence on the efficacy

of either). Or they include an untreated control group but treat the participants before a follow-up comparison can be made (see also point 4, below).

2. *Comorbidity*. Comorbidity is a substantial problem in both treatment
and outcome research; indeed, it is the rule rather than the exception in child
mental health. Despite this fact, until recently, its presence was treated as
grounds for exclusion from studies of treatment effectiveness for any specific
disorder (e.g., comorbid depression would exclude a child from a treatment
trial for conduct disorder). Fortunately, more recent studies now include
children with comorbid diagnoses, and the impact of these complicating concurrent problems is gradually being clarified. This is essential, as the prevalence of comorbidity in clinically referred children had made it very hard to
generalize from much of the outcome research in the field.

3. *Inconsistency between informants*. Assessment of outcome is often inconsistent, as rated from different perspectives: children's internalizing problems
often go unnoticed by adults, whereas externalizing disorders can be denied
by children; furthermore, children can behave very differently in different
contexts. Thus, there is very low agreement among parents, children, teachers, and clinicians on level of symptoms, making the outcome of an intervention difficult to judge decisively. This issue is not fully resolvable, as researchers make pragmatic decisions in the context of a particular trial. For example,
in evaluating the treatment of ADHD, the child's rating of his/her symptoms
might be given less weight than those of adults who observe him/her, and
care should be taken to include ratings from both home and school. However, the need for flexibility about which measures of outcome to use introduces the danger that measures that have been found to show significant differences will be selected for report. To avoid exaggerated claims of efficacy, it
is vital that appropriate measures for a trial are chosen and the analyses
planned in advance of the results.

4. *Developmental issues*. Development creates a constantly changing
background against which a child's functioning and symptomatology are to
be judged. There is a well-documented tendency for one disorder to evolve
into another, with or without treatment; for instance, prepubertal girls who
are disruptive commonly become anxious/depressed adolescents, while for
boys it is the opposite. These normal developmental shifts obscure the effects
of concurrent treatment of the original disorders, especially if the treatment is
medium to long term (which would be normal for entrenched and complex
cases such as those referred to specialist services). When evaluating longer-
term interventions and when conducting follow-up assessments over a period
of at least a year (as is highly desirable), it is therefore necessary to include
well-chosen control groups. Although this may seem obvious, it in fact raises
a difficult ethical problem: a common design is to have a wait-list control
group for the period of the intervention, then to offer the same intervention
to the control-group children during the follow-up period of the first-treated

group (assuming that they improved more than the untreated children during the treatment phase). While this reduces the ethical difficulty of leaving distressed or disruptive children untreated, it creates the problem of evaluating maintenance of gains over follow-up, since there are then no untreated children for a comparison with ordinary developmental changes.

  5. *The need for parents and teachers to participate in treatment.* This need goes far beyond the need to request consent and cooperation from more people. Parents, teachers, and sometimes others in the child's environment are expected to act as therapists in many interventions (e.g., for disruptive behavior). Where this occurs, it is likely to improve maintenance of change, but in clinical settings, families may be unable or unwilling to do what is required. The serious consequence of this for evaluation research is that the results gained with more motivated and cooperative families may not generalize to the range of cases seen in clinics.

  Despite these and other methodological challenges, researchers have become increasingly engaged with providing studies that can be generalized to "real world" settings. Recent research is showing results in certain areas of child mental health treatment. Good examples include efforts to deliver parent training and problem-solving skills training and programs for conduct disorder that increase their effectiveness in clinical settings. The evidence base in other areas remains more sparse, and at this point, there are few studies of treatment for complex emotional disorders and longer-term, more intensive treatments.

  For clarity, we will review the efficacy of different treatment approaches in turn. Across the range of childhood disorders, most outcome studies have focused on behavioral treatment (BT) or CBT. For this reason, we start with a summary of findings regarding these treatment approaches.

  Behavioral techniques are often effective in the treatment of circumscribed phobias, especially in younger children. Older children and adolescents are most often offered a combination of cognitive and behavioral techniques, and there is little evaluation of BT alone for these age groups. OCD can be improved in some cases, though generally not eliminated, by a CBT approach. Certain CBT techniques have been shown to be effective in the treatment of generalized and other anxiety disorders, and those children who improve tend to maintain their gains. There is accumulating evidence that CBT for childhood anxiety disorders can be as successfully delivered in a group as in an individual format. Adding a family component to CBT is often useful for younger children and for families in which parental anxiety is also high. The treatment of PTSD in children is at an early phase of development. A number of studies suggest that trauma-specific CBT improves PTSD symptoms and associated depression and anxiety.

CBT in the treatment of childhood depression appears to be effective, whether provided individually or in a group. However, it has mainly been tested with mildly to moderately impaired adolescents, rather than with severe adolescent cases or preadolescent children. Family factors can reduce treatment response. And providing longer courses of CBT (or booster sessions) may hasten recovery when a standard length of treatment has not succeeded. IPT-A is a promising treatment for adolescent depression.

Psychosocial approaches to anorexia nervosa usually combine operant techniques for weight gain with other treatment techniques aiming to alter irrational beliefs, disturbance of body image, anxiety, poor interpersonal skills, and dysfunctional eating behavior. These approaches have been shown to be effective in short-term weight gain. No particular benefit has been found from CBT over other forms of brief psychotherapy. As yet, there is no evidence of the efficacy of CBT of bulimia in children and adolescents.

Some of the secondary problems associated with autism have been shown to respond to behavioral management, but core social and communicative abnormalities are more resistant. Interventions need to be intensive and bridge both home and school.

Families of children with Tourette syndrome generally report only short-term benefits from behavioral interventions. While psychotherapy or supportive interventions may be useful in helping children and families cope with this syndrome, there have been no controlled studies of their use.

Many therapy programs for children have delivered BT or CBT through the parents, particularly for children with conduct problems. This of course relies on parental availability, motivation, and capacity to act as therapists. For young children with conduct problems, parent training is highly effective. Studies increasingly try to address comorbidity, severity, and parental and social problems, all of which threaten the efficacy of these programs. The variety of programs available and the need to train more therapists in these techniques represent a challenge to dissemination. These interventions have become longer and now include children and teachers, which improves generalization. Problem-solving skills training is particularly effective when offered in combination with parent training, and this combination is the treatment of choice for conduct problems in children between 8 and 12. For adolescents, the strongest evidence of benefit is from multisystemic approaches, which involve working with parents and with the wider community. However because of the complexity and intensity of these approaches, they are not yet widely available.

In cases of ADHD, intensive BT in the presence of comorbid anxiety and higher parental education has been shown to be beneficial. Parent training improves compliance with instructions, but not all families are able to persist with the approach. A number of classroom-based programs have been evaluated. Although these show efficacy, they tend not to generalize to other settings, and their impact is lost after the program is completed. There is some (though limited) evidence that brief eclectic group therapy with the families of adolescents following a suicide attempt can diminish adolescents' feelings of depression and suicidality, and improve family involvement with the adolescent (and hence further compliance with specialist programs).

Although there is clinical consensus that multifaceted treatment programs are effective for eating disorders, there has been little evaluation of the effects of different components of treatment for different patients. Family therapy appears to be somewhat more successful than individual therapy in patients with anorexia with onset before the age of 19 years and whose illness is not chronic. Evidence for the efficacy of family therapy in bulimia is equivocal.

Although there has been some limited research on family therapy (as mentioned above) and other approaches such as individual psychodynamic therapy, in general there is a marked contrast with the amount of work done on evaluating BT and CBT (and psychopharmacology, which is beyond the scope of this book). Family therapy, and parent work in parallel with individual treatment for the child, have rarely been evaluated, despite the fact that these are probably the most frequent psychosocial approaches in routine clinical work. Social skills training and individual child psychotherapy have also been minimally tested as yet, although there is preliminary evidence that psychodynamic psychotherapy may be effective in the treatment of emotional disorders (anxiety and depression, particularly where this is comorbid with other problems). Individual psychodynamic therapy has also been shown to be beneficial in treating late-onset anorexia and may contribute to the prevention of relapses after discharge from hospital treatment. A high priority is the investigation of often used (but rarely evaluated) treatments, such as psychodynamic and family approaches.

Many clinicians point out that when attempting to implement research evidence, they are rarely confronted with a child with a clear-cut psychiatric disorder within a supportive family. This challenge to implementation raises questions about the utility of outcome research for clinical services. Frequently, families seen by child mental health teams present with some combination of social, marital, and mental health problems, with children who are often unhappy or "difficult" and need help with a number of maladaptive symptoms that do not fit neatly into a diagnostic category. This family situation makes it harder for clinicians to apply available treatment research because it is modeled on the adult literature and hence based on identified disorders in single individuals. There is also evidence that the long-term outcome of childhood disorders is a function of children's social background as well as their symptomatology. On this basis, a high priority should be given to developing measures that include family as well as individual functioning and enable assessment of the child's functioning within a social context. A linked issue is that treatment outcome has generally been defined by a change in symptoms and diagnostic status, leading to neglect of other important indices of functioning, such as peer relationships, academic performance, and range of activity and interests. Including these indicators of adaptation, along with symptomatology and diagnosis, would allow more fine-tuned and relevant assessments of the efficacy of treatments for childhood disorders.

Since a diagnostic approach to treatment planning can create barriers to the implementation of an evidence-based approach, it may be helpful, certainly initially, to adopt a broader framework that includes systemic or psychodynamic thinking aimed at understanding what is creating and maintaining stress on the child. This first step does not dictate what form of treatment will be most appropriate. For instance, CBT practitioners could consider systemic and sometimes psychodynamic ideas along with other perspectives, such as educational and biological considerations, to formulate the child's situation and take these into account when deriving a treatment program that maintains broad adherence to the CBT model. This may go part of the way toward interpreting a research literature based on the idea of one treatment for one disorder in one person and restoring the multidimensional and multidisciplinary perspectives essential to working with families. The success of multimodal or multisystemic approaches for young people reflects this reality.

In many respects, the field is at too early a stage to make many evidence-based recommendations about which treatments show the most benefit for which disorders. Conclusions regarding efficacy are limited by the fact that there are not enough large-scale and methodologically rigorous studies for many combinations of treatment and disorder. Even where there is evidence of efficacy, the complexity of presentations in clinical practice is rarely reflected in trials, constraining comments on effectiveness. Moving forward from this conclusion is important, but given the complexity of the task it is not a simple matter of suggesting that more basic research is required, even though this statement is accurate. Equally important is the systematic development of pragmatic trials that can examine the impact of adapting therapeutic strategies based on current knowledge to meet common challenges in clinical practice, such as comorbidity, the parallel implementation of a range of treatments that address difficulties at both individual and systems levels, and the need to ensure that gains are sustainable in the longer term.

CHAPTER 15

EFFECTIVENESS OF PSYCHOLOGICAL INTERVENTIONS WITH OLDER PEOPLE

Robert Woods and Anthony Roth

The literature on psychological interventions with older people "reflects a field still early in its conceptual and research development in which, even in the most explored areas, the research base is suggestive but not definitive" (Smyer et al., 1990, p. 376). A decade or so later, this comment still rings true, perhaps because older people are less likely to receive psychological treatment than younger adults, despite a similar prevalence of psychological problems (such as depression) and a greatly increased prevalence of the dementias, with their well-known impact on immediate family caregivers and the wider community.

PSYCHOLOGICAL PROBLEMS OF LATE LIFE

Definitions

The diagnostic criteria for functional disorders in older people are the same as those used elsewhere in this review. The purpose of treating this group separately rests on two considerations: (1) that the anticipated response to psychological interventions in older people cannot be assumed to be the same as in younger adult samples, in the same way that the efficacy of treatments of childhood disorders is normally considered separately from its impacts with adults; and (2) that the higher prevalence of organic problems, both of central nervous system (CNS) and non–CNS origin, often complicate the application of psychological interventions, and hence necessitates separate evaluation.

Prevalence, Comorbidity, and Natural History

Lindesay et al. (1989) reported the prevalence rates of depression and anxiety in an urban elderly population (Table 15.1). There appears to be a lower prevalence of anxiety disorders in older people than in other age groups. Generalized anxiety disorder (GAD) and specific phobias are the most common diagnoses, each of these conditions being extensively comorbid with depression (Flint, 1994). Obsessive–compulsive disorder is relatively rarely encountered in older people (Stanley & Beck, 2000), and most surveys report very low rates for panic disorders. This may reflect diagnostic criteria requiring three panic attacks in the preceding 3 weeks for the diagnosis to be made; older people may well prevent such attacks by avoidance strategies, but at the expense of greater dependence and disability (Livingston & Hinchliffe, 1993).

In depression, a number of prognostic studies have been reported, although these reflect the usual treatment (nearly always medication) received. Around one-third of patients with depression remain depressed 3 years later, with only around 20% sustaining a complete recovery (Livingston & Hinchliffe, 1993). Denihan et al. (2000) showed that only 10% of older people with depression, identified in a large community-based epidemiological survey, were in complete remission 3 years later. Thirty-five percent were depressed and 25% had other mental health difficulties. Around one-third had died in the follow-up period. In the shorter term, Burvill (1993) suggested that around half (47%) make a complete recovery and do not relapse

TABLE 15.1 Prevalence of Depression and Anxiety Disorders in an Urban Community Sample of Older People

Disorder	Prevalence (%)
Severe depression	4.3
Mild/moderate depression	13.5
Generalized anxiety	3.7
Panic disorder	0.0
Phobic disorders	
Agoraphobia	7.8
Social phobia	1.3
Specific phobia	2.1
Total	10.0
Total without co-occurring depression	6.1

Note. Data from Lindesay et al. (1989).

within a year; 18% recover but then relapse within 12 months; 24% remain depressed or make only a partial recovery; in this study, 11% died within the year. Although there has been much debate regarding the interpretation of such figures (e.g., Baldwin, 1991), it is clear that a substantial number of older people with depression do not recover with the standard treatments, and that relapse is a major issue.

The natural history of anxiety disorders in older people has not been adequately investigated. However, Sullivan et al. (1988) reported a community survey of over 1,000 older people in Liverpool, showing that 12.8% were taking benzodiazepine medication initially; at 3-year follow-up, over 60% of these individuals continued to do so. At follow-up, over 10% of the total sample was taking benzodiazepines as a sleeping medication, reflecting the prevalence of sleep disorders in older people. Morgan (1987) reviewed the prevalence of sleep disorders; surveys suggest that 20% of men and nearly 30% of women age 70 and over report "trouble with sleeping often or all the time." In addition, around a further 25% of both men and women report sometimes having trouble with sleep. These figures are much higher than for younger age groups. They are reflected in studies showing that "on average, about 10–15% of the elderly population living at home consume prescribed hypnotic drugs" (Morgan, 1987, p. 85).

The prevalence of the dementias has been the subject of numerous epidemiological studies internationally. While there are a number of differences between studies, there is broad agreement that the prevalence doubles for each increase of 5 years; 5% of persons over 65 and 20% of those over 80 are widely accepted figures (Livingston & Hinchliffe, 1993; Paykel et al., 1994). The prognosis of the dementias should perhaps, by definition be poor, and this is confirmed by most follow-up studies; however, when early cases are included, a proportion may show little deterioration for up to 4 years (Livingston & Hinchliffe, 1993).

The recognition of dementia as a major source of psychological dysfunction in older people also entails a broadening of the view of psychological treatment from a one-to-one, patient-and-therapist endeavor to include families and other caregivers. Morris et al. (1988) reviewed the impact in terms of strain and depression on family caregivers of older people with dementia, many of whom were themselves over age 65. Estimates of levels of strain and depression in carers do show considerable variation, depending on sample characteristics and measures used. Many samples have comprised those known to services, who may have come to attention through having high stress levels. Estimates from 14 to 40% are reported for depression and 33 to 68% for distress at a level of psychiatric "caseness" (using the General Health Questionnaire [GHQ]). Follow-up studies suggest an increase in GHQ scores, unless the person with dementia is admitted to long-term care (Levin et al., 1989) or receives skilled community support (Woods et al., 2003).

It is worth considering why older people do not receive equitable access to psychological treatment. Taking initial contacts with clinical psychologists in the United Kingdom as a crude index, in 2002–2003, only 11% were with people over 65, despite their forming approximately 16% of the total population; a person age 16–54 was 1.7 times more likely to have an initial contact with a clinical psychologist than someone age 65+ (Department of Health, 2003). Although blame is sometimes attributed to Freud himself for considering psychotherapy with older people inappropriate, other factors may be more relevant. These include a reluctance by therapists themselves to treat older people, perhaps reflecting some of the complexities of their countertransference with older people who may be in poor physical health and be viewed as close to death (Weiss & Lazarus, 1993). In the United States, it is suggested that older people's psychological problems are not identified in primary care, and appropriate referrals are not made (Smyer et al., 1990). There is evidence from three surveys that family physicians in the United Kingdom are reasonably accurate in identifying depression and dementia in their patients. However, cases of depression were sometimes incorrectly identified as dementia, and there were indications of underdiagnosis, low rates of referral to tertiary care, and low use of antidepressant medication (Iliffe et al., 1991; MacDonald, 1986; O'Connor et al., 1988). Finally, older people themselves may be less psychologically minded and less likely to seek to initiate the referral themselves, though we may expect to see changing expectations with future generations of older people.

It is important to reflect that within the arbitrary category of older people (defined in the United Kingdom as over statutory retirement age), we are discussing a broad age band of 30 or so years and a diversity of life experiences and life stages; generalizations must be treated cautiously.

Treatment Approaches

Treatments for Anxiety Disorders

There are now available some well-conducted randomized controlled trials (RCTs) evaluating the effectiveness of psychological therapies with persons with anxiety disorders in later life, though many earlier trials are more problematic. A meta-analytic review by Nordhus and Pallesen (2003) identified 15 studies published between 1975 and 2002. The majority of studies solicited participants rather than utilizing samples of referred patients, and many earlier trials comprise patients seeking help for "subjective anxiety," making it difficult to relate patients' presenting problems to current diagnostic criteria. Six trials focus on GAD, and two on panic disorder. Contrast of psychosocial treatment (almost invariably cognitive-behavioral therapy [CBT]) was made to a control condition or to another treatment, yielding an overall effect size of 0.55. The authors note that while very recent trials report longer follow-up, this is not the case for earlier studies, making it difficult to comment on the durability of treatment effects.

TREATMENTS FOR GENERALIZED ANXIETY DISORDER

Stanley and Novy (2000) reviewed evidence of treatment efficacy for GAD in older adults, noting that most reports comprise case studies or very small trials. However, a small number of RCTs are now available. Stanley et al. (1996) recruited 48 older adults (ages 55–81), allocating them to CBT or supportive therapy, with treatments delivered in group format over 14 weeks. Both interventions resulted in a significant decrease in symptoms—at 6-month follow-up, 50 and 77% of patients receiving CBT and supportive therapy, respectively, were classified as responders. A later trial by this same group (Stanley et al., 2003) contrasted group-based CBT against a minimal-contact (MC) condition in which patients received a weekly monitoring telephone call and were offered a low level of support. There were 85 participants, all age 60 and above (mean age, 66.2), meeting DSM-IV-TR criteria for GAD but, in this study, not receiving any concurrent anxiolytic or antidepressant medication. CBT sessions occurred weekly in small groups over a 15-week period. During the treatment period, 45% of the CBT patients showed a clear response to treatment, compared with 8% of the MC group. At 1-year follow-up, only 19% of the CBT participants still met diagnostic criteria for GAD. Significant gains made by the CBT group during the treatment phase, in worry, anxiety, depression, and quality of life, were maintained or enhanced over the follow-up period.

Wetherell et al. (2003) included a discussion group (addressing topics related to worries and anxieties) and a wait-list control group in their comparison. All 75 participants had a principal diagnosis of GAD, according to DSM-IV-TR criteria; all were age 55 and over (mean age, 67.1); they had been stabilized for at least 2 months on any psychotropic medication. Those in the active conditions attended 12 weekly, 90-minute sessions described as "worry reduction classes" in groups of four to six people, held in a convenient community location. CBT groups included relaxation training, cognitive restructuring, and "worry exposure" (i.e., exposure to worrying thoughts and situations in a graded manner). Discussion groups involved information sharing, peer support, validation, and supportive listening on topics such as health concerns, memory loss, and loss of independence. Participants in both groups were asked to carry out daily, 30-minute homework assignments. Both conditions showed improvements compared with wait-list controls, with CBT participants tending to show greater change. However, at 6-month follow-up, there was no difference between groups. Effect sizes were described as large (0.97) for CBT and medium (0.51) for discussion groups. At follow-up, only 28% of the CBT group still met the diagnostic criteria for GAD (compared with 47% of discussion group participants).

All these trials deliver treatments in group format; an exception is a study by Mohlman et al. (2003), which reports on the effectiveness of two forms of CBT, one adapted to the needs of older adults by the inclusion of learning and memory aids. Although initial results suggest additional gains for the enhanced over standard treatment, a controlled trial is required in order to evaluate its benefits.

TREATMENTS FOR MIXED ANXIETY DISORDERS

Barrowclough et al.'s (2001) study included patients with a range of anxiety disorders and probably reflects better the spectrum of problems encountered in clinical practice. This trial compared individual CBT with supportive counseling (SC), using a 6-week baseline phase before the commencement of therapy to give an indication of the impact of no treatment. There were 55 participants meeting DSM-IV-TR criteria for anxiety disorders; 51% had panic disorders and 19% had GAD. Mean age of the sample was 72, with only one participant between ages 55 and 60. Therapy was usually conducted in the patient's home, as is common practice in the United Kingdom, with patients receiving 8–12 sessions over a 16-week period. All the patients were on anxiolytic or antidepressant medication (or both), but this had been stabilized for at least 3 months. The CBT approach used involved detailed assessment of the anxiety problems and a shared formulation; verbal and behavioral reattribution techniques were used to challenge dysfunctional cognitions and maladaptive behaviors. No changes were evident over the baseline period. At the end of the treatment period, there were significant changes in favor of the CBT group on self-rated measures of anxiety and depression, although the SC group also improved. At 12-month follow-up, 71% of CBT patients met criteria for having responded to treatment, compared with 39% of the SC group. There was also a good treatment response for comorbid depression, although the groups did not show a significant difference on this outcome (59% for CBT, 39% for SC). Effect sizes for CBT were large, averaging 1.3 across anxiety measures at 12 months.

Both Wetherell et al. (2003) and Stanley et al. (2003) comment that, compared with published reports involving younger people, CBT appears to be less effective in these studies of older adults with anxiety disorders. Three issues are relevant here: first, it is probable that group treatment is less effective than individual treatment. Both their studies involved group formats, whereas most of the outcome literature on younger people involves individualized treatment. Barrowclough et al.'s (2001) findings tend to support this position, although a comparative study would be required to confirm it. Second, many of the patients in these studies of older people with anxiety disorders have had anxiety symptoms for many years (an average of 20 years in Barrowclough et al.'s sample; almost 30 years in Wetherell et al.'s [2003] group), which may reduce treatment effectiveness. Finally, many participants had concurrent physical health problems (only 19% of the Barrowclough et al. (2001) sample had no physical health problem; Wetherell et al. (2003) reported an average of 6.8 medical conditions for their population), and this may also be a factor that influences comparative outcomes.

Benzodiazepine Addiction. As noted earlier, a large number of older people (13% in Liverpool, United Kingdom [Sullivan et al., 1988]; 17.3% in Dublin, Ireland [Kirby et al., 1999]) are prescribed benzodiazepine medication, in many cases as an anxiolytic, often for a considerable period of time. Apart from a general concern about their long-term use, there are specific concerns about their use with older people, and possible links with falls and confusion (Higgitt, 1992). Some older people are responding to the widespread publicity and are themselves requesting help to withdraw from benzodiazepine use, and there is some evidence that psychological techniques such as anxiety management, support in gradual withdrawal, and reappraisal of symptoms are helpful to older people in this process. Jones (1990/1991) reported on an RCT in primary care settings; 227 patients completed the study; 39% of treated cases, compared with 20% of controls, succeeded in reducing or stopping their medication over the 9-month period of the trial. Treatment was provided by a practice nurse offering counseling and relaxation therapy, under the supervision of a clinical psychologist. Curran et al. (2003) offered older people who were receiving repeat benzodiazepine prescriptions for sleep problems in primary care the opportunity to withdraw. Of those interviewed, 57% accepted the offer; Curran et al. reported that straightforward advice regarding strategies to promote sleep, together with tapered withdrawal, enabled 80% of those participating in the program to withdraw from their benzodiazepine hypnotics, with no negative impact on sleep quantity or quality, but with some improvement in cognitive function.

Treatments for Depression

Scogin and McElreath (1994) reviewed 17 comparative trials of psychosocial treatments for depression in a total of 765 adults over age 60. All studies included a control condition, which was either no-treatment or delayed treatment, a placebo condition or an alternative psychosocial intervention. However, only four (23%) of these studies included patients with a formal diagnosis of major depressive disorder; 10 (59%) included patients with clinical and subclinical levels of depression, and three (18%) focused only on patients with subclinical levels of depression. At least one study included patients with a diagnosis of dementia.

The mean effect size for any psychosocial treatment versus no treatment or a placebo was 0.78. Comparison of the four studies using only clinically depressed patients with the remaining studies yielded almost exactly equivalent effect sizes (0.76 and 0.79, respectively). Estimates of improvement based on self-report yielded lower effect sizes than those based on clinician's ratings (0.69 vs. 1.15). Because of the small number of studies, only limited exploration of the impact of specific therapies was possible. Cognitive therapy was employed in seven studies, yielding an effect size against no treatment or placebo of 0.85. Based on data from eight trials, reminiscence therapy yielded an effect size of 1.05, again against no treatment or placebo. Comparison between different therapies did not suggest any superiority for any one modality over the other. Subsequent reviews by Cuijpers (1998) and Koder et al. (1996) (who took a stricter definition of cognitive therapy) have reported similarly large effect sizes, with Cuijpers (1998) concluding that CBT is more effective than other psychological therapies in this context.

These effect sizes are clearly comparable with those computed by Robinson et al. (1990) in their broader review of treatments for depression (discussed further in Chapter 4). While it is tempting to compare effect sizes of good RCTs involving participants of different ages, a word of caution is required. Those older people who have participated in the research studies discussed here tend to be "typically healthy, community-residing, white adults in their 60s and 70s" (Karel & Hinrichsen, 2000, p. 723). The high rates of functional disorders in those over age 75, those living in institutions, and those with severe medical problems require treatment studies to focus on these populations also, if they are to do justice to the mental health needs of older people. Within older age groups, Knight (1988), evaluating a range of outpatient therapies, reported that age was negatively related to change but was offset by longer courses of therapy. Thus, an 80-year-old may show as much improvement as a 65-year-old but would probably require more sessions of therapy over a longer period. Newton and Lazarus (1992) suggested that older patients do often require a longer term involvement in therapy, but that after the initial treatment phase, contact can be relatively infrequent.

RELAPSE PREVENTION

A major trial of acute and maintenance therapy for older people with recurrent depression has been reported from the University of Pittsburgh (Reynolds et al., 1999b). Patients ages 60–80 with recurrent, nonpsychotic unipolar depression were treated with the antidepressant nortriptyline combined with weekly sessions of interpersonal psychotherapy (IPT). Once patients showed a good treatment response (defined as a Hamilton Rating Scale for Depression score [HRSD] ≤10), they were assigned to continuation therapy for a further 16 weeks, in which the frequency of sessions was reduced to twice monthly. At this point, patients still in remission were randomized to one of four maintenance therapy conditions: receiving either nortriptyline or placebo, in combination with IPT or alone, over a period of

3 years. One hundred eighty-seven patients entered the open trial of nortriptyline and IPT (mean, age 67), with 107 making a full recovery and randomized into the maintenance trial. Only 20% of those receiving the combination of nortriptyline and monthly IPT sessions relapsed within 3 years, compared with 90% of those receiving the placebo alone. Slightly less relapsed with the medication alone than with IPT plus placebo (43 vs. 64%). The combined approach emerged as the most effective method of relapse prevention. Lenze et al. (2002), in a further analysis from this study, have shown that the combined therapy is more likely to be associated with maintained social adjustment than either therapy alone. They commented that the greatest effect was in relation to interpersonal conflict/friction, which, along with role transitions and abnormal grief, is one of the three most common foci of IPT in older depressed people.

INDIVIDUAL PSYCHOLOGICAL APPROACHES

It has been primarily the cognitive theories and therapies originating from Beck's work that have proved most influential in the development of psychological treatment approaches for older people with depression. Studies emanating from this approach have in turn shed light on other approaches, including psychodynamic psychotherapy.

In the United States, Gallagher-Thompson, Thompson, and colleagues have carried out a systematic series of studies contrasting the efficacy of cognitive, behavioral, and eclectic/psychodynamic psychotherapies in the treatment of 91 older people suffering from depression in an outpatient setting. The behavioral treatment was based on the work of Lewinsohn, which conceptualizes depression as arising from a lack of social reinforcement. Therapy aims to help the person participate again in activities he/she enjoys, and hence to increase his/her level of reinforcement. The brief psychotherapy approach was described as eclectic and dynamic, relying on the use of the therapeutic relationship to help patients gain insight into their problems and formulate plans for change. Generally, no specific skills were taught and, in contrast to the other two modalities, structured homework assignments were not an integral part of the approach.

These three treatment approaches were compared to a wait-list control group (Thompson et al., 1987). Older depressed outpatients received between 16 and 20 individual sessions of one of the three therapy modalities, either immediately or after a 4-month wait-list period. There was a significant treatment effect compared with the wait-list control group, but no differences in efficacy between groups were identified, either immediately after treatment or at 1- and 2-year follow-up. Over half (52%) of the 91 patients in the trial moved out of the depressed range following treatment, with a further 18% showing a substantial improvement on the various measures used (which included observer-rated as well as self-rated depression scales—the HRSD, the Beck Depression Inventory (BDI), and the Geriatric Depression Scale). At 2-year follow-up (Gallagher-Thompson et al., 1990), 70% were no longer in the depressed range. Although far superior in methodology to any other outcome study in this field, as Weiss and Lazarus (1993) pointed out, a number of patients dropped out of treatment; for example, one-fourth of those allocated to cognitive therapy were lost to treatment. Reasons for dropout tended to have as much to do with physical health and transportation problems as with dissatisfaction with the treatment. Further analyses have identified the factor of "patient commitment" (defined as motivation for, and involvement in, therapy) as a key predictor of clinical improvement (Marmar et al., 1989). Levels of the therapeutic alliance did not differ across the groups, with the level of alliance tending to predict improvement in depression better in the behavioral and cognitive therapy groups than in the brief psychotherapy condition (Gaston et al., 1991).

Some efforts have been made to identify the characteristics of those not responding to treatment. Those still depressed at 2 years tended to be those who had not responded initially to treatment. Despite receiving a variety of other treatments in the intervening period, their depression remained intractable. The presence of endogenous symptoms initially predicts poorer outcome (Gallagher & Thompson, 1983), but this is not a good indicator, because a substantial proportion of patients with such symptoms did recover or make significant improvements. Another suggestion is that a coexisting personality disorder may predict poor prognosis (Leung & Orrell, 1993; Thompson et al., 1988). Clearly, there remains a need to develop more effective treatment strategies for these hard-to-treat patients.

This research group (Thompson et al., 2001) has now completed a trial in which CBT (16–20 weekly sessions) was compared with medication (desipramine), and with combined treatment. One hundred patients commenced the trial, with approximately 30% attrition (with greater attrition in those receiving the medication). The level of improvement in those receiving CBT was similar, irrespective of whether they were also receiving desipramine. Although those receiving medication alone also showed improvement, this was less than those receiving CBT.

GROUP THERAPIES

In addition to the studies on group CBT for GAD described earlier, a number of studies on cognitive therapy for depression with this age group have used a group format, with an available detailed treatment manual (Yost et al., 1986). Psychodynamic and CBT group therapies were reported by Steuer et al. (1984) to be equally effective in reducing levels of depression, although there was a 40% dropout rate during the 9-month period of treatment. Of those who completed 9 months of therapy, 40% were in remission and 40% had some symptomatic reduction. In one of the few studies in which CBT has been compared with a pharmacological treatment (Beutler et al., 1987), the attrition rate was lower in the group cognitive therapy condition during the 5 months of treatment. However, the relative effectiveness of CBT is difficult to evaluate, because the drug used, alprazolam, is not widely used as an antidepressant and certainly did not perform well in this trial; those receiving cognitive therapy showed the most evidence of change. In both the Steuer et al. (1984) and the Beutler et al. (1987) studies, beneficial changes related to group cognitive therapy were particularly noted on the self-report BDI rather than on the observer-rated HRSD. Although a comparison of individual and group CBT has yet to be performed, the success rates in bringing older people into the nondepressed range do seem greater in the individual therapy studies. This difference needs to be balanced against the possible greater input of therapeutic time needed in individual therapy.

It is in the sphere of relapse prevention that groups may prove to be most valuable. Several accounts are available of groups that provide long-term support, making use of the peer support available in a group context (Culhane & Dobson, 1991; Ong et al., 1987). For example, in a small randomized controlled study (10 patients in each group) Ong et al. (1987) reported significant differences in rereferral and readmission rates favoring those who attended a weekly support group over a period of a year. Seven of the control patients were rereferred to the hospital and six were readmitted, despite receiving the usual support services available; none of the support group members were rereferred or readmitted.

ORGANIC DISORDERS

Sleep Disorders

Definitions

The essential feature of sleep disorders, as defined by DSM-IV-TR, is a complaint of difficulty maintaining or initiating sleep, or of nonrestorative sleep that lasts for a period of at least 1 month. To meet diagnostic criteria, the level of sleep disturbance needs to result in clinically significant distress or impairment in important areas of functioning. Because the depth and continuity of sleep deteriorate with age, age is always considered a factor in making this diagnosis.

Sleep Problems and Depression

Sleep problems are common in depression. However, in older people, insomnia is not a good diagnostic index of depression (Morgan, 1992), because there are a number of other equally significant etiological factors. Early–morning waking is the classic sleep problem associated with depression;

generally, in older people, problems with broken sleep and in getting to sleep initially are more common.

Treatment Approaches

As described earlier, many older people are prescribed hypnotics (often benzodiazepines) for sleep problems, often over many years. However, a number of psychological approaches are now available to assist with these difficulties (Martin et al., 2000) and may also be of use for those mildly depressed patients for whom sleep disturbance is a major complaint. These approaches include relaxation methods, stimulus–control techniques for enhancing the connection between sleep and bed (Friedman et al., 1991; Pallesen et al., 2003), and CBT approaches. Montgomery and Dennis's (2003) systematic review of the efficacy of cognitive-behavioral interventions for sleep problems in adults over age 60 years identified six randomized trials. Contrasted to wait-list or to placebo control, CBT reduced the amount of wake-time after sleep onset, and increased sleep duration and sleep efficiency (as assessed using polysomnography) both at posttreatment and at follow-up of up to 12 months. Although a promising conclusion, only trials focused on primary insomnia were reviewed, and this may limit generalization to individuals whose insomnia is secondary to other complaints.

Expectations are important here; the well-documented changes in sleep patterns with age imply that individuals who believe that something is wrong unless they are having 8 hours of sleep a night are very likely to be dissatisfied with their sleep, even though it may not be abnormal compared to other people of the same age. Lichstein et al. (2001) reported a trial of "sleep compression" to address this issue. Participants were instructed to reduce their time in bed in a graded fashion, until it reached the level of actual sleep time, recorded in their baseline sleep diary. This approach appeared most useful with those not reporting daytime fatigue; those who did fared better with a relaxation approach geared to extending sleep. Overall, there were no differences between these two treatments. A placebo psychological therapy, which included basic sleep hygiene instructions (rising at the same time each day, avoiding caffeine after noon, etc.), was also associated with some reported improvements in sleep. Objective sleep, assessed using polysomnography in a sleep laboratory, showed no changes with any of the treatments.

Dementias

Definitions

As described by DSM–IV–TR, the dementias are characterized by the development of multiple cognitive deficits (including memory impairment) that are due to the direct physiological effects of a general medical condition, to the persisting effects of a substance, or to multiple etiologies (e.g., the combined effects of cerebrovascular disease and Alzheimer's disease). Specific criteria are given for the diagnosis of dementia of the Alzheimer's type and vascular dementia, with the latter being diagnosed only when there is evidence of cerebrovascular disease. In the last few years, several pharmacological treatments have been licensed for use with people with Alzheimer's disease on the basis of evidence showing, on average, a slower rate of decline in cognition in those patients receiving the medication compared with placebo (Doody et al., 2001).

Psychological Interventions

While there is a long history of psychological "treatments" for older people with dementia, it is only in the past few years that an evidence-based approach has emerged to assist in making sense of a wide-ranging literature (e.g., Kasl-Godley & Gatz, 2000; Woods, 2002). There remains a dearth of rigorous controlled trials, which are especially important in an area where stability of function or slowing of decline may be acceptable goals, against the backdrop of a natural history of progressive decline. These goals are, of course, more difficult for the individual careworker or therapist to discern without the benefit of a control group.

THE CARE ENVIRONMENT

Two models are helpful in understanding the impact of the care environment on older people with dementia (Woods, 1999a). Lawton's "environmental docility" model (Parmelee & Lawton, 1990) suggests that the person with lowered competence and function is more likely to be shaped by and vulnerable to environmental contingencies. Kitwood (1993) proposes that persons with dementia attract and are susceptible to the effects of a "malignant social psychology," where they are devalued, deskilled, and even dehumanized by the care environment. Both concepts lead to a situation in which many people with dementia may be underfunctioning, withdrawing from an unhelpful, perplexing situation that does not support the remaining skills and abilities that the constraints of neurological impairment would allow. Such an understanding has led to attempts to develop more positive, individualized care environments based on psychological principles. Examples of this would include "integrity-promoting care" from Sweden (Brane et al., 1989), and in the United Kingdom, the domus philosophy (Dean et al., 1993).

Evaluations of such approaches are producing promising results. For example, Dean et al. (1993) reported improvements in cognitive function, self-care skills, and communication skills over the first year of operation of a domus for people with dementia. In addition, there were higher levels of activity and interactions in the domus, in comparison with the same patients when residents in a conventional psychogeriatric hospital setting; similar find-ings were reported by Skea and Lindesay (1996). Brane et al. (1989) com-pared patients receiving 3 months of "integrity-promoting care" with a control group receiving conventional care. Improvements were noted in per-formance of motor skills and in mood, with reduced distractibility. Also in Sweden, there have been evaluations of group-living units, where a small number (eight or so) of people with dementia live and are cared for in a small cluster of ordinary housing units, with persons each having their own room, personalized and furnished to their own taste with their own belongings. Annerstedt et al. (1993) reported that 6 months after moving to the unit from institutional care, group-living residents showed enhanced mood and cogni-tion compared with patients remaining in the institution. One year after the move, both groups showed decline, but this was less so in the group-living residents.

Evaluating such "special care" units, in which the whole pattern of care is the intervention, is challenging in several ways (e.g., Sloane et al., 1995). Identifying key components of the care environment, replicating the care environment elsewhere, and identifying appropriate comparison and control groups are far from straightforward. Even a more focused intervention—such as staff training in managing difficult behavior—will interact with aspects of the institutional setting in unpredictable ways. For example, Moniz-Cook et al. (1998) reported a successful training intervention, in which staff in two intervention homes reported reduced difficulty in managing problem behav-ior compared with staff in a control home; the effects were lost at follow-up, in part related to the sociocultural environments of the homes. Large scale multicenter evaluations with cluster randomization (so that the home or ward is the unit of randomization) are required (Woods, 2003) if this problem is to be addressed. Proctor et al. (1999) reported such a study, including 12 care homes, where intervention home staff received a number of training sessions and weekly visits from an experienced mental health nurse, encouraging the development of care-planning skills. Twelve residents reported to show behavioral problems in each home were assessed before and after the inter-vention. Over a 6-month period, depression scores of residents in interven-tion homes improved, as did an index of cognitive impairment, compared with those in the control homes.

SENSORY STIMULATION

This group of approaches may be applicable to those with the most severe degree of dementia, even those who appear to be unresponsive to most external stimuli. Types of stimulation have included music, hand massage, pet animals, and physical exercise (Woods, 1999c). For example, using an ABAB design, Goddaer and Abraham (1994) showed a 63.4% reduction in agitation during mealtimes when relaxing music was played for patients with moderate to severe dementia. Burns et al. (2002) reviewed promising evidence from three RCTs for the impact of aromatherapy (using lemon balm or lavender oil) on agitation. They also indicated that bright-light treatment has some empirical support; it would be expected to be most helpful with those patients who show clear "sundowning" (i.e., an increase in agitation and restlessness in the evening), which may be hypothesized to reflect a disturbed circadian rhythm. Multisensory stimulation (often known as *Snoezelen*, and which includes various components such as calming music, visual stimulation from fiber optics and lava lamps, tactile stimulation, and aromatherapy) has been shown in one RCT (Baker et al., 1997, 2001) to be associated with improvements in mood and behavior, and reduced behavioral disturbance; an activity group (also for eight sessions) served as the control group. Physical exercise has been associated with cognitive changes, including increased alertness in an RCT of 6 months of twice-weekly "psychomotor activation" sessions (Hopman-Rock et al., 1999); little change on behavioral measures was reported.

REALITY ORIENTATION AND COGNITIVE REHABILITATION

Reality orientation (RO) is the most extensively evaluated of the psychological approaches to dementia. It has two main forms: (1) RO sessions involving small, structured group meetings, which use a variety of activities and materials to engage the patients with their surroundings and to maintain contact with the wider world, and (2) 24-hour RO involving environmental changes, with clear sign posting and extensive use of memory aids, and a consistent approach by all staff in interacting with the person with dementia. There are concerns that, when used insensitively, RO can have negative effects, with an emphasis on "reality confrontation," and Holden and Woods (1995) emphasize the need for RO to be applied in the context of an individualized, person-centered approach to care.

Spector et al. (2000) presented a systematic review and meta-analysis of the RO literature, focusing on RO sessions. Six studies, including a total of 125 patients with dementia, were included; there was a significant effect of RO on both cognitive function (effect size = 0.59; confidence interval = 0.22–0.95) and behavioral function (effect size = 0.66; confidence interval = 0.05–1.3). Spector et al. (2003) reported outcomes from a cognitive stimulation program developed on the basis of this review, comprising elements of RO and reminiscence, drawn from studies showing the most positive outcomes (Spector, 2001). Two hundred and one older people with dementia, drawn from 23 care homes and day centers, were randomized to standard care or to receive 14 biweekly sessions of the active intervention. Contrasted to control, at posttherapy, significant improvements in measures of memory functioning and quality-of-life measures were evident, suggesting generalized cognitive benefits from participation in the program. The size of the effect on cognition proved comparable to those reported in published studies on the most frequently used medications for people with Alzheimer's disease (the acetylcholinesterase inhibitors). Quayhagen et al. (1995) reported a comparison of three types of cognitive stimulation (memory, problem solving, and conversation) with a placebo control (involving passive exposure to the activity) and a wait-list control. The active intervention groups showed some cognitive benefits and declined less than the control groups in a follow-up period.

Twenty-four-hour RO has been the subject of fewer evaluations; improvements in spatial orientation (Reeve & Ivison, 1985) and significant cognitive and behavioral improvements (Williams et al., 1987) have been reported. There have been several studies, typically using single-case designs, demonstrating the efficacy of specific training sessions in helping disoriented patients find their way around the ward or home, often using sign posting (e.g., Lam & Woods, 1986; McGilton et al., 2003). This approach, using training procedures to achieve specific cognitive or behavioral goals, reflects a change of emphasis from cognitive stimulation toward cognitive rehabilitation (Clare & Woods, 2001). Learning techniques such as spaced retrieval (Camp et al., 1996) have proved useful, especially in the context of an errorless learning environment, where the aim is to avoid potentially interfering errors during the learning process (Clare et al., 1999). A number of single cases have demonstrated how these methods can be used to achieve carefully selected, clinically relevant goals, and it is likely that there will be a rapid increase in the outcome research in this area in the near future.

REMINISCENCE

Reminiscence therapy has been widely used with individuals and small groups, and has proved a popular approach, although there has often been a lack of clarity regarding its aims (Woods & McKiernan, 1995). Photographs, music, archive recordings, and items from the past are used to stimulate a variety of personal memories. Spector et al. (1998) carried out a Cochrane review and identified only one RCT that could be included; the results of this small study (Baines et al., 1987) were inconclusive. Several studies have examined the immediate impact of involvement in a reminiscence group, with participants acting as their own controls. Head et al. (1990) found an increase in interaction in one group, compared with an alternative activity, but a group in another day center failed to show a differential benefit from involvement in reminiscence activities. Brooker and Duce (2000) showed higher levels of well-being during reminiscence groups, compared with other activities and unstructured time, in people with dementia attending three day hospitals. Head et al. (1990) pointed out that the relative efficacy of reminiscence work will depend on the alternative activities offered. Further studies are needed regarding the outcomes of different types of reminiscence work in relation to aspects such as well-being and autobiographical memory, where it might be expected to have most impact.

VALIDATION THERAPY

Dissatisfaction with RO, which, as mentioned earlier, can be applied in a rather rigid, unfeeling fashion if too much emphasis is put on "correcting" the person rather than seeking to understand his/her attempts at communication (Dietch et al., 1989), has led to increasing interest in validation therapy (Feil, 1993), where attempts are made to discern and respond to the emotional content of what the person says rather than focusing on the factual content. A Cochrane review (Neal & Briggs, 1999) identified only two studies—both of validation therapy group-work—that could be included, with a total of 87 participants. The larger of these studies (Toseland et al., 1997) ensured that the validation approach was used appropriately, with training and supervision backed up by random sampling and monitoring of tape recordings of group sessions. The results of the review were inconclusive, although some trends (e.g., on depression) favored validation.

PSYCHOTHERAPY AND COGNITIVE-BEHAVIORAL THERAPY

Depression and anxiety are increasingly recognized as common co-morbidities of dementia (Ballard et al., 1996a, 1996b). Earlier recognition and diagnosis means that some patients with dementia will present knowing that something is wrong (e.g., they may be aware that they are not able to function as they did previously, or may know of others—often their relatives— who have had dementia). Sharing the diagnosis with such individuals provides a therapeutic opportunity to assist with adjustment, discuss misconceptions, and plan for the future (Husband, 1999). Attempts are being made to apply psychotherapeutic (Cheston, 1998; Kasl-Godley & Gatz, 2000) and CBT approaches (Scholey & Woods, 2003; Teri & Gallagher-Thompson, 1991) to older people with dementia, in the individual therapy context. Clearly, the presence of cognitive impairment must lead to some adaptations, with perhaps greater emphasis on "here and now" concerns, but early case reports suggest this is an area worthy of further development. Teri et al. (1997) described an intervention taught to family caregivers of people with dementia experiencing significant depression, involving problem solving and increasing involvement in pleasurable activities. In a controlled trial, significant improvements in the level of depression in the person with dementia were noted, accompanied by improvements in caregiver mood also, in relation to the interventions. An RCT of relaxation training (Suhr et al., 1999) showed reduced anxiety and behavioral problems for those receiving training in progressive muscle relaxation, compared with control patients who were taught imaginal relaxation techniques. The former approach presumably makes use of the relative preservation of procedural memory in dementia.

BEHAVIORAL MANAGEMENT

Despite being recommended as the first line of approach to behavioral problems in dementia, there are few reports of the successful application of behavioral approaches, either to reducing problem behavior or to promoting maintenance or relearning of skills (Allen-Burge et al., 1999; Woods, 1999b). Successful interventions aimed at promoting independence include a large study of 90 nursing home residents with severe cognitive impairment (Beck et al., 1997), in which nursing assistants used simple behavioral and problem-solving techniques to increase residents' degree of independence in dressing. Reducing incontinence has been the aim of the "prompted voiding procedure" described by Schnelle et al. (1989) and Burgio et al. (1988). Nursing home residents are simply asked on a regular schedule, say hourly, whether they wish to use the toilet, and continence is systematically reinforced. Results have been so dramatic that the intervention should be considered as a change in environmental contingency rather than a relearning procedure. The aim here is not independent toileting; in fact, self-initiated toileting became less frequent in the latter study. Unfortunately, when the research team leaves, staff seem to prefer to change residents when they become incontinent rather than continue with this preventive approach (Schnelle et al., 1993), suggesting that contingencies for staff also need to be carefully considered (Burgio & Burgio, 1990).

There have been some successful interventions reported in relation to problem behaviors. These include a 23% reduction in disruptive vocalizations, when white-noise was played to the patient on an audiotape through headphones (Burgio et al., 1996), and a 24% reduction in physical aggression during bathing, following hands-on training for staff in verbal and nonverbal communication (Hoeffer et al., 1997). However, as Woods and Bird (1999) argued, individualized approaches will always be required, rather than the application of standard therapies, to reflect the complexity of the types and functions of behavioral problems encountered. This viewpoint is illustrated by a number of single cases using rigorous designs, tackling a variety of difficulties, including aggression, inappropriate urination, sexual disinhibition and wandering reported by Moniz-Cook et al. (2001, 2003), Bird et al. (1995) and Bird (2000). The latter work illustrated the use of cognitive retraining methods to learn important rules or associations serving to prevent or reduce behavioral problems.

Teri et al. (2000) reported a large-scale RCT in which agitation in people with dementia living at home with a family caregiver was the target of intervention. A commonly used medication (trazodone) was compared with advice to the caregiver on behavioral management, with a placebo control group. Although the behavioral management was no less effective than the medication, unfortunately, neither was more effective than the placebo in reducing agitation. Although there is no doubt that tranquilizing medication is often overused in dementia care (McShane et al., 1997), further work is required to develop alternative interventions that have less negative effects and proven efficacy.

Interventions for Family Caregivers

Many of those providing care for older people with physical or mental health problems are older people themselves, looking after their partner or other relative, or a parent in advanced old age. A number of studies have shown that levels of strain and depression are high, particularly in those caregivers in contact with service providers (Morris et al., 1988), and that this may impact on the caregiver's physical health and life expectancy (Schulz & Beach, 1999). This tends to be particularly the case where the cared-for person suffers from a dementia, perhaps reflecting the experience of loss, or "living bereavement," experienced by the caregiver, as well as behavioral problems (Donaldson et al., 1998).

There is now a large literature on interventions with family caregivers in the context of dementia. Brodaty et al. (2003) report a meta-analysis of "psychosocial" interventions; 30 studies were included, with a positive effect size of 0.31 (CI = 0.13–0.50) for psychological distress. In four out of seven studies including time to nursing home placement as an outcome measure, placement was delayed by the intervention. The key elements of successful interventions could not be delineated, but it appeared that interventions in which the person with dementia was also involved tended to be more effective. Other systematic reviews have emphasized the diversity of results reported, but have examined in more detail the nature of interventions offered. Pusey and Richards (2001) concluded that individualized interventions, utilizing problem solving and behavior management were most effective; Cooke et al. (2001) similarly identified problem solving as important but also highlighted the role of social support.

It is likely that most studies have included a variety of interventions; for example, Marriott et al. (2000) reported a successful intervention program described as a "cognitive-behavioral family intervention," which probably included an educational component, as well as problem-solving skills and relaxation; Mittelman et al. (1995) described the impact of a "comprehensive support program" on depression in spouse caregivers, which included family counseling sessions and encouragement to join peer support groups. The available strategies, used to varying degrees in the various programs are as follows:

- Behavioral management of the problems being experienced (i.e., to make the caregiving less stressful).
- Direct reduction of negative affect and anxiety through stress-reduction techniques such as relaxation, anger management, and/or therapy for depressed mood.
- Education regarding dementia, symptoms, and management, including addressing attributions and perceptions regarding the problems experienced and developing problem-solving skills. This may take place in a peer support context, with a group of other family caregivers sharing ideas and experiences.
- Mobilizing family resources, and enhancing social support and networks; identifying and making use of possible sources of help.

The majority of studies have recruited any caregivers willing to take part rather than targeting those with clinical levels of depression or anxiety. Exceptions include the Marriott et al. (2000) study mentioned earlier, in which caregivers were selected on the basis of "psychiatric caseness," and a larger study reported by Gallagher-Thompson and Steffen (1994), who contrasted cognitive-behavioral and brief psychodynamic treatments in 66 clinically depressed caregivers of frail, elderly relatives (some, but not all, had dementia). At posttreatment, the two therapies were equally effective overall; 71% of patients no longer met clinical criteria for depression. However, there was an interaction between outcome and longevity of caretaking. Patients who had been caretakers for a shorter period had a greater response to psychodynamic therapy, while those who had been caring for their relative for more than 3.5 years responded better to CBT. This interaction was less evident at 3- and 12-month follow-up. It is possible that more "chronic" caregivers have a greater need for support and structure (which CBT offers) and a corresponding difficulty in exploring problems that may have left them emotionally depleted.

SUMMARY AND CLINICAL IMPLICATIONS

Prevalence rates of most functional disorders in older people are similar (although, in some studies, somewhat elevated), contrasted to younger age groups, though their natural history is less favorable, with relapse being a major problem in depression. Older people appear to be less likely to be in receipt of psychological treatment. This may be a reflection of both patients' and clinicians' expectations of treatment outcome, and might also reflect problems in the detection of these disorders.

There is relatively little research into the specific efficacy of treatments for functional disorders in older people. There is some evidence from RCTs that CBT in group and individual formats is effective in treating anxiety disorders in older people, but its differential effectiveness compared with other treatments is less clear. Treatment of anxiety with anxiolytics, although common, appears to be problematic.

Data from controlled trials suggest that cognitive therapy, behavior therapy, and brief psychodynamic psychotherapy appear to be equally effective treatment modalities for depression in older people, with the effect size for cognitive therapy being comparable to that in younger people. A combined approach, using medication and monthly sessions of IPT, has been shown to be particularly helpful in preventing relapse for patients in this age group. As many as 30% of patients with depression fail to respond to any type of treatment; a number of these have been described as having a personality disorder. The long-term effects of traumatic experiences in the person's life may also be relevant. Work on applying approaches to personality disorders, developed with younger people, to this population would be helpful.

There is growing evidence from controlled trials that sleep problems in older people respond well to a variety of psychological approaches, including CBT. With the exception of reality orientation, there has been little systematic evaluation of interventions for people with dementia. A number of techniques have been employed to improve functioning in people with dementia (including modification of the care environment, reminiscence therapy, validation therapy, psychodynamic psychotherapy, cognitive therapy, and behavior management). Though many of these techniques show promise in case reports and open trials, the absence of controlled studies makes it difficult to draw unequivocal conclusions about the efficacy of these interventions. Cognitive stimulation, as provided in reality orientation, shows significant benefits on measures of cognition and verbal orientation, with some evidence of improvements in function and quality of life. The benefits in cognitive function are of the same order as those associated with current medications for Alzheimer's disease.

Reducing strain and depression in caregivers of dementia sufferers is an important goal given that these are known complications of an increasingly common family circumstance. Interventions aimed at improving coping strategies have been examined; these include increasing knowledge concerning the disorder through psychoeducation, psychodynamic and cognitive-behavioral treatments addressing depression, training in behavioral management, and coping skills training (stress reduction, assertiveness, and problem-solving skills). Programs are often multifaceted, and though studies of these interventions show overall effectiveness, they do not identify any single intervention as the treatment of choice. Unfortunately, many trials suffer from methodological problems, including a failure to target caregivers most needing input, a failure to offer intervention to caregivers at an early stage, use of group rather than individualized interventions, use of interventions that are too brief, and a lack of long-term follow-up. Overall there are encouraging indications that psychosocial interventions of sufficient intensity may have an impact in delaying institutionalization of the person with dementia.

Demographic, epidemiological, and financial imperatives highlight the need to encourage research into the psychotherapeutic care of older people; older people continue to be excluded from this endeavor for no good reason. There is a continuing need for more studies that directly assess the effectiveness of treatments for functional disorders as applied to older adults, and which consider whether and how therapies need to be adapted to meet the needs of this population. There is also little systematic study of interventions for common issues and challenges in later life (particularly issues arising from physical health problems and bereavement). Finally, few trials compare the use of psychological approaches with commonly used medical regimens for functional disorders, and the adjunctive use of psychological approaches with pharmacological treatment.

Further research is required to address the most effective ways to maximize functioning in people with dementias, and to carefully examine the suggestions in the literature that early intervention for the person with dementia is particularly important. Earlier detection of organic problems may help the person with dementia to cope and adjust better, and caregivers are more likely to manage and to provide effective care if emergent psychological problems are more rapidly identified and treated.

In applying some of these interventions, it may be especially important to consider the education of care staff and other professionals. Many approaches to dementia take a broad view and require the involvement of hard-pressed direct care staff. Further work on ways of supporting positive attitudes and behavior in such staff in the context of the unit in which they work may be necessary for the widespread application of approaches that might benefit the function and well-being of many people with dementia.

There is justification for specialist psychotherapeutic services for older people, both to meet the need created by mental health problems in these individuals and to support, advise, and treat those who are involved in their care. Adequate services for this population will require specialist post-qualification training of mental health practitioners because of the particular obstacles faced in the treatment of functional disorders (such as lower response rates), the special problems presented by comorbid organic disorders, and the specific difficulties faced by those involved in the care of older people.

CHAPTER 16

THE CONTRIBUTIONS OF THERAPISTS AND PATIENTS TO OUTCOME

Up to this point, we have focused on the effectiveness of *specific* techniques with *particular* groups of psychiatric disorders. However, psychotherapy research over the past decades has demonstrated repeatedly that a substantial proportion of the variability in therapeutic outcomes is not explained by differences between formally defined therapeutic procedures, differences between client groups, or (though less well examined) the interaction between these two factors (e.g., Beutler et al., 1994, 2004; Clarkin & Levy, 2004; Garfield, 1994). In this chapter, we examine the contribution therapists make to treatment outcome, in terms of what they bring to the treatment situation by virtue of their training and experience, the techniques they apply, and the degree to which variation from the technique specified by their particular orientation has implications for effectiveness. In addition, we review the impact of patient characteristics beyond those immediately associated with diagnosis.

THERAPISTS' CONTRIBUTIONS TO EFFECTIVENESS

Schaffer (1982) differentiates the therapist's contributions into three conceptual dimensions—the techniques they employ, their "skillfulness," and their personal qualities (e.g., warmth, empathy, and perceived sincerity). Disentangling the impacts of each aspect is a challenge: Although many practitioners espouse a view that outcomes depend on therapists as much as techniques, evidence to support or refute this position is difficult to come by. As noted by a number of authors (e.g., Carroll, 2001; Elkin, 1999), methodological issues make it hard to disentangle therapists from therapies. Trials are usually designed to identify the impact of therapies; the use of manualization is intended to reduce variability attributable to individual therapists, and exploratory analyses for therapist effects are almost invariably conducted post hoc. Most studies contain relatively small patient numbers and rarely include a sufficient number of therapists to make analysis of therapist effects viable. Randomization of patients is to treatment rather than to therapist, leading to inevitable and complex interactions between patient and therapist characteristics. Since research designs in which the therapist is an independent variable are unlikely to receive funding, there is a necessary reliance on underpowered trials with limited capacity to detect and interpret between-therapist differences.

Detecting Variance Attributable to Therapists

Luborsky et al. (1986) computed the variance accounted for by therapists in four major studies of psychotherapy, and found that this was often larger than that claimed for between-treatment differences (even though all therapists in these trials were experienced). The analysis examined differences between outcomes for each therapist and also explored any special patient–therapist matches that might account for this difference. Significant differences in therapist efficacy were found in all four studies on various measures. For some (but not all) therapists, the initial level of functioning of the patient influenced outcome, though this was a strong positive predictor for some and a negative predictor for others. Although some therapists appeared to achieve consistently better outcomes, even those who performed poorly overall had some patients with good outcomes. More detailed examination suggested that individual therapists achieved better effects in some domains than others—for example, some therapists achieved better impacts on target symptoms, whereas others were more successful at increasing levels of interpersonal functioning. A further study (Luborsky et al., 1997) examined outcomes from 22 therapists working across seven samples of substance-abusing and depressed patients (derived from a number of research trials). Differences in rates of improvement across therapists were found that did not appear to relate to patient severity or to patient attributes. Furthermore, three therapists took part in more than one study, showing similar levels of efficacy with different patient samples, even when they applied different manualized techniques.

Although few in number, other studies of therapist effects tended to focus on the relationship between experience and outcome, and these are described below.

Impact of Specific Therapist Characteristics

Beutler et al. (1994, 2004) carefully reviewed a number of studies exploring the impact of therapist characteristics on outcome, though there are rather few substantive findings. While studies vary in their findings, most reports suggest that there is little overall impact of therapist age, gender, or ethnicity, or differences in outcome when therapist and client are matched on these variables. Assessment of the impact of therapist personality variables is limited, with some studies attempting post hoc atheoretical analysis, and others a more theory-driven approach, with no consistent or robust findings. There are indications that therapists with better levels of adjustment have better outcomes, though there is some inconsistency across studies.

The power of therapist characteristics per se to explain outcome differences may be rather limited. For example, although there have been suggestions that therapist effects are more striking in treatments of substance abuse (e.g., Najavits & Weiss, 1994), no such impacts were discernible in analysis of therapist effects in Project MATCH, a very large-scale trial in which 80 therapists offered cognitive-behavioral therapy (CBT), motivational interviewing, or 12-step programs to 1,726 clients (Project MATCH Research Group, 1998b). Some basic differences in therapist characteristics were evident, partly reflecting the fact that (by definition) the 12-step program is less professionalized than the other treatments. Where therapist effects did emerge, inspection of the data suggested that these were attributable to "outlier" therapists, suggesting a statistical anomaly rather than meaningful pattern.

Rather than looking at therapist characteristics *sui generis*, it may be more profitable to examine therapist in-session behaviors. For example, Lafferty et al. (1989) contrasted outcomes from 30 trainee therapists. Two patients from each therapist's caseload were selected at random; on the basis of residualized gain scores, therapists were divided into two groups—those whose patients improved, and those whose patients did not. Though measures of therapist attitudes and dispositions were included in the analysis, the best predictors of therapist efficacy were in-therapy experiences. Less effective therapies were characterized by lower levels of therapist empathy, less patient involvement, and higher levels of therapist directiveness. Although their patients felt less well understood by them, when contrasted to more effective therapist, less effective therapists saw their patients as more involved in therapy.

Impact of Therapist Experience and Training

Though professional and lay opinion assume the benefits of experience and training, evidence for this is surprisingly hard to find. Some early reviews suggested a clear relationship between outcome and experience, but recent studies have been more equivocal. Bergin (1971) coded studies according to the level of therapist experience in 48 studies of psychotherapy; 53% demonstrated positive results for more experienced therapists, while only 18% of trials using inexperienced therapists showed clear improvement. Smith and Glass's (1977) large-scale meta-analysis yielded a correlation of zero between experience and outcome, though because most therapists were rather inexperienced, few contrasts were available for analysis. Shapiro and Shapiro (1982b) obtained a similar result, noting that, on average, therapists had only 2.9 years of training plus experience. This restriction on experience level limits the degree to which meta-analytic results can be meaningfully generalized.

A number of reviews have examined the impact of different levels of experience both directly and within (rather than across) studies. Anthony and Carkhuff (1977) concluded that therapist experience was not associated with better outcomes, though the review appears to have been based on studies of poor internal validity. Durlak (1979) reviewed 40 studies, again containing a high proportion of studies of poor methodological quality (Fisher & Nietzel, 1980, cited in Stein & Lambert, 1984). Auerbach and Johnson (1977) examined a narrower subset of comparative outcome studies. Professional trainees and novice therapists were contrasted with more senior psychotherapists; a modest but weak relationship was found between outcome and experience. Hattie et al. (1984) concluded that paraprofessionals were more likely than professionals to achieve therapeutic success. However, the systems they used for coding of therapists as "professionals" and "paraprofessionals" may have led to some blurring of the distinction between the two groups, making their results difficult to interpret. Thus, definitions of professionals did not differentiate between professional training and psychotherapeutic training, and in their coding of paraprofessionals, some therapists were included who may indeed have received some psychotherapy training (e.g., nurses and social workers).

Berman and Norton (1985) carried out a meta-analysis of 32 studies of training, excluding those with poor methodology. Despite this greater selectivity, contrasting professionals with paraprofessionals yielded effect sizes close to zero, both at posttherapy and at follow-up.

Lyons and Woods (1991) reported a meta-analysis of 70 studies of rational–emotive therapy; defining experience in terms of professional degree, therapist training was significantly correlated with treatment effects ($r = .3$). Balestrieri et al. (1988) examined studies contrasting outcomes in psychiatric patients after treatment by family physicians or specialist mental health workers, such as psychiatrists, psychologists, or social workers. Though all patients received medication (hence reducing likely differences between groups), better outcomes were achieved by specialist workers (effect size = 0.22).

In a careful review, Stein and Lambert (1984) sampled 41 studies, restricting their analysis to trials in which patients had clinically significant problems (hence excluding studies of interventions such as vocational and academic counseling, and analogue interviews), and including enough therapists in each trial to enable meaningful comparison to be made. Again, therapists tended to have limited experience—most having no more than 5 years in practice. Experience level was operationalized in a complex manner; three systems were employed to tap the impact of different codings:

1. A score based on training plus experience.
2. A "difference in experience" score, obtained by subtracting the years of experience of the experienced group from that of the inexperienced group.
3. A 5-point rating system on which, for example, 1 represented a lay person with no training and 5, a clinician with 3 or more years of postgraduate training.

Overall, the mean effect size for experience was zero. Regression analysis indicated that for some comparisons, there was an association between experience and outcome, though for one comparison, this favored experience, while in another, less-experienced therapists obtained better results. This rather confusing result may reflect methodological differences between studies.

Contrasting experience using the 5-point rating scale and examining the impact of increasing distance between therapist groups and the overall effect size yielded a significant but modest correlation ($r = .11$). In addition, the "difference in years of experience" measure was a significant predictor of more positive outcomes for more experienced therapists. Finally, there was a trend for outcomes to be better for more experienced therapists when more disturbed patients were being seen (though, of some interest in this debate, rather few studies included more distressed patients).

A further meta-analysis by Stein and Lambert (1995) reached more definitive conclusions than earlier studies. As in their earlier study (1984), Stein and Lambert restricted their analysis to trials of therapy for clinically relevant problems. These authors noted that the codings of experience used by most studies make it difficult to distinguish between experience and training—for example, researchers frequently classify experience using global criteria, such as the type of degree held by a therapist. However, this may be misleading, since categorizing in this way will treat as homogeneous both newly degreed therapists and those who have been practicing for many years. These classificatory problems are likely to reduce the variance attributable to experience. Nonetheless, on the basis of 36 studies, moderate effect sizes were found for the relationship between experience and outcome, as measured both by pre- and posttherapy measures of symptoms (0.3) and by clients (0.27).

A small number of pertinent studies postdate these reviews. Huppert et al. (2001) examined therapist differences in a trial of manualized CBT for panic disorder delivered by 14 well-trained therapists treating 183 patients. Although the level of training and the use of a manualized therapy would be likely to reduce between-therapist variances, and overall most patients showed some benefit from treatment, it was possible to rank therapists into three bands—those with consistently good outcomes, those with a mix of outcomes, and those with consistently poor outcomes. Ratings of competence and adherence to the CBT model did not account for these differences, nor were they attributable to differences in patient presentation. However, there was evidence that greater therapist experience (measured in years of practice rather than specific experience with the CBT model) was associated with better outcomes.

Franklin et al. (2003) contrasted outcomes from experienced and inexperienced therapists treating 86 consecutively admitted patients with obsessive–compulsive disorder (OCD) using exposure and response prevention. Although participants were recruited and treated in a research unit, they had either refused randomization to trials or failed to meet criteria for eligibility, and were subsequently treated on a fee-for-service basis. Therapists were either doctoral-level clinical psychologists ($n = 11$) or interns ($n = 16$), with interns receiving supervision (which tended to be offered with greater intensity for those with least experience of OCD treatments). Case allocation was nonrandom and reflected case complexity. Experience was operationalized as low if therapists had less than 1 year of experience with OCD, moderate if this amounted to 2–8 years, and high if greater than 8 years. Overall, patients exhibited high levels of clinically significant improvement, with no differences in relation to the experience level of therapists. However, since the most severe cases were allocated to the most experienced therapists, the greatest pre- to posttherapy change was evident in this group. Although this could suggest the relevance of experience to outcome, these patients may have fared as well with less experienced therapists. The absence of randomized allocation makes interpretation difficult.

Lambert et al. (2003) reported on outcomes in the context of three studies of case tracking, in which therapists were given feedback about the progress of their patients (a technology discussed in more detail below). Patients were treated either by qualified or by graduate trainees, and trainees appeared to have somewhat better outcomes than trained staff. However, allocation to treatment was not random, making it plausible that the complexity of case mix may have determined this pattern of results. The case-tracking system alerted therapists when patients were failing to make gains at the expected rate; a greater proportion of trainees were subject to this alert than were experienced therapists.

While evidence for a relationship between therapist experience and outcome seems to be modest, this may reflect poor definitions of experience, a restriction in the range of experience in therapists surveyed, and (as indicated particularly by Stein & Lambert's [1984] study) methodological issues in the coding of experience. Stein and Lambert (1995) note that, given these problems, it is surprising that studies should attribute any variance to therapist experience. It may also be the case that experience is less relevant than expertise, and (as discussed below) a number of studies have linked this variable to outcomes. It also needs to be borne in mind that in many studies, less experienced therapists were supervised. This factor—frequently covert in terms of reporting—needs to be emphasized, since answering research questions about the efficacy of naive therapists requires evidence of their impacts when operating independent of supervision.

Therapist Experience and Dropout from Treatment

The notion of premature dropout from therapy can be hard to define; for example, dropout immediately after assessment is different from dropout of a patient who leaves a planned, long-term therapy after 6 months. Despite this methodological problem, the association between lower attrition and greater experience is reasonably consistent in the literature (e.g., Burlingame et al., 1989; Crits-Christoph et al., 1991; Fiester, 1977; Levitz & Stunkard, 1974; Slipp & Kressel, 1978) and is particularly evident with more psychodynamic therapies (e.g., Betz & Shullman, 1979; Epperson, 1981; Krauskopf et al., 1981). Sue et al. (1976) reported dropout rates for 13,000 patients in 17 community mental health centers. They found that patients were less likely to return after their initial interview or to terminate prematurely if seen by paraprofessionals (defined as therapists with less than graduate level training). This effect was evident even after statistical control for a variety of client factors. Data from Stein and Lambert's (1995) meta-analysis suggest that while there is no or little relationship between experience and dropout within university counseling centers (frequently the site for studies in this area), such effects become more prominent in other mental health settings. This observation may be relevant to Wierzbicki and Pekarik's (1993) meta-analysis of 125 studies, which found no correlation between dropout and either the number of years of therapist experience or the professional degree gained by the therapist.

It is important to note that different rates of attrition between more and less experienced therapists make it more difficult to interpret research that attempts to estimate the link between therapist experience and outcomes. As pointed out by Stein and Lambert (1995), the apparent efficacy of less experienced therapists will be increased if their clients drop out of treatment earlier (clients remaining in therapy may be unrepresentative of the original pool of untreated patients). An example of this is offered by Kopoian (1981, cited by Stein & Lambert, 1995), who contrasted therapists with graduate degrees and those with postgraduate degrees. Though the two groups achieved comparable outcomes, almost half the clients treated by less experienced therapists left the trial prematurely. This suggests that experienced and inexperienced therapists are best contrasted in terms of the probability that they will have a good outcome, rather than the absolute outcomes achieved—in other words, focusing on outcomes derived from intention-to-treat (ITT) rather than completer samples.

Professional Training and Outcome

As noted earlier, possession of a professional qualification is (at best) only weakly associated with better outcomes, a conclusion that—if robust—would have obvious and profound implications for training and accreditation. However, this is a difficult area to survey, since different levels of professional qualification are often conflated with level of experience. Furthermore (and as noted by Atkins and Christensen, 2001), the criteria used to distinguish between professionals and paraprofessionals vary across studies and reviews, and classification as a paraprofessional often indicates the absence of a formal qualification rather than a lack of experience, training, or skillfulness. Rather few studies of this issue have been published since Stein and Lambert's (1995) review, resulting in little opportunity for clarification of this issue.

Bright et al. (1999) contrasted the impacts of professional and paraprofessional therapists offering group CBT or a mutual support group for 98 depressed patients. Prior to the study, professional therapists were reasonably proficient in CBT, and paraprofessionals, in running support groups. All received brief training to enable them to run a group in the modality with which they were unfamiliar, as well as running a group using techniques with which they were familiar. Though patients in all groups showed statistically significant improvement, a categorical analysis that classified patients in relation to clinically significant improvement indicated that the greatest gains were evident in CBT groups run by professional, rather than paraprofessional, therapists. Gains from mutual support groups were equivalent, whether conducted by professional or paraprofessional therapists. Fals-Stewart and Birchler (2002) found that while bachelor's and master's level therapists were equivalent in their adherence to manualized behavior couple therapy for alcoholic men and their partners, master's-level therapists were judged to be more competent, and their clients had better outcomes.

Howard (1999) contrasted 20 specialists and 27 nonspecialists treating 86 patients with anxiety disorders using CBT. A "specialist" was defined as an individual who had training not only in CBT but also in the specific application of CBT to anxiety disorders (on which basis the term nonspecialists may be misleading, since it does not imply that these therapists are untrained). Results were clear: Patients seen by the specialist group were seen for a shorter period of time, had better posttherapy outcomes and lower relapse rates over 2 years, and fewer sought additional treatment after therapy had ended. One caution on this interpretation is the additional finding that therapists who used CBT techniques had better outcomes, suggesting a possible confound between the notion of specialism and the use of ineffective technique.

An alternative approach to this question would be the demonstration of advantage of training in novice entrants to a profession, or the benefits of trained over novice therapists, though only a small number of trials directly examine this. As part of their meta-analysis of behavioral treatments for agoraphobia, Trull et al. (1988) found that doctoral-level therapists achieved better results than nondoctoral practitioners. Burns and Nolen-Hoeksema (1992) analyzed therapist effects in an open trial of 185 depressed patients treated with CBT; the 13 therapists ranged in experience from untrained "novices" to senior therapists (defined as those with more than 4 years' clinical experience with CBT). Measures were taken of the level of patient disturbance, compliance with homework tasks, and degree of therapist empathy. Controlling for these factors, the patients of novice therapists improved significantly less than did the patients of those with more experience.

Henry et al. (1993a, 1993b) studied the impact of training therapists in short-term dynamic therapy, as a part of which therapist adherence was measured; hence, measures of transference interpretation were taken. Some specific effects related to technique were found; overall training seemed to increase the rate of interpretation, though at the expense of decreasing supportive interventions and the therapeutic alliance. As part of the design, therapists were assigned to one of two supervisors. Post hoc analysis indicated that allocation to supervisor was associated with significantly different rates of adherence, suggesting that even the notion of training may be amenable to finer grained analysis; it may be the outputs from training, rather than the training itself, that deserve attention. Rather few studies assess this directly. Two reports suggest that training in cognitive therapy is associated with improvement (Freiheit & Overholser, 1997; Milne et al., 1999). Both indicated that competence in delivery of therapy increased (on the basis of self-report and ratings by independent judges, respectively), though the specific link between increasing competence and outcome is not clearly established in either study. Hilsenroth et al. (2002) randomized 68 patients to receive short-term psychodynamic therapy either from a trainee receiving highly structured supervision, or from a trainee receiving "supervision-as-usual." Though alliance levels were high in both groups, there was significant additional benefit to structured training in relation to the alliance. A potential confound is that while only one supervisor therapist offered the structured supervision, "supervision-as-usual" was offered by 14 supervisors; findings from Henry et al. (1993a, 1993b; cited earlier), suggest that generalization beyond the impacts of particular supervisors carries some risk.

Overall, evidence for the impact of training is suggestive rather than substantive, yet we need such evidence in order to bypass what has hitherto been a rather unproductive debate regarding the benefits of professional training or experience. Reframing this debate, a more rigorous and relevant question would be to determine whether a therapist has acquired relevant and specific competencies in the course of his/her training or experience, and whether this process of acquisition is linked to better therapeutic outcomes. An even more challenging question is whether training enhances therapists' capacity to generalize their learning—for example, to apply their knowledge to novel clinical situations, or to acquire novel therapeutic skills at a faster rate. Questions about the impact of training often assume that it is procedural knowledge rather than a capacity for learning that is relevant, and at present, researchers inappropriately equate skills acquisition with the mantle of professional accreditation. By way of example, though "trainees" in Milne et al.'s (1999) study already possessed a relevant professional qualification, they demonstrated wide differences in their competences at the end of training (James et al., 2001). Bein et al. (2000) conducted an examination of training in short-term psychodynamic therapy, contrasting outcomes from two patients treated pretraining with those of two patients treated after training. No evidence of additional benefit from training was obtained, but—more pertinent—only a minority of therapists in the study were judged to have acquired basic levels of competence. From evidence reviewed below, there is reason to believe that competence is pertinent to outcome; whether training enhances competence is therefore a critical question.

IMPACT OF ADHERENCE TO TECHNIQUE AND OF THERAPIST COMPETENCE ON OUTCOME

Carrying out a treatment as intended and described in a manual ("adherence") is not necessarily the same as delivering the therapy in a competent or skilful manner. Measuring competence is harder than measuring adherence, because it usually rests on judgments about what constitutes skilled performance; quite apart from different viewpoints among therapists, this will often be linked to the theoretical underpinnings of the therapy. On this basis, procedures for rating competence often vary in important ways from therapy to therapy (e.g., O'Malley et al., 1988; Vallis et al., 1986). There is also the risk of conflating these two concepts, since the criteria employed in measures of competence sometimes imply—but do not necessarily assess—adherence to technique.

Impact of Adherence to Manuals

The main aim of Crits-Christoph et al.'s (1991) meta-analysis was to determine whether the use of manualized therapies would decrease the variance attributable to therapists. Fifteen outcome studies were selected for examination, employing either CBT or psychodynamic therapy in the treatment of a range of presenting problems. Along with use of a manual, the analysis also considered the interrelationships between therapist experience, and type and length of therapy. Outcome variance attributable to differences between therapists was smaller when therapy was manualized, and when more experienced therapists conducted the therapy. Logically, between-therapist variance increased when inexperienced therapists conducted therapies without a manual. Overall, therapist-related impacts were equivalent to a medium effect size, though the size of this effect varied widely across studies. Some caution in interpretation is appropriate, however. CBT studies tended to make more use of manuals, and there are no within-study contrasts of manualized or nonmanualized approaches.

There seem to be rather few direct contrasts of manualized or nonmanualized approaches to therapy. Emmelkamp et al. (1994) randomized 22 patients with OCD to manualized exposure therapy or to a "tailor-made" therapy of the therapists' choice. Though outcomes were broadly equivalent, nearly all those receiving "tailor-made" therapy received some form of cognitive therapy. In contrast Schulte et al. (1992) found benefit for manualized treatment (which included *in vivo* exposure) over "individualized" therapy for specific phobia, though when individualized treatment also included *in vivo* exposure, no differences in efficacy were evident. However, bearing in mind the fact that the efficacy of *in vivo* exposure for specific phobias is well established, this result may speak as much to the benefits of manual-guided therapy as it does to the capacity of therapists to select nonefficacious treatments.

Studies suggest that therapists vary considerably in their ability to adhere to therapy protocols. Rounsaville et al. (1988) examined adherence to the interpersonal psychotherapy (IPT) manual in 11 psychologists and psychiatrists, with an average of 15 years' experience. The average level of adherence did not change significantly throughout the study, which involved two or three training cases, and an additional 5–10 cases in the efficacy phase of the study. Although the severity of patients' pretreatment symptoms did not relate to adherence, there was a strong relationship between patient hostility and therapist adherence. More hostile patients with negative pretherapy expectations made adherence to the IPT protocol more difficult. General therapist qualities such as greater warmth and lower expectations correlated both with therapist adherence to IPT and patient outcome. The authors suggested that this may represent a "good therapist" factor, in which the competent therapist is more capable of adapting techniques to conform to the dictates of the training manual.

Similarly, while Luborsky et al. (1985) found that personal qualities of the therapist (the level of personal adjustment and interest in helping the patient) and the quality of the helping alliance related significantly to therapy outcome, they also found that the extent to which therapists adhered to the techniques of either supportive–expressive therapy or CBT ("purity") related to positive outcome. The authors argued that a good helping alliance may make adherence to a manualized treatment possible, either because the therapist who is able to establish an alliance can execute the intended therapy, or because a good alliance enables the therapist to implement his/her intended technique.

Other studies find lower correlations between adherence to a manual and therapist skills, such as overall competence, use of language, attunement to the patient, timing and meaningfulness of intervention, openness to feedback, and avoidance of blaming (e.g., Henry et al., 1993a, 1993b). Winston et al. (1987) reported no significant association between adherence to the techniques of short-term psychodynamic psychotherapy or brief adaptational psychotherapy and outcome.

Impact of Therapist Competence

Two trials reported on the contribution of therapist competence to outcome in the IPT and CBT arms of the NIMH Treatment of Depression Collaborative Research Program (Elkin, 1994). O'Malley et al. (1988) examined the performance of 11 IPT therapists who treated 35 patients between them. Tape recordings of the fourth session of therapy were examined, together with therapist reports and ratings from supervisors. A correlation between competence and outcome was found for patient-rated change. However, there was also an association between patients' pretreatment social adjustment and change (in that the more maladjusted patients derived greater benefit). Controlling for this through regression analysis, initial patient functioning predicted 34% of outcome variance; the addition of therapist performance measures added a further 23% of variance beyond initial patient characteristics. A median split between therapists high and low in skill indicated significantly greater patient change in the more skilled group. Although therapist competence was associated with patient-rated change, there was no evidence of such a relationship on measures of social adjustment, and only weak evidence of association on measures of depression. It should be noted that all therapists in this trial were chosen for their competence in delivering their therapy, reducing the variance attributable to this factor (though, in contrast to most such studies, in the direction of a uniformly higher level of competence).

Shaw et al. (1999) undertook an analogous study focused on the CBT therapist in the NIMH trial, examining the adherence and competence in the therapies of 36 patients treated by eight therapists. Ratings of competence were made using the Cognitive Therapy Scale (CTS), which has two factor-based components, one reflecting specific CBT skills and general therapy skills, and the other, the capacity of the therapist to structure CBT (e.g., to create an agenda, or to assign and review homework). Ratings were made on nine of the 20 sessions of therapy, and an average score was derived for each therapy. Simple correlation of the CTS with outcome suggested that it contributed little to outcome variance. However, CTS scores were highly correlated with measures of adherence to CBT technique and general facilitative conditions. Controlling for this by partial correlation yielded a more substantive effect (accounting for 19% of the variance in Hamilton Rating Scale of Depression [HRSD] scores). This suggests that aspects of the CTS associated with outcome are those not associated with adherence to CBT or to basic therapy skills. Further analysis indicated that it is the structure (rather than the skill) factor of the CTS that accounts for this impact, and that the degree to which therapists structured treatment distinguished between patients who improved and those who did not. However, these associations were evident only on the HRSD (and not on the Beck Depression Inventory [BDI]).

Frank et al. (1991) examined the relationship between outcome and competence in 38 patients treated using IPT as part of a long-term maintenance study of depression (reviewed in detail in Chapter 4). Briefly, patients who had recovered from their index episode of depression received monthly sessions of IPT over 3 years. Competence of delivery of IPT was defined as the extent to which the therapist maintained the patient's focus on interpersonal issues (a measure that also taps adherence to the IPT protocol). Sessions were divided into those above and below the median of competence. On this basis, patients in receipt of more competently delivered therapy had a median survival time to relapse of 2 years; in contrast, those receiving less competently delivered therapy had a median time to relapse of 5 months. Since therapists showed some variation between patients in their ability to deliver "competent" therapy, this finding may not be a reflection of therapist competence per se; rather, it relates to the capacity of therapists to establish an interpersonal focus with particular clients. A similar "interactive" pattern was reported by Foley et al. (1987). Although (as discussed earlier) competence of delivery of IPT was associated with greater patient change in the NIMH trials (O'Malley et al., 1988), more "difficult" patients were found significantly to decrease therapists' performance. Taken together, these studies suggest that both patient and therapist factors, in interaction one with the other, will need to be considered in any assessment of the relationship between therapist competence and therapeutic efficacy.

Svartberg and Stiles (1994) examined the influence of both the therapeutic alliance and therapist competence on outcome in Sifneos's (1987) short-term anxiety-provoking therapy (STAP). Seven experienced therapists worked with 13 patients using STAP; on measures of symptomatic change, there was a negative correlation between competence and outcome but a positive relationship between alliance and change. It is possible that these results reflect the nature of the techniques employed, which emphasize confrontation and might therefore increase the salience of the alliance in relation to their successful application.

Barber et al. (1996) employed a measure that assessed both adherence and competence in a 16-week trial of delivery of supportive–expressive therapy to 29 depressed patients. Assessment of adherence–competence was made at the third session. Analyses partialed out initial intake scores and any improvement in symptoms between intake and the third session. On this basis, adherence did not predict improvement, but there was an association between outcome and competence in delivery of expressive (but not of supportive) techniques. Adherence—but not competence—was greater for therapies in which patients showed improvement earlier in therapy, suggesting that it is easier for therapists to adhere to technique with patients who show benefit. The link between competence and outcome appeared to be robust in the face of several subanalyses, suggesting the importance of the way in which expressive techniques were delivered rather than the frequency with which they were used.

In summary, there appears to be a complex relationship between adherence, competence, and outcome. The relationship between adherence (the implementation of technical training) and outcome is probably weak (e.g., Rounsaville et al., 1981) and may depend on the prior establishment of a helping alliance (Luborsky et al., 1985).

There is better evidence that greater competence is related to better outcome, though the specific competencies that create this association probably require greater elaboration. There is also an indication that more competent therapists are able to deviate appropriately from technical recommendations with more difficult patients (Rounsaville et al., 1988), and that these individuals are rated as more competent by their supervisors and produce greater improvement in their patients (O'Malley et al., 1988). This suggests that extensive training may be necessary not only in specific techniques, but also to indicate where deviations from prescriptive technique are desirable. These observations may be important in explaining some of the paradoxical associations between training, experience, and outcome, to be reviewed below.

The frequent use of experienced rather than inexperienced or novice therapists limits the implications for training that can be drawn from these studies. Conclusions from experienced therapists may not generalize, since novice therapists are far more amenable to suggestions regarding technique and style than experienced practitioners, who are likely to be quite comfortable with their approach. It should also be noted that many of the recommendations that emerge from these studies, such as the importance of establishing a working alliance with a patient, are hard to translate into specific skills that can be taught (Strupp et al., 1988). Adequate levels of personal adjustment and clinical sensitivity are also likely to be essential therapist characteristics, though there appears to be little evidence that personal therapy has the capacity to "teach" therapists appropriately to deal with chronic hostility and negativism from patients (Henry et al., 1986).

THE THERAPEUTIC ALLIANCE

The importance of the therapist–client relationship is widely recognized, and the findings of psychotherapy research have identified this factor as perhaps of the greatest importance, alongside therapeutic technique. In this section, we review the evidence concerning the importance of establishing a good helping alliance and the qualities of both client and therapist that are likely to maximize the chances of a successful therapeutic relationship. This literature has implications not only for training but also for the selection of good practitioners, and in the appraisal of the quality of psychotherapeutic services.

The notion of the therapeutic alliance originates from within a psychodynamic perspective. Freud (1964) underscored the importance of the "pact" between the analyst and the patient, who "band themselves together" with a common goal based on the demands of external reality. The term "therapeutic alliance" was coined by Zetzel (1956), who argued that in a successful therapy there is a conscious collaborative, rational agreement between therapist and client. Others (e.g., Bowlby, 1988) maintain that this alliance may in itself have a curative aspect in providing the patient with a new "healthier," positive relationship than he/she may have experienced in the past (see Gittleson, 1962). This emphasis is even stronger in the humanistic tradition, where the therapist's willingness to be empathic, congruent, and unconditionally accepting of the client is seen as a sufficient condition for therapeutic success (Rogers, 1951). From a more behavioral, social learning perspective, LaCrosse (1980) and Strong (1968) point to the importance of the client's perception of the therapist as expert, attractive, and trustworthy. These perceptions will strengthen the therapist's influence and thus predict the degree to which the patient is likely to benefit from therapy.

The importance of the therapeutic alliance is also emphasized by authors who adopt a less "school-based," more generic approach to psychotherapeutic treatment (e.g., Bordin, 1979). Horvath et al. (1993) distinguish three aspects of the therapeutic alliance from a pantheoretical point of view:

1. The client's perception that the interventions offered are both relevant and potent.
2. Congruence between the client and therapists' expectations of the short- and medium-term goals of therapy.
3. The client's ability to forge a personal bond with the therapist and the therapist's ability to present him/herself as a caring, sensitive, and sympathetic, helping figure.

While the forgoing account might suggest some stability in alliance level once it has developed, in reality, variations from session to session are likely and common. For some researchers, these variations in alliance level are in themselves important, since the process of "repairing" significant challenge to, and deterioration in, the alliance (denoted as alliance rupture) could be seen as therapeutic in its own right (e.g., Safran & Muran, 2000; Safran et al., 1990). Though this notion is interesting and potentially important, rather few studies have directly examined this possibility (e.g., Bennett, 1998; Safran & Muran, 1996).

Therapeutic Alliance and Outcome

In recent years, an increasing number of research reports have been published on the relationship between the alliance and outcome, with qualitative reviews by Gaston (1990) and Horvath et al. (1993), and quantitative reviews by Horvath and Symonds (1991) and Martin et al. (2000) The first meta-analysis by Horvath and Symonds (1991) included 24 studies. Calculation of effect sizes was hampered by the fact that some studies that found non-significant correlations between the alliance and outcome did not cite the actual value of the statistic; in such cases, Horvath and Symonds assigned an r value of zero. This means that their estimated average effect size (0.26) linking quality of alliance to therapy outcome may be somewhat conservative. Martin et al. (2000) adopted the same inclusion criteria and coding procedure as Horvath and Symonds (1991), identifying a further 55 published and unpublished trials. Meta-analysis of this much larger sample (which included all those in the Horvath and Symonds review) yielded a weighted correlation with outcome of .22, confirming a moderate but consistent association between alliance and outcome. The reliability of the various alliance scales in common use was high, though disaggregation of outcomes by alliance measure suggested that while the Working Alliance Inventory, Penn, Vanderbilt, and California scales were correlated with outcome, the Toronto scale was not. Horvath and Symonds' review suggested that outcome was better predicted by client-based ratings than by therapist or observer ratings, and that effect size estimates linking alliance to outcome were somewhat higher if the alliance was measured early in therapy, as opposed to a measure based on averaging alliance ratings across sessions. Martin et al.'s (2000) more substantive review did not support these observations: No further variance was accounted for by type of rater (patient, therapist, or observer), time or type of alliance rating (early, middle, late, or averaged across sessions), type of therapy or methodological quality. However, there were some indications that patient-rated alliance is stable over sessions, whereas therapist- or observer-rated alliance is more variable.

Although there are variations across individual studies, the majority of trials confirm a robust, if modest, link between alliance and outcome across different intervention methods. Exemplifying this are three post hoc analyses of major trials for depression, all of good methodological quality. Krupnick et al. (1996) analyzed data from the 225 completer patients who participated in the NIMH trial for depression (Elkin, 1994), which contrasted CBT, IPT, clinical management combined with imipramine, and clinical management combined with placebo. Therapy sessions were rated using the Vanderbilt scales (an observer-based measure that distinguishes between patient and therapist contributions to the alliance). Alliance levels were equivalent across all treatment conditions. Mean patient and total alliance scores were significantly associated with outcome, accounting for approximately 20% of the variance in outcome scores; furthermore, there was a significant association between the strength of the alliance and probability of remission. These associations were evident whether analysis was based on a single measure of the alliance early in therapy, or on a mean figure based on early, middle, and late sessions. Therapist contribution to the alliance did not emerge as a predictor of outcome, though; since there was little variance in this factor across therapists, statistical analysis would not be a helpful test of any putative relationship.

Castonguay et al. (1996) examined sessions from 30 of the 32 patients who completed CBT treatment for depression in the Pittsburgh trial (which contrasted CBT for depression against pharmacotherapy; Hollon et al., 1992). The alliance was assessed using the Working Alliance Inventory, and a process measure used to monitor the degree to which therapists drew attention to unhelpful intrapersonal processes (such as cognitive distortions)—in a sense, the extent to which they applied aspects of basic CBT technique. Higher levels of the alliance were associated with better outcomes both midtreatment and at posttherapy. Unexpectedly, there was a significant association between therapist focus on intrapersonal issues and poorer outcome, though statistical control for alliance level removes this link. This suggests that (for example) focusing on dysfunctional thoughts in the context of a negative alliance was unhelpful. Descriptive analysis of sessions in which this took place indicated that attempts by therapists to restore a poor alliance through adherence to technique led to further strain on the alliance, and hence to poorer results.

Stiles et al. (1998) used the Agnew Relationship Measure (ARM) to assess alliance levels in the therapies of 79 participants in the Sheffield Psychotherapy Project (Shapiro et al., 1994, 1995), which contrasted CBT and psychodynamic–interpersonal therapy). Residual gain scores were correlated with scores on the ARM, a rating scale completed independently by patient and therapist, which has five factor-based scales. Alliance levels were positive and (essentially) equivalent across both forms of therapy, and were significantly correlated with posttherapy outcome. The association between outcome and the alliance was broadly similar whether the alliance was measured early or late in therapy, or whether it was rated by clients or therapists.

Overall, and across a range of therapies, the therapeutic alliance appears to make a small but consistent contribution to outcome. There can be a tendency for this relationship to be treated uncritically as a causal one, when in fact it is most commonly accepted that alliance acts as a moderating variable—a catalytic mode of action that makes treatment more effective. An alternative view is that it acts as an effector variable—in other words, that it operates in a complex relationship with technique and other processes, with these variables acting and reacting in a temporal sequence. However, it is also clear that disentangling the alliance from other process factors is very difficult, simply because these measures are not independent of one another. Nonetheless, the studies described below have attempted to examine this issue systematically.

Therapist and Patient Factors Contributing to the Alliance

Ackerman and Hilsenroth (2001, 2003) identified a number of therapist characteristics associated with the development of the alliance, noting that these are consistent across therapeutic orientations. Positive alliances tend to be fostered by therapist empathy, warmth and understanding, perceived trustworthiness, experience and confidence, and perceived investment in the treatment relationship. Perhaps unsurprisingly, therapists perceived to be rigid, uncertain, critical, and uninvolved are more likely to have negative alliances. Because different orientations employ different techniques, it follows that identification of a "list" of in-session activities associated with positive or negative alliances highlights activities of varying salience to different orientations. Nonetheless, there is evidence for the positive benefits of support, attention to patient experience, reflection and exploration, facilitation of affect, and accurate interpretation. Techniques linked to poorer alliances include overstructuring therapy, inappropriate use of self-disclosure, silence, and high intensity of transference interpretation.

Client factors contributing to the alliance include motivation, psychological status and quality of object relations, quality of social and family relations, and indices of stressful life events. Both intrapersonal and interpersonal factors appear to play a part. At the intrapersonal level, lack of hope, poor intrapsychic representations of others, and lack of psychological mindedness are often associated with poor outcome in terms of treatment alliance and therapeutic efficacy (Piper et al., 1991b; Ryan & Cicchetti, 1985). Difficulty in maintaining relationships and poor family relations are both associated with poor alliance and poor outcome (Kokotovic & Tracey, 1990; Moras & Strupp, 1982), and there is some evidence for the influence of attachment style—for example, individuals rated as securely attached had higher scores on the goal subscale of the Working Alliance Inventory (Satterfield & Lyddon, 1998). While anxiety about intimacy may impede the development of the alliance, the impact of specific attachment patterns on the alliance is probably complex (e.g., Eames & Roth, 2000; Malinckrodt et al., 1995), and may be partly dependent on the interaction between therapist and patient attachment styles (e.g., Dozier et al., 1994; Rubino et al., 2000; Tyrell et al., 1999). This (admittedly limited) work implies that patient and therapist contributions to the alliance cannot be reduced to a simple factor, such as the capacity to form relationships, and points toward a multiplicity of relational processes. It may be (for example) that concordance between attachment patterns is a better predictor of the working relationship than security of attachment, or that the combination of a therapist and patient with (respectively) preoccupied and dismissive attachment patterns might have different consequences to a dismissing therapist and a preoccupied patient.

Patient Expectancy, Credibility, and the Alliance

A number of studies have examined patient expectancies of treatment, with some evidence to suggest that expectations of improvement predict treatment response—for example, in depression (e.g., Sotsky et al., 1991) or social phobia (Safren et al., 1997). Joyce and Piper (1998) and Meyer et al. (2002) both found that the link between expectancy and outcome is mediated through the therapeutic alliance. Meyer et al.'s analysis suggests that effects are limited to patients' specific expectations of treatment rather than to global expectations.

Patients' appraisal of the credibility of the treatments they are offered is not equivalent to expectancy, but it is at least conceptually related. Hardy et al. (1995a) reported an analysis of the Sheffield trial for depression, which employed CBT and psychodynamic therapy. Prior to randomization, patients completed a questionnaire tapping the credibility of CBT and psychodynamic principles. Results were somewhat complex; while outcomes in CBT were not related to credibility, those receiving psychodynamic therapy had better outcomes if they saw either CBT or psychodynamic therapy as credible. This lack of specificity suggests that some form of psychological mindedness, rather than credibility as such, is pertinent to outcome in psychodynamic therapy.

Temporal Relationships between the Therapeutic Alliance and Symptomatic Change

Modeling the link between symptomatic change and variations in the alliance is an important issue. It might be that early improvement in therapy results in patients viewing their therapists and their therapy more positively, and that early improvement also predicts continued improvement (an issue discussed below, and for which there is some evidence); in other words, the observed links between alliance and outcome could reflect symptomatic improvement, or an interplay between improvement and the alliance. On this basis the notion of the alliance as a "common factor" acting independently of technique could be both methodologically and theoretically unsound. Because most trials examine the association between the alliance (measured at varying points through the therapy) and change in symptom status between intake and termination, they cannot speak directly to this issue. Evidence is restricted to those few trials whose analyses exert statistical control for symptomatic change that occurred prior to the measurement of the alliance.

Gaston et al. (1991) examined outcomes from a study of depression in 54 older adults (Thompson et al., 1987), which contrasted behavior therapy, CBT, psychodynamic therapy, or a wait-list control. Measures of the alliance were taken at sessions 5, 10, and 15, with therapy lasting between 16 and 20 sessions. They sought to determine whether the alliance uniquely accounted for additional variance in outcome after controlling for pretreatment symptom severity and for symptomatic change that had taken place prior to measurement of the alliance. On this basis no significant association was found between alliance and outcome, but the alliance did account for increasing levels of variance as therapy progressed, an effect which was more marked in behavioral and cognitive than psychodynamic therapy.

DeRubeis and Feeley (1990) explored the relationship between the alliance, technique, and outcome in 25 depressed patients treated with CBT, with therapies lasting from 10 to 60 weeks (with a median of 42). Four sessions were monitored through the first 12 weeks of therapy. Taking account of prior symptomatic change, they found no relationship between the alliance and subsequent outcome, and that prior symptomatic change predicted the alliance. In addition, the use of CBT-specific techniques in session 2 was associated with better outcomes, though this relationship did not extend to subsequent sessions. These techniques related to more concrete aspects of CBT (e.g., setting an agenda or assigning homework) as opposed to a more abstract focus (e.g., exploration of assumptions and beliefs).

Feeley et al. (1999) partially replicated these findings with data from a further group of 25 patients treated with a fixed duration of CBT (a subset of the same patients analyzed by Castonguay et al. (1996; reviewed earlier). In this study, the previous findings in relation to the alliance were only weakly replicated. Thus, while there was a trend (at the $p < .06$ level) for the alliance to be predicted by prior symptom change in the third quadrant of therapy, in the last quadrant, there was no relationship. More robustly, the same relationship was found between outcome and the use of concrete CBT techniques in session 2. These two reports raise important questions about the relationship between technique and alliance, though an obvious concern is that findings in the later study are at variance with Castonguay et al. This might reflect differences in both the number of patients sampled and their analytic procedures. A major difference is the use of residualized subsequent scores in Feeley et al. (1999), in contrast to Castonguay et al. (1996), who employed the posttherapy score.

Barber et al. (1999) examined links between the alliance and outcome in 252 cocaine-dependent individuals treated using CBT, psychodynamic therapy, or drug counseling. Therapies were offered over approximately 6 months; the alliance was measured at sessions 2 and 5 (which, because initial sessions were biweekly, occurred at week 1 and just after week 2), and most symptom measures were taken monthly. Analysis of temporal relationships related alliance level at session 5 with outcome at 1 month (based on measures of cocaine use, essentially because this was assessed weekly rather than monthly, allowing analysis to control for change between intake and session 5). On this basis, and accounting for earlier improvements, the association between the alliance and outcome was just outside statistical significance. It should be noted that when using psychiatric symptom measures (and without control for prior change), there was only a weak associations between the alliance and outcome in this study.

In contrast to the forgoing trials, two studies suggest that alliance level is indeed predictive of subsequent symptom change. Barber et al. (2000) extracted data from four open trials of supportive–expressive therapy, which included 88 patients with varying diagnostic presentations: depression/dysthmic disorder ($n = 11$); generalized anxiety disorder ($n = 44$); avoidant ($n = 19$) or obsessive–compulsive personality disorder ($n = 14$). Patients completed measures of alliance and depression at sessions 2, 5, and 10, and received between 16 and 52 sessions of therapy (though only patients with personality disorders were seen beyond 20 weeks). With the exception of session 2 (perhaps reflecting the very early point in therapy), greater change in depressive symptomatology from intake to the point at which the alliance is measured was associated with higher alliance level. Alliance level at sessions 2, 5, or 10 predicted symptomatic change subsequent to the point at which the alliance was measured. Partialing out prior improvement, alliance at each of these measurement points predicted subsequent change in depression—that is, considering patients with an equivalent level of symptomatic improvement, those who reported a higher level of alliance improved more.

Klein et al. (2003) analyzed data from a large trial of cognitive-behavioral analysis system of psychotherapy for 445 depressed individuals (Keller et al., 2000; discussed in Chapter 4), who either received therapy alone or in combination with nefazodone over 12 weeks. Symptom measures were available at weekly or biweekly intervals, and measures of the alliance at weeks 2, 6, and 12. Growth-curve modeling was used to determine the influence of the early alliance on subsequent levels of depression after controlling for prior symptomatic change. These techniques indicated that higher alliance level continued to be predictive of improvement and also permitted control for patient variables, such as prior and concurrent level of symptomatology, comorbidity, and a range of interpersonally relevant factors that might be expected to influence alliance level (e.g., personality disorder, level of social functioning, and history of neglect or abuse).

These studies are somewhat inconsistent in their findings. It may be that further trials with equivalent statistical power to Klein et al. (2003) would resolve this issue, though it is also possible that different patient populations and diagnostic grouping might result in different pattern of associations. While it would be misleading to reduce the alliance to a proxy for improvement, equally the notion of the alliance as a common relationship factor, exerting impact independent of therapeutic progress, may be an oversimplification. At the very least, it seems appropriate to question the assumption that the alliance represents a homogeneous variable. It might be more useful to think of it as a complex set of processes that vary across stages of therapy, especially because the limited available literature on temporal relationship suggests that at different points in the therapy, it acts in different ways. Perhaps a failing with these studies is that their definition of "stages of therapy" relates to time rather than to therapeutic context—for example, some sense of the progression or challenge faced by the therapy. By way of illustration, the procedures used to engage a client in the initial stages of therapy are very different from those deployed in the management of alliance ruptures, and these shifts in focus and process are difficult for statistical techniques to capture and to explain. Examining whether the alliance operates in different ways across therapies may illuminate this point, as discussed in the next section.

The Therapeutic Alliance in Different Therapies

Although most studies do not find differences in alliance level between therapies, inspection of subscales of measurement instruments sometimes suggests differences, perhaps reflecting more the impact of technique on the various components of the alliance than a fundamental variation in alliance level. Two analyses of alliance based on the Sheffield study reflect this. Using data from all participants in the trial, Agnew-Davies et al. (1998) reported that measures of "partnership" were rated significantly more highly by patients receiving CBT than by those receiving psychodynamic therapy. Raue et al. (1997) examined possible links between the alliance and "session impact," defined as the therapists' sense of the session having been "greatly helpful" or "greatly hindering." Two sessions from each therapy were selected for examination on the basis that they represented the sessions having most and least impact, respectively. Significantly higher alliance levels for CBT than for psychodynamic–interpersonal therapy were found, though this statistical difference only obtained for low-impact sessions.

Raue et al. (1993) also contrasted alliance levels in CBT and psychodynamic therapies. They identified therapists by asking experts in the field to nominate individuals whom they saw as especially competent. Thirty-one therapists agreed to participate, 18 of whom practiced using CBT, and 13 using psychodynamic approaches. Therapists were asked to submit an audiotape of a session in which (in their view) significant change had occurred. Overall alliance levels were high for both therapies, though they were higher in CBT than in psychodynamic therapy. This study is difficult to interpret, in that the criteria used by therapists for selecting sessions may have differed. For example (and as discussed further below), focusing on relationship issues is a basic technique in psychodynamic therapy, and therapists may positively connote (and therefore submit) sessions in which the alliance is challenged and subsequently repaired. This would inevitably result in lower within-session ratings of the alliance. In contrast, CBT tends to foster and to value explicit collaboration between therapist and client, again creating some bias in likely session selection.

Gaston et al. (1998) examined outcomes from Thompson et al. (1987; described earlier) As well as rating the alliance, therapist technique was assessed using an inventory that identified the degree to which exploratory or supportive strategies were employed. Alliance and outcome were positively correlated, though with a stronger association for behavioral and cognitive therapy than for psychodynamic therapy. However, this study also indicated the potential complexity of associations between alliance, technique, therapy type, and outcome, suggesting a differential impact of different strategies, at different points in therapy for different therapies.

Although evidence is sparse, it seems at least plausible that the meaning and application of processes associated with the alliance varies across orientations. Most research reflects an expectation that the alliance should be a common underlying factor (and correlational studies could be seen as broadly confirming this picture), However, the few studies that directly explore this issue hint at the possibility that the moderating effects of the alliance vary with different types of therapy, perhaps because of the different emphases they place on processes associated with the alliance. As an example, within CBT, explicit collaboration is part and parcel of the way in which technical aspects of the therapy are delivered. Although exemplars of collaborative behavior occur in other therapies, their frequency, as well as the context in which they arise, might well be expected to be different from their occurrence in CBT. This would not only influence the apparent (measured) level of the alliance but also (more subtly and less well detected by research) the moderating effect of behaviors associated with the alliance.

MATCHING PATIENTS TO THERAPIES

The ability to match patients to therapies would be a major advance in efficacy and efficiency, but as has been noted in other chapters, there is rather little consistent evidence to guide researchers or clinicians. It may be that this reflects the low statistical power common to psychotherapy trials, which would render them unable to detect potential matches, though even analyses from three large-scale trials (Crits-Christoph et al., 1999; Project MATCH Research Group, 1997a, 1998a; Rohsenow et al., 2000; all described in Chapter 12) have failed to detect patient–therapy interaction effects. Beutler et al. (2004) reported a meta-analytic review of 16 trials, all of which—bar these three—suggested patient coping style may be relevant. Specifically, self-reflective and introspective individuals appeared to benefit more from insight-oriented therapies, while impulsive and aggressive patients responded better to symptom-focused procedures.

Despite the general lack of relevant findings in this area, a number of studies have examined the impact on outcome of patients' "quality of object relations" and psychological mindedness. Horowitz et al. (1984) describe outcomes in 52 patients receiving 12 sessions of short-term psychodynamic therapy for bereavement. Patients with higher levels of motivation for psychodynamic therapy and a more stable and coherent sense of self responded better to dynamic exploration of their difficulties; in contrast, those with low levels of these qualities appeared to respond better to more supportive interventions. Adopting a rather different strategy, Jones et al. (1988) examined transcripts of completed therapies from 40 patients, also undergoing 12 sessions of brief therapy following bereavement. A psychotherapy Q sort was used, in effect, to analyze the content of sessions and, in particular, the contributions of the therapist. Patients who showed the greatest distress and disturbance appeared to respond best to expressive techniques, whereas those with less distress had better outcomes with more supportive interventions. Horowitz et al. (1988, 1993) also presented data suggesting that patients who describe their problems more in terms of interpersonal difficulties than symptoms tend to have better outcomes in psychodynamic psychotherapy.

Piper and colleagues have conducted a series of studies which have explored the link between patient characteristics, technique and outcome. Broadly, "quality of object relations" (QOR) refers to the maturity and stability of an individual's interpersonal relationships, and is assessed by standardized interview. Psychological mindedness is assessed by asking patients to comment on videotaped scenarios, with scoring reflecting the degree of psychological complexity in responses (McCallum & Piper, 1997). Piper et al. (1990, 1991a, 1991b) presented data from 64 individuals with mixed diagnoses who completed a trial of short-term dynamic therapy. Patients with high QOR had better outcomes than those with low QOR; the proportion meeting criteria for clinically significant change across three measures was 70–83% and 12–32%, respectively. Further analyses explored the relationship between interpretation and outcome, distinguishing between the number of interpretations made in a session ("concentration") and the degree to which these interpretations "correspond" to therapists' formulations (or, in the specific sense of fidelity to formulation, the extent to which interpretation was accurate). Correspondence was assessed using the core conflictual relationship theme method (Luborsky & Crits-Christoph, 1990), a technique for systematically and reliably formulating patients' difficulties. Findings were complex, but overall, there was an inverse relationship between the number of interpretations made per session and both outcome and the patient-rated alliance, an effect seen most clearly for patients with a high QOR. The impact of the correspondence (or accuracy) of interpretations differed according to the patient's QOR rating. While patients with high QOR appeared to benefit from correspondent interpretation, their use was associated with poorer outcome for patients with low QOR. Correspondence and concentration were not correlated, suggesting that effects noted earlier were not simply a product of a high frequency of inaccurate interpretation. Regression analysis indicated an interaction between these factors and outcome in high-QOR patients, such that the best outcomes were seen in these patients when their therapist made fewer, but accurate, interpretations. Piper et al. (1994) explored outcomes in the context of a day-treatment program, with 165 patients with mixed affective and personality disorders treated using psychodynamic group treatments. Better outcome was associated with higher levels of QOR and psychological mindedness; higher QOR was also associated with lower attrition.

On the basis of forgoing studies Piper et al. (1998) matched patient pairs on the basis of their QOR score, level of psychological mindedness, use of medication, and (where possible) their gender and age. On the basis of this match, one of each pair was randomized to a more interpretive, and the other to a more supportive therapy. One hundred seventy-one patients started treatment, with therapy offered over a 20-week period. Overall, both therapies had similar impacts, but as in earlier trials, QOR differentiated outcome in interpretive therapy, but not in supportive therapy. Though there were some issues relating to its measurement, higher levels of psychological mind-edness were associated with better outcomes for both forms of therapy. At 6- and 12-month follow-up (Piper et al., 1999), the pattern of results for QOR continued to obtain, though psychological mindedness was no longer associ-ated with differential benefit. A further trial explored these factors in the con-text of interpretive or supportive group therapy for individuals with compli-cated grief reactions (Ogrodniczuk et al., 2002; Piper et al., 2001). QOR was associated with better outcome for interpretive therapy and lower QOR with greater success in supportive therapy; psychological mindedness was associated with more improvement in both therapies.

Two further studies presented data relevant to this issue. Hoglend (1993) examined the frequency of transference interpretation in 43 patients receiving psychodynamic therapy of (quite widely varying) length, reporting (as in Piper et al., 1991a) that rate of interpretation was inversely related to out-come for individuals with higher QOR. Connolly et al. (1999) reported out-comes from 29 depressed patients treated with supportive–expressive therapy, examining the use of transference interpretation in early sessions (up to ses-sion 9 of a 16-week therapy). Interpersonal functioning was assessed using a measure based on current rather than lifelong functioning (as in the QOR measure). Though, overall, rather few transference interpretations were made, their greater use was associated with poorer outcomes for patients with poorer interpersonal functioning, while outcomes for patients with better interpersonal functioning were not related to frequency of interpretation. Connolly et al. noted that (apart from methodological differences between studies), transference interpretations occurred at approximately one-fifth the rate in the Piper et al. (1991a) study. They suggest that differences between studies reflect the fact that interpretations are toxic to patients with low QOR at all but very low frequency, while individuals with higher QOR benefit from low to moderate levels of interpretation. On this basis, low QOR patients in Piper et al.'s trial showed no differential impact from inter-pretation, because they had already been exposed beyond threshold, while those with high QOR showed worsening outcomes as the concentration increased from moderate to high. This ingenious resolution of somewhat variant results requires further research.

Overall, these studies suggest that individuals with a history of difficulties relating to others in a stable and consistent manner may react badly to the interpersonal challenge that transference interpretations can pose. If a mini-mal maturity of mental function is essential to make use of insight-oriented psychodynamic psychotherapy, then some caution and care should be taken in the use of psychodynamic techniques with such individuals. However, whether this finding generalizes to all forms of psychodynamic approaches is not so clear. For example, patients with borderline personality disorder—who would presumably score low on QOR—do appear responsive to struc-tured psychodynamic techniques (as described in Chapter 11). It may be that some of the interventions employed with these patients (aimed at facilitating mentalization and clarifying mental states) would be coded as supportive rather than interpretive by Piper's group. Although this is a matter of technical concern when viewed from a research perspective, it would be of pragmatic value when considering ways in which appropriate modifications of technique might be made for patients low in QOR.

PREDICTION OF OUTCOME
FROM PRIOR RESPONSE TO TREATMENT

Research data offer general rather than specific prognostic indicators; they cannot predict the trajectory of change for an individual patient. Because outcome reflects an interaction between patient, therapist, and technique, it may be more fruitful to use a patient's initial response to therapy as an indicator of later benefit, rather than attempting to do this at the stage of pretherapy assessment.

There is evidence that patients exposed to more treatment derive more benefit than those receiving less therapy (Orlinsky et al., 1994), though it is less clear what the optimum treatment might be for any different condition. Howard et al. (1986) sought to determine how many sessions were required to produce clinically significant change by meta-analyzing 15 data sets in which 2,431 patients received therapy of varying length. After 2, 8, 26, and 52 sessions, 30%, 53%, 75%, and 85%, respectively, of patients showed improvement, suggesting that the measurable rate of change is fastest in the earlier stages of therapy, with diminishing returns in relation to increasing treatment length. A limitation of this study is that it relied on pre- to posttherapy data to estimate the likely "shape" of change across sessions rather than examining session-by-session change directly. Recent reports have employed survival analysis to derive a more direct estimate of the number of sessions required to achieve clinically significant change. Anderson and Lambert (2001) tracked outcomes for 75 clients, estimating the number of sessions required for 50% of clients to achieve clinically significant change. For their sample, a median of 11 sessions was required. Combining this with a sample of 47 patients from Kadera et al. (1996) indicated that while less distressed individuals required a median of 12 sessions, more distressed patients required 20. A larger trial by Hansen and Lambert (2003) examined outcomes for 4,761 patients seen in standard treatment settings (including HMOs, employee assistance programs, and community mental health centers). These individuals required a median of between 15 and 19 sessions to achieve this level of change, dependent on setting.

Based on the dose–response relationship, Howard et al. (1993) developed a pantheoretical model of change, which suggests that therapy has three distinct phases—a restoration of subjective well-being, followed by resolution

of symptoms, and finally a period addressing maladaptive aspects of life functioning. This implies a sequential progression through therapy, a proposition
for which there is mixed evidence (e.g., Barkham et al., 1996b; Hilsenroth et
al., 2001; Joyce et al., 2002; Kopta et al., 1994). There are also indications
from recent studies that improvement in at least some patients may be better
characterized as a process of sudden but stable gains rather than linear
improvement (e.g., Stiles et al., 2003; Tang & DeRubeis, 1999; Tang et al.,
2002). Nonetheless, the dose–response model suggests a lawful and predictable course of recovery, and the possibility that "profiling" outcomes for a
very large number of patients would yield an average course of recovery. On
this basis, the gains made by an individual patient could be contrasted against
those made by the "average" patient at each stage of therapy, with clinicians
afforded an actuarial rather than clinical judgment of their progress.

Two research groups have developed conceptually similar, though
methodologically distinct, procedures for determining patient profiles. Both
use assessment information to yield an expected trajectory of response that
varies depending on the initial severity of patient presentation, with slower
rates of change predicted for those with more severe problems. Built into
both systems are a series of confidence limits that warn therapists when
expected change is not occurring, and especially when there is evidence of
deterioration (prompting case review). Equally, they can indicate when the
patient has made rapid change and (in effect) has already achieved benefit
from therapy, prompting earlier discharge. Howard's group utilized a battery
of instruments that assess symptoms and life functioning and well-being, as
well as considering patients' views of their problems and their expectations of
therapy (e.g., Lueger et al., 2001; Lutz et al., 1999). Lambert's group adopt a
simpler procedure, using a relatively short, 45-item questionnaire that covers
symptomatic state, social role functioning, and interpersonal relationships
(e.g., Finch et al., 2001; Lambert et al., 2001a, 2001b). Lambert et al. (2001b)
demonstrated the potential utility of this system by randomizing therapists to
receive, or not to receive, feedback regarding the progress of their patients
relative to expected trajectories. Although this system resulted in a small
improvement in overall outcomes, of particular interest is the subgroup of
patients whose trajectories indicated that they were not responding to treatment. In these instances, feedback led to a significant reduction in those who
had poor outcomes. Contrasted to patients whose therapists did not receive
feedback, 6% and 26% of these patients, respectively, showed significant deterioration at the end of therapy. A similar pattern of outcomes was found by
Whipple et al. (2003).

As yet, it is unclear how these "case-tracking" systems will perform in
client groups representative of standard clinical populations. Leon et al.
(1999) contrasted the predicted and actual trajectories of change in 890
patients, classifying them according to the predictability or unpredictability of

their outcomes. Discriminant function analysis indicated that patients with lower levels of symptomatology and better functioning had more predictable trajectories, raising some question about the utility of this approach in more disturbed populations. The only study to examine this to date (Hawkins et al., 2004) was conducted in a hospital outpatient unit, and addressed the question of how feedback would impact on outcome rather than predictability. In line with studies described earlier, feedback improved outcomes, despite the fact that in almost 50% of cases, therapists received warning of deterioration, a frequency that might have been expected to reduce the salience of the feedback system.

The utility of these systems for enhancing clinical practice has yet to be adequately explored. However, they represent a potentially powerful aid for service planners, because they make it more likely that patients with severe and complex presentations are offered treatments of a length likely to result in benefit, avoiding the cost-inefficiencies of inappropriately brief treatments. Equally, they limit the provision of lengthy therapies for those with responsive presentations. For clinicians, they represent an aid to decision making and to supervision, since they can help to focus particular attention on those cases in which expected change is not happening at an expected rate.

SUMMARY AND CLINICAL IMPLICATIONS

Although variance in outcome attributable to therapists appears to be large and reasonably consistent across studies, it is surprisingly hard to account for these differences. Although practitioners (and, indeed, managers and patients) might expect experience and training to be relevant to efficacy, findings are equivocal, and—at first glance—do not offer strong support for the benefit of these factors. However, the methodologies used to detect these associations are invariably correlational and analysis is post hoc, and in most trials, each therapist sees so few patients that attributing outcomes to therapist characteristics is an unreliable exercise. Furthermore, many studies confound issues of patient difficulty and complexity with therapist seniority, because naturalistic allocation means that more difficult patients are usually allocated to more senior therapists.

There is some evidence that experience becomes a more important predictor of outcome with patients who are more disturbed. The tendency for more experienced therapists both to have less dropout and to retain more difficult patients in therapy may lead them to show apparently poorer average outcomes relative to inexperienced therapists. Experience may therefore be important in dealing with cases in which the patient's attitude is predominantly negative to the therapy. This effect may make it harder to detect differences attributable to experience in studies that do not control for the impact of attrition. Given the importance of understanding sources of variance in therapist performance, it is surprising that this issue is invariably explored as a secondary analysis. An ideal trial would categorize therapists as part of the design, recruiting an appropriate number of therapists at differing levels of assumed skillfulness and—crucially—randomizing patients to therapists.

Studies that examine therapists' behavior rather than their backgrounds tend to underscore the importance of manualized treatments, suggesting an association (even if also a confound) among outcome, adherence, and competence, though the latter appears more pertinent than the former. This suggests that it would be more productive to detect the impact of competence as enacted in the context of therapy, rather than assuming it to be "gifted" through experience or training. Notwithstanding this point, there are indications that some therapists are more competent than others, though even this does not guarantee that they will be competent in all their therapies, or that they will always be able (as it were) to do the right thing at the right time. In this sense, competence is really a reference to competence of delivery rather than being (straightforwardly) an attribute of an individual.

The foregoing suggests that manuals of psychotherapy have much to contribute to the training of psychotherapists, and that models of good training practice would include formally assessing their capacity to adhere to these. However, it also suggests that while good knowledge of the key components of a technique is an important foundation for effective practice, expert practitioners may be those who are able to use technical recommendations flexibly, and deviate and go beyond them at times, when the clinical situation seems to require this.

The tools used to measure competence tend to reflect something of the central tenets of the therapy being delivered; there is no pantheoretical measurement system (beyond the assessment of basic skills nor is there likely to be). Since there are indications that the level and type of skills defining competence vary across therapies, it difficult to know whether studies that consider the impact of skillfulness in delivering different therapies are commensurate. This further complicates discussion of competence, because it indicates that judgments of skillfulness are determined—at least in part—by parameters such as the type of therapy, and also the complexity of the therapeutic intervention. It seems reasonable to assume that the more demanding the therapy, the more critical issues of competence are likely to be. As an example, it seems unlikely that performing exposure therapy for a specific phobia requires the same skill level as delivering complex CBT to individuals with multiple disabilities (e.g., implementing schema-focused work, or CBT focused on the modification of delusional beliefs). It is at least an interesting possibility that studies finding an apparent lack of difference between simpler and more elaborate therapies may be detecting the wider variation in competence associated with the latter—an issue which is rarely specifically examined.

Whatever their technical differences, most models of therapy recognize the importance of the therapeutic alliance, treating it as a moderating variable without which no therapy would succeed. This proposition has high face validity and empirical support from a large number of studies showing small but significant correlations between alliance level and outcome. This sort of result appeals to clinical intuition; psychological therapy is an interpersonal process, and it seems reasonable that relationship factors should be important to its success. Any kind of therapy asks patients to undertake something they had been reluctant to do in the past, making it probable that some form of social exchange is needed to tolerate this. However, research over recent years has complicated this picture. An important question is whether the alliance precedes or reflects symptomatic improvement, an issue that is difficult to settle because it requires measures of symptom change and alliance level at multiple points throughout therapy. Rather few studies with appropriate data are available, and results are not completely consistent. While some larger studies suggest that alliance remains a robust indicator of outcome, even when prior change is accounted for, others suggest that symptom change may precede improvement in the alliance. Were this to be so, it would challenge assumptions about the mutative power of the alliance as a process factor *sui generis*. This repositioning would represent a considerable challenge to our thinking about the alliance, particularly for those who have contrasted the lack of evidence for differential efficacy for different treatments with consistent evidence for the impact of the alliance, and concluded that common "relationship" factors are more important to therapy outcome than considerations of technique.

Some of the complications of this area may reflect the tendency to treat the alliance as a singular concept, when, in fact, it may better be seen as a proxy for different therapeutic processes operating at different stages in therapy, influenced by the therapeutic context and implemented rather differently across therapeutic modalities. Attempts to research the alliance may have blurred these issues in favor of a uniform—hence, measurable—concept. As a result, qualitative research, which does account for the meaning and context of activities associated with the alliance, is somewhat isolated from quantitative approaches to this subject. Bringing these two approaches together might help identify that part of the alliance that is specifically therapeutic, and the processes that contribute to this.

Being able to match patients to treatments prospectively would be an obvious benefit for clients, therapists, and managers alike. Unfortunately, relevant findings are few, and though some of this may relate to the fact that matching effects are often sought on a post hoc basis, even large trials that have set out to explore this issue have been disappointing. However, attempts to identify a demographic or characteristic that enables prospective assignment may be unproductive. The most interesting studies in this area tend to describe the impact of a process rather than a category (e.g., variations in QoR seem a more powerful predictor of treatment response than qualities such as gender, class, ethnicity, etc.). This observation also applies to issues such as the therapist's or patient's contribution to outcome, where it seems less likely that the characteristics of each party will emerge as obvious determinants of outcome than the way these factors operate in therapy.

Case-tracking methods make few assumptions about patient or therapist characteristics other than those that are derived empirically and contribute to the screening systems used to predict likely trajectories of change. However, they do reflect an approach to issues of treatment matching based entirely on client responsiveness, and in this way sidestep not only concerns about the capacity of therapists to allocate patients to appropriate treatment but also one of the central problems of therapy research—the fact that we know little about how an individual patient will respond even when there is evidence for the efficacy of a treatment. Case-tracking research is still developing, but studies already indicate the feasibility of its methodology, though few trials have as yet been conducted in routine settings. Available evidence indicates that the feedback systems inherent to these techniques result in improved outcomes, most particularly in relation to patients whose initial responses to therapy are poor.

Our review of process factors suggests to us that questions about the therapist's contribution to effectiveness are more likely to be answered by examination of the emerging dynamics of a therapy than by attempts to consider these prior to therapy. This is a far from abstract issue. By creating anchor points that indicate whether therapy is making appropriate headway, outcome tracking techniques could help to focus attention on such issues as alliance, adherence to technique and competence, as well as issues of client–treatment match. Combining case tracking with appropriate supervision, even of experienced therapists, may be an especially potent system both for improving outcomes and avoiding adverse events, as well as for generating ideas about the ways in which process factors contribute to the trajectory of therapy.

CHAPTER 17

CONCLUSIONS AND IMPLICATIONS

Previous chapters have presented an appraisal of research into psychological therapies for a range of conditions. Attempting to integrate our findings so that they can be applied constructively in service settings is a challenge. In the introductory chapters of this book, we drew attention to the fact that efficacy, as reported in research trials, is not equivalent to (and does not guarantee) clinical effectiveness in everyday practice. In Chapter 3, we discussed a model in which evidence-based practice emerges from a mix of psychotherapy research and professional consensus, with clinical guidelines guiding clinical practice, and with clinical judgment informing the applicability of guidelines to the individual case. We hope this will support practice that is rooted in empirical findings but not circumscribed by them.

Increasingly, systematic reviews of treatment outcomes are used to derive a list of "validated" or "empirically supported" treatments. Although this approach has the benefit of providing a summary of the evidence, it can easily be misinterpreted as a list of "facts" about treatment effects. Ignoring the cautions necessary to interpret such lists opens them to abuse. This is especially so when the absence of a therapy from a list is used to justify its exclusion from service provision, without recognition that while absence of evidence for efficacy can indeed indicate absence of treatment effects, this cannot be assumed.

Although we start this chapter with a list of treatments with demonstrated efficacy, we follow it with a reminder of why such a summary should be treated with caution. Oversimplification of complex issues will do little service to achieving truly evidence-based practice, and attempting to isolate this list from our caveats and concerns (which reflect issues raised at many points throughout this volume) would be an error.

FOR WHICH TREATMENTS IS THERE EVIDENCE OF EFFICACY?

Reducing evidence to a binary option of supported or not supported is not an adequate representation of the research literature, and the criteria used to judge whether a treatment has evidence of efficacy will always be to some degree arbitrary. Notions of efficacy beg the question of what is considered sufficient evidence, and what degree of change may be regarded as appropriate or significant. Nonetheless, a summary of evidence for treatment efficacy is helpful, and in approaching this issue, we identified the following criteria as important:

- Replicated demonstration of superiority to a control condition or another treatment condition, or a single, high-quality randomized control trial.
- The availability of a clear description of the therapeutic method (preferably but not necessarily in the form of a therapy manual) of sufficient clarity to be usable as the basis for training.
- A clear description of the patient group to whom the treatment was applied.

Our requirement for replicated superiority does not distinguish between contrast to a bona fide alternative therapy and contrast to a control condition, the former being a more challenging test than the latter. Although it is feasible to make this distinction, it also complicates any attempt at summarizing the evidence, and on balance, we have chosen to elide this issue.

Rather than restricting our summary only to those interventions that meet all our criteria, we have also included some treatments for which there is only limited evidence of efficacy. This allows us to identify innovative techniques, where promising but restricted evidence reflects their stage of development, and to include approaches commonly used in treatment settings, but where research is limited by methodological constraints. Where such treatments appear in the list below, we have added a comment to justify their inclusion. We recognize that, for some readers this could be seen as an inappropriately liberal approach to the research evidence, but we feel that there is a balance to be struck between rigorous application of methodological criteria and exclusion of comment on clinically relevant approaches.

The list that follows is a simplification of a complex set of findings, and it should not be considered a substitute for the more detailed appraisals of treatments found in the relevant chapters dealing with each disorder. It describes techniques largely at the level of approaches rather than identifying specific manual-based interventions. In our view, this is a more helpful way of summarizing the evidence, largely because it maps research therapies onto the families of treatments out of which they emerged and of which they are exemplars. It also avoids creating what can often be an illusory degree of specification of therapeutic approaches. However, there are risks attached to our decision. As techniques are devolved into clinical settings, they could depart from some of the successful elements that make them effective. This issue applies strongly to cognitive-behavioral therapy (CBT), where it needs to be remembered that modern applications of this model are underpinned by several theoretical approaches, and that a range of specific clinical procedures need to be applied in relation to specific clinical populations. Finally, this list makes the assumption that it is the specific (theoretically derived) technique that is the effective component, rather than the context in which it is applied (which is usually unspecified).

The following annotations are used in the sections that follow:

Interventions for which there is clear evidence of efficacy: indicated by ▲

Interventions for which there is some, but limited support for efficacy: indicated by *italicized text*

Major Depressive Disorder

▲ Cognitive-behavioral approaches
▲ Interpersonal psychotherapy
Short-term structured psychodynamic psychotherapy

Comment: *Although this is a widely used technique, there is clear support from only one large-scale randomized controlled trial (RCT). There is some additional support from small and nonrandomized trials, and (indirectly) from trials with diagnostically heterogeneous populations.*

Dysthymic Disorder

Comment: *The only available large-scale trials contrast psychological therapy (usually problem solving, CBT or interpersonal psychotherapy [IPT]), medication, and their combination. Most studies suggest that little advantage is conferred by the addition of psychological therapy to medication, and that medication alone is usually more effective than psychological therapy alone. There are only small-scale, usually nonrandomized trials of CBT and IPT alone. Although techniques applied successfully for patients with major depressive disorder may be applicable to this group, this observation relies on clinical judgment rather than research evidence.*

Bipolar Disorder

Psychoeducation
Cognitive-behavioral therapy aimed at relapse prevention and the management of depressive symptomatology, usually combined with cognitive techniques aimed at stabilizing the patient's lifestyle

Interpersonal and social rhythm therapy
Family interventions, particularly for families with higher levels of expressed emotion

Comment: *All these interventions show promise, but at this stage, evidence is limited by small sample sizes, or a lack of replication. The results of a number of large-scale trials already in progress will enable more conclusive statements to be made about the efficacy of these approaches.*

Specific Phobia

▲ Exposure therapy (*in vivo*)
Applied tension and exposure for blood–injury phobia

Comment: *Although research support for applied tension for blood–injury phobia is consistent (and reflects clinical experience), results are available from only one research group.*

Social Phobia

▲ Exposure therapy
▲ Cognitive therapy in combination with exposure

Comment: *While the benefits of exposure-based approaches are clear, evidence for the additive benefit of cognitive techniques to exposure therapy is not always strong. However, some more recent trials that include specific adaptations for social phobia indicate more substantive benefits.*

Generalized Anxiety Disorder

▲ Cognitive-behavioral therapy
▲ Applied relaxation

Panic Disorder with and without Agoraphobia

▲ Exposure therapy
▲ Cognitive-behavioral therapy
▲ Panic control therapy

Obsessive–Compulsive Disorders

▲ Exposure and response prevention
Cognitive restructuring and rational–emotive therapy, in combination with exposure

Comment: *There is mixed evidence for the benefit of adding cognitive therapy to exposure and response prevention (ERP) in standard treatment. There may be stronger evidence for this combination when patients have failed to respond to intensive ERP treatments alone, and in the management of ruminations.*

Posttraumatic Stress Disorder

▲ Cognitive-behavioral approaches
▲ Eye movement desensitization and reprocessing
Structured psychodynamic psychotherapy

Comment: *There are a number of CBT approaches to posttraumatic stress disorder (PTSD), all of which imply an exposure element, and this technique is also evident in eye movement desensitization and reprocessing (EMDR). The balance between behavioral and cognitive-behavioral techniques varies across studies, and also in relation to the specific needs of the patient. The impact of psychodynamic techniques has been explored in a small number of trials, but methodological problems make it hard to discern a clear benefit.*

Anorexia Nervosa

Inpatient contingency management (in relation to short-term weight gain)
Family therapy (particularly when offered to younger patients with anorexia)
Cognitive-behavioral approaches
Focal psychodynamic therapy
Cognitive analytic therapy

Comment: *There are rather few studies available on which to base conclusions. Psychological treatments invariably include dietary advice. Inpatient contingency management seems effective in ensuring immediate—but not sustained—weight gain. Family therapy, focal psychodynamic therapy, and cognitive analytic therapy (CAT) show benefit over standard care or no treatment. There is little evidence for the benefit of cognitive therapy in younger patients with anorexia, though one trial indicates its potential in relapse prevention with older women. For younger anorexics (under the age of 18), there is some evidence of advantage to family over individual therapy.*

Bulimia Nervosa

▲ Cognitive-behavioral therapy, including dietary management, for patients with bulimia nervosa
▲ Interpersonal psychotherapy for bulimic patients

Binge-Eating Disorder

Comment: *Studies of treatments for binge-eating disorder have increased in recent years, but evidence is still limited. Some studies have suggested that CBT is an effective approach, but further work is required to reach firmer conclusions.*

Schizophrenia

▲ Family intervention programs
Cognitive therapy for delusions
Psychoeducation in combination with psychological intervention

Comment: *There is mixed evidence regarding the capacity of cognitive therapy to shorten initial episodes or to ameliorate specific symptoms, and no indication that it reduces relapse rates. However, this rapidly developing area of work and future research should clarify the benefits of this approach. Psychoeducation shows best results in combination with techniques recognizable as psychological intervention; there is little therapeutic gain from psychoeducation alone, apart from increases in knowledge and short-term increases in compliance.*

Personality Disorders

▲ Dialectical behavior therapy for borderline personality disorder
▲ Psychodynamic psychotherapy for borderline personality disorder
Social skills training for avoidant personality disorder

Comment: *There are few substantive findings for the treatment of personality disorders other than borderline personality disorder (BPD) and (to a lesser degree) avoidant personality disorder (APD). There should be clear regard for the fact that nonspecific factors may be integral in treating individuals with BPD (but by extension any cluster B personality disorder); successful approaches emphasize the importance of structure in treatment implementation and a coherent theoretical base.*

Alcohol Abuse

▲ Brief educational interventions, including motivational interviewing (particularly for patients with lower initial severity of alcohol abuse and an absence of comorbid psychiatric problems)
▲ Social skills training, relapse prevention, cue exposure, coping skills training, contingency management, motivational interviewing, and marital therapy, usually offered adjunctively and in various combinations as part of a broader package of treatment
▲ 12-step approaches
▲ Community reinforcement approaches

Comment: *Treatments for alcohol abuse (and cocaine and opiate abuse) are often administered adjunctively and in a number of combinations, meaning that judgments about efficacy need to consider the context in which any single "stand-alone" treatment is likely to be delivered.*

Cocaine Abuse

▲ Contingency management and community reinforcement approaches
12-step approaches
Cognitive-behavioral therapy (focused on relapse prevention)
Behavioral marital therapy

Opiate Abuse

Supportive–expressive therapy

Comment: *Treatments are most usually researched in the context of a program that includes methadone maintenance. There is some limited evidence for supportive–expressive therapy, based on only one trial.*

Sexual Dysfunctions

▲ Behavioral and cognitive-behavioral treatment approaches aimed at reducing sexual anxiety and improving communication for erectile dysfunction
▲ Exposure-based behavioral techniques for vaginismus
Specific behavioral techniques for premature ejaculation

Interventions with Children

Cognitive-behavioral therapy for depression
Interpersonal psychotherapy adapted for adolescents with depression
Psychodynamic therapy for mixed anxiety and depression
▲ Exposure techniques for phobias
▲ Cognitive-behavioral therapy for obsessive–compulsive disorder and generalized anxiety disorder
▲ Contingency management treatment of undesirable behavior in autism
▲ Parent training programs and cognitive-behavioral therapy for conduct problems
▲ Multisystemic therapy for adolescent conduct problems
Long-term multimodal therapy for attention-deficit/hyperactivity disorder

Comment: *In general, the development of an evidence base for interventions with children lags behind that for adult disorders, with a higher proportion of single-case or small-scale studies and rather few large-scale controlled randomized trials. As a consequence, rather few treatments can be listed in this section. This means that great caution is required before interpreting the absence of an approach from this list as an indicator of a lack of efficacy.*

For many specific disorders (e.g., PTSD, eating disorders, and deliberate self-harm), there are rather few studies focused specifically on outcomes for children/adolescents. Although this necessarily limits conclusions, it seems reasonable for treatment choice in these areas to be guided by the adult literature.

Interventions with Older People

▲ Behavioral, cognitive-behavioral, and structured psychodynamic psychotherapy for depression

Cognitive-behavioral therapy for anxiety disorders

Cognitive-behavioral therapy for sleep disorders

Psychoeducational and psychotherapeutic interventions for caregivers

Reality orientation for people with dementia, including cognitive stimulation offered as part of reality orientation

Comment: *Although psychological approaches show benefit for older adults with functional presentations, there is only limited research on which conclusions can be based. While a number of approaches to the management of dementia show benefit, again, the strength of evidence limits the conclusions that can be drawn.*

METHODOLOGICAL CAVEATS AND CAUTIONS

Efficacy and Effectiveness

At various points in our review, we have cautioned that the clinical impact of treatments may not reflect the promise of research. The very techniques that are used to distinguish therapy effects from other sources of variance restrict generalization: The use of diagnostically homogeneous patient samples, well-trained and well-supervised therapists, extensive monitoring of the patient's progress, and careful adherence to treatment protocols may serve to increase the apparent effectiveness of psychotherapeutic interventions. Though recent years have seen the emergence of studies benchmarking the effectiveness of therapies in routine practice against efficacy in research contexts, these are still few in number. We are also seeing the emergence of techniques for service profiling and benchmarking (e.g., Barkham et al., 2001), and the next few years should bring greater clarity about the relative effect sizes obtained in research and clinical contexts. Although Weisz et al.'s (1995a) meta-analytic contrast of outcomes in research and clinical contexts was based on a very limited number of trials, it still stands as a helpful caution on generalization, indicating as it does a much larger impact for treatments in research settings than in clinical ones.

It follows that whatever the efficacy of an intervention, its effectiveness in the framework of everyday service provision cannot be guaranteed. This means that the interests of clients are not met simply by claiming to practice a treatment of "known efficacy." There is also a risk that the broadly favorable tone of this and other reviews could be used to shield ineffective practice and practitioners from scrutiny. Our interpretation of the evidence is that a variety of techniques in the hands of well-trained and supervised practitioners, operating within a structured and controlled framework, are likely to be both safe and effective. The context within which these studies were carried out should not be overlooked in interpreting these findings. The high level of training of diagnosticians and therapists in many of these trials, and the systematic way in which adherence to treatment protocols was assured may, in and of themselves, be factors critical to the efficacy of the treatment procedures under scrutiny.

Limitations Imposed by the Use of the DSM

As noted in Chapter 2, most outcome research is organized in relation to diagnosis, and overwhelmingly the DSM is used as a framework for patient selection. Inevitably, this shapes the way in which reviews such as our own are structured, and pragmatic considerations overrule whatever philosophical concerns there might be about the use of diagnosis in general, and the DSM in particular. Nonetheless, use of the DSM can obscure several pertinent issues.

1. By definition, diagnostic homogeneity assures a uniformity of symptom presentation, but the problems that underpin patients' presentations are likely to be diverse. Developmental psychopathology indicates not only that different life experiences can result in the same diagnostic end point, but also that exposure to the same event can lead to different diagnostic outcomes, and we do not know whether response to treatment is substantially affected by such diversity. The likely heterogeneity of biology and psychosocial experience reflected within any one diagnosis is increasingly seen as relevant (Gottesman & Gould, 2003), and can become obvious in the course of guideline development, when the heterogeneity of results seems quite likely to reflect definitional ambiguities. By way of example, a guideline for depression produced by the U.K. National Institute for Clinical Excellence (2004) notes that " 'depression' may be too heterogeneous in biological, psychological and social terms to enable clarity on which specific interventions, for which problem, for which person, and in which context, will be effective" (p. 17).

2. At several points in this book, we have referred to the problem of comorbidity between DSM disorders, which in clinical populations ranges from 50 to 90%, depending on the primary condition (Kessler et al., 1996, 1999; Newman et al., 1998). Attempts to reduce comorbidity in research

samples make it more difficult to be clear about both the likely process of therapy and its outcome in clinical samples, especially when personality disorder is a significant part of a patient's presentation.

3. One virtue of DSM is that diagnosis is only made when a clear pattern of symptoms is present. A consequence is the exclusion of individuals with "subthreshold" presentations from many trials, and there is a risk that researchers and those responsible for service provision make the criteria for treatment of emotional distress synonymous with a DSM diagnosis. In fact, it is clear that high levels of distress can occur in the absence of a diagnosable condition. Some studies suggest that between 30 and 50% of patients seeking help for mental health problems cannot be diagnosed using the DSM because their problems are "subthreshold" (e.g., Howard et al., 1996). This means that there is rather less evidence than is desirable regarding outcomes for individuals with milder or subthreshold forms of mental health problems. Indeed, in some areas—for example, eating disorders—the prevalence of subthreshold cases means that there are appropriate questions about the utility of research focused only on diagnosable cases. Quite appropriately, there is ongoing debate about the degree to which DSM-V should acknowledge this issue (e.g., Kessler et al., 2003), especially when psychological treatment for a milder disorder may prevent the emergence of more serious difficulties at a later stage.

4. A number of studies are excluded from this book because they employ mixed patient samples (with heterogeneous diagnoses), and this places them outside the structure we have adopted. This impacts rather more severely on reports of psychodynamic therapies than on other orientations, because although some quite large research programs have been conducted (reflecting the traditions of this approach), these are not focused on links between treatment and specific symptomatic presentation. This inevitably renders them "silent" in relation to a review based on DSM, and further reduces the already rather small pool of available trials for this orientation. Of course, the structure of this book is not arbitrary—it is shaped by the trials available for review, and diagnostically homogenous samples have become increasingly normative. However, it is worth acknowledging that this trend only partly reflects shifts in "scientific" standards. Pragmatic considerations have also been important; it has become harder for researchers to obtain funding for samples based on other criteria, further reinforcing the skew in the literature.

5. RCTs may produce different outcomes depending on the patient mix, defined in terms of comorbidity, chronicity, and severity, which can often be influenced by contextual factors, such as the manner in which patients have been recruited to a trial (e.g., Brent et al., 1998).

6. The sheer number of disorders makes it improbable that disorder-specific, manualized treatments will become a generally viable way of orga-

nizing services, except in the cases of a relatively small number of the most common disorders (Beutler et al., 2002).

While in our view, none of the limitations of DSM, singly or in combination, invalidate our conclusions, they do imply that we should be cautious in interpreting and implementing the findings of research based exclusively on DSM.

The "File Drawer" Problem and the Problem of Unpublished Trials

Researchers usually submit papers to journals when their trials show positive benefits for patients, though an exception is when null findings fit into a research context. Only very rarely are findings presented that yield clear evidence of deterioration or positive damage to patients. Overall, there is the potential for a skew in the literature, with the possibility that selective publication introduces a bias into our general picture of both the relative efficacy of therapies and also their potential to harm as well as to help. One way of addressing this problem is by the systematic registration of all trials before commencement (e.g., Easterbrook, 1992). Making this compulsory may be onerous, but it would carry the advantage of ensuring the availability of a more complete picture of expected outcomes.

The Absence of Long-Term Follow-Up Data

Throughout this book, we have highlighted the long-term nature of many psychological disorders. Unfortunately, few studies have investigated the capacity of psychological therapies to influence the long-term course of these disorders; hence, estimates of efficacy frequently relate only to short- or medium-term outcomes. It is important to recognize that there are practical as well as conceptual problems in improving our knowledge. Longer follow-up requires the expenditure of considerable effort and resources. Patient attrition inevitably increases over time, leading to problems of data interpretation. Additionally, longer follow-up periods are not necessarily informative of treatment effects, unless there is some control on any additional therapies patients receive, and only rarely is this likely to be possible.

A further problem is that there is little consensus in the literature about how indicators of progress are to be defined and measured, though we noted in Chapter 2 that there are moves toward consistent use of terms such as "relapse," "recurrence," and "remission." However, there is little sign of agreement over conventions that guide both how data is analyzed and how good outcomes are defined over follow-up—both factors that can alter the apparent efficacy of a trial. The significance of these issues is highlighted by Brown and Barlow (1995; reviewed in Chapter 6), who present 2-year outcomes for patients with panic disorder. First, aggregated data suggested good results for a high percentage of patients, but this obscured shifts in symptomatic status by individual patients; because some patients improved and others deteriorated, overall outcomes appeared more stable than was in fact the case. Second, decisions about the criteria for declaring high end-state functioning markedly altered apparent efficacy; long-term outcomes appeared much poorer when a criterion of "no panic attacks in the past year" was employed, contrasted to one of "no panic attacks in the past month."

The natural history of many mental health problems is both long-term and (in some cases) cyclic, and it is against this background that measures of improvement should be judged. Equally, however, the natural course of many disorders might suggest that overstringent criteria for high end-state functioning may be inappropriate; for example, improvement might be judged less by the presence or absence of symptoms than by the speed of improvements or the latency to relapse. Further work is required to agree on realistic standards by which longer term outcomes may be judged.

Representation and Meta-Analysis

For a number of reasons (and as discussed in Chapter 2), some meta-analytic reviews may not be representative of the field they claim to cover. As the availability of clinical trials increases, fewer meta-analyses include analog rather than clinical populations, but where this occurs, their inclusion usually leads to larger effect sizes. Given the tendency for reviewers to be based in English-speaking countries, studies published in foreign-language journals are less likely to be evaluated adequately. If studies present data in a way that makes it impossible to calculate an effect sizes, they will be excluded from meta-analyses. Although this follows logically, their invisibility in the subsequent review will reflect statistical rather than clinical considerations. In some areas, this means that rather few trials are available to meta-analysis, with the consequence that conclusions rest on an inappropriately narrow base. Classification of therapies within analyses can also present a problem, especially when an approach straddles domains or adopts an explicitly integrative framework. This can lead to reviews of the same area arriving at somewhat disparate estimates of effect sizes that, on closer scrutiny, relate to their decisions about how to locate a therapy within a class of approaches. Critically, inclusion in a meta-analysis does not guarantee that the trial is of good quality; review of individual studies may reveal many detailed concerns, but these are usually lost to sight. Although reviews can attempt to consider such factors, for example, some examine the impact of methodological features on effect-size, and it is now routine to consider the homogeneity of the sample, this may not overcome problems that reside in the studies themselves, on occasion leading to reviews with poor face validity.

ISSUES IN EVIDENCE-BASED PRACTICE

Can Absence of Evidence Be Taken as Evidence for Ineffectiveness?

Although the inclusion of a therapy on a list of evidence-based approaches suggests its positive benefit, there are two broad reasons why an intervention may be absent. If it was adequately tested and found ineffective, then its status is unambiguous, but when it has not been subject to adequate evaluation, interpretation becomes more difficult. We have noted at several points that psychodynamic therapies are underresearched when contrasted to their prominence in clinical settings. It may be that this links to the intellectual climate associated with this orientation, but the relative absence of empirical data means that debates regarding the status of this approach are likely to intensify rather than to diminish. This is especially likely if the grounds for debate relate to a critique of, rather than an engagement with, a quantitative approach. Thus Holmes (2002) has argued that CBT could be adopted by default because of its research and marketing strategy rather than its intrinsic superiority, pointing to weaknesses in its theory, gaps in the evidence, lack of long-term follow-up, and exaggeration of effect sizes by contrast to wait-list control rather than active treatment. He also notes the emergence of "post-cognitive behavior therapy" approaches (e.g., Segal et al., 2002; Young, 1999) that could be seen to overlap with psychodynamic ideas. This critique would, of course, be stronger if backed by direct evidence of efficacy for psychodynamic therapy, and it is unsurprising that a number of therapist–researchers have been quick to rebut this analysis (e.g., Sensky & Scott, 2002; Tarrier et al., 2002).

Many of its practitioners continue to view psychoanalysis as incompatible with research, because its focus is on meaning, and narrative is not easily reduced to measures of symptoms or suffering (e.g., Whittle, 2000). It is easy to appreciate that this approach is less easy to manualize, or that adapting technique to conform to the rigor of a research trial represents a challenge. However, the limits to this argument are demonstrated by the publication record of a number of researchers committed to psychodynamic method. In the United States alone, individuals such as Jacques Barber, Jeffrey Binder, John Clarkin, Paul Crits-Christoph, Leonard Horowitz, Mardi Horowitz, Lester Luborsky, William Piper, Hans Strupp, Drew Westen, and others have published good-quality controlled trials of psychodynamic approaches, suggesting that there is no inherent discontinuity between this method and empirical investigation (and also indicating the potential effectiveness of this method). Returning to our starting point, while an absence of evidence does not preclude the possibility of efficacy, the credibility of a treatment is much reduced if an evidential vacuum reflects the reluctance of its practitioners to explore its impact.

These observations imply that the reasons behind a lack of research out-

put need to be considered carefully, especially where practitioners are committed to conducting research but meet significant obstacles to the development of a program. At a basic level, restrictions on funding may prevent a
trial taking place—an issue discussed in more detail below. There might also
be pragmatic issues that restrict research effort. An important example of this
comes from the field of mental retardation, where practitioners increasingly
employ psychotherapeutic interventions despite the almost complete absence
of randomized trials with this client group (Beail, 2003; Prout & Nowak-
Drabik, 2003). Most research in this area has utilized open trials or case series,
which places it lower in the hierarchy of evidence adopted in this (and many
other) reviews. However, this may reflect genuine methodological and ethical problems in establishing the conditions for research trials with this client
group (e.g., Beail, 2003; Oliver et al., 2002, 2003). It follows that a demand
that practice be based on evidence would be unhelpfully restrictive if that
demand equates evidence only with randomized trials and neglects to note
any specific issues that restrict the range of available methodologies. The hierarchy of evidence adopted in this book reflects a progression in scientific
rigor but does not imply that one design should automatically be privileged
over another, without consideration of the context from which such evidence could be drawn.[1] When the reasons for an absence of evidence are logically based and persuasive, as they seem to be in this and other cases, it
would be consonant with our model of evidence-based practice for professionals to interpret available research, and to consider its likely generalization
to their own field.

The Role of Adjunctive Pharmacological
and Psychological Treatments

As detailed in the relevant sections of this book, our knowledge of the relative impact of pharmacological and psychological therapies delivered alone or
in combination differs according to the condition under examination. This
reflects not only variations in the clarity of outcomes from trials but also the
paucity of available research for some presentations, which makes conclusions
unreliable. Obviously, where research is available, it should guide practice,

---

[1] A further example is offered by personal construct therapy (PCT). Practitioners of this
approach tend to eschew psychiatric diagnosis, which means that an already small literature is
usually based on mixed patient samples. In addition, most reports are of single-case studies or
uncontrolled trials, using measures that are designed to detect shifts in process and meaning,
rather than shifts in symptomatic functioning (e.g., Winter, 2003). This compounds the fact of
a small evidence base with the problem that what is available is philosophically at variance with
a conventional review such as this one. This latter point could be used to argue that the
absence of reports of evidence for PCT in this book reflects our selection bias rather than a real
absence of evidence, and this would be a reasonable point for debate (e.g., Viney, 1998).

but for many conditions there is little compelling evidence routinely to dictate a preference for one form of treatment over another in the individual case.

Many patients seen in clinical settings will be in receipt of pharmacotherapy at the point of referral. Whether such individuals are or are not representative of research populations is a moot point. Among trials ostensibly examining outcomes for psychological therapy alone, there is inconsistency in whether patients are required to be drug-free, an issue that is difficult systematically to account for when reviewing the literature. Trials that include medication do not always ensure that patients are medication-compliant (e.g., by using blood testing). Even where there is clarity about the pharmacological status of patients in a trials, it is quite likely that patients presenting in clinical settings will be taking medications that have never been specifically tested in combination with any particular psychological therapy; there are simply too many potential combinations for this to be feasible. All this means that, in most instances, adjunctive treatment with pharmacotherapy and psychotherapy will usually represent adherence to general principles rather than to specific treatment recommendations.

Clearly, the role of medication varies across conditions. For example, most research indicates that medication is integral to the treatment of individuals with psychotic presentations, but this level of certainty does not apply to the management of patients with other disorders. Nonetheless, some broad conclusions are possible. Although, in general, there is little evidence to suggest that concurrent medication will reduce the impact of psychological therapy, it is worth noting that in some areas (e.g., anxiety disorders or bulimia), findings point to a negative impact of pharmacotherapy on outcomes or treatment acceptability. Usually, however, combination treatments appear to be more helpful than one or the other modality offered alone. Medication and psychological therapy offered alone are often broadly equivalent in their outcomes. However, cessation of pharmacological treatment is often associated with relapse, and while it is possible to overstate the prophylactic benefit of psychological therapy, there are indications that patients are more likely to maintain gains when this is part of their treatment.

These observations suggest that patients are likely to benefit when both psychological and pharmacological modes of intervention are available, which suggests the need for integration between the services offering these modalities. This makes it more likely that clients showing a poor response to the treatment they are offered—be it adjunctive, or one or the other therapy offered alone—can be switched to an alternative approach without a major disruption of treatment. This implies that clinicians have some sense of the effectiveness of their initial treatment, which in turn relies on careful monitoring and some sense of the likely trajectory of change—an issue discussed elsewhere in this chapter.

The Role of Maintenance Treatments

It seems clear that there is an important role for short-term structured treatments. There is evidence of benefit for a range of disorders, with follow-up suggesting low or, at worst, moderate rates of relapse (e.g., with phobias, panic disorder, PTSD, or obsessive–compulsive disorder). Individuals with more acute and less severe presentations of many other disorders might also be expected to do well following brief interventions, using a variety of psychotherapeutic techniques.

The situation may be somewhat different for long-term and severe disorders marked by a natural history indicating the probability of relapse, particularly when these conditions present in individuals with poor adaptation and a high level of comorbidity (especially when this includes many of the diagnoses within Axis II). For these patients, the longer term outcome following brief treatments may be poor (even if their initial response is good). However, there is evidence that offering "maintenance" treatments (offered subsequent to acute treatment, at lower intensity and over prolonged periods) is especially helpful to individuals vulnerable to relapse. This observation almost certainly applies to patients who have a history of recurrent depression or to individuals with dysthymic disorder, but it may be equally applicable to other groups and is consistent with findings from the phase model of psychotherapy (discussed in Chapter 16), which suggest that while symptom relief occurs within 16 sessions, enduring rehabilitation requires more extended treatment.

Service models that assume interventions to be "curative" may not be appropriate when patients present with chronic and potentially recurrent disorders. Although interventions can improve an individual's adaptation, reduce symptomatology, and improve quality of life, the expectation that a one-time treatment should necessarily lead to stable improvement may be unrealistic, especially when epidemiological evidence shows that the natural history of a disorder is characterized by relapse–remission cycling. Rather than a surgical metaphor, treatment in these cases might better follow the model offered in the treatment of diabetes, or other conditions in which the hope is not only to stabilize the presenting condition but also to monitor the individual, allow for continued contact, and expect that the patient will return at times of crisis.

It follows that even when psychotherapy services primarily offer short-term therapies, they need to recognize and plan for the likelihood of recurrence after brief treatment for certain disorders. Furthermore, relapse after recovery following psychotherapy should not necessarily contraindicate the appropriateness of further psychological intervention. In some cases, relapse could be seen as a predictable aspect of the disorder, and relapse prevention and management as an important component within a treatment package.

Especially for chronic and severe cases, long-term maintenance therapy may be an appropriate and necessary treatment model.

TRANSLATING RESEARCH INTO PRACTICE
Dissemination via Manualized Treatments

It may be tempting to assume that transporting a manualized treatment into clinical practice is equivalent to ensuring evidence-based practice. However, as detailed in Chapter 2, manuals are not usually designed to serve as the foundation of either practice or training (Westen, 2002); they were developed in the context of research, in large part as attempts to ensure independence from other approaches under test (hence, to improve the capacity of researchers to draw causal inferences from trials). It follows that the conditions under which they are implemented in a research trial differ in many respects from those obtaining in clinical settings, meaning that there are good reasons to be cautious about the belief that direct transportation can guarantee clinical effectiveness.

At present, there is only limited evidence bearing on this debate. Some have suggested that manuals can and should be implemented directly into community practice (e.g., Addis et al., 1999; Wilson, 1998), and a number of studies have demonstrated certain manualized treatments to be quite "transportable" in the sense of achieving comparable results to those observed in treatment trials (see Chambless & Ollendick, 2001, for a review; Franklin et al., 2000; Stuart et al., 2000). However, other studies suggest these assessments may be overoptimistic. For example, as reviewed in Chapter 15, in relation to childhood depression, while implementing a research-based treatment protocol can improve outcomes relative to routine practice, this is not to the same level as that achieved in efficacy studies (Weersing & Weisz, 2002).

As is evident at many points in this review and from our model of evidence-based practice, in general, we are cautious about the likely benefits of implementing "protocol-driven" therapies as though these can be operated without the filter of clinical judgment, or where clinicians do not have the capacity to implement alternative strategies (where such deviations from technique appear justified by their assessment and formulation of the individual case). It needs to be remembered that most clinical practice is much more heterogeneous than any manual would credit, and that manuals themselves are essentially ideal prototypes that embody the principles of complex interventions that have taken many decades to evolve in the field (Westen, 2002). These facts are easily overlooked if the techniques embodied in a manual are reified as *the* way to practice a treatment, rather than *a* way in which it could be practiced. Attempting to "legislate" the form in which a treatment is delivered runs the risk of ossification, and of stifling appropriate creativity.

None of the forgoing implies that manuals cannot be used as the basis for service implementation, but it seems appropriate to suggest that this be done as part of a "systemic" process, in which the impact of the manual is itself part of a research cycle. For example, differences in the efficacy and effectiveness of a manualized therapy could be attributed to a variety of causes—most obviously differences in patient samples (comorbidity, chronicity, or social disadvantage) or the quality of treatments delivered (or, indeed, both). These issues have different implications. If a manualized intervention is less effective because it is being applied to more challenging samples, it might suggest further treatment development that takes the reality of clinical caseloads into full consideration. Equally, if deficiencies in treatment delivery are an issue, the need for further therapist training and supervision would be highlighted. As much as anything else, these are "local" issues defined by the capacity of a particular service to monitor the delivery of an approach for which there is general evidence of efficacy, but where the specific evidence of benefit for the clients of that service rests on practice-based evidence rather than appeal to the research literature.

Dissemination via Clinical Guidelines

Researchers cannot assume that their findings are readily absorbed into practice. Surveys repeatedly demonstrate that clinicians are often ill-informed about, and have limited interest in, findings from psychotherapy research (e.g., Cohen et al., 1986; Morrow-Bradley & Elliot, 1986). On the whole, research has only limited impact on services, perhaps for understandable reasons. Clinicians are experts in their field, but there is a tendency for them to limit their interest to the studies that apply directly to their current practice and to selectively disregard findings that would require of them substantial modification of their mode of work. This appears to be as true of CBT therapists as of psychodynamic clinicians (e.g., Raw, 1993; Suinn, 1993). On this basis it is clear that evidence cannot be expected to speak for itself (Chilvers et al., 2002; Higgitt & Fonagy, 2002).

In response to this problem, the past decade has seen an increasing availability of professional (or, more rarely, national) clinical guidelines. Though many of these are uniprofessional, ideally these are drawn up by multidisciplinary panels, with individual members selected for their expertise and their capacity to appraise therapeutic approaches in an even-handed manner. Just as important, they should also have an awareness of the vicissitudes of everyday clinical practice, and use this to shape the tone of any recommendations. Increasingly, guidelines also include the views of individuals whose expertise is as users and carers. This is important and appropriate, because professionals largely judge outcomes in relation to changes in symptomatic or functional status. Both of these will be important to "consumers," but their concerns frequently extend to "nonspecifics," such as the acceptability of a treatment or the clinical context in which it is delivered (e.g., any restrictions on equity or speed of access).

Unfortunately, the existence of a guideline, no matter how well constructed, does not guarantee a change in service delivery. In addressing the process by which change can be influenced, it is useful to differentiate between "diffusion," "dissemination," and "implementation" (Palmer & Fenner, 1999). Publication in a journal article (diffusion) is a passive form of communication, untargeted and seemingly insufficient to achieve much in the way of change. The development of practice guidelines is more active and targeted to an intended audience (dissemination). Implementation is yet more dynamic, with monitoring and adjustment to local needs, and potentially incentives, as well as sanctions. As noted by Chilvers et al. (2002), the pharmaceutical industry eschews passive techniques in favor of implementation, with personal and material resources targeted to individual practitioners, with clear evidence of the impact of these techniques on prescribing practice. On this basis, the use of multiple pathways to dissemination seems a plausible, if untested, recommendation. Unfortunately, there is little research on the extent to which guidance on psychological therapy is utilized by practitioners. Based largely on intuition, there is a sense that the impact of a guideline is likely to be greater if it is shorter, carefully targeted, and initiated at a local level, but this has not been tested.

Dissemination of Information to Patients

The problem of dissemination is even greater when it comes to users of psychotherapy services. Currently, it is unlikely that the majority of patients have adequate information about the demonstrated efficacy of psychological treatments they may be offered. Some steps have been taken to remedy this, with both professional organizations and public bodies ensuring that many guidelines are produced in versions both appropriate to and accessible by clients. However, it is worth bearing in mind that patient-oriented guidelines are prone to the same risks as those aimed at clinicians—for example, of being overinterpreted and used rigidly rather than flexibly, or of becoming out of date through failure to observe the usual maxims regarding regular revision.

Information for patients is also provided through the media (particularly the press and television), and increasingly through the Internet, though both routes are potentially haphazard. The Internet is an increasingly powerful mode of transmission, though its uncontrolled nature means that while some of its content will be accurate and helpful, some will be unbalanced and mis-leading. Some sites created by patient organizations concerned with specific disorders include clear and helpful explanations of treatment options, though not all organizations adopt a neutral stance in relation to the evidence. This means that there is a particular need for the websites of professional and gov-ernmental organizations to include unbiased and clear information accessible to patients.[2] However, there is always scope for "experts" to disagree among themselves, making some variance in opinion even across "official" sites quite likely. Though some of this disagreement will reflect legitimate differences of interpretation, it does risk yet further confusion for the public.

Whatever the challenges, it is clearly important that the public be pro-vided with high-quality and readily comprehensible information concerning the availability and likely effectiveness of psychological help. The steps already taken toward this (some of which we have referred to in Chapter 3) need to continue in order to ensure that users can make a genuinely informed choice about their treatment.

Determining Outcomes within Services

Case Tracking, Service Benchmarking, and Service Profiling

Here, we note, the developing role and potential importance of case tracking. Along with service profiling and benchmarking of outcomes, this gives the possibility of generating an evidence base in relation to a service and to indi-vidual practitioners. While this is an exciting and potentially creative devel-opment, there are different ways in which it could be implemented. To polarize these positions, on the one hand, monitoring could be seen as part of reflective practice, spurred by therapists' interest in the impact of their work, and a concern for self-improvement where this appears to be necessary. On the other hand, monitoring might be perceived as a coercive exercise, oper-ated by a management system with little regard for the vicissitudes of clinical practice, with the consequence that therapists become alienated from (and suspicious of) the process of data collection. While there is no justification for practice that falls below an expected standard, there is a question about how routine outcome measurement can be a productive rather than a persecutory endeavor—a systemic dilemma common in many areas of health care deliv-ery, and not confined to psychotherapy.

---

[2] An example would be a guideline developed for the English Department of Health (available at *http://www.doh.gov.uk/mentalhealth/talkingtherapies.pdf*), which aims to help patients to make informed choices about their treatment. Based on a professional guideline (*Treatment Choice in Psychological Therapies and Counselling: Evidence-Based Clinical Guideline*; Department of Health, 2001), it translates research and information about service availability into a form accessible to users and caregivers.

Case tracking may be a helpful approach to this issue. We know that change is most likely and most speedy in patients with lower levels of initial symptoms and higher levels of functioning, with the implication that without profiling of a service and of individual therapist caseloads within it, contrast to other therapists, services, or indeed to research is unhelpful at best, and meaningless at worst. For example, senior therapists working with more challenging patients will probably have poorer outcomes than novice therapists working with less complex cases, but penalizing therapists for working with more difficult individuals would not be a way to build high-quality services. The screening systems employed by case-tracking systems link greater severity to slower trajectories of change and the necessity for longer therapies to achieve improvement. Using these systems, the focus of interest when monitoring outcomes shifts from a concern with absolute levels of change to the therapist's capacity to maintain an expected rate of progress. In terms of the cautions noted earlier, deviations from this path should then be a prompt to case review, rather than assumptions regarding therapeutic competence.

Case-tracking systems are developing rapidly, and it seems likely that they will find a place in routine practice over the next few years. Currently, there are some obvious caveats to their use, partly based on the resources required to implement them, the dearth of research on how these methods work in routine clinical settings, and the need to consider how clinicians can best integrate feedback from these systems with their clinical judgment. One way of achieving this would be to link feedback systems to supervision (hence, to continuing professional training). Since the particular benefit of case tracking may lie in avoiding deterioration, supervision is the obvious and appropriate arena for careful consideration of remedial strategies.

Case tracking could also be used to generate broader information about outcomes across a service, especially because case mix and complexity are automatically accommodated through the screening instruments integral to this technology. By considering factors relevant to variations in outcome, this would link case tracking (largely the preserve of the individual therapist) to service profiling and benchmarking (where outcomes are monitored at a service level).

Benchmarking outcomes against results obtained in research settings, or against the results obtained by other clinical services, would be a way of indicating the effectiveness and perhaps the efficiency of a unit. In order for this to be meaningful, however, the profile of patients seen by the service needs to be considered, since case mix will obviously influence outcomes. In one of the few studies to consider this issue directly, Barkham et al. (2001) profiled the level of patient distress among attendees to a large sample of mental health services in the United Kingdom. They found wide variation in the severity of patient presentations. This suggests that simple comparisons of outcomes of services will almost certainly result in a confound with patient difficulty. The use of benchmarking and profiling gives a service and its therapists the opportunity for self-appraisal, with scrutiny anchored to an external reference point. The degree to which this can be systematized will vary, but, as described next, the possibility of locally based research initiatives is potentially a fruitful way to generate research information directly relevant to a service.

Pragmatic Trials

"Pragmatic trials" may be a further way to bridge the efficacy–effectiveness divide. In essence, these trials are conducted within a service setting and usually take the form of randomized allocation to alternative methods of care. For example, a service seeing patients with acute onset might wonder whether at least some benefit from their treatment reflects a trajectory of natural recovery. They might investigate this systematically by randomizing patients to receive immediate treatment or to a wait list of a specified duration, which would enable them to contrast outcomes after a standardized period of time had elapsed from referral. Another example would be to explore whether there is benefit to adding additional sessions for individuals who do not respond to treatment by randomizing such patients to standard treatment or to a set number of further sessions. A final example would be to examine the variance accounted for by the way treatment services are delivered and organized (rather than the impact of offering different therapeutic modalities). This would enable exploration of systemic factors that might be viewed as nonspecific but may be highly pertinent to effectiveness.

These trials enable services to ask questions of direct relevance to their service by systematically manipulating practice; patients who participate naturally reflect clinical (as opposed to research) populations, exclusion criteria are kept to a minimum, and there are minimal constraints on how patients are managed. Pragmatic trials could be an important additional source of information for evidence-based practice. In combination with more rigorous RCTs (particularly relevant to new treatments) and the judicious use of observational data, they could provide evidence of sufficient richness to advance standards of care significantly. Their inclusion in the hierarchy of evidence would add to the family of methods that inform technique.

"Systemic" Conditions Fostering Evidence-Based Practice

Implementing research-based therapies into services is usually done in the absence of any evidence about the infrastructure required to ensure a reasonable chance that treatments will be effective. The usual focus of concerns about implementation is the way in which variability among clients might reduce efficacy. Equally worthy of consideration is the influence of service organization on therapists' capacity to deliver effective therapy.

The Role of Supervision

In most major studies, treatment fidelity is monitored, and therapists are supervised to ensure that treatments are delivered competently. This is clearly reported in journal articles, but its significance is rarely commented on when considering how a research-based treatment should be implemented in routine settings. Logically, estimates of treatment efficacy are based on the therapist's skillfulness in the context of expert support, but this is rarely noted explicitly and can lead to an assumption that the technique is transportable in the absence of the support structures available to research therapists. Unfortunately, we do not know whether this is, or is not, the case. Direct evidence of the efficacy of supervision is sparse, and although there is evidence that competence is linked to better outcomes, it is not clear that this is an inevitable consequence of supervision. We also need to admit that evidence of a link between training, professional qualification, and outcome is far from compelling. Equally, because the nesting of supervision (and in effect, training) within trials makes it invisible in most analyses, it is unclear how well an "evidence-based" treatment can be expected to perform in a routine service where therapists are not supervised. Indeed, it could be argued that removal of the supervisory element means that the treatment is no longer evidence-based, since its absence could represent a substantive deviation from the original protocol under which it was tested. It seems reasonable to suggest that therapeutic impact is influenced by the supportive context within which therapy is practiced—which includes supervision but also extends to the climate within which a therapist works. On this basis, it would seem prudent to ensure that these elements are integral to service implementation.

The Role of Therapist Competence

Most trials—particularly those conducted more recently—attempt to ensure that the therapists they recruit and train are competent in the therapy they are delivering. The assumption is that greater competence is associated with better outcome and, as discussed earlier, some presumption that supervision enhances the probability of this; both notions are backed by at least some supportive evidence.

Many pronouncements on evidence-based therapies focus on the therapy rather than the therapist who delivers it, as though the fundamentally interpersonal context of psychotherapy can be ignored. This is often justified by appeal to the application of therapies for which there is a "protocol," with the implication that this can be implemented by individuals of variable skill

levels. However, a reasonable question would be to ask how skillful a therapist needs to be in order for an evidence-based therapy to show effectiveness.
As with supervision, research is sparse; because few, if any, trials randomize
patients in relation to therapists (rather than seeking therapist effects in post
hoc analyses), the few available studies are methodologically weak.

One challenge to this line of argument is that there is some evidence of
the successful use of computerized, protocol-driven therapies, particularly for
anxiety and depression. In the main, these are sophisticated programs, structured carefully and implemented thoroughly, but the point remains that such
studies demonstrate that therapeutic strategies can have impact when offered
independent of therapists. However, this still leaves open the question of
which patients are suited to such an approach; indeed, many studies of low
contact therapy (whether delivered in computerized form or via bibliotherapy) suggest advantage to therapist contact as patient severity and complexity increases.

It seems reasonable to caution against the assumption that the availability
of a protocol for therapy entitles a service to implement it either in the
absence of careful checks relating to fidelity of practice, or in the absence of
supervision—both of these being issues of training. It also seems inappropriate to allow therapists with low skill levels to operate independently of a
structure that allows them access to individuals with greater experience and
(presumed) expertise.

Respecting the Lack of Evidence for Evidence-Based Practice

There is irony in the fact that although there is an increasing requirement for
practice to be based on evidence, we are not aware of systematic evidence
demonstrating the benefit of this process. At present, implementation is
largely based on an appeal to face validity. Although not inappropriate, this
untested assumption ignores our lack of knowledge regarding the specificity
of any recommendation (the likelihood of falsely identifying a treatment as
effective), as well as its sensitivity (the chance of misclassifying an effective
treatment as ineffective). This implies a continuing role for clinical judgment;
ignoring this consideration by implementing or imposing guidelines naively
risks invoking an unhelpful skepticism and reactance among clinicians, as witnessed by the intense debates surrounding the publication of professional
guidelines.

It should be remembered that, whatever the strength of evidence,
method accounts for only a proportion of the variance in outcome. While
factors related to the client and to the interaction of therapist and client are
also pertinent, therapist judgment and skill should not be ignored. Implementing the science of evidence-based practice while ignoring the "art"

of therapy risks reducing creativity, and with it, potential advances in technique.

FUNDING AND PSYCHOTHERAPY RESEARCH

Since there is no commercial value in proving the efficacy of psychotherapy, funding for psychotherapy research is almost exclusively dependent on government, academic or charitable bodies. The monies available from these sources appear to be increasingly restricted, creating an obvious inequity when contrasted to the resources of the pharmaceutical industry. In a field of practice where a failure to demonstrate efficacy has consequences for the availability of treatments, there is an obvious risk that bias in funding skews the process of research.

Given the difficulty of obtaining funding, the extent of available research into psychotherapy is remarkable and stands as a testament to the commitment of many practitioners. However, much of this research focuses on one form of therapy—CBT. This is no accident, and it reflects the fact that proponents of CBT tend to be enthusiasts for research, probably resulting in better preparation of research proposals, more sophisticated research designs, and more mature research programs within which to contextualize proposed studies. Success can become its own virtue, and there is a risk that funding bodies, impressed by the sense that CBT is a "treatment of choice," will be less willing to support proposals from alternative therapies. This would be unfortunate. First, while the evidence for CBT is strong, there is room for question about its benefit relative to other bona fide therapies. Second, it is evident that both clinical practice and theory have evolved at a fairly high rate, in part fueled by a dialectic between different orientations. Privileging one approach over another removes this tension, with the risk that public challenge to accepted practice becomes restricted. It would also compound the reluctance of some practitioners to demonstrate the benefits of their approach, since it would become reasonable to point to a lack of funding as the basis for a lack of evidence. In the worst case, we could arrive at a monoculture in which CBT became eponymous with evidence-based practice.

These risks should not be overstated. CBT has shown a capacity to reinvent itself when exploring its application to different areas, suggesting that innovation within the model is likely to continue. Also, as it attempts to apply cognitive ideas to challenging areas (such as the problem of treating personality disorders, or of preventing relapse in depression), its theoretical base has broadened to incorporate ideas that mirror those seen in psychodynamic or interpersonal models—in this sense, creating the basis for a rapprochement or an integration across approaches. Nonetheless, it is critical for the development of the field that funding is seen to be even-handed and to encourage innovation.

ISSUES FOR CLINICAL PRACTICE
The Organization of Services

In the first edition of this book, we commented on the ways that services could be organized to maximize likely benefit to clients. We focused on the potential benefit of trying to match clients to psychological therapy services located at different levels of the health system, across primary, secondary, and tertiary care. This model assumed that patients with relatively mild and acute disorders without comorbidity may be amenable to the briefer and more generic (though theory-based) therapies usually offered in primary care settings. In contrast, individuals with more severe and chronic disorders seem to require more specialized and possibly more lengthy treatments, and hence were best treated in secondary or tertiary settings.

Although this suggestion probably strikes most readers as logical and unsurprising, our concern lay in the fact that many services are not organized in a way that allows for pathways of care to match to patient need. Referral across and between services can delay access to appropriate care, and unless explicit steps are taken to ensure that there is equity of access to a range of therapies, it is possible for client choice to be restricted to the therapy offered by an individual therapist. On this basis, we suggested that referral systems across different levels of mental health should be integrated, that psychological therapy services themselves should ensure access both to pharmacological and psychological care, and that the quality of a service should be reflected by its capacity to ensure the delivery of therapies tailored as far as possible to client need rather than to service availability.

In more recent years, the notion of "stepped care" has been widely discussed. This procedure is variously interpreted but essentially focuses on matching treatments to patients in relation to the minimum therapeutic effort required to achieve clinical change. To some extent, there is a presumption of "doing more with less" (Davison, 2000), often by initially offering more restricted therapies (such as bibliotherapy), monitoring the response of the client, and moving to more intensive treatments only if the problem persists. This referral process may or may not relate to the location where treatment actually takes place, but it certainly echoes some of the concern for rational organization of resources that we were attempting to highlight.

The stepped-care model has risks as well as benefits. As is usual with any procedure, it can be implemented without regard for individual need, such that minimal interventions are used as a simple screening tool. Though there may be some benefit to this, especially where resources are limited and access to treatment is problematic, there may be issues about not only delaying access to therapy for those in more serious need but also ensuring the management of attrition among those fail to respond at this level of input. There is also the need for some clarity about the criteria that indicate when a particular phase of therapy is ineffective, and the procedures available to move to another approach—an issue that may relate as much to the organization of therapy services as to the actions of individual therapists.

Perhaps the most appealing application of stepped care is its use as a heuristic that guides treatment using evidence-based principles in combination with clinical judgment, and determines progression through the levels of care on the basis of the client's response (e.g., Sobell & Sobell, 2000). Within this model, care is offered not only in relation to the presenting problem but also in relation to the client's beliefs, resources, and the available treatment options. The basis for offering treatments is that they reflect the current state of knowledge about efficacy (not, of course, the same as insisting that only evidence-based approaches are used), and because continuous assessment of outcomes is linked to its implementation, it creates helpful conditions for a form of practice-based evidence.

Training and Education

Training in Specific Applications or for Broad Competencies

Our review provides some evidence for the efficacy of specific treatments for particular disorders. We can see this as implying two possible, and equally valid, models of training. One would emphasize the need to learn specific techniques to a high standard for application to particular groups, an exemplar of which would be the training of nurse therapists in specific cognitive-behavioral techniques for the management of anxiety disorders. In this model, the hope is that more specific training and greater familiarity with particular problems are likely to result in more competent delivery of treatment, though this has the limitation that such therapists may be less competent when the patient's presentation is unusual or complex. On this basis, we can also see the virtue—and the importance—of training directed toward the acquisition and integration of more generic metacompetencies, on the assumption that a broader understanding of therapeutic principles will allow therapists to learn new skills more rapidly and adapt technique to match client characteristics. Examples of this approach would be a training in more than one intervention (e.g., both supportive and exploratory techniques), or one in which therapists emerge with a deep and broad understanding of a specific therapy, allowing them to implement it across a spectrum of presentations.

Most services with a broad case mix could benefit from individuals with both forms of training, and in this sense, it is not obvious that one form of training should be privileged over another.

Linking the Evidence to the Structure of Training Programs

It is a matter of observation that the curricula of many programs often include teaching on approaches for which there is rather little evidence. There is some justification for this. The strength of evidence of treatment effectiveness varies across diagnoses, which means that there is scope for debate about the appropriateness of imposing current research findings to shape training programs. Nonetheless, it seems appropriate to suggest that, at minimum, training programs for psychological therapists should include material concerning the efficacy of interventions. Certainly, there is little justification for the exclusion of teaching interventions of known efficacy, especially when the evidence for such interventions is robust. This could be facilitated if relevant professional bodies' accreditation criteria emphasized the inclusion of treatment programs of demonstrated validity, indicated that practitioners should be competent at administering these treatments to acceptable criteria, and required qualified individuals to know not only for whom their techniques were of demonstrable value, but also for whom they would be ill-advised.

Role of Direct Observation in Training

We are clear that training should require trainees to be directly observed conducting therapy with a number of patients. This follows because our review of attempts to link therapist characteristics and successful outcome suggests that it is only when the actual performance of a therapist is appraised that any such links emerge. The fact that this draws attention to the interpersonal context within which therapy takes place is hardly novel, but it does imply that reliance on trainees' reports of what they have done results in a weaker training procedure than observation of their actual behavior.

Role of Continuing Professional Development

A model of evidence-based practice implies that clinicians have access to continuing postqualification training in order to apply their current clinical skills to the maximum benefit of patients and to acquire competence in newer approaches as these appear. Our review makes it clear that techniques are evolving quite rapidly, and any service that lays claim to being evidence-based needs explicitly to integrate the training needs of its practitioners into its service planning.

Access to Training

If researchers developing new and empirically validated treatment methods find that a therapy has evidence of efficacy, it seems reasonable that they should ensure that their techniques are accessible to those involved in the training of clinicians, and that any restriction on training in that method should be justifiable on pedagogic rather than commercial grounds. We note that some recently developed approaches limit certification to specific (usually commercial) courses, and justify this by concerns that training by noncertified staff will result in the "dilution" of the therapy. To a large degree, this is a moral issue, based not on the entitlement of training organizations to charge for their services, but more on the rationale for so doing. Clearly, it is to the disadvantage of patients and services alike if access to training is narrowed by a motivation to enhance profit rather than ensure quality training.

DIRECTIONS FOR PSYCHOTHERAPY RESEARCH

For all that, the volume of psychotherapy research is almost overwhelming; it remains the case that some areas remain much more poorly researched than others. There is some risk that we will know increasingly more about areas in which knowledge is already fairly extensive but continue to remain in the dark where our understanding is limited. Research volume broadly reflects the prevalence of a disorder, but there does seem to be some link between the availability of a guiding principle or model and the amount of available research. As an example, comparison of our current and previous chapters on work with people with schizophrenia and especially bipolar disorder shows a remarkable growth in the number of trials, presumably reflecting the enthusiasm generated when clinicians detect the possibility of intervening to alleviate problems previously ill-understood or resistant to change. This suggests an important principle, since the developments that seem to us most exciting are those in which speculation about the processes underpinning psychopathology informs treatment innovation, which in turn is subject to empirical investigation.

This approach is unusual, because much of what we have learned from psychotherapy research applies generally rather than specifically, and even where we have some certainty about therapeutic impact, we are often much less certain about the processes that bring about change. A formal response to this state of affairs comes from Kazdin (2004), who has outlined a radical and rigorous program for psychotherapy research. The first stage follows from the proposition that treatment should reflect what we know about the processes that directly bear on the onset and course of a clinical problem. This contrasts the present position, in which treatment principles are often based on general processes (e.g., distorted cognitions) that are applicable across disorders, rather than being testable hypotheses that can be linked to a specific dysfunction. In Kazdin's model, demonstrating the presence of a specific process in a sizable proportion of individuals with a specific presentation would be the basis of treatment development. Furthermore, rather than assuming that all individuals with the same presentation would be equally responsive to treatment, further work would aim to detect subtypes of a dysfunction, multiple pathways to the same presentation, as well as risk and protective factors.

The second step would be to ask questions about the processes by which a treatment method achieves change, first by specifying the processes or factors responsible for change, then developing measures of these processes, and finally showing that these processes change before therapeutic change occurs. On this basis, manualization becomes feasible, on the presumption that the manual now includes a high dosage of "effective" ingredients. Evaluation of outcome can then follow (using the hierarchy of evidence detailed in Chapter 2), along with process–outcome studies that aim to examine moderator variables (helping us to discover more about what actually does work for whom).

A key difference between this and current models is that it sets out not only to establish the hypothesized processes and mechanisms of therapy through experimental rather than post hoc correlational findings, but also to identify patient and environmental characteristics that promote or undermine the effectiveness of a therapy. The promise of identifying key, mutative psychological processes is especially attractive given its potential to bring order to the current proliferation of therapeutic approaches, and to identify what is, or is not, both effective and common across orientations.

The promise of this program is great, though its realization is more challenging. In outline, however, there are already indications of how a focus on process would enable psychotherapists to integrate biological, psychological, and social factors in the context of a model of psychological problems based on developmental psychopathology.

Future psychotherapy research will almost certainly become more firmly rooted in developmental psychopathology, essentially because it is increasingly clear that many adult psychiatric disorders are rooted in abnormalities already observable in childhood or adolescence (e.g., Kim-Cohen et al., 2003). The prospective gain from increasing links between psychotherapy research, neuroscience, and molecular biology is particularly exciting. As molecular genetic findings unfold, it is likely that particular types of biological markers will be linked to expression in the form of psychological vulnerabilities, though this relationship will almost certainly be complex (Plomin & McGuffin, 2003). As an example, serotonin is presumed to play a role in depression and in the mediation of stressful experiences (Nemeroff, 1996). Genes responsible for its production exist in two forms, one of which is associated with lower levels of serotonin in the brain. A recent longitudinal study demonstrated that individuals with different forms of these genotypes responded differently to environmental factors. Depending on genetic make-up, and when exposed to three or more life events, rates of diagnosed major depression were approximately 30% contrasted to 10%. Similarly, rates of major depressive disorder in the context of severe childhood maltreatment doubled from 30 to 60% (Caspi et al., 2003). This raises interesting questions about the mechanisms that result in this differential vulnerability, and intriguingly suggests that preventive interventions aimed at managing adverse events would be expected to exert their impact on only a subset of the population. At this stage such considerations are highly speculative, but the integration of biological indicators into treatment planning would represent a major shift in current thinking, particularly if it enabled specific psychosocial interventions to assist individuals with known genetic vulnerabilities. While such developments could bring benefit, especially if they allowed more targeted therapeutic effort, they would bring with them ethical concerns regarding both the screening of individuals and any decisions regarding access to, or denial of, treatment.

CONCLUDING COMMENTS

We have tried to present an overview of current findings from psychotherapy research and consider their implications for practice. We have attempted to interpret evidence from a clinical perspective, and this has meant balancing a demand for methodological rigor with the need to keep a focus on the application of research in real-world settings. Throughout, we have tried to maintain an open and neutral position, and attempted to appraise the evidence without privileging any one method over another. Doubtless, at least some of our conclusions could be open to challenge, but our hope is that any differences of opinion between ourselves and our readers are based on differences in interpretation rather than prejudice on our part.

We believe that an open examination of the evidence regarding methods of psychological intervention—both favorable and unfavorable—should lead to improvements in patient care. This is an idea that has taken root in recent years, and at least in broad outline, few would disagree with the sentiment of this position. As ever, the devil is in the detail. The success of this enterprise depends on the thoughtful and reflective application of research, applying its findings in formats applicable in the field and in a form that preserves the role of clinical judgment, thus safeguarding the possibility of further innovation and development.

The first edition of this book ended as follows:

> . . . though we have aimed to present the current state of the art, there is a para-
> dox inherent in this goal. In writing this book we became aware of the rapid
> growth of the field, which over time will modify the validity of our conclusions
> and recommendations. Yet this is as it should be—our model of evidence-based
> practice implies that the best results will be achieved through a process of con-
> tinuous and reflexive refinements to technique and procedure. (Roth &
> Fonagy, 1996, p. 378)

For us at least, the degree of revision required to produce this second edition
confirms this point, and the wisdom of ensuring that the relationship
between researchers, managers, and practitioners is one of dynamic dialogue.

APPENDIX I

Converting Effect Sizes to Percentiles

Effect sizes are computed using the formula

$$\text{Effect size} = \frac{M_1 - M_2}{SD}$$

where M_1 is the mean of the treatment group, M_2 is the mean of the control group, and SD is the pooled standard deviation. Converting scores to effect sizes assumes that the scores of the control group and the treatment group correspond to a normal distribution. It is assumed that, in all the contributing studies, patient scores will be distributed in this way.

As long as this assumption is correct, this equation gives a numerical answer to the question, "How far apart are the means of the control group and the treated group?" on a common metric—the common metric being a standard score (known as a Z score). Data from many different studies can then be combined; effect sizes from each individual study contribute to a final overall effect size for the variable being examined.

As an example, imagine that the effect size is being used to indicate the position of the average treated client relative to that of untreated clients. Figure A.1 shows the (hypothetical) distributions of scores for treated and untreated patient groups and Table A.1 the relationship of effect sizes to percentile scores.

If there were no difference between the treated and untreated group, the distribution of scores would be exactly the same; this would be indicated by an effect size of 0.0. This could be expressed in terms of percentiles; the average treated client would be at the 50th percentile of scores for the untreated client group.

An effect size of 1.0 indicates that the average treated patient will be placed at the 84th percentile of the scores for the untreated group. Similarly, an effect size of 2.0 would indicate that the average client had a score at the 97th percentile of scores for the untreated group.

Effect Size = 0

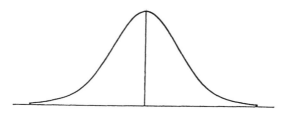

Effect Size = 1

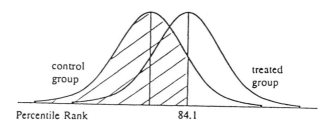

Effect Size = 2

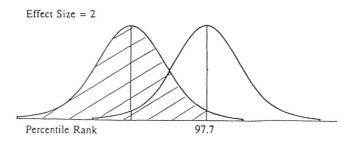

FIGURE A.1. Hypothetical distributions of scores.

TABLE A.1. Converting Effect Sizes into Percentiles

Effect size	Percentile	Effect size	Percentile	Effect size	Percentile
0.0	50.0	0.3	61.8	1.0	84.1
0.1	54.0	0.5	69.1	1.5	93.3
0.2	57.9	0.7	75.8	2.0	97.7

An Illustration of Commonly Used "Clinically Intuitive" Ways of Representing the Outcome of Trials

A hypothetical study of a treatment of alcohol abuse randomized 50 participants to the experimental group and 53 to the control group. At follow-up, the number of participants "recovered" (no longer drinking) was 38 in the experimental group and 20 in the controls. The numbers relapsed (drinking again) were 12 in the experimental group and 33 in the control group.

If relapse is taken as the outcome of interest:

The *experimental event rate* (EER) is (12/50) = 24%

The *control event rate* (CER) is (33/53) = 62%

The odds of relapse in

The experimental group is 12/(50 − 12) = 0.32

The control group is 33/(53 − 33) = 1.65

	Calculated as	Calculation for this example	
Absolute risk reduction (ARR)	CER − EER	62 − 24	38% (or 0.38)
Number needed to treat (NTT)	1/ARR	1/0.38	2.6 (in practice NNTs are often rounded—in this case to 3)
Relative risk (RR)	EER/CER	24%/62%	0.39
Relative risk reduction (RR)	ARR/CER	38%/62%	61%
Odds ratio (OR)	Odds of event in experimental group/odds of event in control group	0.32/1.65	0.19

Contrast between 1-Year Prevalence Rates for Adults Ages 18–54 Derived from the Epidemiologic Catchment Area Survey, the National Comorbidity Survey, and Recomputed Rates by Narrow et al. (2002; see Chapter 4)

	ECA uncorrected prevalence (corrected for clinical significance)	NCS uncorrected prevalence (corrected for clinical significance)	Combined ECA + NCS estimate after correction for clinical significance
Major depressive disorder	5.4 (4.6)	8.9 (5.4)	4.5
Dsythymia	5.7 (1.7)	2.5 (1.8)	1.6
Bipolar disorder	1.2 (0.6)	1.3 (1.3)	0.6
Specific phobia	8.5 (8.5)	8.6 (4.4)	4.4
Social phobia	2.0 (2.0)	7.4 (3.7)	3.7
Generalized anxiety disorder	Not cited	3.4 (2.8)	2.8
Agoraphobia	5.0 (5.0)	3.7 (2.2)	2.2
Panic disorder	1.6 (1.6)	2.2 (1.7)	1.7
Posttraumatic stress disorder	Not cited	3.6 (3.6)	3.6

REFERENCES

Abel, J. (1993). Exposure with response prevention and serotonergic antidepressants in the treatment of obsessive–compulsive disorder: A review and implications for interdisciplinary treatment. *Behaviour Research and Therapy, 31,* 463–478.

Abikoff, H., Ganeles, D., Reiter, G., Blum, C., Foley, C., & Klein, G. R. (1988). Cognitive training in academically deficient ADDH boys receiving stimulant medication. *Journal of Abnormal Child Psychology, 16,* 411–432.

Abikoff, H., & Gittelman, R. (1985). Hyperactive children treated with stimulants: Is cognitive training a useful adjunct? *Archives of General Psychiatry, 42*(10), 953–961.

Abikoff, H. B., & Hechtman, L. (1996). Multimodal therapy and stimulants in the treatment of children with attention deficit hyperactivity disorder. In P. S. Jensen & E. D. Hibbs (Eds.), *Psychosocial treatments for child and adolescent disorders: Empirically based strategies for clinical practice* (pp. 341–369). Washington, DC: American Psychological Association.

Abramowitz, I., & Coursey, R. (1989). Impact of an educational support group of family participants who take care of their schizophrenic relatives. *Journal of Consulting and Clinical Psychology, 57,* 232–236.

Abramowitz, J. S. (1996). Variants of exposure and response-prevention in the treatment of obsessive–compulsive disorder: A meta-analysis. *Behavior Therapy, 27,* 583–600.

Abramowitz, J. S. (1997). Effectiveness of psychological and pharmacological treatments for obsessive–compulsive disorder: A quantitative review. *Journal of Consulting and Clinical Psychology, 65*(1), 44–52.

Abramowitz, J. S. (1998). Does cognitive behavioral therapy cure obsessive–compulsive disorder?: A meta-analytic evaluation of clinical significance. *Behavior Therapy, 29,* 339–355.

Abramowitz, J. S., & Foa, E. B. (2000). Does comorbid major depressive disorder influence outcome of exposure and response prevention for OCD? *Behavior Therapy, 31,* 795–800.

Abramowitz, J. S., Foa, E. B., & Franklin, M. E. (2003). Exposure and ritual prevention for obsessive–compulsive disorder: Effects of intensive versus twice-weekly sessions. *Journal of Consulting and Clinical Psychology, 71*(2), 394–398.

Abramowitz, J. S., Franklin, M. E., Street, G. P., Kozak, M. J., & Foa, E. B. (2000). Effects of comorbid depression on response to treatment for obsessive–compulsive disorder. *Behavior Therapy, 31,* 517–528.

Abramowitz, S., & Sewell, H. (1980). Marital adjustment and sex therapy outcome. *Journal of Sex Research, 16,* 325–337.

Acierno, R., Hersen, M., Van Hasselt, V., & Tremont, G. (1994). Review of the validation and dissemination of eye-movement desensitization and re-processing: A scientific and ethical dilemma. *Clinical Psychology Review, 14*, 287–299.

Ackerman, S. J., & Hilsenroth, M. J. (2001). A review of therapist characteristics and techniques negatively impacting the therapeutic alliance. *Psychotherapy: Theory, Research, Practice, Training, 38*, 171–185.

Ackerman, S. J., & Hilsenroth, M. J. (2003). A review of therapist characteristics and techniques positively impacting the therapeutic alliance. *Clinical Psychology Review, 23*, 1–33.

Addis, M., Wade, W., & Hatgis, W. (1999). Barriers to dissemination of evidence based practices: Addressing practitioners' concerns about manual based psychotherapies. *Clinical Psychology: Science and Practice, 6*, 430–411.

Addis, M. E. (1997). Evaluating the treatment manual as a means of disseminating empirically validated psychotherapies. *Clinical Psychology: Science and Practice, 4*, 1–11.

Agnew-Davies, R., Stiles, W. B., Hardy, G. E., Barkham, M., & Shapiro, D. A. (1998). Alliance structure assessed by the Agnew Relationship Measure (ARM). *British Journal of Clinical Psychology, 37*(2), 155–172.

Agosti, V., & Ocepek-Welikson, K. (1997). The efficacy of imipramine and psychotherapy in early-onset chronic depression: A reanalysis of the National Institute of Mental Health Treatment of Depression Collaborative Research Program. *Journal of Affective Disorders, 43*(3), 181–186.

Agras, W. S., Crow, S. J., Halmi, K. A., Mitchell, J. E., Wilson, G. T., & Kraemer, H. C. (2000a). Outcome predictors for the cognitive behavior treatment of bulimia nervosa: Data from a multisite study. *American Journal of Psychiatry, 157*(8), 1302–1308.

Agras, W. S., Rossiter, E., Arnow, B., Telch, C., Raebum, S., Bruce, B., et al. (1994a). One year follow-up of psychosocial and pharmacologic treatments for bulimia. *Journal of Clinical Psychiatry, 55*, 179–183.

Agras, W. S., Rossiter, E., Arnow, B., Telch, C. F., Raeburn, S. D., Schneider, et al. (1992). Pharmacologic and cognitive-behavioral treatment for bulimia nervosa: A controlled comparison. *American Journal of Psychiatry, 149*, 82–87.

Agras, W. S., Schneider, J. A., Arnow, B., Raeburn, S. D., & Telch, C. F. (1989). Cognitive-behavioral and response prevention treatments for bulimia nervosa. *Journal of Consulting and Clinical Psychology, 57*, 215–221.

Agras, W. S., Telch, C. F., Amow, B., Eldredge, K., Wilfley, D. E., Raebum, S. D., et al. (1994b). Weight loss, cognitive-behavioral, and desipramine treatments in binge eating disorder: An additive design. *Behavior Therapy, 25*, 225–238.

Agras, W. S., Telch, C. F., Arnow, B., Eldredge, K., Detzer, M. J., Henderson, J., et al. (1995). Does interpersonal therapy help patients with binge eating disorder who fail to respond to cognitive-behavioral therapy? *Journal of Consulting and Clinical Psychology, 63*(3), 356–360.

Agras, W. S., Telch, C. F., Arnow, B., Eldredge, K., & Marnell, M. (1997). One-year follow-up of cognitive-behavioral therapy for obese individuals with binge eating disorder. *Journal of Consulting and Clinical Psychology, 65*(2), 343–347.

Agras, W. S., Walsh, T., Fairburn, C. G., Wilson, G. T., & Kraemer, H. C. (2000b). A multicenter comparison of cognitive-behavioral therapy and interpersonal psychotherapy for bulimia nervosa. *Archives of General Psychiatry, 57*(5), 459–466.

Alanen, Y., Rakkozainen, Y., Riija, R., et al. (1985). Psychotherapeutically oriented treatment of schizophrenia: Results of a five year follow-up. *Acta Psychiatrica Scandinavica, 71*, 31–49.

Alden, L. E. (1989). Short term structured treatment for avoidant personality disorder. *Journal of Consulting and Clinical Psychology, 56*, 756–764.

Alden, L. E., & Capreol, M. J. (1993). Avoidant personality disorder: Interpersonal problems as predictors of treatment response. *Behavioural Therapy, 24*, 357–376.

Alexander, F., & French, T. (1946). *Psychoanalytic therapy: Principles and applications.* New York: Ronald Press.

Al-Kubaisy, T., Marks, I., Logsdail, S., Marks, M., Lovell, K., Sungur, M., et al. (1992). Role of exposure homework in phobia reduction: A controlled study. *Behavior Therapy, 23*, 599–621.

Allard, R., Marshall, M., & Plante, M. C. (1992). Intensive follow-up does not decrease the risk of repeat suicide attempts. *Suicide and Life-Threatening Behavior, 22*(3), 303–314.

Allen-Burge, R., Stevens, A. B., & Burgio, L. D. (1999). Effective behavioral interventions for decreasing dementia-related challenging behavior in nursing homes. *International Journal of Geriatric Psychiatry, 14*(3), 213–232.

Alterman, A. I., Rutherford, M. J., Cacciola, J. S., McKay, J. R., & Woody, G. E. (1996). Response to methadone maintenance and counseling in antisocial patients with and without major depression. *Journal of Nervous and Mental Disease, 184*(11), 695–702.

Althof, S., Turner, L., Levine, S., Risen, C., Bodner, D., Kursh, E., et al. (1991). Sexual psychological and marital impact of self-injection of papaverine and phentolamine: A long-term prospective study. *Journal of Sex and Marital Therapy, 17*, 101–112.

Amenson, C. S., & Liberman, R. P. (2001). Dissemination of educational classes for families of adults with schizophrenia. *Psychiatric Services, 52*(5), 589–592.

American Academy of Child and Adolescent Psychiatry. (1998a). Practice parameters for the assessment and treatment of children and adolescents with depressive disorders. *Journal of the American Academy of Child and Adolescent Psychiatry, 37*(10, Suppl.), 63S–83S.

American Academy of Child and Adolescent Psychiatry. (1998b). Practice parameters for the assessment and treatment of children and adolescents with obsessive–compulsive disorder. *Journal of the American Academy of Child and Adolescent Psychiatry, 37*(10, Suppl.), 27S–45S.

American Academy of Child and Adolescent Psychiatry. (1999). Practice parameters for the assessment of children, adolescents and adults with autism and other pervasive developmental disorders. *Journal of the American Academy of Child and Adolescent Psychiatry, 38*(12, Suppl.), 32S–54S.

American Psychiatric Association. (1993a). Practice guideline for eating disorders. *American Journal of Psychiatry, 150*, 207–228.

American Psychiatric Association. (1993b). Practice guidelines for major depressive disorder in adults. *American Journal of Psychiatry, 150*, 1–26.

American Psychiatric Association. (2000). *Diagnostic and statistical manual of mental disorders* (4th ed., text rev.). Washington, DC: Author.

American Psychiatric Association. (1997). Practice guideline for the treatment of patients with schizophrenia. *American Journal of Psychiatry, 154*, 1–63.

Anastopoulos, A. D., Barkley, R. A., & Shelton, T. L. (1996). Family-based treatment: Psychosocial intervention for children and adolescents with attention deficit hyperactivity disorder. In E. D. Hibbs & P. S. Jensen (Eds.), *Psychosocial treatments for child and adolescent disorders: Empirically based strategies for clinical practice* (pp. 267–284). Washington, DC: American Psychological Association.

Anastopoulos, A. D., Shelton, T. L., DuPaul, G. J., & Guevremont, D. C. (1993). Parent training for attention-deficit hyperactivity disorder: Its impact on parent functioning. *Journal of Abnormal Child Psychology, 21*, 581–596.

Anderson, E. M., & Lambert, M. J. (2001). A survival analysis of clinically significant change in outpatient psychotherapy. *Journal of Clinical Psychology, 57*(7), 875–888.

Anderson, S. R., Avery, D. L., DiPeitro, E. K., Edwards, G. L., & Christian, W. P. (1987). Intensive home based early intervention with autistic children. *Education and Treatment of Children, 10*, 352–366.

André, C., Lelord, F., Legeron, P., Reignier, A., & Delattre, A. (1997). Etude controlée sur l'efficacité à 6 mois d'une prise en charge précoce de 132 conducteurs d'autobus victimes d'aggression [Effectiveness of early intervention on 132 bus drivers who have been victims of aggression: A controlled study]. *Encephale, 23*(1), 65–71.

Angst, J. (1992). Epidemiology of depression. *Psychopharamacology, 106*, 571–574.

Angst, J., Dobler-Mikola, A., & Schbniedegger, P. (1985). The Zurich study: Anxiety and phobia in young adults. *European Archives of Psychiatric and Neurological Sciences, 235*, 171–178.

Angst, J., & Dobler-Mikola, A. (1983). Anxiety states, panic and phobia in a young general population. In P. Pichot, R. Beiner, R. Wolf, & K. Thaw (Eds.), *Psychiatry: The state of the art* (Proceedings of the World Psychiatry Congress, Vienna). New York: Plenum Press.

Annerstedt, L., Gustafson, L., & Nilsson, K. (1993). Medical outcome of psychosocial intervention in demented patients: One-year clinical follow-up after relocation into group living units. *International Journal of Geriatric Psychiatry, 8*, 833–841.

Anthony, W., & Carkhuff, R. (1977). The functional professional therapeutic agent. In A. Gurman & A. Razin (Eds.), *Effective psychotherapy*. Elmsford, NY: Pergamon Press.

Antikainen, R., Hintikka, J., Lehtonen, J., Koponen, H., & Arstila, A. (1995). A prospective three-year follow-up study of borderline personality disorder inpatients. *Acta Psychiatrica Scandinavica, 92*(5), 327–335.

Anton, R. F., Moak, D. H., Waid, L. R., Latham, P. K., Malcolm, R. J., & Dias, J. K. (1999). Naltrexone and cognitive behavioral therapy for the treatment of outpatient alcoholics: Results of a placebo-controlled trial. *American Journal of Psychiatry, 156*(11), 1758–1764.

Antony, M. M., & Barlow, D. H. (2002). Specific phobias. In D. H. Barlow, *Anxiety and its disorders: The nature and treatment of anxiety and panic* (2nd ed., pp. 380–417). New York: Guilford Press.

Apfelbaum, B. (1984). The ego-analytic approach to individual body-work sex therapy: Five case examples. *Journal of Sex Research, 20*, 44–70.

Argyle, M., Bryant, B., & Trower, P. (1974). Social skills training and psychotherapy: A comparative study. *Psychological Medicine, 4*, 435–443.

Arntz, A. (2003). Cognitive therapy versus applied relaxation as treatment of generalized anxiety disorder. *Behaviour Research and Therapy, 41*(6), 633–646.

Aronson, T. (1987). Follow-up of two panic disorders–agoraphobic study populations. *Journal of Nervous and Mental Disease, 175*, 595–598.

Asarnow, J. R., Jaycox, L. H., & Tompson, M. C. (2001). Depression in youth: psychosocial interventions. *Journal of Clinical Child Psychology, 30*(1), 33–47.

Atkins, D. C., & Christensen, A. (2001). Is professional training worth the bother?: A review of the impact of psychotherapy training on client outcome. *Australian Psychologist, 36*, 122–130.

Auerbach, A., & Johnson, M. (1977). Research on the therapist's level of experience. In A. Gurman & A. Razin (Eds.), *Effective psychotherapy*. New York: Pergamon Press.

Auerbach, R., & Kilmann, P. (1977). The effects of group systematic desensitization on secondary erectile failure. *Behavior Therapy, 8*, 330–339.

Austad, C., & Berman, W. (1991). Managed health care and the evolution of psychotherapy. In C. Austad & W. Berman (Eds.), *Psychotherapy in managed health care* (pp. 3–18). Washington DC: American Psychological Association.

Avants, S. K., Margolin, A., Sindelar, J. L., Rounsaville, B. J., Schottenfeld, R., Stine, S., et al. (1999). Day treatment versus enhanced standard methadone services for opioid-dependent patients: A comparison of clinical efficacy and cost. *American Journal of Psychiatry, 156*(1), 27–33.

Ayllon, T., Garber, S., & Pisor, K. (1975). The elimination of discipline problems through a combined school–home motivational system. *Behaviour Therapy, 6*, 616–626.

Azrin, N. (1976). Improvements in the community reinforcement approach to alcoholism. *Behaviour Research and Therapy, 6*, 7–12.

Azrin, N., Sisson, R., Meyers, R., & Godley, M. (1982). Alcoholism treatment by disulfiram and community reinforcement therapy. *Journal of Behavior Therapy and Experimental Psychiatry, 13*, 105–112.

Azrin, N. H., & Peterson, A. L. (1988). Habit reversal for the treatment of Tourette syndrome. *Behaviour Research and Therapy, 11*, 347–355.

Azrin, N. H., & Peterson, A. L. (1990). Treatment of Tourette syndrome by habit reversal: A waiting-list control group comparison. *Behaviour Therapy, 21*, 305–318.

Bacaltchuk, J., Hay, P., & Trefiglio, R. (2001). Antidepressants versus psychological treatments and their combination for bulimia nervosa (Cochrane Review). In *The Cochrane Library*, Issue 4, 2002. Oxford, UK: Update Software.

Bacaltchuk, J., Trefiglio, R. P., Oliveira, I. R., Hay, P., Lima, M. S., & Mari, J. J. (2000). Combination of antidepressants and psychological treatments for bulimia nervosa: A systematic review. *Acta Psychiatrica Scandinavica, 101*(4), 256–264.

Bachar, E., Latzer, Y., Kreitler, S., & Berry, E. M. (1999). Empirical comparison of two psychological therapies: Self psychology and cognitive orientation in the treatment of anorexia and bulimia. *Journal of Psychotherapy Practice and Research, 8*(2), 115–128.

Baguley, I., Butterworth, A., Fahy, K., Haddock, G., Lancashire, S., & Tarrier, N. (2000). Bringing into clinical practice skills shown to be effective in research settings: A follow-up of "Thorn Training" in psychosocial family interventions for psychosis. In B. Martindale, A. Bateman, M. Crowe, & F. Margison (Eds.), *Psychosis: Psychological approaches and their clinical effectiveness* (pp. 96–117). London: Royal College of Psychiatrists, Gaskell.

Baines, S., Saxby, P., & Ehlert, K. (1987). Reality orientation and reminiscence therapy: A controlled cross-over study of elderly confused people. *British Journal of Psychiatry, 151*, 222–231.

Baker, R. (2001). Is it time to review the idea of compliance with guidelines? *British Journal of General Practice, 51*, 7.

Baker, R., Bell, S., Baker, E., Gibson, S., Holloway, J., Pearce, R., Dowling, et al. (2001). A randomized controlled trial of the effects of multi-sensory stimulation (MSS) for people with dementia. *British Journal of Clinical Psychology, 40*, 81–96.

Baker, R., Dowling, Z., Wareing, L. A., Dawson, J., & Assey, J. (1997). Snoezelen: its long-term and short-term effects on older people with dementia. *British Journal of Occupational Therapy, 60*(5), 213–218.

Bakker, A., van Balkom, A. J., Spinhoven, P., Blaauw, B. M., & van Dyck, R. (1998). Follow-up on the treatment of panic disorder with or without agoraphobia: A quantitative review. *Journal of Nervous and Mental Disease, 186*(7), 414–419.

Baldwin, B. (1991). The outcome of depression in old age. *International Journal of Geriatric Psychiatry, 6*, 395–400.

Balestrieri, M., William, P., & Wilkinson, G. (1988). Specialist mental health treatment in general practice: A meta-analysis. *Psychological Medicine, 18*, 711–717.

Ballard, C. G., Boyle, A., Bowler, C., & Lindesay, J. (1996a). Anxiety disorders in dementia sufferers. *International Journal of Geriatric Psychiatry, 11*, 987–990.

Ballard, C. G., Bannister, C., & Oyebode, F. (1996b). Depression in dementia sufferers. *International Journal of Geriatric Psychiatry, 11*(6), 507–515.

Bancroft, J., & Coles, L. (1976). Three years experience in a sexual problems clinic. *British Medical Journal, 1976*(1), 1575–1577.

Bancroft, J., Dickerson, M., Fairburn, C., Gray, J., Greenwood, J., Stevenson, N., et al. (1986). Sex therapy outcome research: A reappraisal of methodology. *Psychological Medicine, 16*, 851–863.

Bank, L., Marlowe, J. H., Reid, J. B., Patterson, G. R., & Weinrott, M. R. (1991). A comparative evaluation of parent-training interventions for families of chronic delinquents. *Journal of Abnormal Child Psychology, 19*, 15–33.

Barbato, A., & D'Avanzo, B. (2000). Family interventions in schizophrenia and related disorders: A critical review of clinical trials. *Acta Psychiatrica Scandinavica, 102*, 81–97.

Barber, J. P., Connolly, M. B., Crits-Christoph, P., Gladis, L., & Siqueland, L. (2000). Alliance predicts patients' outcome beyond in-treatment change in symptoms. *Journal of Consulting and Clinical Psychology, 68*(6), 1027–1032.

Barber, J. P., Crits-Christoph, P., & Luborsky, L. (1996). Effects of therapist adherence and competence on patient outcome in brief dynamic therapy. *Journal of Consulting and Clinical Psychology, 64*(3), 619–622.

Barber, J. P., Luborsky, L., Crits-Christoph, P., Thase, M. E., Weiss, R., Frank, A., et al.

(1999). Therapeutic alliance as a predictor of outcome in treatment of cocaine dependence. *Psychotherapy Research, 9*, 54–73.

Barber, J. P., Morse, J. Q., Krakauer, I. D., Chittams, J., & Crits-Christoph, K. (1997). Change in obsessive–compulsive and avoidant personality disorders following time-limited supportive–expressive therapy. *Psychotherapy, 34*(2), 133–143.

Barber, J. P., & Muenz, L. R. (1996). The role of avoidance and obsessiveness in matching patients to cognitive and interpersonal psychotherapy: Empirical findings from the treatment for depression collaborative research program. *Journal of Consulting and Clinical Psychology, 64*(5), 951–958.

Barbui, C., & Hotopf, M. (2001). Amitriptyline v. the rest: Still the leading antidepressant after 40 years of randomized controlled trials. *British Journal of Psychiatry, 178*, 129–144.

Bark, N., Revheim, N., Huq, F., Khalderov, V., Watras Ganz, Z., & Medalia, A. (2003). The impact of cognitive remediation on psychiatric symptoms of schizophrenia. *Schizophrenia Research, 63*, 229–235.

Barker, W., Scott, J., & Eccleston, D. (1987). The Newcastle chronic depression study: Results of a treatment regime. *International Clinical Psychopharmacology, 2*, 261–272.

Barkham, M., Lucock, M., Leach, C., Evans, C., Margison, F., Mellor-Clark, J., et al. (2001). Service profiling and outcomes benchmarking using the CORE OM: Toward practice based evidence in the psychological therapies. *Journal of Consulting and Clinical Psychology, 69*, 184–196.

Barkham, M., Rees, A., Shapiro, D. A., Stiles, W. B., Agnew, R. M., Halstead, J., et al. (1996a). Outcomes of time-limited psychotherapy in applied settings: Replicating the Second Sheffield Psychotherapy Project. *Journal of Consulting and Clinical Psychology, 64*(5), 1079–1085.

Barkham, M., Rees, A., Stiles, W. B., Shapiro, D. A., Hardy, G. E., & Reynolds, S. (1996b). Dose–effect relations in time-limited psychotherapy for depression. *Journal of Consulting and Clinical Psychology, 64*(5), 927–935.

Barkley, R. A., Shelton, T. L., Crosswait, C. C., Moorehouse, M., Fletcher, K., Barrett, S., et al. (2000). Multi-method psycho-educational intervention for preschool children with disruptive behavior: Preliminary results at post-treatment. *Journal of Child Psychology and Psychiatry, 41*, 319–332.

Barley, W., Buie, S., Peterson, E., Hollingsworth, A., et al. (1993). Development of an inpatient cognitive-behavioral treatment program for borderline personality disorder. *Journal of Personality Disorders, 7*(3), 232–240.

Barlow, D. H. (1988). *Anxiety and its disorders: The nature and treatment of anxiety and panic.* New York: Guilford Press.

Barlow, D. H. (1996). The effectiveness of psychotherapy: Science and policy. *Clinical Psychology: Science and Practice, 3*, 236–240.

Barlow, D. H., Craske, M., Cemy, J., & Klosko, J. (1989). Behavioral treatment of panic disorder. *Behavior Therapy, 20*, 261–282.

Barlow, D. H., Gorman, J. M., Shear, M. K., & Woods, S. W. (2000). Cognitive-behavioral therapy, imipramine, or their combination for panic disorder: A randomized controlled trial. *Journal of the American Medical Association, 283*(19), 2529–2536.

Barlow, D. H., Rapee, R. M., & Brown, T. A. (1992). Behavioral treatment of generalized anxiety disorder. *Behavior Therapy, 23*, 551–570.

Barrett, J. E., Williams, J. W., Jr., Oxman, T. E., Frank, E., Katon, W., Sullivan, M., et al. (2001). Treatment of dysthymia and minor depression in primary care: A randomized trial in patients aged 18 to 59 years. *Family Practice, 50*(5), 405–412.

Barrett, P. M., Dadds, M. R., & Rapee, R. M. (1996). Family treatment for childhood anxiety: A controlled trial. *Journal of Consulting and Clinical Psychology, 64*, 333–342.

Barrowclough, C., King, P., Colville, J., Russell, E., Burns, A., & Tarrier, N. (2001). A randomized trial of the effectiveness of cognitive-behavioral therapy and supportive counseling for anxiety symptoms in older adults. *Journal of Consulting and Clinical Psychology, 69*(5), 756–762.

Barrowclough, C., & Tarrier, N. (1984). Psychosocial intervention with families and their effects on the course of schizophrenia: A review. *Psychological Medicine, 14*, 629–642.

Barrowclough, C., Tarrier, N., Lewis, S., Sellwood, W., Mainwaring, J., Quinn, J., et al. (1999). Randomised controlled effectiveness trial of a needs-based psychosocial intervention service for carers of people with schizophrenia. *British Journal of Psychiatry, 174*, 505–511.

Barrowclough, C., Tarrier, N., Watts, S., Vaughn, C., Bamrah, J., & Freeman, H. (1987). Assessing the functional value of relatives knowledge about schizophrenia: A preliminary report. *British Journal of Psychiatry, 151*, 1–8.

Barry, A., & Lippman, B. (1990). Anorexia nervosa in males. *Postgraduate Medicine, 87*, 161–165.

Basoglu, M., Lax, T., Kasvikis, Y., & Marks, I. (1988). Predictors of improvement in obsessive–compulsive disorder. *Journal of Anxiety Disorders, 2*, 299–231.

Basoglu, M., Marks, I., Kilic, C., Swinson, R., Noshirvani, H., Kuch, K., et al. (1994). Relationship of panic, anticipatory anxiety, agoraphobia and global improvement in panic disorder with agoraphobia treated with alprazolam and exposure. *British Journal of Psychiatry, 164*, 647–652.

Bateman, A., & Fonagy, P. (1999). The effectiveness of partial hospitalization in the treatment of borderline personality disorder—a randomized controlled trial. *American Journal of Psychiatry, 156*, 1563–1569.

Bateman, A., & Fonagy, P. (2001). Treatment of borderline personality disorder with psychoanalytically oriented partial hospitalization: An 18-month follow-up. *American Journal of Psychiatry, 158*(1), 36–42.

Bateman, A., & Fonagy, P. (2003). Health service utilization costs for borderline personality disorder patients treated with psychoanalytically oriented partial hospitalization versus general psychiatric care. *American Journal of Psychiatry, 160*(1), 169–171.

Bateman, A., & Fonagy, P. (2004). *Psychotherapy for borderline personality disorder: Mentalization based treatment*. Oxford, UK: Oxford University Press.

Baucom, D. H., Shoham, V., Mueser, K. T., Daiuto, A. D., & Stickle, T. R. (1998). Empirically supported couple and family interventions for marital distress and adult mental health problems. *Journal of Consulting and Clinical Psychology, 66*(1), 53–88.

Bauer, M. S. (2002). A review of quantitative studies of adherence to mental health clinical practice guidelines. *Harvard Review of Psychiatry, 10*, 138–153.

Beach, S. R., Fincham, F. D., & Katz, J. (1998). Marital therapy in the treatment of depression: Toward a third generation of therapy and research. *Clinical Psychology Review, 18*(6), 635–661.

Beach, S. R. H., & O'Leary, K. D. (1992). Treating depression in the context of marital discord: Outcome and predictors of response for marital therapy vs. cognitive therapy. *Behavior Therapy, 23*, 507–528.

Beail, N. (2003). What works for people with mental retardation?: Critical commentary on cognitive-behavioral and psychodynamic psychotherapy research. *Mental Retardation, 41*, 468–472.

Beardslee, W. R., Wright, E. J., Salt, P., Drezner, K., Gladstone, T. R., Versage, E. M., et al. (1997). Examination of children's responses to two preventive intervention strategies over time. *Journal of the American Academy of Child and Adolescent Psychiatry, 36*(2), 196–204.

Bebbington, P., & Kuipers, L. (1994). The positive utility of expressed emotion in schizophrenia: An aggregate analysis. *Psychological Medicine, 24*, 707–707.

Bebbington, P. E., Brugha, T. S., Meltzer, H., Jenkins, R., Ceresa, C., Farrell, M., et al. (2000a). Neurotic disorders and the receipt of psychiatric treatment. *Psychological Medicine, 30*, 1369–1376.

Bebbington, P. E., Meltzer, H., Brugha, T. S., Farrell, M., Jenkins, R., Ceresa, C., et al. (2000b). Unequal access and unmet need: Neurotic disorders and the use of primary care services. *Psychological Medicine, 30*, 1359–1367.

Beck, A., Sokol, L., Clark, D., Berchick, R., & Wright, F. (1992). A crossover study of focused cognitive therapy for panic disorder. *American Journal of Psychiatry, 149,* 778–783.

Beck, A. T. (1976). *Cognitive therapy and the emotional disorders.* New York: International Universities Press/Meriden.

Beck, A. T., Rush, A., Shaw, B., & Emery, G. (1979). *Cognitive therapy of depression.* New York: Guilford Press.

Beck, A. T., Hollon, S. D., Young, J. E., et al. (1985). Treatment of depression with cognitive therapy and amitriptyline. *Archives of General Psychiatry, 42,* 142–148.

Beck, C. K., Heacock, P., Mercer, S. O., Walls, R., Rapp, C. G., & Vogelpohl, T. S. (1997). Improving dressing behavior in cognitively impaired nursing home residents. *Nursing Research, 46*(3), 126–132.

Beck, J., Stanley, M., Baldwin, L., Deagle, E., & Averill, P. (1994). Comparison of cognitive therapy and relaxation training for panic disorder. *Journal of Consulting and Clinical Psychology, 62,* 818–826.

Becker, R., Heimberg, R., & Bellack, A. (1987). *Social skills training treatment for depression.* New York: Pergamon Press.

Beidel, D. C., & Turner, S. M. (1997). At risk for anxiety: I. Psychopathology in the offspring of anxious parents. *Journal of the American Academy of Child and Adolescent Psychiatry, 36*(7), 918–924.

Beidel, D. C., Turner, S. M., & Morris, T. L. (1999). Psychopathology of childhood social phobia. *Journal of the American Academy of Child and Adolescent Psychiatry, 38,* 643–650.

Beidel, D. C., Turner, S. M., & Morris, T. L. (2000). Behavioral treatment of childhood social phobia. *Journal of Consulting and Clinical Psychology, 68*(6), 1072–1080.

Bein, E., Anderson, T., Strupp, H. H., Henry, W. P., Schacht, T. E., Binder, J. L., et al. (2000). The effects of training in time-limited dynamic psychotherapy: Changes in therapeutic outcome. *Psychotherapy Research, 10,* 119–132.

Beitchman, J. H., Zucker, K. J., Hood, J. E., daCosta, G. A., & Akman, D. (1991). A review of the short-term effects of child sexual abuse. *Child Abuse and Neglect, 15,* 537–556.

Beitchman, J. H., Zucker, K. J., Hood, J. E., daCosta, G. A., Akman, D., & Cassavia, E. (1992). A review of the long-term effects of child sexual abuse. *Child Abuse and Neglect, 16,* 101–118.

Bell, M., Bryson, G., Greig, T., Corcoran, C., & Wexler, B. E. (2001). Neurocognitive enhancement therapy with work therapy: Effects on neuropsychological test performance. *Archives of General Psychiatry, 58*(8), 763–768.

Bellack, A., Hersen, M., & Himmelhoch, J. (1981). Social skills training compared with pharmacotherapy and psychotherapy for depression. *American Journal of Psychiatry, 138,* 1562–1567.

Bellack, A. S., Weinhardt, L. S., Gold, J. M., & Gearon, J. S. (2001). Generalization of training effects in schizophrenia. *Schizophrenia Research, 48*(2–3), 255–262.

Bell-Dolan, D. J., Last, C. G., & Strauss, C. C. (1990). Symptoms of anxiety disorders in normal children. *Journal of the American Academy of Child Psychiatry, 29,* 759–765.

Bellucci, D., Glaberman, K., & Haslam, N. (2002). Computer-assisted cognitive rehabilitation reduces negative symptoms in the severely mentally ill. *Schizophrenia Research, 59,* 225–232.

Bemis, K. M. (1987). The present status of operant conditioning for the treatment of anorexia nervosa. *Behaviour Modification, 11,* 432–463.

Bender, D. S., Dolan, R. T., Skodol, A. E., Sanislow, C. A., Dyck, I. R., McGlashan, T. H., et al. (2001). Treatment utilization by patients with personality disorders. *American Journal of Psychiatry, 158*(2), 295–302.

Bennett, D. E. (1998). Deriving a model of therapist competence from good and poor outcome cases in the psychotherapy of borderline personality disorder. PhD thesis Sheffield University, Sheffield, UK.

Benson, R. (1975). The forgotten treatment modality in bipolar illness: Psychotherapy. *Diseases of the Nervous System, 36,* 634–638.

Benton, M., & Scroeder, H. (1990). Social skills training with schizophrenics: A meta-analytic evaluation. *Journal of Consulting and Clinical Psychology, 58,* 741–747.

Berelowitz, M., & Tarnopolsky, A. (1993). The validity of borderline personality disorder: An updated review of recent research. In P. Tyrer & G. Stein (Eds.), *Personality disorder reviewed* (pp. 90–112). London: Gaskell, Royal College of Psychiatrists.

Bergin, A. E. (1971). The evaluation of therapeutic outcomes. In A. E. Bergin & S. L. Garfield (Eds.), *Handbook of psychotherapy and behavior change* (pp. 217–270). New York: Wiley.

Berkowitz, R., Eberlein-Friess, R., Kuipers, L., & Leff, J. (1984). Educating relatives about schizophrenia. *Schizophrenia Bulletin, 10,* 418–429.

Berman, J., & Norton, N. C. (1985). Does professional training make a therapist more effective? *Psychological Bulletin, 98,* 401–407.

Berman, S. L., Kurtines, W. M., Silverman, W. K., & Serafini, L. T. (1996). The impact of exposure to crime and violence on urban youth. *American Journal of Orthopsychiatry, 66*(3), 329–336.

Berman, S. R., Weems, C., Silverman, W., & Kurtines, W. (2000). Predictors of outcome in exposure-based cognitive and behavioural treatments for phobic and anxiety disorders in children. *Behavior Therapy, 31,* 713–731.

Bernstein, G. A., & Borchardt, C. M. (1991). Anxiety disorders of childhood and adolescence: A critical review. *Journal of the American Academy of Child and Adolescent Psychiatry, 30,* 519–532.

Bernstein, G. A., Borchardt, C. M., Perwien, A. R., Crosby, R. D., Kushner, M. G., Thuras, P. D., et al. (2000). Imipramine plus cognitive-behavioral therapy in the treatment of school refusal. *Journal of the American Academy of Child and Adolescent Psychiatry, 39*(3), 276–283.

Betz, N., & Shullman, S. (1979). Factors related to client return following intake. *Journal of Counselling Psychology, 26,* 542–545.

Beutler, L., Engle, D., Mohr, D., Daldrup, R., et al. (1991). Predictors of differential response to cognitive, experiential, and self-directed psychotherapeutic procedures. *Journal of Consulting and Clinical Psychology, 59*(2), 333–340.

Beutler, L., Machado, P., & Neufeldt, S. (1994). Therapist variables. In A. Bergin & S. Garfield (Eds.), *Handbook of psychotherapy and behavior change* (4th ed., pp. 229–269). New York: Wiley.

Beutler, L., Scogin, F., Kirkish, P., Schretlen, D., Corbishley, A., Hamblin, D., et al. (1987). Group cognitive therapy and alprazolam in the treatment of depression in older adults. *Journal of Consulting and Clinical Psychology, 55,* 550–556.

Beutler, L. E., Malik, M., Alimohamed, S., Harwood, T. M., Talebi, H., Noble, S., et al. (2004). Therapist variables. In M. J. Lambert (Ed.), *Bergin and Garfield's handbook of psychotherapy and behavior change* (pp. 227–306). New York: Wiley.

Beutler, L. E., Moleiro, C., & Talebi, H. (2002). How practitioners can systematically use empirical evidence in treatment selection. *Journal of Clinical Psychology, 58*(10), 1199–1212.

Bhugra, D., & Cordle, C. (1988). A case control study of sexual dysfunction in Asian and non-Asian couples 1981–1985. *Sexual and Marital Therapy, 3,* 71–76.

Bickel, W. K., Amass, L., Higgins, S. T., Badger, G. J., & Esch, R. A. (1997). Effects of adding behavioral treatment to opioid detoxification with buprenorphine. *Journal of Consulting and Clinical Psychology, 65*(5), 803–810.

Bien, T. H., Miller, W. R., & Tonigan, J. C. (1993). Brief interventions for alcohol problems: A review. *Addiction, 88,* 315–336.

Bird, M. (2000). Psychosocial rehabilitation for problems arising from cognitive deficits in dementia. In R. D. Hill, L. Backman, & A. S. Neely (Eds.), *Cognitive rehabilitation in old age* (pp. 249–269). New York: Oxford University Press.

Bird, M., Alexopoulos, P., & Adamowicz, J. (1995). Success and failure in five case studies: Use of cued recall to ameliorate behaviour problems in senile dementia. *International Journal of Geriatric Psychiatry, 10,* 305–311.

Birmaher, B., Brent, D. A., Kolko, D., Baugher, M., Bridge, J., Holder, D., et al. (2000). Clinical outcome after short-term psychotherapy for adolescents with major depressive disorder. *Archives of General Psychiatry, 57*(1), 29–36.

Birmaher, B., Ryan, N. D., Williamson, D., Brent, D. A., Kaufman, J., Dahl, R. E., et al. (1996a). Childhood and adolescent depression: A review of the past 10 years: Part I. *Journal of the American Academy of Child and Adolescent Psychiatry, 35*, 1427–1439.

Birmaher, B., Ryan, N. D., Williamson, D. E., Brent, D. A., & Kaufman, J. (1996b). Childhood and adolescent depression: A review of the past 10 years: Part II. *Journal of the American Academy of Child and Adolescent Psychiatry, 35*, 1575–1583.

Birnbrauer, J. S., & Leach, D. J. (1993). The Murdoch early intervention program after two years. *Behavior Change, 10*, 63–74.

Bisson, J. I. (2003). Single-session early psychological interventions following traumatic events. *Clinical Psychology Review, 23*(3), 481–499.

Bisson, J. I., Jenkins, P. L., Alexander, J., & Bannister, C. (1997). Randomised controlled trial of psychological debriefing for victims of acute burn trauma. *British Journal of Psychiatry, 171*, 78–81.

Black, D. W., Monahan, P., Gable, J., Blum, N., Clancy, G., & Baker, P. (1998). Hoarding and treatment response in 38 nondepressed subjects with obsessive–compulsive disorder. *Journal of Clinical Psychiatry, 59*, 420–425.

Black, D. W., Wesner, R., Bowers, W., & Gabel, J. (1993). A comparison of fluvoxamine, cognitive therapy, and placebo in the treatment of panic disorder. *Archives of General Psychiatry, 50*, 44–50.

Black, D. W., Wesner, R. B., Gabel, J., Bowers, W., & Monahan, P. (1994). Predictors of short-term treatment response in 66 patients with panic disorder. *Journal of Affective Disorders, 30*(4), 233–241.

Blackburn, I., Bishop, S., Glen, A., Whalley, L., & Christie, J. (1981). The efficacy of cognitive therapy in depression: A treatment trial using cognitive therapy and pharmacotherapy, each alone and in combination. *British Journal of Psychiatry, 139*, 181–189.

Blackburn, I., Eunson, K., & Bishop, S. (1986). A two-year naturalistic follow-up of depressed patients treated with cognitive therapy, pharmacotherapy and a combination of both. *Journal of Affective Disorders, 10*, 65–75.

Blackburn, I. M., & Moore, R. G. (1997). Controlled acute and follow-up trial of cognitive therapy and pharmacotherapy in out-patients with recurrent depression. *British Journal of Psychiatry, 171*, 328–334.

Blagg, N. R., & Yule, W. (1984). The behavioural treatment of school refusal: A comparative study. *Behaviour Research and Therapy, 22*, 119–127.

Blanchard, E. B., Hickling, E. J., Devineni, T., Veazey, C. H., Galovski, T. E., Mundy, E., et al. (2003). A controlled evaluation of cognitive behavioural therapy for posttraumatic stress in motor vehicle accident survivors. *Behaviour Research and Therapy, 41*(1), 79–96.

Bland, R., Newman, S., & Orn, H. (1988). Age of onset of psychiatric disorders. *Acta Psychiatrica Scandinavica, 77*, 43–49.

Blatt, S. J., Quinlan, D. M., Zuroff, D. C., & Pilkonis, P. A. (1996). Interpersonal factors in brief treatment of depression: Further analyses of the National Institute of Mental Health Treatment of Depression Collaborative Research Program. *Journal of Consulting and Clinical Psychology, 64*(1), 162–171.

Blazer, D., Hughes, D., George, L., Swartz, M., & Boyer, R. (1991). Generalized anxiety disorder. In L. Robins & D. Regier (Eds.), *Psychiatric disorders in America: The Epidemiological Catchment Area Study.* New York: Free Press.

Blazer, D., Kessler, R., McGonagle, K., & Swartz, M. (1994). The prevalence and distribution of major depression in a national community sample: The National Comorbidity Survey. *American Journal of Psychiatry, 151*, 979–986.

Blomhoff, S., Haug, T. T., Hellstrom, K., Holme, I., Humble, M., Madsbu, H. P., et al. (2001). Randomised controlled general practice trial of sertraline, exposure therapy and combined treatment in generalised social phobia. *British Journal of Psychiatry, 179*, 23–30.

Blum, N., Pfohl, B., John, D. S., Monahan, P., & Black, D. W. (2002). STEPPS: A cognitive-behavioral systems-based group treatment for outpatients with borderline personality disorder—a preliminary report. *Comprehensive Psychiatry, 43*(4), 301–310.

Boersma, K., den Hengst, S., Dekker, J., & Emmelkamp, P. (1976). Exposure and response prevention in the natural environment: A comparison with obsessive compulsive patients. *Behaviour Research and Therapy, 14,* 19–24.

Bohus, M., Haaf, B., Simms, T., Limberger, M. F., Schmahl, C., Unckel, C., et al. (2004). Effectiveness of inpatient dialectical behavioral therapy for borderline personality disorder: A controlled trial. *Behaviour Research and Therapy, 42,* 487–499.

Bohus, M., Haaf, B., Stiglmayr, C., Pohl, U., Bohme, R., & Linehan, M. (2000). Evaluation of inpatient dialectical-behavioral therapy for borderline personality disorder—a prospective study. *Behaviour Research and Therapy, 38*(9), 875–887.

Boland, F., Mellor, C., & Revusky, S. (1978). Chemical aversion treatment of alcoholism: Lithium as the aversive agent. *Behaviour Research and Therapy, 16,* 401–409.

Bolton, P., Bass, J., Neugebauer, R., Verdeli, H., Clougherty, K. F., Wickramaratne, P., et al. (2003). Group interpersonal psychotherapy for depression in rural Uganda: A randomized controlled trial. *Journal of the American Medical Association, 289*(23), 3117–3124.

Bolwig, T. G. (1998). Editorial: Debriefing after psychological trauma. *Acta Psychiatrica Scandinavica, 98*(3), 169–170.

Bond, A. J., Wingrove, J., Valerie Curran, H., & Lader, M. H. (2002). Treatment of generalised anxiety disorder with a short course of psychological therapy, combined with buspirone or placebo. *Journal of Affective Disorders, 72*(3), 267–271.

Bordin, E. (1979). The generalizability of the psychoanalytic concept of the working alliance. *Psychotherapy, 16,* 252–260.

Borduin, C. M. (1999). Multisystemic treatment of criminality and violence in adolescents. *Journal of the American Academy for Child and Adolescent Psychiatry, 38,* 242–249.

Borduin, C. M., Mann, B. J., Cone, L. T., Henggeler, S. W., Fucci, B. R., Blaske, D. M., et al. (1995). Multisystemic treatment of serious juvenile offenders: Long-term prevention of criminality and violence. *Journal of Consulting and Clinical Psychology, 63,* 569–578.

Borkovec, T., Abel, J., & Newman, H. (1995). Effects of psychotherapy on comorbid conditions in generalized anxiety disorder. *Journal of Consulting and Clinical Psychology, 63,* 479–483.

Borkovec, T., & Costello, E. (1993). Efficacy of applied relaxation and cognitive-behavioral therapy in the treatment of generalized anxiety disorder. *Journal of Consulting and Clinical Psychology, 61,* 611–619.

Borkovec, T. D. (1997, July). *Limitations of cognitive behavioral treatment of generalized anxiety disorder.* Paper presented to the meeting of the British Association for Cognitive and Behavioral Psychotherapy, Canterbury, UK.

Borkovec, T. D., & Castonguay, L. G. (1998). What is the scientific meaning of empirically supported therapy? *Journal of Consulting and Clinical Psychology, 66*(1), 136–142.

Borkovec, T. D., & Newman, M. G. (1998). Worry and generalized anxiety disorder. In P. Salkovskis, A. S. Bellack, & M. Hersen (Eds.), *Comprehensive clinical psychology: Vol. 6. Adults: Clinical formulation and treatment* (pp. 439–459). New York: Pergamon Press.

Borkovec, T. D., Newman, M. G., Pincus, A. L., & Lytle, R. (2002). A component analysis of cognitive-behavioral therapy for generalized anxiety disorder and the role of interpersonal problems. *Journal of Consulting and Clinical Psychology, 70*(2), 288–298.

Borkovec, T. D., & Ruscio, A. M. (2001). Psychotherapy for generalized anxiety disorder. *Journal of Clinical Psychiatry, 62*(Suppl. 11), 37–42; discussion, 43–45.

Boudewyns, P., & Hyer, L. (1990). Physiological response to combat memories and preliminary treatment outcome in Vietnam veteran PTSD patients treated with direct therapeutic exposure. *Behavior Therapy, 21,* 63–87.

Boudewyns, P., & Hyer, L. A. (1996). Eye-movement desensitization and reprocessing (EMDR) as a treatment for posttraumatic stress disorder (PTSD). *Clinical Psychology and Psychotherapy, 3,* 185–195.

Boudewyns, P., Hyer, L., Woods, M., Harrison, W., & McCranie, E. (1990). PTSD among Vietnam veterans: An early look at treatment outcome using direct therapeutic exposure. *Journal of Traumatic Stress, 3,* 359–368.

Boudewyns, P., Stwertka, L., Hyer, J., Albrecht, X., & Sperr, E. (1993). Eye-movement desensitization for PTSD of combat: A treatment outcome pilot study. *Behavior Therapist, 16,* 29–33.

Boulougouris, J. (1977). Variables affecting outcome in obsessive–compulsive patients treated by flooding. In J. Bolouglouris & A. Rabevillas (Eds.), *Treatment of phobic and obsessive–compulsive disorders.* Oxford, UK: Pergamon Press.

Bowen, G., & Lambert, J. (1986). Systematic desensitization therapy with PTSD cases. In C. Figley (Ed.), *Trauma and its wake II* (pp. 280–291). New York: Brunner/Mazel.

Bower, P., Byford, S., Barber, J., Beecham, J., Simpson, S., Friedli, K., et al. (2003a). Meta-analysis of data on costs from trials of counselling in primary care: Using individual patient data to overcome ample size limitations in economic analyses. *British Medical Journal, 326,* 1247–1250.

Bower, P., Rowland, N., & Hardy, R. (2003b). The clinical effectiveness of counselling in primary care: A systematic review and meta-analysis. *Psychological Medicine, 33*(2), 203–215.

Bowers, T. G., & Al-Redha, M. R. (1990). A comparison of outcome with group/marital and standard/individual therapies with alcoholics. *Journal of Studies on Alcohol, 51*(4), 301–309.

Bowers, W. (1990). Treatment of depressed in-patients: Cognitive therapy plus medication, relaxation plus medication and medication alone. *British Journal of Psychiatry, 156,* 73–78.

Bowers, W., Stuart, S., MacFarlane, R., & Gorman, L. (1993). Use of computer-administered CBT with depressed inpatients. *Depression, 1,* 294–299.

Bowlby, J. (1988). *A secure base: Clinical applications of attachment theory.* London: Routledge.

Bradley, S., Brody, J., Landy, S., Tallett, S., Watson, W., Shea, B., et al. (1999). *Brief psychoeducational parenting program: An evaluation.* Paper presented at the 46th Annual Meeting of the American Academy of Child and Adolescent Psychiatry, Chicago, IL.

Brandsma, J., Maultsby, M., & Welsh, R. (1980). *The outpatient treatment of alcoholism: A review and a comparative study.* Baltimore: University Park Press.

Brane, G., Karlsson, I., Kihlgren, M., & Norberg, A. (1989). Integrity-promoting care of demented nursing home patients: Psychological and biochemical changes. *International Journal of Geriatric Psychiatry, 4,* 165–172.

Brent, D. A., Holder, D., Kolko, D., Birmaher, B., Baugher, M., Roth, C., et al. (1997). A clinical psychotherapy trial for adolescent depression comparing cognitive, family and supportive therapy. *Archives of General Psychiatry, 54,* 877–885.

Brent, D. A., Kolko, D., Birmaher, B., Baugher, M., & Bridge, J. (1999). A clinical trial for adolescent depression: Predictors of additional treatment in the acute and follow-up phases of the trial. *Journal of the American Academy of Child and Adolescent Psychiatry, 38,* 263–270.

Brent, D. A., Kolko, D., Birmaher, B., Baugher, M., Bridge, J., Roth, C., et al. (1998). Predictors of treatment efficacy in a clinical trial of three psychosocial treatments for adolescent depression. *Journal of the American Academy of Child and Adolescent Psychiatry, 37,* 906–914.

Breslau, N., & Davis, G. (1985). DSM-III generalized anxiety disorder: An empirical investigation of more stringent criteria. *Psychiatry Research, 14,* 231–238.

Breslau, N., Davis, C., Andreski, P., & Peterson, E. (1991). Traumatic events and PTSD in an urban population of young adults. *Archives of General Psychiatry, 40,* 216–222.

Brestan, E. V., Eyberg, S. M., Boggs, S. R., & Algina, J. (1997). Parent–child interaction therapy: Parents' perceptions of untreated siblings. *Child and Family Behaviour Therapy, 19,* 13–28.

Breuer, J., & Freud, S. (1955). Studies on hysteria. In J. Strachey (Ed. and Trans.), *The standard edition of the complete psychological works of Sigmund Freud* (Vol. 2, pp. 1–311). London: Hogarth Press. (Original work published 1893–1895)

Brewer, D. D., Catalano, R. F., Haggerty, K., Gainey, R. R., & Fleming, C. B. (1998). A meta-analysis of predictors of continued drug use during and after treatment for opiate addiction. *Addiction, 93*(1), 73–92.

Brewin, C. R. (2001). A cognitive neuroscience account of posttraumatic stress disorder and its treatment. *Behaviour Research and Therapy, 39*(4), 373–393.

Brewin, C. R., Andrews, B., & Valentine, J. D. (2000). Meta-analysis of risk factors for post-traumatic stress disorder in trauma-exposed adults. *Journal of Consulting and Clinical Psychology, 68,* 748–766.

Brewin, C. R., & Bradley, C. (1989). Patient preferences and randomised clinical trials. *British Medical Journal, 299,* 313–315.

Briggs, A. (2000). Economic evaluation and clinical trials: Size matters. *British Medical Journal, 321,* 1362–1363.

Bright, J. I., Baker, K. D., & Neimeyer, R. A. (1999). Professional and paraprofessional group treatments for depression: A comparison of cognitive-behavioral and mutual support interventions. *Journal of Consulting and Clinical Psychology, 67*(4), 491–501.

Brinkley, J., Beitman, B., & Friedal, R. (1979). Low-dose neuroleptic regimens in the treatment of borderline patients. *Archives of General Psychiatry, 36,* 319–326.

Brock, G. B., & Bochinski, D. (2001). Modern pharmacotherapy for erectile dysfunction: Evolving concepts with central and peripheral acting agents. *Current Opinion in Urology, 11,* 625–630.

Brodaty, H., Green, A., & Koschera, A. (2003). Meta-analysis of psychosocial interventions for caregivers of people with dementia. *Journal of American Geriatrics Society, 51,* 657–664.

Brom, D., Kleber, R., & Defares, P. (1989). Brief psychotherapy for PTSD. *Journal of Consulting and Clinical Psychology, 57,* 607–612.

Brooker, C., Falloon, I., Butterworth, A., Goldberg, D., Graham-Hole, V., & Hillier, V. (1994). The outcome of training community psychiatric nurses to deliver psychosocial interventions. *British Journal of Psychiatry, 165,* 222–230.

Brooker, C., Tarrier, N., Barrowclough, C., Butterworth, A., & Goldberg, D. (1992). Training community psychiatric nurses for psychosocial intervention: Report of a pilot study. *British Journal of Psychiatry, 160,* 836–844.

Brooker, D., & Duce, L. (2000). Wellbeing and activity in dementia: A comparison of group reminiscence therapy, structured goal-directed group activity and unstructured time. *Aging and Mental Health, 4*(4), 354–358.

Brooner, R. K., King, V. L., Kidorf, M., Schmidt, C. W., & Bigelow, G. E. (1997). Psychiatric and substance use comorbidity among treatment seeking opiate users. *Archives of General Psychiatry, 54,* 71–80.

Brown, E. J., Heimberg, R. G., & Juster, H. R. (1995). Social phobia subtype and avoidant personality disorder: Effect on severity of social phobia, impairment and outcome of cognitive behavioral treatment. *Behavior Therapy, 26,* 467–486.

Brown, G., Birley, J., & Wing, J. (1972). Influence of family life on the course of schizophrenic disorders: Replication. *British Journal of Psychiatry, 121,* 241–258.

Brown, R. T., Wynne, M. E., Borden, K. A., Clingerman, S. R., Geniesse, R., & Spunt, A. L. (1986). Methylphenidate and cognitive therapy in children with attention deficit disorder: A double-blind trial. *Journal of Developmental and Behavioral Pediatrics, 7*(3), 163–174.

Brown, T., Antony, M., & Barlow, D. (1995). Diagnostic comorbidity in panic disorder: Effect on treatment outcome and course of comorbid diagnoses following treatment. *Journal of Consulting and Clinical Psychology, 63,* 408–418.

Brown, T., & Barlow, D. (1992). Comorbidity among anxiety disorders: Implications for treatment and DSM-IV. *Journal of Consulting and Clinical Psychology, 60,* 835–844.

Brown, T., & Barlow, D. (1995). Long-term outcome in cognitive-behavioral treatment of panic disorder: Clinical predictors and alternative strategies for assessment. *Journal of Consulting and Clinical Psychology, 63,* 754–765.

Brown, T. A., Campbell, L. A., Lehman, C. L., Grisham, J. R., & Mancill, R. B. (2001). Current and lifetime comorbidity of the DSM-IV anxiety and mood disorders in a large clinical sample. *Journal of Abnormal Psychology, 110*(4), 585–599.

Browne, G., Steiner, M., Roberts, J., Gafni, A., Byrne, C., Dunn, E., et al. (2002). Sertraline and/or interpersonal psychotherapy for patients with dysthymic disorder in primary care: 6-month comparison with longitudinal 2-year follow-up of effectiveness and costs. *Journal of Affective Disorders, 68*(2–3), 317–330.

Bryant, R. A., Moulds, M. L., Guthrie, R. M., Dang, S. T., & Nixon, R. D. (2003). Imaginal exposure alone and imaginal exposure with cognitive restructuring in treatment of post-traumatic stress disorder. *Journal of Consulting and Clinical Psychology, 71*(4), 706–712.

Bryant, R. A., Sackville, T., Dang, S. T., Moulds, M., & Guthrie, R. (1999). Treating acute stress disorder: An evaluation of cognitive behavior therapy and supportive counseling techniques. *American Journal of Psychiatry, 156*(11), 1780–1786.

Bryant-Waugh, R. (1993). Anorexia nervosa in young boys. *Neuropsychiatre de l'Enfance et de l'Adolescence, 41*, 287–290.

Bryant-Waugh, R., Knibbs, J., Fosson, A., Kaminski, Z., & Lask, B. (1988). Long term follow up of patients with early onset anorexia nervosa. *Archives of Disease in Childhood, 63*, 5–9.

Bryant-Waugh, R., & Lask, B. (1995). Annotation: Eating disorders in children. *Journal of Child Psychology and Psychiatry, 36*(2), 191–202.

Bryson, S. (1997). Epidemiology of autism: Overview and issues outstanding. In D. J. Cohen & F. R. Volkmar (Eds.), *Handbook of autism and pervasive developmental disorders* (pp. 41–46). New York: Wiley.

Buchkremer, G., Klingberg, S., Holle, R., Schulze Monking, H., & Hornung, W. P. (1997). Psychoeducational psychotherapy for schizophrenic patients and their key relatives or care-givers: Results of a 2-year follow-up. *Acta Psychiatrica Scandinavica, 96*(6), 483–491.

Buchkremer, G., Schulze Monking, H., Holle, R., & Hornung, W. P. (1995). The impact of therapeutic relatives' groups on the course of illness of schizophrenic patients. *European Psychiatry, 10*, 17–27.

Bulik, C. M., Sullivan, P. F., Carter, F. A., McIntosh, V. V., & Joyce, P. R. (1998b). The role of exposure with response prevention in the cognitive-behavioural therapy for bulimia nervosa. *Psychological Medicine, 28*(3), 611–623.

Bulik, C. M., Sullivan, P. F., Carter, F. A., McIntosh, V. V., & Joyce, P. R. (1999). Predictors of rapid and sustained response to cognitive-behavioral therapy for bulimia nervosa. *International Journal of Eating Disorders, 26*(2), 137–144.

Bulik, C. M., Sullivan, P. F., Fear, J., & Pickering, A. (1998a). Predictors of the development of bulimia nervosa in women with anorexia nervosa. *Journal of Nervous and Mental Disease, 185*, 704–707.

Burgio, L., Engel, B., McCormick, K., Hawkins, A., & Scheve, A. (1988). Behavioral treatment for urinary incontinence in elderly inpatients: Initial attempts to modify prompting and toileting procedures. *Behavior Therapy, 19*, 345–357.

Burgio, L. D., & Burgio, K. L. (1990). Institutional staff training and management: A review of the literature and a model for geriatric, long-term care facilities. *International Journal of Aging and Human Development, 30*(4), 287–302.

Burgio, L. D., Scilley, K., Hardin, J. M., Hsu, C., & Yancey, J. (1996). Environmental "white noise": An intervention for verbally agitated nursing home residents. *Journal of Gerontology, 51*, 364–373.

Burke, K., Burke, J., Rae, D., & Regier, D. (1991). Comparing age at onset of major depression and other psychiatric disorders by birth cohorts in five US community populations. *Archives of General Psychiatry, 48*, 789–795.

Burke, M., Drummond, L. M., & Johnston, D. W. (1997). Treatment choice for agoraphobic women: Exposure or cognitive-behaviour therapy? *British Journal of Clinical Psychology, 36*(3), 409–420.

Burlingame, G., Fuhriman, A., Paul, S., & Ogles, B. (1989). Implementing a time-limited therapy program: Differential effects of training and experience. *Psychotherapy, 26*, 303–313.

Burls, A., Gold, L., & Clark, W. (2001). Systematic review of randomised controlled trials of sildenafil (Viagra) in the treatment of male erectile dysfunction. *British Journal of General Practice, 51*, 1004–1012.

Burnand, Y., Andreoli, A., Kolatte, E., Venturini, A., & Rosset, N. (2002). Psychodynamic psychotherapy and clomipramine in the treatment of major depression. *Psychiatric Services*, *53*(5), 585–590.

Burns, A., Byrne, J., Ballard, C., & Holmes, C. (2002). Sensory stimulation in dementia. *British Medical Journal*, *325*, 1312–1313.

Burns, D. D., & Nolen-Hoeksema, S. (1992). Therapeutic empathy and recovery from depression in cognitive-behavioral therapy: A structural equation model. *Journal of Consulting and Clinical Psychology*, *60*, 441–449.

Burns, L., & Teesson, M. (2002). Alcohol use disorders comorbid with anxiety, depression and drug use disorders: Findings from the Australian National Survey of Mental Health and Well Being. *Drug and Alcohol Dependence*, *68*, 299–307.

Burvill, P. (1993). Prognosis of depression in the elderly. *International Review of Psychiatry*, *5*, 437–443.

Butler, G., Cullington, A., Mumby, M., Amies, P., & Gelder, M. (1984). Exposure and anxiety management in the treatment of social phobia. *Journal of Consulting and Clinical Psychology*, *52*, 642–650.

Butler, G., Fennell, M., Robson, P., & Gelder, M. (1991). Comparison of behavior therapy and cognitive behavior therapy in the treatment of generalized anxiety disorder. *Journal of Consulting and Clinical Psychology*, *59*, 167–175.

Butzlaff, R. L., & Hooley, J. M. (1998). Expressed emotion and psychiatric relapse: A meta-analysis. *Archives of General Psychiatry*, *55*(6), 547–552.

Byford, S., Knapp, M., Greenshields, J., Ukoumunne, O. C., Jones, V., Thompson, S., et al. (2003a). Cost-effectiveness of brief cognitive behaviour therapy versus treatment as usual in recurrent deliberate self-harm: A decision-making approach. *Psychological Medicine*, *33*(6), 977–986.

Byford, S., McCrone, P., & Barrett, B. (2003b). Developments in the quantity and quality of economic evaluations in mental health. *Current Opinion in Psychiatry*, *16*, 703–707.

Cadogan, D. (1973). Marital group therapy in the treatment of alcoholism. *Quarterly Journal of Studies on Alcohol*, *34*, 1187–1194.

Cahill, S. P., Carrigan, M. H., & Frueh, B. C. (1999). Does EMDR work? And if so, why?: A critical review of controlled outcome and dismantling research. *Journal of Anxiety Disorders*, *13*, 5–33.

Calabrese, J. R., Shelton, M. D., Rapport, D. J., Kimmel, S. E., & Elhaj, O. (2002). Long-term treatment of bipolar disorder with lamotrigine. *Journal of Clinical Psychiatry*, *63*(Suppl. 10), 18–22.

Calhoun, K. S., Moras, K., Pilkonis, P. A., & Rehm, I. P. (1998). Empirically supported treatments: Implications for training. *Journal of Consulting and Clinical Psychology*, *66*, 151–162.

Callahan, A. M., & Bauer, M. S. (1999). Psychosocial interventions for bipolar disorder. *Psychiatric Clinics of North America*, *22*, 675–688.

Camp, C. J., Foss, J. W., O'Hanlon, A. M., & Stevens, A. B. (1996). Memory interventions for persons with dementia. *Applied Cognitive Psychology*, *10*, 193–210.

Campbell, M., Schopler, E., Cueva, J. E., & Hallin, A. (1996). Treatment of autistic disorder. *Journal of the American Academy of Child and Adolescent Psychiatry*, *35*, 134–143.

Cannon, D., & Baker, T. (1981). Emetic and electric shock aversion therapy: Assessment of conditioning. *Journal of Consulting and Clinical Psychology*, *49*, 20–33.

Cannon, D., Baker, T., & Wehl, C. (1981). Emetic and electric shock aversion therapy: Six and twelve month follow-up. *Journal of Consulting and Clinical Psychology*, *49*, 360–368.

Cappe, R., & Alden, L. (1986). A comparison of treatment strategies for clients functionally impaired by extreme shyness and social avoidance. *Journal of Consulting and Clinical Psychology*, *54*, 796–801.

Cardena, E. (2000). Hypnosis in the treatment of trauma: A promising, but not yet fully supported, efficacious intervention. *International Journal of Clinical and Experimental Hypnosis*, *48*, 225–238.

Cardin, V., McGill, C., & Falloon, I. (1986). An economic analysis: Costs benefits and effectiveness. In I. Falloon (Ed.), *Family management of schizophrenia* (pp. 115–123). Baltimore: Johns Hopkins University Press.

Carlson, J. G., Chemtob, C. M., Rusnak, K., Hedlund, N. L., & Muraoka, M. Y. (1998). Eye movement desensitization and reprocessing (EMDR) treatment for combat-related post-traumatic stress disorder. *Journal of Traumatic Stress, 11*(1), 3–24.

Carpenter, W., Gunderson, J., & Strauss, J. (1977). Considerations of the borderline syndrome: A longitudinal comparative study of borderline and schizophrenic patients. In P. Hartocollis (Ed.), *Borderline personality disorders.* New York: International Universities Press.

Carrion, V. G., Weems, C. F., Ray, R., & Reiss, A. L. (2002). Toward an empirical definition of pediatric PTSD: The phenomenology of PTSD symptoms in youth. *Journal of the American Academy of Child and Adolescent Psychiatry, 41*(2), 166–173.

Carroll, K., Rounsaville, B., & Gawin, F. (1991). A comparative trial of psychotherapies for ambulatory cocaine abusers: Relapse prevention and interpersonal psychotherapy. *American Journal of Drug and Alcohol Abuse, 17,* 229–247.

Carroll, K., Rounsaville, B., Gordon, L., Nich, C., Jatlow, P., Bisighini, R., et al. (1994a). Psychotherapy and pharmacotherapy for ambulatory cocaine abusers. *Archives of General Psychiatry, 51,* 177–187.

Carroll, K., Rounsaville, B., Nich, C., Gordon, L., Wirtz, P., & Gawin, F. (1994b). One-year follow-up of psychotherapy and pharmacotherapy for cocaine dependence: Delayed emergence of psychotherapy effects. *Archives of General Psychiatry, 51,* 989–997.

Carroll, K. M. (1996). Relapse prevention as a psychosocial treatment: A review of controlled clinical trials. *Experimental and Clinical Psychopharmacology, 4,* 46–54.

Carroll, K. M. (1999). Old psychotherapies for cocaine dependence revisited. *Archives of General Psychiatry, 56*(6), 505–506.

Carroll, K. M. (2001). Constrained, confounded and confused: Why we really know so little about therapists in treatment outcome research. *Addiction, 96*(2), 203–206.

Carroll, K. M., Ball, S. A., Nich, C., O'Connor, P. G., Eagan, D. A., Frankforter, T. L., et al. (2001). Targeting behavioral therapies to enhance naltrexone treatment of opioid dependence: Efficacy of contingency management and significant other involvement. *Archives of General Psychiatry, 58*(8), 755–761.

Carter, F. A., & Bulik, C. M. (1994). Exposure treatments for bulimia nervosa: Procedure, efficacy, and mechanisms. *Advances in Behavior Research and Therapy, 16,* 77–129.

Carter, F. A., McIntosh, V. V., Joyce, P. R., Sullivan, P. F., & Bulik, C. M. (2003). Role of exposure with response prevention in cognitive-behavioral therapy for bulimia nervosa: Three-year follow-up results. *International Journal of Eating Disorders, 33*(2), 127–135.

Carter, J. C., & Fairburn, C. G. (1998). Cognitive-behavioral self-help for binge eating disorder: A controlled effectiveness study. *Journal of Consulting and Clinical Psychology, 66*(4), 616–623.

Carter, J. C., Olmsted, M. P., Kaplan, A. S., McCabe, R. E., Mills, J. S., & Aime, A. (2003). Self-help for bulimia nervosa: A randomized controlled trial. *American Journal of Psychiatry, 160*(5), 973–978.

Casacalenda, N., Perry, J. C., & Looper, K. (2002). Remission in major depressive disorder: A comparison of pharmacotherapy, psychotherapy, and control conditions. *American Journal of Psychiatry, 159*(8), 1354–1360.

Caspi, A., Sugden, K., Moffitt, T. E., Taylor, A., Craig, I. W., Harrington, H., et al. (2003). Influence of life stress on depression: Moderation by a polymorphism in the 5–HTT gene. *Science, 301*(5631), 386–389.

Castle, D. J., Deane, A., Marks, I. M., Cutts, F., Chadboury, Y., & Stewart, A. (1994). Obsessive–compulsive disorder: Prediction of outcome from behavioral psychotherapy. *Acta Psychiatrica Scandinavica, 89,* 393–398.

Castonguay, L., Eldredge, K. L., & Agras, W. S. (1995). Binge eating disorder: Current state and future directions. *Clinical Psychology Review, 15,* 865–890.

Castonguay, L. G., Goldfried, M. R., Wiser, S., Raue, P. J., & Hayes, A. M. (1996). Predicting the effect of cognitive therapy for depression: A study of unique and common factors. *Journal of Consulting and Clinical Psychology, 64*(3), 497–504.

Catalan, J., Hawton, K., & Day, A. (1990). Couples referred to a sexual dysfunction clinic: Psychological and physical morbidity. *British Journal of Psychiatry, 156,* 61–67.

Celiberti, D. A., & Harris, S. L. (1993). Behavioral intervention for siblings of children with autism: A focus on skills to enhance play. *Behavior Therapy, 24*(4), 573–599.

Cerbone, M., Mayo, J., Cuthbertson, B., & O'Connell, R. (1992). Group therapy as an adjunct to medication in the management of affective disorder. *Group, 16,* 174–187.

Cermele, J. A., Melendez-Pallitto, L., & Pandina, G. J. (2001). Intervention in compulsive hoarding: A case study. *Behavior Modification, 25,* 214–232.

Chadwick, P., Sambrooke, S., Rasch, S., & Davies, E. (2000). Challenging the omnipotence of voices: Group cognitive behavior therapy for voices. *Behaviour Research and Therapy, 38*(10), 993–1003.

Chakos, M., Lieberman, J., Hoffman, E., Bradford, D., & Sheitman, B. (2001). Effectiveness of second-generation antipsychotics in patients with treatment-resistant schizophrenia: A review and meta-analysis of randomized trials. *American Journal of Psychiatry, 158,* 518–526.

Chamberlain, P., & Reid, J. B. (1998). Comparison of two community alternatives to incarceration for chronic juvenile offenders. *Journal of Consulting and Clinical Psychology, 66,* 624–633.

Chamberlain, P., & Rozicky, J. G. (1995). The effectiveness of family therapy in the treatment of adolescents with conduct disorders and delinquency. *Journal of Marital and Family Therapy, 21,* 441–459.

Chambless, D. L., & Gillis, M. M. (1993). Cognitive therapy of anxiety disorders. *Journal of Consulting and Clinical Psychology, 61,* 248–260.

Chambless, D. L., & Hollon, S. D. (1998). Defining empirically supported therapies. *Journal of Consulting and Clinical Psychology, 66,* 7–18.

Chambless, D. L., & Ollendick, T. H. (2001). Empirically supported psychological interventions: Controversies and evidence. *Annual Review of Psychology, 52,* 685–713.

Chambless, D. L., Renneberg, B., Goldstein, A., & Gracely, E. J. (1992). MCMI-diagnosed personality disorders among agoraphobic outpatients: Prevalence and relationship to severity and treatment outcome. *Journal of Anxiety Disorders, 6,* 193–211.

Chambless, D. L., Sanderson, W. C., Shoham, V., Johnson, S. B., Pyne, J., Pope, K. S., et al. (1996). An update on empirically validated therapies. *Clinical Psychologist, 49,* 5–18.

Chambless, D. L., Tran, G. Q., & Glass, C. R. (1997). Predictors of response to cognitive-behavioral group therapy for social phobia. *Journal of Anxiety Disorders, 11*(3), 221–240.

Chaney, E. F., O'Leary, M. R., & Marlatt, G. A. (1978). Skill training with alcoholics. *Journal of Consulting and Clinical Psychology, 46,* 1092–1104.

Channon, S., DeSilva, P., Hemsley, D., & Perkins, R. (1989). A controlled trial of cognitive-behavioral and behavioral treatment of anorexia nervosa. *Behaviour Research and Therapy, 27,* 529–535.

Chapman, P. L. H., & Huygens, I. (1988). An evaluation of three-month treatment programmes for alcoholism: An experimental study with 6 and 18 month follow-ups. *British Journal of Addiction, 83,* 67–81.

Charlop-Christy, M. H., Carpenter, M., Le, L., LeBlanc, L. A., & Kellet, K. (2002). Using the picture exchange communication system (PECS) with children with autism: Assessment of PECS acquisition, speech, social–communicative behavior, and problem behavior. *Journal of Applied Behavior Analysis, 35*(3), 213–231.

Chemtob, C. M., Nakashima, J., & Carlson, J. G. (2002a). Brief treatment for elementary school children with disaster-related posttraumatic stress disorder: A field study. *Journal of Clinical Psychology, 58*(1), 99–112.

Chemtob, C. M., Nakashima, J. P., & Hamada, R. S. (2002b). Psychosocial intervention for postdisaster trauma symptoms in elementary school children: A controlled community field study. *Archives of Pediatric and Adolescent Medicine, 156*(3), 211–216.

Chemtob, C. M., Tolin, D. F., van der Kolk, B. A., & Pitman, R. K. (2000). Eye movement desensitization and reprocessing. In E. B. Foa, T. M. Keane, & M. J. Friedman (Eds.), *Effective treatments for PTSD* (pp. 139–154). New York: Guilford Press.

Cheston, R. (1998). Psychotherapeutic work with people with dementia: A review of the literature. *British Journal of Medical Psychology, 71,* 211–231.

Chevron, E. S., & Rounsaville, B. J. (1983). Evaluating the clinical skills of psychotherapists: A comparison of techniques. *Archives of General Psychiatry, 40,* 1129–1132.

Chick, J., Lloyd, G., & Crombie, E. (1985). Counselling problem drinkers in medical wards: A controlled study. *British Medical Journal, 290,* 965–967.

Chick, J., Ritson, B., Connaughton, J., Stewart, A., & Chick, J. (1988). Advice versus extended treatment for alcoholism: A controlled study. *British Journal of Addictions, 83,* 159–170.

Chiesa, M., & Fonagy, P. (2000). Cassel Personality Disorder Study: Methodology and treatment effects. *British Journal of Psychiatry, 176,* 485–491.

Chiesa, M., & Fonagy, P. (2003). Psychosocial treatment for severe personality disorder: 36-month follow-up. *British Journal of Psychiatry, 183,* 356–362.

Chiles, J. A., Lambert, M. J., & Hatch, A. L. (1999). The impact of psychological interventions on medical cost offset: A meta-analytic review. *Clinical Psychology: Science and Practice, 6,* 204–220.

Chilvers, R., Harrison, G., Sipos, A., & Barley, M. (2002). Evidence into practice: Application of psychological models of change in evidence-based implementation. *British Journal of Psychiatry, 181,* 99–101.

Chisholm, D., Diehr, P., Knapp, M., Patrick, D., Treglia, M., & Simon, G. (2003). Depression status, medical co-morbidity and resource costs: Evidence from an international study of major depression in primary care. *British Journal of Psychiatry, 183,* 121–131.

Chisholm, D., Healey, A., & Knapp, M. (1996). QALYs in mental health care. *Social Psychiatry and Psychiatric Epidemiology, 32,* 68–75.

Christensen, H., Hadzi, P., Andrews, G., & Mattick, R. (1987). Behavior therapy and tricyclic medication in the treatment of obsessive–compulsive disorder: A quantitative review. *Journal of Consulting and Clinical Psychology, 55,* 701–711.

Chung, T., Langenbucher, J., Labouvie, E., Pandina, R. J., & Moos, R. H. (2001). Changes in alcoholic patients' coping responses predict 12-month treatment outcomes. *Journal of Consulting and Clinical Psychology, 69*(1), 92–100.

Churchill, R., Hunot, V., Corney, R., Knapp, M., McGuire, H., Tylee, A., et al. (2001). A systematic review of controlled trials of the effectiveness and cost-effectiveness of brief psychological treatments for depression. *Health Technology Assessment, 5*(35).

Chutuape, M. A., Silverman, K., & Stitzer, M. (1999a). Contingent reinforcement sustains post-detoxification abstinence from multiple drugs: A preliminary study with methadone patients. *Drug and Alcohol Dependence, 54*(1), 69–81.

Chutuape, M. A., Silverman, K., & Stitzer, M. L. (1999b). Use of methadone take-home contingencies with persistent opiate and cocaine abusers. *Journal of Substance Abuse Treatment, 16*(1), 23–30.

Clare, L., Wilson, B. A., Breen, K., & Hodges, J. R. (1999). Errorless learning of face–name associations in early Alzheimer's disease. *Neurocase, 5,* 37–46.

Clare, L., & Woods, B. (2001). Editorial: A role for cognitive rehabilitation in dementia care. *Neuropsychological Rehabilitation, 11*(3/4), 193–196.

Clark, D. B., & Agras, W. S. (1991). The assessment and treatment of performance anxiety in musicians. *American Journal of Psychiatry, 148,* 598–605.

Clark, D. M., Ehlers, A., McManus, F., Hackmann, A., Fennell, M., Campbell, H., et al. (2003). Cognitive therapy versus fluoxetine in generalized social phobia: A randomized placebo-controlled trial. *Journal of Consulting and Clinical Psychology, 71*(6), 1058–1067.

Clark, D. M., & McManus, F. (2002). Information processing in social phobia. *Biological Psychiatry, 51*(1), 92–100.

Clark, D. M., Salkovskis, P. M., & Chalkey, A. J. (1985). Respiratory control as a treatment for panic attacks. *Journal of Behavior Therapy and Experimental Psychiatry, 16,* 23–30.

Clark, D. M., Salkovskis, P. M., Hackmann, A., Middleton, H., Anastasiades, P., & Gelder, M. (1994). A comparison of cognitive therapy, applied relaxation and imipramine in the treatment of panic disorder. *British Journal of Psychiatry, 164,* 759–769.

Clark, D. M., Salkovskis, P. M., Hackmann, A., Wells, A., Ludgate, J., & Gelder, M. (1999). Brief cognitive therapy for panic disorder: A randomized controlled trial. *Journal of Consulting and Clinical Psychology*, *67*(4), 583–589.

Clark, D. M., & Wells, A. (1995). A cognitive model of social phobia. In R. Heimberg, G. Richard, & M. R. Liebowitz (Eds.), *Social phobia: Diagnosis, assessment, and treatment* (pp. 69–93). New York: Guilford Press.

Clarke, G. N., Rohde, P., Lewinsohn, P. M., Hops, H., & Seeley, J. R. (1999). Cognitive-behavioral treatment of adolescent depression: Efficacy of acute group treatment and booster sessions. *Journal of the American Academy of Child and Adolescent Psychiatry*, *38*, 272–279.

Clarkin, J. F., Carpenter, D., Hull, J., Wilner, P., & Glick, I. (1998). Effects of psychoeducational intervention for married patients with bipolar disorder and their spouses. *Psychiatric Services*, *49*, 531–533.

Clarkin, J. F., Foelsch, P. A., Levy, K. N., Hull, J. W., Delaney, J. C., & Kernberg, O. F. (2001). The development of a psychodynamic treatment for patients with borderline personality disorder: A preliminary study of behavioral change. *Journal of Personality Disorders*, *15*(6), 487–495.

Clarkin, J. F., Glick, I. D., Haas, G. L., Spencer, J. H., Lewis, A. B., Peyser, J., DeMane, et al. (1990). A randomized clinical trial of inpatient family intervention: V. Results for affective disorders. *Journal of Affective Disorders*, *18*(1), 17–28.

Clarkin, J. F., & Kendall, P. C. (1992). Comorbidity and treatment planning: Summary and future directions. *Journal of Consulting and Clinical Psychology*, *60*, 904–908.

Clarkin, J. F., & Levy, K. N. (2004). The influence of client variables on psychotherapy. In M. J. Lambert (Ed.), *Bergin and Garfield's handbook of psychotherapy and behavior change* (5th ed., pp. 194–226). New York: Wiley.

Clement, U., & Schmidt, G. (1983). The outcome of couple therapy for sexual dysfunctions using three different formats. *Journal of Sex and Marital Therapy*, *9*, 67–78.

Clum, G. A. (1989). Psychological interventions vs. drugs in the treatment of panic. *Behavior Therapy*, *20*, 429–457.

Clum, G. A., & Surls, R. (1993). A meta-analysis of treatments for panic disorder. *Journal of Consulting and Clinical Psychology*, *61*, 317–326.

Coatsworth, J. D., Santisteban, D. A., McBride, C. K., & Szapocznik, J. (2001). Brief strategic family therapy versus community control: Engagement, retention, and an exploration of the moderating role of adolescent symptom severity. *Family Process*, *40*(3), 313–332.

Cobham, V. E., Dadds, M. R., & Spence, S. H. (1998). The role of parental anxiety in the treatment of childhood anxiety. *Journal of Consulting and Clinical Psychology*, *66*, 893–905.

Coccaro, E. F., & Kavoussi, R. J. (1997). Fluoxetine and impulsive aggressive behavior in personality disordered subjects. *Archives of General Psychiatry*, *54*, 1081–1088.

Cochran, S. (1984). Preventing medical non-compliance in the out-patient treatment of bipolar affective disorder. *Journal of Consulting and Clinical Psychology*, *52*, 873–878.

Cogher, L. (1999). The use of non-directive play in speech and language therapy. *Child Language Teaching and Therapy*, *15*(1), 7–15.

Cohen, J. (1962). The statistical power of abnormal social psychological research: A review. *Journal of Abnormal and Social Psychology*, *65*, 145–153.

Cohen, J. (1988). *Statistical power analysis for the behavioural sciences* (2nd ed.). Hillsdale, NJ: Erlbaum.

Cohen, J. A., & Mannarino, A. P. (1996). A treatment outcome study for sexually abused preschool children: Initial findings. *Journal of the American Academy of Child and Adolescent Psychiatry*, *35*(1), 42–50.

Cohen, J. A., & Mannarino, A. P. (1997). A treatment study for sexually abused preschool children: Outcome during a one-year follow-up. *Journal of the American Academy of Child and Adolescent Psychiatry*, *36*(9), 1228–1235.

Cohen, J. A., & Mannarino, A. P. (1998). Interventions for sexually abused children: Initial treatment outcome findings. *Child Maltreatment: Journal of the American Professional Society on the Abuse of Children*, *3*(1), 17–26.

Cohen, L. H., Sargenet, M. M., & Sechrest, L. B. (1986). Use of psychotherapy research by professional psychologists. *American Psychologist, 41,* 198–206.

Cohen, P., Cohen, J., Kasen, S., Velez, C., Hartmark, C., Johnson, J., et al. (1993). An epidemiological study of disorders in late childhood and adolescence: I. Age- and gender-specific prevalence. *Journal of Child Psychology and Psychiatry, 34,* 851–865.

Coldwell, S. E., Getz, T., Milgrom, P., Prall, C. W., Spadafora, A., & Ramsay, D. S. (1998). CARL: A LabVIEW 3 computer program for conducting exposure therapy for the treatment of dental injection fear. *Behaviour Research and Therapy, 36,* 429–441.

Cole, M. (1986). Socio-sexual characteristics of men with sexual problems. *Sexual and Marital Therapy, 1,* 89–108.

Collings, S., & King, M. (1994). Ten year follow-up of 50 patients with bulimia nervosa. *British Journal of Psychiatry, 164,* 80–87.

Colom, F., Vieta, E., Martinez-Aran, A., Reinares, M., Goikolea, J. M., Benabarre, A., et al. (2003). A randomized trial on the efficacy of group psychoeducation in the prophylaxis of recurrences in bipolar patients whose disease is in remission. *Archives of General Psychiatry, 60*(4), 402–407.

Comings, D. E., & Comings, B. G. (1985). Tourette syndrome: Clinical and psychological aspects of 250 cases. *American Journal of Human Genetics, 37,* 435–450.

Condelli, W. S., & Dunteman, G. H. (1993). Exposure to methadone programs and heroin use. *American Journal of Drug and Alcohol Abuse, 24,* 1–16.

Conklin, C. A., & Tiffany, S. T. (2002). Applying extinction research and theory to cue-exposure addiction treatments. *Addiction, 97*(2), 155–167.

Connolly, J., Hallam, R. S., & Marks, I. (1976). Selective association of fainting with blood–injury–illness fear. *Behavior Therapy, 7,* 8–13.

Connolly, M. B., Crits-Christoph, P., Shappell, S., Barber, J. P., Luborsky, L., & Shaffer, C. (1999). Relation of transference interpretations to outcome in the early sessions of brief supportive–expressive psychotherapy. *Psychotherapy Research, 9,* 485–495.

Connors, G. J., Walitzer, K. S., & Dermen, K. H. (2002). Preparing clients for alcoholism treatment: Effects on treatment participation and outcomes. *Journal of Consulting and Clinical Psychology, 70*(5), 1161–1169.

Conte, H. R., Plutchik, R., Wild, K. V., & Karasu, T. B. (1986). Combined psychotherapy and pharmacotherapy for depression. *Archives of General Psychiatry, 43,* 471–479.

Cook, T. D., & Campbell, D. T. (Eds.). (1979). *Quasi-experimentation: Design and analysis issues for field settings.* Chicago: Rand McNally.

Cooke, D. D., McNally, L., Mulligan, K. T., Harrison, M. G. J., & Newman, S. P. (2001). Psychosocial interventions for caregivers of people with dementia: A systematic review. *Aging and Mental Health, 5*(2), 120–135.

Cooper, A. J. (1969). Clinical and therapeutic studies in premature ejaculation. *Comprehensive Psychiatry, 10,* 285–295.

Cooper, N. A., & Clum, G. A. (1989). Imaginal flooding as a supplementary treatment for PTSD in combat veterans: A controlled study. *Behavior Therapy, 20,* 381–391.

Cooper, P., Coker, S., & Fleming, C. (1996). An evaluation of the efficacy of supervised cognitive behavioral self-help for bulimia nervosa. *International Journal of Psychosomatic Research, 40,* 281–287.

Cooper, P. J., Coker, S., & Fleming, C. (1994). Self-help for bulimia nervosa: A preliminary report. *International Journal of Eating Disorders, 16,* 401–404.

Corder, B. F., Corder, R. F., & Laidlaw, N. D. (1972). An intensive treatment program for alcoholics and their wives. *Quarterly Journal of Studies on Alcohol, 33,* 1114–1146.

Cormac, I., Jones, C., & Campbell, C. (2002). Cognitive behaviour therapy for schizophrenia (Cochrane Review). In *The Cochrane Library,* Issue 4. Oxford, UK: Update Software.

Cornelius, J. R., Soloff, P. H., Perel, J. M., & Ulrich, R. F. (1993). Continuation pharmacotherapy of borderline personality disorder with haloperidol and phenelzine. *American Journal of Psychiatry, 150,* 1843–1848.

Corney, R. H. (1987). Marital problems and treatment outcome in depressed women: A clinical trial of social work intervention. *British Journal of Psychiatry, 151,* 652–659.

Coryell, W., Endicott, J., Andreason, N. C., Keller, M. B., Clayton, P. J., Hirsclifeld, R. M. A., et al. (1988). Depression and panic attacks: The significance of overlaps as reflected in follow-up and family study data. *American Journal of Psychiatry, 145*, 293–300.

Coryell, W., & Noyes, R. (1988). Placebo response in panic disorder. *American Journal of Psychiatry, 145*, 1138–1140.

Cotgrove, A. J., Zirinsky, L., Black, D., & Weston, D. (1995). Secondary prevention of attempted suicide in adolescence. *Journal of Adolescence, 18*, 569–577.

Cottraux, J. (1989). Behavioural psychotherapy for obsessive–compulsive disorder. *International Review of Psychiatry, 1*, 227–234.

Cottraux, J., Messy, P. M., Marks, I. M., Mollard, E., & Bouvard, M. (1993). Predictive factors in the treatment of obsessive–compulsive disorders with fluvoxamine and or behavior therapy. *Behavioural Psychology, 21*, 45–50.

Cottraux, J., Mollard, E., Bouvard, M., Marks, I., Sluys, M., Nury, A. M., et al. (1990). A controlled study of fluvoxamine and exposure in obsessive–compulsive disorder. *International Journal of Clinical Pharmacotherapy, 5*, 17–30.

Cottraux, J., Note, I., Albuisson, E., Yao, S. N., Note, B., Mollard, E., et al. (2000). Cognitive behavior therapy versus supportive therapy in social phobia: A randomized controlled trial. *Psychotherapy and Psychosomatic, 69*(3), 137–146.

Cousins, L. S., & Weiss, G. (1993). Parent training and social skills training for children with attention-deficit hyperactivity disorder: How can they be combined for greater effectiveness? *Canadian Journal of Psychiatry, 38*, 449–457.

Covi, L., & Lipman, R. S. (1987). Cognitive-behavioral group psychotherapy combined with imipramine in major depression. *Psychopharmacology Bulletin, 23*, 173–176.

Cowdrey, R. W., & Gardener, D. L. (1988). Pharmacotherapy of borderline personality disorder: Alprazolam, carbamazepine, trifluoperazine and tranylcypromine. *Archives of General Psychiatry, 45*, 111–119.

Cox, B. J., Endler, N. S., & Lee, P. S. (1992). A meta-analysis of treatments for panic disorder with agoraphobia: Imipramine, alprazolam and in vivo exposure. *Journal of Behavior Therapy and Experimental Psychiatry, 23*, 175–182.

Cozolino, L. J., Goldstein, M. J., Nuechterlein, K. H., West, K. L., & Synder, K. S. (1988). The impact of education about schizophrenia on relatives varying in expressed emotion. *Schizophrenia Bulletin, 14*, 675–687.

Craighead, L. W., & Agras, W. S. (1991). Mechanisms of action in cognitive-behavioral and pharmacological interventions for obesity and bulimia nervosa. *Journal of Consulting and Clinical Psychology, 59*, 115– 125.

Craske, M. G., Brown, T. A., & Barlow, D. H. (1991). Behavioral treatment of panic disorder: A two year follow-up. *Behavior Therapy, 22*, 289–304.

Craske, M. G., DeCola, J. P., Sachs, A. D., & Pontillo, D. C. (2003). Panic control treatment for agoraphobia. *Journal of Anxiety Disorders, 17*, 321–333.

Craske, M. G., Maidenberg, E., & Bystritsky, A. (1995). Brief cognitive-behavioral versus nondirective therapy for panic disorder. *Journal of Behavior Therapy and Experimental Psychiatry, 26*(2), 113–120.

Craske, M. G., Rowe, M., Lewin, M., & Noriega-Dimitri, R. (1997). Interoceptive exposure versus breathing retraining within cognitive-behavioural therapy for panic disorder with agoraphobia. *British Journal of Clinical Psychology, 36*(1), 85–99.

Crawford, A. M., & Manassis, K. (2001). Familial predictors of treatment outcome in childhood anxiety disorders. *Journal of the American Academy Child and Adolescent Psychiatry, 40*, 1182–1189.

Creamer, M. (1987). Cognitive interventions in the treatment of obsessive compulsive disorder. *Behavior Change, 4*, 20–27.

Crisp, A. H. (2002). Treatment of anorexia nervosa: Is "where" or "how" the main issue? *European Eating Disorders Review, 10*, 233–240.

Crisp, A. H., Norton, K., Gowers, S., Halek, C., Bowyer, C., Yeldham, D., et al. (1991). A controlled study of the effect of therapies aimed at adolescent and family psychopathology in anorexia nervosa. *British Journal of Psychiatry, 159*, 325–333.

Crisp, A. H., Palmer, R. L., & Kalucy, R. S. (1976). How common is anorexia nervosa?: A prevalence study. *British Journal of Psychiatry, 128,* 549–554.

Crits-Christoph, P. (1992). The efficacy of brief dynamic psychotherapy: A meta-analysis. *American Journal of Psychiatry, 149,* 151–158.

Crits-Christoph, P. (1996). The dissemination of efficacious psychological treatments. *Clinical Psychology: Science and Practice, 3,* 260–263.

Crits-Christoph, P., Baranackie, K., Kurcias, J., Beck, A., Carroll, K., Perry, K., et al. (1991). Meta-analysis of therapist effects in psychotherapy outcome studies. *Psychotherapy Research, 1,* 81–91.

Crits-Christoph, P., Connolly, M. B., Azarian, K., Crits-Christoph, K., & Shappell, S. (1996). An open trial of brief supportive–expressive psychotherapy in the treatment of generalized anxiety disorder. *Psychotherapy, 33,* 418–430.

Crits-Christoph, P., Cooper, A., & Luborsky, L. (1988). The accuracy of therapists' interpretations and the outcome of dynamic psychotherapy. *Archives of General Psychiatry, 56,* 490–495.

Crits-Christoph, P., Siqueland, L., Blaine, J., Frank, A., Luborsky, L., Onken, L. S., et al. (1997). The National Institute on Drug Abuse Collaborative Cocaine Treatment Study: Rationale and methods. *Archives of General Psychiatry, 54*(8), 721–726.

Crits-Christoph, P., Siqueland, L., Blaine, J., Frank, A., Luborsky, L., Onken, L. S., et al. (1999). Psychosocial treatments for cocaine dependence: National Institute on Drug Abuse Collaborative Cocaine Treatment Study. *Archives of General Psychiatry, 56*(6), 493–502.

Crits-Christoph, P., Siqueland, L., McCalmont, E., Weiss, R. D., Gastfriend, D. R., Frank, A., et al. (2001). Impact of psychosocial treatments on associated problems of cocaine-dependent patients. *Journal of Consulting and Clinical Psychology, 69*(5), 825–830.

Crowe, M. J., Gillan, P., & Golombok, S. (1981). Form and content in the conjoint treatment of sexual dysfunction: A controlled study. *Behaviour Research and Therapy, 19,* 47–54.

Crumbach, J. C., & Carr, G. L. (1979). Treatment of alcoholics with logotherapy. *International Journal of the Addictions, 14,* 847–853.

Cryer, L., & Beutler, L. (1980). Group therapy: An alternative approach for rape victims. *Journal of Sex and Marital Therapy, 6,* 40–46.

Csillag, E. R. (1976). Modification of penile erectile response. *Journal of Behavior Therapy and Experimental Psychiatry, 7,* 27–29.

Cuffe, S. P., Addy, C. L., Garrison, C. Z., Waller, J. L., Jackson, K. L., McKeown, R. E., et al. (1998). Prevalence of PTSD in a community sample of older adolescents. *Journal of the American Academy of Child and Adolescent Psychiatry, 37*(2), 147–154.

Cuijpers, P. (1997). Bibliotherapy in unipolar depression: A meta-analysis. *Journal of Behavior Therapy and Experimental Psychiatry, 28*(2), 139–147.

Cuijpers, P. (1998). Psychological outreach programmes for the depressed elderly: A meta-analysis of effects and drop-out. *International Journal of Geriatric Psychiatry, 13,* 41–48.

Culhane, M., & Dobson, H. (1991). Groupwork with elderly women. *International Journal of Geriatric Psychiatry, 6,* 415–418.

Cummings, N. A. (1987). The future of psychotherapy: One psychologist's perspective. *American Journal of Psychotherapy, 41,* 349–360.

Cummings, N. A. (1991). Brief intermittant therapy throughout the life cycle. In C. S. Austad & W. H. Berman (Eds.), *Psychotherapy in managed health care: The optimal use of time and resources* (pp. 35–45). Washington, DC: American Psychological Association.

Cunningham, C. E., Bremner, R., & Boyle, M. (1995). Large group community-based parenting programs for family of preschoolers at risk for disruptive behavior disorders: Utilization, cost-effectiveness and outcome. *Journal of Child Psychology and Psychiatry, 36,* 1141–1159.

Cunningham Owens, D. G., Carroll, A., Fattah, S., Clyde, Z., Coffey, I., & Johnstone, E. C. (2001). A randomized, controlled trial of a brief interventional package for schizophrenic out-patients. *Acta Psychiatrica Scandinavica, 103*(5), 362–369.

Curran, H. V., Collins, R., Fletcher, S., Kee, S. C., Woods, B., & Iliffe, S. (2003). Older adults and withdrawal from benzodiazepine hypnotics in general practice: Effects on cognitive function, sleep, mood and quality of life. *Psychological Medicine, 33*(7), 1223–1237.

Curran, P. S., Bell, P., Murray, G., Loughrey, G., Roddy, R., & Rocke, L. G. (1990). Psychological consequences of the Enniskillen bombing. *British Journal of Psychiatry, 156*, 478–482.

Curson, D. A., Barnes, T. R. E., Bamber, R. W., et al. (1985). Long term depot maintenance of chronic schizophrenic outpatients. *British Journal of Psychiatry, 146*, 464–480.

Curson, D. A., Patel, M., Liddle, P. F., et al. (1988). Psychiatric morbidity of a long stay hospital population with chronic schizophrenia and implications for future community care. *British Medical Journal, 297*, 819–822.

Cusack, K., & Spates, C. R. (1999). The cognitive dismantling of eye movement desensitization and reprocessing (EMDR) treatment of posttraumatic stress disorder (PTSD). *Journal of Anxiety Disorders, 13*(1–2), 87–99.

Dadds, M. R., Schwartz, S., & Sanders, M. R. (1987). Marital discord and treatment outcome in behavioural treatment of child conduct disorders. *Journal of Consulting and Clinical Psychology, 55*, 396–403.

Dadds, M. R., Spence, S. H., Holland, D. E., Barrett, P. M., & Laurens, K. R. (1997). Prevention and early intervention for anxiety disorders: A controlled trial. *Journal of Consulting and Clinical Psychology, 65*(4), 627–635.

Daniels, L. (1998). A group cognitive-behavioural and process-oriented approach to treating the social impairment and negative symptoms accossiated with chronic mental illness. *Journal of Psychotherapy Practice and Research, 7*, 167–176.

Danziger, Y., Carcl, C. A., Varsono, I., Tyano, S., & Mimouni, M. (1988). Parental involvement in treatment of patients with anorexia nervosa in a paediatric day-care unit. *Paediatrics, 81*, 159–162.

Dar, R., Serlin, R. C., & Omer, H. (1994). Misuse of statistical tests in three decades of psychotherapy research. *Journal of Consulting and Clinical Psychology, 62*, 75–82.

Dare, C., Eisler, I., Russell, G., Treasure, J., & Dodge, L. (2001). Psychological therapies for adults with anorexia nervosa: Randomised controlled trial of out-patient treatments. *British Journal of Psychiatry, 178*, 216–221.

Dare, C., & Szmukler, G. (1991). The family therapy of short history early onset anorexia nervosa. In D. B. Woodside & L. Shekter-Wolfson (Eds.), *Family approaches to eating disorders* (pp. 25–47). Washington, DC: American Psychiatric Press.

Darke, S., & Ross, J. (1997). Polydrug dependence and psychiatric comorbidity among heroin injectors. *Drug and Alcohol Dependence, 48*(2), 135–141.

Dauw, D. C. (1988). Evaluating the effectiveness of the SECS surrogate-assisted sex therapy model. *Journal of Sex Research, 24*, 269–275.

Davanloo, H. (Ed.). (1978). *Basic principles and techniques in short-term dynamic therapy.* New York: SP Medical and Scientific Books.

Davenport, Y., Ebert, M., Adland, M., & Goodwin, F. (1977). Couples group therapy as an adjunct to lithium maintenance in the manic patient. *Journal of Orthopsychiatry, 47*, 495–502.

Davidson, J. R., Hughes, D., Blazer, D. G., & George, L. K. (1991). Post-traumatic stress disorder in the community: An epidemiological study. *Psychological Medicine, 21*, 713–721.

Davidson, K. M., & Tyrer, P. (1996). Cognitive therapy for antisocial and borderline personality disorders: Single case study series. *British Journal of Clinical Psychology, 35*(3), 413–429.

Davidson, P. R., & Parker, K. C. (2001). Eye movement desensitization and reprocessing (EMDR): A meta-analysis. *Journal of Consulting and Clinical Psychology, 69*(2), 305–316.

Davis, R., McVey, G., Heinmaa, M., Rockert, W., & Kennedy, S. (1999). Sequencing of cognitive-behavioral treatments for bulimia nervosa. *International Journal of Eating Disorders, 25*(4), 361–374.

Davis, R., Olmsted, M., Rockert, W., Marques, T., & Dolhanty, J. (1997). Group psychoeducation for bulimia nervosa with and without additional psychotherapy process sessions. *International Journal of Eating Disorders, 22*(1), 25–34.

Davis, R., Olmsted, M. P., & Rockert, W. (1992). Brief group psychoeducation for bulimia nervosa: II. Prediction of clinical outcome. *International Journal of Eating Disorders, 11*, 205–211.

Davison, G. C. (2000). Stepped care: Doing more with less? *Journal of Consulting and Clinical Psychology, 68*, 580–585.

Dawe, S., Powell, J., Richards, D., Gossop, M., Marks, I., Strang, J., et al. (1993). Does post-withdrawal cue exposure improve outcome in opiate addiction?: A controlled trial. *Addiction, 88*(9), 1233–1245.

Dawe, S., Rees, V. W., Mattick, R., Sitharthan, T., & Heather, N. (2002). Efficacy of moderation-oriented cue exposure for problem drinkers: A randomized controlled trial. *Journal of Consulting and Clinical Psychology, 70*(4), 1045–1050.

De Amicis, L. A., Goldberg, D. C., LoPiccolo, J., Friedman, J., & Davies, L. (1985). Clinical follow-up of couples treated for sexual dysfunction. *Archives of Sexual Behavior, 14*, 467–489.

Dean, C., Surtees, P. G., & Sashisharan, S. P. (1983). Comparison of research diagnostic systems in an Edinburgh community sample. *British Journal of Psychiatry, 142*, 247–256.

Dean, R., Briggs, K., & Lindesay, J. (1993). The Domus philosophy: A prospective evaluation of two residential units for the elderly mentally ill. *International Journal of Geriatric Psychiatry, 8*, 807–817.

Deblinger, E., Lippmann, J., & Steer, R. (1996). Sexually abused children suffering post traumatic stress symptoms. *Child Maltreatment, 1*, 310–321.

Deblinger, E., Stauffer, L. B., & Steer, R. A. (2001). Comparative efficacies of supportive and cognitive behavioral group therapies for young children who have been sexually abused and their nonoffending mothers. *Child Maltreatment: Journal of the American Professional Society on the Abuse of Children, 6*(4), 332–343.

Deblinger, E., Steer, R. A., & Lippmann, J. (1999). Two-year follow-up study of cognitive behavioral therapy for sexually abused children suffering post-traumatic stress symptoms. *Child Abuse and Neglect, 23*(12), 1371–1378.

De Giacomo, P., Pierri, G., Santoni Rugiu, A., Buonsante, M., Vadruccio, F., & Zavoianni, L. (1997). Schizophrenia: A study comparing a family therapy group following a paradoxical model plus psychodrugs and a group treated by the conventional clinical approach. *Acta Psychiatrica Scandinavica, 95*(3), 183–188.

de Haan, E., van Oppen, P., van Balkom, A. J. L. M., Spinhoven, P., Hoogduin, K. A. L., & Van Dyck, R. (1997). Prediction of outcome and early vs. late improvement in OCD patients treated with cognitive behaviour therapy and pharmacotherapy. *Acta Psychiatrica Scandinavica, 96*, 354–361.

Deitz, S. M. (1985). Good Behaviour Game. In A. S. Bellack & M. Hersen (Eds.), *Dictionary of behaviour therapy techniques* (pp. 131–132). New York: Pergamon Press.

De Jong, R., Treiber, R., & Henrich, G. (1986). Effectiveness of two psychological treatments for inpatients with severe and chronic depressions. *Cognitive Therapy and Research, 10*, 645–663.

De Jongh, A. D., Muris, P., Horst, G. T., Van Zuuren, F., Schoenmakers, N., & Makkes, P. (1995). One-session cognitive treatment of dental phobia: Preparing dental phobics for treatment by restructuring negative cognitions. *Behaviour Research and Therapy, 33*, 947–954.

de Jonghe, F., Kool, S., van Aalst, G., Dekker, J., & Peen, J. (2001). Combining psychotherapy and antidepressants in the treatment of depression. *Journal of Affective Disorders, 64*(2–3), 217–229.

Dekker, J., Dronkers, J., & Staffeleu, J. (1985). Treatment of sexual dysfunctions in male-only groups: Predicting outcome. *Journal of Sex and Marital Therapy, 11*, 80–90.

Delaney-Black, V., Covington, C., Ondersma, S. J., Nordstrom-Klee, B., Templin, T., Ager, J., Janisse, J., et al. (2002). Violence exposure, trauma, and IQ and/or reading deficits among urban children. *Archives of Pediatric and Adolescent Medicine, 156*(3), 280–285.

DeLeon, P. H., Uyeda, M. K., & Welch, B. (1985). Psychology and HMOs: New partnership or new adversary? *American Psychologist, 40*, 1122–1124.

de Mello, M. F., Myczcowisk, L. M., & Menezes, P. R. (2001). A randomized controlled trial comparing moclobemide and moclobemide plus interpersonal psychotherapy in the treatment of dysthymic disorder. *Journal of Psychotherapy Practice and Research, 10*(2), 117–123.

Denihan, A., Kirby, M., Bruce, I., Cunningham, C., Coakley, D., & Lawlor, B. A. (2000). Three-year prognosis of depression in the community-dwelling elderly. *British Journal of Psychiatry, 176*, 453–457.

Department of Health. (1996). *A review of strategic policy on NHS psychotherapy services in England*. NHS Executive.

Department of Health. (2001). *Treatment choice in psychological therapies and counselling evidence based clinical practice guideline*. London: Author.

Department of Health. (2003). Summary of clinical psychology services. Form KT24, DH Statistics Division (SD3G). Retrieved 5 January 2004, from *http://www.doh.gov.uk/public/kt240203/#tables*

Depression Guideline Panel. (1993a). *Depression in primary care: Vol. 1. Diagnosis and detection* (Clinical Practice Guideline No. 5, AHCPR Publication No. 93-0550). Rockville, MD: U.S. Department of Health and Human Services Public Health Service Agency for Health Care Policy and Research.

Depression Guideline Panel. (1993b). *Depression in primary care: Vol. 2. Treatment of major depression* (Clinical Practice Guideline No. 5, AHCPR Publication No. 93-0551). Rockville, MD: U.S. Department of Health and Human Services Public Health Service Agency for Health Care Policy and Research.

Depression Guideline Panel. (1993c). *Depression in primary care: Detection, diagnosis and treatment: Quick reference guide for clinicians* (Clinical Practice Guideline No. 5, AHCPR Publication No. 93-0552). Rockville, MD: U.S. Department of Health and Human Services Public Health Service Agency for Health Care Policy and Research.

Derogatis, L. R. (1977). *SCL-90: Administration and procedure manual for the revised version*. Baltimore: Clinical Psychometrics Research.

DeRubeis, R. J., & Amsterdam, J. D. (2002, June 25). *Acute effects of cognitive therapy, pharmacotherapy, and placebo in severely depressed outpatients*. Paper presented at 33rd annual meeting of the Society for Psychotherapy Research, Santa Barbara, CA.

DeRubeis, R. J., & Feeley, M. (1990). Determinants of change in cognitive therapy for depression. *Cognitive Therapy and Research, 14*, 469–482.

DeRubeis, R. J., & Feeley, M. (1991). Determinants of change in cognitive therapy for depression. *Cognitive Therapy and Research, 14*, 469–482.

DeRubeis, R. J., Gelfand, L. A., Tang, T. Z., & Simons, A. D. (1999). Medications versus cognitive behavior therapy for severely depressed outpatients: Mega-analysis of four randomized comparisons. *American Journal of Psychiatry, 156*, 1007–1013.

DeRubeis, R. J., & Stirman, S. W. (2001). Determining the pertinence of psychotherapy outcome research findings for clinical practice: Comment on Westen and Morrison (2001). *Journal of Consulting and Clinical Psychology, 69*(6), 908–909.

de Ruiter, C., Rijken, H., Garssen, B., & Kraaimaat, F. (1989). Breathing retraining, exposure and a combination of both in the treatment of panic attacks with agoraphobia. *Behaviour Research and Therapy, 27*, 647–665.

DeVeaugh-Geiss, J., Moroz, G., Biederman, J., Cantwell, D. P., Fontaine, R., Greist, J. H., et al. (1992). Clomipramine in child and adolescent obsessive–compulsive disorder: A multicenter trial. *Journal of the American Academy of Child and Adolescent Psychiatry, 31*, 45–49.

Devilly, G. J., & Foa, E. B. (2001). The investigation of exposure and cognitive therapy: Comment on Tarrier et al. (1999). *Journal of Consulting and Clinical Psychology, 69*(1), 114–116.

Devilly, G. J., & Spence, S. H. (1999). The relative efficacy and treatment distress of EMDR and a cognitive-behavior trauma treatment protocol in the amelioration of posttraumatic stress disorder. *Journal of Anxiety Disorders, 13*(1–2), 131–157.

Devilly, G. J., Spence, S. H., & Rapee, R. M. (1998). Statistical and reliable change with eye movement desensitization and reprocessing (EMDR): Treating trauma within a veteran population. *Behavior Therapy, 29*, 435–455.

Dew, M. A., Bromet, E. J., Brent, D., & Greenhouse, J. B. (1987). A quantitative literature review of the effectiveness of suicide prevention centers. *Journal of Consulting and Clinical Psychology, 55*, 239–244.

Diamond, G. S., Reis, B. F., Diamond, G. M., Siqueland, L., & Isaacs, L. (2002). Attachment-based family therapy for depressed adolescents: A treatment development study. *Journal of the American Academy of Child and Adolescent Psychiatry, 41*, 1190–1196.

Dickerson, F. B. (2000). Cognitive behavioral psychotherapy for schizophrenia: A review of recent empirical studies. *Schizophrenia Research, 43*(2–3), 71–90.

Diekstra, R. F. W., Kienhorst, C. W. M., & de Wilde, E. J. (1995). Suicide and suicidal behaviour among adolescents. In M. Rutter & D. J. Smith (Eds.), *Psychosocial disorders in young people: Time trends and their causes* (pp. 686–761). Chichester, UK: Wiley.

Dietch, J. T., Hewett, L. J., & Jones, S. (1989). Adverse effects of reality orientation. *Journal of the American Geriatrics Society, 37*, 974–976.

Diguer, L., Barber, J. P., & Luborsky, L. (1993). Three concomitants: Personality disorders, psychiatric severity and outcome of dynamic psychotherapy of major depression. *American Journal of Psychiatry, 150*, 1246–1248.

Dimeff, L. A., & Marlatt, G. A. (1998). Preventing relapse and maintaining change in addictive behaviors. *Clinical Psychology: Science and Practice, 5*(4), 513–525.

Dinwiddie, S. H., Cottler, L., Compton, W., & Ben Abdallah, A. (1996). Psychopathology and HIV risk behaviors among injection drug users in and out of treatment. *Drug and Alcohol Dependence, 43*, 1–11.

Dishion, T. J., & Andrews, D. W. (1995). Preventing escalation in problem behaviors with high-risk young adolescents: Immediate and 1-year outcomes. *Journal of Consulting and Clinical Psychology, 63*, 538–548.

Dixon, L., Lyles, A., Scott, J., Lehman, A., Postrado, L., Goldman, H., et al. (1999). Services to families of adults with schizophrenia: From treatment recommendations to dissemination. *Psychiatric Services, 50*(2), 233–238.

Dixon, L., Stewart, B., Burland, J., Delahanty, J., Lucksted, A., & Hoffman, M. (2001). Pilot study of the effectiveness of the family-to-family education program. *Psychiatric Services, 52*(7), 965–967.

Dobson, K. S. (1989). A meta-analysis of the efficacy of cognitive therapy for depression. *Journal of Consulting and Clinical Psychology, 57*, 414–419.

Dodge, E., Hodes, M., Eisler, I., & Dare, C. (1995). Family therapy for bulimia nervosa in adolescents: An exploratory study. *Journal of Family Therapy, 17*, 59–77.

Dolan, B., Warren, F., & Norton, K. (1997). Change in borderline symptoms one year after therapeutic community treatment for severe personality disorder. *British Journal of Psychiatry, 171*, 274–279.

Donahoe, C. P., & Driesenga, S. A. (1989). A review of social skills training with chronic mental patients. *Progress in Behavior Modification, 21*, 131–164.

Donaldson, C., Tarrier, N., & Burns, A. (1998). Determinants of carer stress in Alzheimer's disease. *International Journal of Geriatric Psychiatry, 13*(4), 248–256.

Doody, R. S., Stevens, J. C., Beck, C., Dubinsky, R. M., Kaye, J. A., Gwyther, L., et al. (2001). Practice parameter: Management of dementia (an evidence-based review): Report of the Quality Standards Subcommittee of the American Academy of Neurology. *Neurology, 56*, 1154–1166.

Dorer, C., Feehan, C., Vostanis, P., & Winkley, L. (1999). The overdose process—adolescents' experience of taking an overdose and their contact with services. *Journal of Adolescence, 22*, 413–417.

Dorus, W., Ostrow, D. G., Anton, R., Cushman, P., Collins, P. F., Schaefer, M., et al. (1989). Lithium treatment of depressed and non-depressed alcoholics. *Journal of the American Medical Association, 262,* 1646–1652.

Dowrick, C., Dunn, G., Ayuso-Mateos, J. L., Dalgard, O. S., Page, H., Lehtinen, V., et al. (2000). Problem solving treatment and group psychoeducation for depression: Multicentre randomised controlled trial: Outcomes of Depression International Network (ODIN) Group. *British Medical Journal, 321*(7274), 1450–1454.

Dozier, M., Cue, K., & Barnett, L. (1994). Clinicians as caregivers: Role of attachment organization in treatment. *Journal of Consulting and Clinical Psychology, 62,* 793–800.

Drake, R. E., & Sederer, L. I. (1986). The adverse effects of intensive treatment of schizophrenia. *Comprehensive Psychiatry, 27,* 313–326.

Dreessen, L., & Arntz, A. (1998). The impact of personality disorders on treatment outcome of anxiety disorders: Best-evidence synthesis. *Behaviour Research and Therapy, 36*(5), 483–504.

Dreessen, L., Arntz, A., Luttels, C., & Sallaerts, S. (1994). Personality disorders do not influence the results of cognitive behavior therapies for anxiety disorders. *Comprehensive Psychiatry, 35,* 265–274.

Dreessen, L., Hoekstra, R., & Arntz, A. (1997). Personality disorders do not influence the results of cognitive and behavior therapy for obsessive compulsive disorder. *Journal of Anxiety Disorders, 11*(5), 503–521.

Drew, A., Baird, G., Baron-Cohen, S., Cox, A., Slonims, V., Wheelwright, S., et al. (2002). A pilot randomised control trial of a parent training intervention for pre-school children with autism: Preliminary findings and methodological challenges. *European Journal of Child and Adolescent Psychiatry, 11*(6), 266–272.

Drummond, D. C., & Glautier, S. (1994). A controlled trial of cue exposure treatment in alcohol dependence. *Journal of Consulting and Clinical Psychology, 62*(4), 809–817.

Drury, V., Birchwood, M., & Cochrane, R. (2000). Cognitive therapy and recovery from acute psychosis: A controlled trial: III. Five-year follow-up. *British Journal of Psychiatry, 177,* 8–14.

Drury, V., Birchwood, M., Cochrane, R., & Macmillan, F. (1996a). Cognitive therapy and recovery from acute psychosis: A controlled trial: I. Impact on psychotic symptoms. *British Journal of Psychiatry, 169*(5), 593–601.

Drury, V., Birchwood, M., Cochrane, R., & Macmillan, F. (1996b). Cognitive therapy and recovery from acute psychosis: A controlled trial: II. Impact on recovery time. *British Journal of Psychiatry, 169*(5), 602–607.

Ducharme, J. M., Atkinson, L., & Poulton, L. (2000). Success-based, noncoercive treatment of oppositional behavior in children from violent homes. *Journal of the American Academy of Child and Adolescent Psychiatry, 39*(8), 995–1004.

Dugas, M. J., Ladouceur, R., Leger, E., Freeston, M. H., Langlois, F., Provencher, M. D., et al. (2003). Group cognitive-behavioral therapy for generalized anxiety disorder: Treatment outcome and long-term follow-up. *Journal of Consulting and Clinical Psychology, 71*(4), 821–825.

Dumas, J. E., & Albin, J. B. (1986). Parent training outcome: Does active parental involvement matter? *Behaviour Research and Therapy, 24,* 227–230.

Dunlap, G., Koegel, R., Johnson, J., & O'Neill, R. (1987). Maintaining performance of autistic clients in community settings with delayed contingencies. *Journal of Applied Behaviour Analysis, 20,* 185–191.

Dunn, C., Deroo, L., & Rivara, F. (2001). The use of brief interventions adapted from motivational interviewing across behavioral domains: A systematic review. *Addiction, 96*(12), 1725–1742.

Dunner, D. L., Schmaling, K. B., Hendrickson, H., Becker, J., Lehman, A., & Bea, C. (1996). Cognitive therapy versus fluoxetine in the treatment of dysthymic disorder. *Depression, 4*(1), 34–41.

Durham, R. C., & Allan, T. (1993). Psychological treatment of generalized anxiety disorder: A review of the clinical significance of outcome studies since 1980. *British Journal of Psychiatry, 163,* 19–26.

Durham, R. C., Allan, T., & Hackett, C. A. (1997). On predicting improvement and relapse in generalized anxiety disorder following psychotherapy. *British Journal of Clinical Psychology, 36,* 101–119.

Durham, R. C., Chambers, J. A., MacDonald, R. R., Power, K. G., & Major, K. (2003a). Does cognitive-behavioural therapy influence the long-term outcome of generalized anxiety disorder?: An 8–14 year follow-up of two clinical trials. *Psychological Medicine, 33*(3), 499–509.

Durham, R. C., Fisher, P. L., Treliving, L. R., Hau, C. M., Richard, K., & Stewart, J. B. (1999). One year follow-up of cognitive therapy, analytic psychotherapy and anxiety management training for generalized anxiety disorder: Symptom change, medication usage and attitudes to treatment. *Behavioural and Cognitive Psychotherapy, 27,* 19–35.

Durham, R. C., Guthrie, M., Morton, R. V., Reid, D. A., Treliving, L. R., Fowler, D., et al. (2003b). Tayside–Fife clinical trial of cognitive-behavioural therapy for medication–resistant psychotic symptoms: Results to 3-month follow-up. *British Journal of Psychiatry, 182,* 303–311.

Durham, R. C., Murphy, T., Allan, T., Richard, K., Treliving, L. R., & Fenton, G. W. (1994). Cognitive therapy, analytic psychotherapy and anxiety management training for generalised anxiety disorder. *British Journal of Psychiatry, 165,* 315–323.

Durham, R. C., & Turvey, A. A. (1987). Cognitive therapy vs. behavior therapy in the treatment of chronic general anxiety. *Behaviour Research and Therapy, 25,* 229–234.

Durlak, J. A. (1979). Comparative effectiveness of paraprofessional and professional helpers. *Psychological Bulletin, 86,* 80–92.

Dush, D. M., Hirt, M. L., & Schroeder, H. E. (1989). Self-statement modification in the treatment of child behavior disorders: A meta-analysis. *Psychological Bulletin, 106,* 97–106.

Eames, V., & Roth, A. D. (2000). Patient attachment orientation and the early working alliance—a study of patient and therapist reports of alliance quality and ruptures. *Psychotherapy Research, 10,* 421–434.

Easterbrook, P. J. (1992). Directory of registries of clinical trials. *Statistics in Medicine, 11,* 345–359.

Eaton, W. W., Dryman, A., & Weissman, M. M. (1991). Panic and phobia. In L. N. Robins & I. D. A. Regier (Eds.), *Psychiatric disorders in America: The Epidemiologic Catchment Area Study.* New York: Free Press.

Eckert, E. D., Goldberg, S. C., Halmi, K. A., Casper, R. C., & Davis, J. M. (1979). Behaviour therapy in anorexia nervosa. *British Journal of Psychiatry, 134,* 55–59.

Eddy, D. M., Hasselbad, V., & Schacter, R. (1990). A Bayesian method for synthesizing evidence: The confidence profile method. *International Journal of Technology Assessment in Health Care, 6,* 31–55.

Edwards, G., Orford, J., Egert, S., Guthrie, S., Hawker, A., Hensman, C., et al. (1977). Alcoholism: A controlled trial of "treatment" and "advice." *Journal of Studies on Alcohol, 38,* 1004–1031.

Eells, T. D. (Ed.). (1997). *Handbook of psychotherapy case formulation.* New York: Guilford Press.

Ehlers, A., & Clark, D. (2000). A cognitive model of posttraumatic stress disorder. *Behaviour Research and Therapy, 38,* 319–345.

Ehlers, A., & Clark, D. (2003). Early psychological interventions for adult survivors of trauma: A review. *Biological Psychiatry, 53*(9), 817–826.

Ehlers, A., Clark, D. M., Hackmann, A., McManus, F., Fennell, M., Herbert, C., & Mayou, R. (2003). A randomized controlled trial of cognitive therapy, a self-help booklet, and repeated assessments as early interventions for posttraumatic stress disorder. *Archives of General Psychiatry, 60*(10), 1024–1032.

Eikeseth, S., Smith, T., Jahr, E., & Eldevik, S. (2002). Intensive behavioral treatment at school for 4- to 7-year-old children with autism: A 1-year comparison controlled study. *Behavior Modification, 26*(1), 49–68.

Eisler, I. (1988). Family therapy approaches to anorexia. In D. Scott (Ed.), *Anorexia and bulimia nervosa: Practical approaches* (pp. 95–107). New York: New York University Press.

Eisler, I., Dare, C., Hodes, M., Russell, G., Dodge, E., & Le Grange, D. (2000). Family therapy for adolescent anorexia nervosa: The results of a controlled comparison of two family interventions. *Journal of Child Psychology and Psychiatry, 41*(6), 727–736.

Eisler, I., Dare, C., Russell, G. F., Szmukler, G., le Grange, D., & Dodge, E. (1997). Family and individual therapy in anorexia nervosa: A 5-year follow-up. *Archives of General Psychiatry, 54*(11), 1025–1030.

Eldredge, K. L., Stewart Agras, W., Arnow, B., Telch, C. F., Bell, S., Castonguay, L., et al. (1997). The effects of extending cognitive-behavioral therapy for binge eating disorder among initial treatment nonresponders. *International Journal of Eating Disorders, 21*(4), 347–352.

Elkin, I. (1994). The NIMH Treatment of Depression Collaborative Research Program: Where we began and where we are. In A. E. Bergin & S. L. Garfield (Eds.), *Handbook of psychotherapy and behavior change* (4th ed., pp. 114–142). New York: Wiley.

Elkin, I. (1999). A major dilemma in psychotherapy outcome research: Disentangling therapists from therapies. *Clinical Psychology: Science and Practice, 6,* 10–32.

Elkin, I., Gibbons, R. D., Shea, M. T., & Shaw, B. F. (1996). Science is not a trial (but it can sometimes be a tribulation). *Journal of Consulting and Clinical Psychology, 64,* 92–103.

Elkin, I., Gibbons, R. D., Shea, M. T., Sotsky, S. M., Watkins, J. T., Pilkonis, P. A., et al. (1995). Initial severity and differential treatment outcome in the National Institute of Mental Health Treatment of Depression Collaborative Research Program. *Journal of Consulting and Clinical Psychology, 63,* 841–847.

Elkin, I., Pilkonis, P. A., Docherty, J. P., & Sotsky, S. M. (1988a). Conceptual and methodological issues in comparative studies of psychotherapy and pharmacotherapy: I. Active ingredients and mechanisms of change. *American Journal of Psychiatry, 145,* 909–917.

Elkin, I., Pilkonis, P. A., Docherty, J. P., & Sotsky, S. M. (1988b). Conceptual and methodological issues in comparative studies of psychotherapy and pharmacotherapy. II. Nature and timing of treatment effects. *American Journal of Psychiatry, 145,* 1070–1076.

Elkin, I., Shea, M. T., Watkins, J. T., Imber, S. D., Sotsky, S. M., Collins, J. F., et al. (1989). National Institute of Mental Health Treatment of Depression Collaborative Program: General effectiveness of treatments. *Archives of General Psychiatry, 46,* 971–982.

Elkins, R. L. (1980). Covert sensitization treatment of alcoholism: Contributions of successful conditioning to subsequent abstinence maintenance. *Addictive Behaviors, 5,* 67–89.

Elkins, R. L., & Murdoch, R. P. (1977). The contribution of successful conditioning to abstinence maintenance following covert sensitization (verbal aversion) treatment of alcoholism. *IRCS Medical Science: Psychology and Psychiatry: Social and Occupational Medicine, 5,* 167–169.

Elliott, R. (1998). Editor's introduction: A guide to the empirically supported treatments controversy. *Psychotherapy Research, 8,* 115–125.

Elvy, G. A., Wells, J. E., & Baird, K. A. (1988). Attempted referral as intervention for problem drinking in the general hospital. *British Journal of Addiction, 83,* 83–89.

Emanuels-Zuurveen, L., & Emmelkamp, P. M. (1996). Individual behavioural-cognitive therapy v. marital therapy for depression in maritally distressed couples. *British Journal of Psychiatry, 169*(2), 181–188.

Emmelkamp, P., Bouman, T. K., & Blaauw, E. (1994). Individualized versus standardized therapy: A comparative evaluation with obsessive–compulsive patients. *Clinical Psychology and Psychotherapy, 1,* 95–100.

Emmelkamp, P. M., Krijn, M., Hulsbosch, A. M., de Vries, S., Schuemie, M. J., & van der Mast, C. A. (2002). Virtual reality treatment versus exposure *in vivo*: A comparative evaluation in acrophobia. *Behaviour Research and Therapy, 40*(5), 509–516.

Emmelkamp, P. M., van den Heuvell, C., Rüphan, M., & Sanderman, R. (1989). Home-based treatment of obsessive–compulsive patients: Intersession interval and therapist involvement. *Behaviour Research and Therapy, 27,* 89–93.

Emmelkamp, P. M. G. (1982). *Phobic and obsessive–compulsive disorders: Theory, research and practice.* New York: Plenum Press.

Emmelkamp, P. M. G. (1994). Behavior therapy with adults. In A. E. Bergin & S. L. Garfield (Eds.), *Handbook of psychotherapy and behavior change* (4th ed., pp. 379–427). New York: Wiley.

Emmelkamp, P. M. G., & Beens, H. (1991). Cognitive therapy with obsessive–compulsive disorder: A comparative evaluation. *Behaviour Research and Therapy, 29,* 293–300.

Emmelkamp, P. M. G., & Giesselbach, P. (1981). Treatment of obsessions: Relevant vs. irrelevant exposure. *Behavioural Psychotherapy, 9,* 322–329.

Emmelkamp, P. M. G., & Kwee, K. (1977). Obsessional ruminations: A comparison between thought-stopping and prolonged exposure in imagination. *Behaviour Research and Therapy, 15,* 441–444.

Emmelkamp, P. M. G., Mersch, P. P. A., Vissia, E., & Van der Helm, M. (1985). Social phobia: A comparative evaluation of cognitive and behavioural interventions. *Behaviour Research and Therapy, 23,* 365–369.

Emmelkamp, P. M. G., & van der Hayden, H. (1980). Treatment of harming obsessions. *Behavior Analysis Modification, 4,* 28–35.

Emmelkamp, P. M. G., van der Helm, M., van Zanten, B. L., & Plocgh, I. (1980). Treatment of obsessive–compulsive patients: The contribution of self-instructional training to the effectiveness of exposure. *Behaviour Research and Therapy, 18,* 61–66.

Emmelkamp, P. M. G., Visser, S., & Hoekstra, R. J. (1988). Cognitive therapy vs. exposure in-vivo in the treatment of obsessive–compulsive disorder. *Cognitive Therapy and Research, 12,* 103–114.

Ends, E. J., & Page, C. W. (1957). Group therapy and concomitant psychological change. *Psychological Monographs, 73*(Serial No. 480).

Enright, S. J. (1991). Group treatment for obsessive–compulsive disorder: An evaluation. *Behavioral Psychotherapy, 19,* 183–192.

Epperson, D. L. (1981). Counsellor gender and early premature termination from counselling: A replication and extension. *Journal of Counselling Psychology, 28,* 349–356.

Epstein, D. H., Hawkins, W. E., Covi, L., Umbricht, A., & Preston, K. L. (2003). Cognitive-behavioral therapy plus contingency management for cocaine use: Findings during treatment and across 12-month follow-up. *Psychology of Addictive Behaviors, 17,* 73–82.

Erwin, B. A., Heimberg, R. G., Juster, H., & Mindlin, M. (2002). Comorbid anxiety and mood disorders among persons with social anxiety disorder. *Behaviour Research and Therapy, 40*(1), 19–35.

Esbensen, F. A., & Osgood, D. W. (1999). Gang resistance education and training (GREAT): Results from the national evaluation. *Journal of Research in Crime and Delinquency, 36,* 194–225.

Evans, C., Margison, F., & Barkham, M. (1998). The contribution of reliable and clinically significant change methods to evidence-based mental health. *Evidence Based Mental Health, 1,* 70–72.

Evans, K., Tyrer, P., Catalan, J., Schmidt, U., Davidson, K., Dent, J., et al. (1999). Manual-assisted cognitive-behaviour therapy (MACT): A randomized controlled trial of a brief intervention with bibliotherapy in the treatment of recurrent deliberate self-harm. *Psychological Medicine, 29*(1), 19–25.

Evans, M. D., Hollon, S. D., DeRubeis, R. J., Piasecki, J. M., Grove, W. M., Garvey, M. J., et al. (1992). Differential relapse following cognitive therapy and pharmacotherapy for depression. *Archives of General Psychiatry, 49,* 802–808.

Everaerd, W., & Dekker, J. (1985). Treatment of male sexual dysfunction: Sex therapy compared with systematic desensitisation and rational emotive therapy. *Behaviour Research and Therapy, 23,* 13–25.

Everaerd, W., et al. (1982). Treatment of homosexual and heterosexual sexual dysfunction in male-only groups of mixed sexual orientation. *Archives of Sexual Behavior, 11*, 1–10.

Eyberg, S. M., Boggs, S. R., & Algina, J. (1995). Parent–child interaction therapy: A psychosocial model for the treatment of young children with conduct problem behaviour and their families. *Psychopharmacology Bulletin, 31*, 83–91.

Eyberg, S. M., Funderburk, B. W., Hembree Kigin, T. L., McNeil, C. B., Querido, J. G., & Hood, K. K. (2001). Parent–child interaction therapy with behavior problem children: One and two year maintenance of treatment effects in the family. *Child and Family Behavior Therapy, 23*(4), 1–20.

Fadden, G. (1997). Implementation of family interventions in routine clinical practice following staff training programs: A major cause for concern. *Journal of Mental Health, 6*, 599–612.

Fairburn, C. G. (1985). Cognitive-behavioral treatment for bulimia. In D. M. Garner & P. E. Garfinkel (Eds.), *Handbook of psychotherapy for anorexia and bulimia* (pp. 160–192). New York: Guilford Press.

Fairburn, C. G., & Beglin, S. J. (1990). Studies of the epidemiology of bulimia nervosa. *American Journal of Psychiatry, 147*, 401–408.

Fairburn, C. G., Cooper, Z., Doll, H. A., Norman, P., & O'Connor, M. (2000). The natural course of bulimia nervosa and binge eating disorder in young women. *Archives of General Psychiatry, 57*(7), 659–665.

Fairburn, C. G., & Harrison, P. J. (2003). Eating disorders. *Lancet, 361*(9355), 407–416.

Fairburn, C. G., Jones, R., Peveler, R., Carr, S., Hope, R. A., & O'Connor, M. (1993). Psychotherapy and bulimia nervosa: Longer term effects of interpersonal psychotherapy, behavior therapy, and cognitive behavior therapy. *Archives of General Psychiatry, 50*, 419–428.

Fairburn, C. G., Jones, R., Peveler, R., Cart, S., et al. (1991). Three psychological treatments for bulimia nervosa: A comparative trial. *Archives of General Psychiatry, 48*, 463–469.

Fairburn, C. G., Kirk, J., O'Connor, M., & Cooper, P. J. (1986). A comparison of two psychological treatments for bulimia nervosa. *Behaviour Research and Therapy, 24*, 629–643.

Fairburn, C. G., Norman, P. A., Welch, S. L., O'Connor, M. E., Doll, H. A., & Peveler, R. C. (1995). A prospective study of outcome in bulimia nervosa and the long term effects of three psychological treatments. *Archives of General Psychiatry, 52*, 304–312.

Falloon, I. R. H., Boyd, J., & McGill, C. (1984). *Family care of schizophrenia: A problem-solving approach to the treatment of mental illness.* New York: Guilford Press.

Falloon, I. R. H., Boyd, J. L., McGill, C. W., Williamson, M., Ranzini, J., Moss, H. B., et al. (1985). Family management in the prevention of morbidity of schizophrenia: Clinical outcome of a two year longitudinal study. *Archives of General Psychiatry, 42*, 887–896.

Falloon, I. R. H., Boyd, J. L., McGill, C. W., Ranzini, J., Moss, H. B., & Gilderman, A. M. (1982). Family management in the prevention of exacerbation in schizophrenia: A controlled study. *New England Journal of Medicine, 306*, 1437–1440.

Falloon, I. R. H., McGill, C. W., Boyd, J. L., & Pederson, J. (1987). Family management in the prevention of morbidity of schizophrenia: Social outcome of a two year longitudinal study. *Psychological Medicine, 17*, 59–66.

Fals-Stewart, W., & Birchler, G. R. (2002). Behavioral couples therapy with alcoholic men and their intimate partners: The comparative effectiveness of bachelor's and master's level counselors. *Behavior Therapy, 33*, 123–147.

Fals-Stewart, W., Birchler, G. R., & O'Farrell, T. J. (1996). Behavioral couples therapy for male substance-abusing patients: Effects on relationship adjustment and drug-using behavior. *Journal of Consulting and Clinical Psychology, 64*, 959–972.

Fals-Stewart, W., & Lucente, S. (1993). An MCMI cluster typology of obsessive–compulsives: A measure of personality characteristics and its relationship to treatment participation, compliance and outcome in behavior therapy. *Journal of Psychiatric Research, 27*(2), 139–154.

Fals-Stewart, W., & O'Farrell, T. J. (2003). Behavioral family counseling and naltrexone for male opioid-dependent patients. *Journal of Consulting and Clinical Psychology, 71*(3), 432–442.

Fals-Stewart, W., O'Farrell, T. J., & Birchler, G. R. (2001). Behavioral couples therapy for male methadone maintenance patients: Effects on drug-using behavior and relationship adjustment. *Behavior Therapy, 32,* 391–411.

Fals-Stewart, W., O'Farrell, T. J., Feehan, M., Birchler, G. R., Tiller, S., & McFarlin, S. K. (2000). Behavioral couples therapy versus individual-based treatment for male substance-abusing patients: An evaluation of significant individual change and comparison of improvement rates. *Journal of Substance Abuse Treatment, 18*(3), 249–254.

Farmer, E. M., Compton, S. N., Burns, B. J., & Robertson, E. (2002). Review of the evidence base for treatment of childhood psychopathology: Externalizing disorders. *Journal of Consulting and Clinical Psychology, 70*(6), 1267–1302.

Farrell, A. D., & Bruce, S. E. (1997). Impact of exposure to community violence on violent behavior and emotional distress among urban adolescents. *Journal of Clinical Child Psychology, 26*(1), 2–14.

Fava, G. A., Grandi, S., Rafanelli, C., Ruini, C., Conti, S., & Belluardo, P. (2001a). Long-term outcome of social phobia treated by exposure. *Psychological Medicine, 31*(5), 899–905.

Fava, G. A., Grandi, S., Zielezny, M., Canestrari, R., & Morphy, M. A. (1994). Cognitive behavioral treatment of residual symptoms in primary major depressive disorder. *American Journal of Psychiatry, 151,* 1295–1299.

Fava, G. A., Rafanelli, C., Grandi, S., Canestrari, R., & Morphy, M. A. (1998a). Six-year outcome for cognitive behavioral treatment of residual symptoms in major depression. *American Journal of Psychiatry, 155*(10), 1443–1445.

Fava, G. A., Rafanelli, C., Grandi, S., Conti, S., & Belluardo, P. (1998b). Prevention of recurrent depression with cognitive behavioral therapy: Preliminary findings. *Archives of General Psychiatry, 55*(9), 816–820.

Fava, G. A., Rafanelli, C., Grandi, S., Conti, S., Ruini, C., Mangelli, L., et al. (2001b). Long-term outcome of panic disorder with agoraphobia treated by exposure. *Psychological Medicine, 31*(5), 891–898.

Fava, G. A., Zielezny, M., Savron, G., & Grandi, S. (1995). Long-term effects of behavioural treatment for panic disorder with agoraphobia. *British Journal of Psychiatry, 166*(1), 87–92.

Fawcett, J., Zajecka, M., & Kravitz, M. (1989). Fluoxetine vs. amitryptiline in adult outpatients with major depression. *Current Therapy Research, 46,* 821–832.

Febbraro, G. A. R., Clum, G. A., Roodman, A. A., & Wright, J. H. (1999). The limits of bibliotherapy: A study of the differential effectiveness of self-administered interventions in individuals with panic attacks. *Behavior Therapy, 30,* 209–222.

Fecteau, G., & Nicki, R. (1999). Cognitive behavioural treatment of post traumatic stress disorder after motor vehicle accident. *Behavioural and Cognitive Psychotherapy, 27,* 201–214.

Fedoroff, I. C., & Taylor, S. (2001). Psychological and pharmacological treatments of social phobia: A meta-analysis. *Journal of Clinical Psychopharmachology, 21*(3), 311–324.

Feeley, M., DeRubeis, R. J., & Gelfand, L. A. (1999). The temporal relation of adherence and alliance to symptom change in cognitive therapy for depression. *Journal of Consulting and Clinical Psychology, 67*(4), 578–582.

Feil, N. (1993). *The validation breakthrough: Simple techniques for communicating with people with "Alzheimer's type dementia."* Baltimore: Health Professions Press.

Feinberg, M. (1992). Comment: Subtypes of depression and response to treatment. *Journal of Consulting and Clinical Psychology, 60,* 670–674.

Feindler, E. L., Marriott, S. A., & Iwata, M. (1984). Group anger control training for junior high school delinquents. *Cognitive Therapy and Research, 8,* 299–311.

Feinman, J. A., & Dunner, D. L. (1996). The effect of alcohol and substance abuse on the course of bipolar affective disorder. *Journal of Affective Disorders, 37,* 43–49.

Fennel, M. J., & Teasdale, J. D. (1982). Cognitive therapy with chronic drug refractory depressed outpatients: A note of caution. *Cognitive Therapy and Research, 6,* 455–460.

Ferrell, W. L., & Galassi, J. P. (1981). Assertion training and human relations training in the treatment of chronic alcoholics. *International Journal of the Addictions, 16,* 959–968.

Feske, U., & Chambless, D. L. (1995). Cognitive behavioral versus exposure only treatment for social phobia: A meta-analysis. *Behavior Therapy, 26,* 695–720.

Feske, U., & Goldstein, A. J. (1997). Eye movement desensitization and reprocessing treatment for panic disorder: A controlled outcome and partial dismantling study. *Journal of Consulting and Clinical Psychology, 65*(6), 1026–1035.

Feske, U., Perry, K. J., Chambless, D. L., Renneberg, B., & Goldstein, A. J. (1996). Avoidant personality disorder as a predictor for treatment outcome among generalized social phobics. *Journal of Personality Disorders, 10,* 174–184.

Fichten, C. S., Libman, E., & Brender, W. (1986). Measurement of therapy outcome and maintenance of gains in the behavioral treatment of secondary orgasmic dysfunction. *Journal of Sex and Marital Therapy, 12,* 22–34.

Field, R., Woodside, D. B., Kaplan, A. S., Olmstead, M., & Carter, J. C. (2001). Pretreatment motivated enhancement therapy for eating disorders: A pilot study. *International Journal of Eating Disorders, 29,* 393–400.

Field, T., Sanders, C., & Nadel, J. (2001). Children with autism display more social behaviors after repeated imitation sessions. *Autism, 5*(3), 317–323.

Fiester, A. (1977). Clients' perceptions of therapists with high attrition rates. *Journal of Consulting and Clinical Psychology, 43,* 528–535.

Finch, A. E., Lambert, M. J., & Schaalje, B. G. (2001). Psychotherapy quality control: The statistical generation of expected recovery curves for integration into an early warning system. *Clinical Psychology and Psychotherapy, 8,* 231–242.

Fine, S., Forth, A., Gilbert, M., & Haley, G. (1991). Group therapy for adolescent depressive disorder: A comparison of social skills and therapeutic support. *Journal of the American Academy of Child and Adolescent Psychiatry, 30,* 79–85.

Fink, H. A., MacDonald, R., Rutks, I. R., Nelson, D. B., & Wilt, T. J. (2002). Sildenafil for male erectile dysfunction: A systematic review and meta-analysis. *Archives of Internal Medicine, 162,* 1349–1360.

Finney, J. W., & Monahan, S. C. (1996). The cost-effectiveness of treatment for alcoholism: A second approximation. *Journal of Studies on Alcohol, 57*(3), 229–243.

Firth-Cozens, J. (1993). *Audit in mental health services: A guide to carrying out clinical audits for clinical psychologists, nurses, occupational therapists, psychiatrists, psychotherapists, social workers and all health professionals involved in mental health, learning difficulties, and the elderly.* Hillsdale, NJ: Erlbaum.

Fisher, P. L., & Durham, R. C. (1999). Recovery rates in generalized anxiety disorder following psychological therapy: An analysis of clinically significant change in the STAI-T across outcome studies since 1990. *Psychological Medicine, 29*(6), 1425–1434.

Flament, M. F., Koby, E., Rapoport, J. L., Berg, C. J., Zahn, T., Cox, C., Denckla, M., et al. (1990). Childhood compulsive disorder: A prospective follow-up study. *Journal of Child Psychology and Psychiatry, 31,* 363–380.

Flannery-Schroeder, E. C., & Kendall, P. C. (2000). Group and individual cognitive-behavioral treatments for youth with anxiety disorders: A randomized controlled trial. *Cognitive Therapy and Research, 24*(3), 251–278.

Fleiger, D. L., & Zingle, H. W. (1973). Covert sensitisation treatment with alcoholics. *Canadian Counsellor, 7,* 269–277.

Fleming, M. F., Mundt, M. P., French, M. T., Manwell, L. B., Stauffacher, E. A., & Barry, K. L. (2002). Brief physician advice for problem drinkers: Long-term efficacy and benefit–cost analysis. *Alcoholism: Clinical and Experimental Research, 26*(1), 36–43.

Flick, S. N. (1988). Managing attrition in clinical research. *Clinical Psychology Review, 8,* 499–515.

Flint, A. J. (1994). Epidemiology and comorbidity of anxiety disorders in the elderly. *American Journal of Psychiatry, 151,* 640–649.

Foa, E. B. (1979). Failure on treating obsessive–compulsives. *Behaviour Research and Therapy, 17,* 169–176.

Foa, E. B. (2000). Psychosocial treatment of posttraumatic stress disorder. *Journal of Clinical Psychiatry, 61*(Suppl. 5), 43–48; discussion 49–51.

Foa, E. B., Abramowitz, J. S., Franklin, M. E., & Kozak, M. J. (1999a). Feared consequences, fixity of belief, and treatment outcome in patients with obsessive–compulsive disorder. *Behavior Therapy, 30*, 717–724.

Foa, E. B., Amir, N., Bogert, K. V. A., Molnar, C., & Przeworski, A. (2001). Inflated perception of responsibility for harm in obsessive–compulsive disorder. *Journal of Anxiety Disorders, 15*, 259–275.

Foa, E. B., Dancu, C. V., Hembree, E. A., Jaycox, L. H., Meadows, E. A., & Street, G. P. (1999b). A comparison of exposure therapy, stress inoculation training, and their combination for reducing posttraumatic stress disorder in female assault victims. *Journal of Consulting and Clinical Psychology, 67*(2), 194–200.

Foa, E. B., Davidson, J., & Rothbaum, B. O. (1995). Treatment of post-traumatic stress disorder. In G. O. Gabbard (Ed.), *Treatments of psychiatric disorders: The DSM-IV edition* (2nd ed., Vol. 1). Washington, DC: American Psychiatric Press.

Foa, E. B., Grayson, J. B., Steketee, G. S., Doppelt, H. G., Turner, R. M., & Latimer, P. R. (1983a). Success and failure in the behavioral treatment of obsessive–compulsives. *Journal of Consulting and Clinical Psychology, 51*, 287–297.

Foa, E. B., Keane, T. M., & Friedman, M. J. (Eds.). (2000). *Effective treatments for PTSD: Practice guidelines from the International Society for Traumatic Stress Studies.* New York: Guilford Press.

Foa, E. B., & Kozac, M. J. (1996). Obsessive–compulsive disorder: Long-term outcome of psychological treatment. In M. R. Mavissakalian & R. F. Prien (Eds.), *Long-term treatments of anxiety disorders* (pp. 285–309). Washington, DC: American Psychiatric Press.

Foa, E. B., Kozac, M. J., Steketee, G. S., & McCarthy, P. R. (1992). Treatment of depressive and obsessive–compulsive symptoms in OCD by imipramine and behaviour therapy. *British Journal of Clinical Psychology, 31*, 279–292.

Foa, E. B., & Meadows, E. A. (1997). Psychosocial treatments for posttraumatic stress disorder: A critical review. *Annual Review of Psychology, 48*, 449–480.

Foa, E. B., & Rothbaum, B. O. (1988). *Treating the trauma of rape: Cognitive-behavioural therapy for PTSD.* New York: Guilford Press.

Foa, E. B., Rothbaum, B. O., Riggs, D. S., & Murdoch, T. B. (1991). Treatment of PTSD in rape victims: A comparison between cognitive-behavioral procedures and counselling. *Journal of Consulting and Clinical Psychology, 59*, 715–723.

Foa, E. B., Steketee, G., Grayson, J. B., & Doppelt, H. G. (1983b). Treatment of obsessive–compulsives: When do we fail? In E. B. Foa & P. M. G. Emmelkamp (Eds.), *Failures in behavior therapy* (pp. 55–81). New York: Wiley.

Foa, E. B., Steketee, G., Grayson, J. B., & Latimer, P. R. (1984). Deliberate exposure and blocking of obsessive–compulsive rituals: Immediate and long-term effects. *Behavior Therapy, 15*, 450–472.

Foa, E. B., Steketee, G., & Milby, J. B. (1980). Differential effects of exposure and response prevention in obsessive–compulsive washers. *Journal of Consulting and Clinical Psychology, 48*, 71–79.

Foley, S. H., O'Malley, S., Rounsaville, B., Prusoff, B. A., & Weissman, M. M. (1987). The relationship of patient difficulty to therapist performance in interpersonal psychotherapy of depression. *Journal of Affective Disorders, 12*, 207–217.

Foley, S. H., Rounsaville, B. J., Weissman, M. M., Sholomskas, D., & Chevron, E. (1989). Individual versus conjoint interpersonal therapy for depressed patients with marital disputes. *International Journal of Family Psychiatry, 10*, 29–42.

Fombonne, E. (1994). Increased rates of depression: Update of epidemiological findings and analytical problems. *Acta Psychiatrica Scandinavica, 90*, 145–156.

Fombonne, E. (1998a). Epidemiology of autism and related conditions. In F. R. Volkmar (Ed.), *Autism and pervasive developmental disorders* (pp. 32–63). Cambridge, UK: Cambridge University Press.

Fombonne, E. (1998b). Increased rates of psychosocial disorders in youth. *European Archives of Psychiatry and Clinical Neuroscience, 248,* 14–21.

Fonagy, P., & Higgitt, A. (1989). Evaluating the performance of departments of psychotherapy. *Psychoanalysis and Psychotherapy, 4,* 121–153.

Fonagy, P., & Kurtz, A. (2002). The treatment of disturbance of conduct. In P. Fonagy, M. Target, D. Cottrell, J. Phillips, & Z. Kurtz, *What works for whom?: A critical review of treatments for children and adolescents* (pp. 106–192). New York: Guilford Press.

Fonagy, P., & Moran, G. S. (1993). Selecting single case designs for clinicians. In N. Miller, L. Luborsky, J. P. Barber, & J. P. Docherty (Eds.), *Psychodynamic treatment research: A handbook for clinical practice* (pp. 62–95). New York: Basic Books.

Fonagy, P., & Target, M. (1994). The efficacy of psychoanalysis for children with disruptive disorders. *Journal of the American Academy of Child and Adolescent Psychiatry, 33,* 45–55.

Fonagy, P., Target, M., Cottrell, D., Phillips, J., & Kurtz, Z. (2002). *What works for whom?: A critical review of treatments for children and adolescents.* New York: Guilford Press.

Forehand, R., & Long, N. (1988). Outpatient treatment of the acting out child: Procedures, long-term follow-up data, and clinical problems. *Advances in Behaviour Research and Therapy, 10,* 129–177.

Forgatch, M. S., & Patterson, G. R. (1989). *Parents and adolescents living together: Part 2. Family problem solving.* Eugene, OR: Castalia.

Foulkes, S. H. (1975). *Group analytic psychotherapy.* London: Gordon & Breach.

Fowler, D., Garety, P. A., & Knipers, L. (1995). *Cognitive behaviour therapy for people with psychosis: A clinical handbook.* Chichester, UK: Wiley.

Frank, A. F., & Gunderson, J. G. (1990). The role of the therapeutic alliance in the treatment of schizophrenia: Relationship to course and outcome. *Archives of General Psychiatry, 47,* 228–238.

Frank, E., Anderson, B., Stewart, B. D., Dancu, C., et al. (1988). Efficacy of behavior therapy and systematic desensitization in the treatment of rape trauma. *Behavior Therapy, 19,* 403–420.

Frank, E., Grochocinski, V. J., Spanier, C. A., Buysse, D. J., Cherry, C. R., Houck, P. R., et al. (2000). Interpersonal psychotherapy and antidepressant medication: evaluation of a sequential treatment strategy in women with recurrent major depression. *Journal of Clinical Psychiatry, 61*(1), 51–57.

Frank, E., Hlastala, S., Ritenour, A., Houck, P., Tu, X. M., Monk, T. H., et al. (1997). Inducing lifestyle regularity in recovering bipolar disorder patients: Results from the maintenance therapies in bipolar disorder protocol. *Biological Psychiatry, 41*(12), 1165–1173.

Frank, E., & Kupfer, D. J. (1976). In every marriage there are two marriages. *Journal of Sex and Marital Therapy, 2,* 137–143.

Frank, E., & Kupfer, D. J. (1994). Reply to G. J. Barnes and Q. Jones. Maintenance therapy in depression. *Archives of General Psychiatry, 51,* 504–505.

Frank, E., Kupfer, D. J., & Perel, J. M. (1989). Early recurrence in unipolar depression. *Archives of General Psychiatry, 46,* 397–400.

Frank, E., Kupfer, D. J., Perel, J. M., Jarrett, D. B., Mallinger, A. G., Thase, M. E., et al. (1990). Three year outcomes for maintenance therapies in recurrent depression. *Archives of General Psychiatry, 47,* 1093–1099.

Frank, E., Kupfer, D. J., Wagner, E. F., McEachern, A. B., & Comes, C. (1991). Efficacy of interpersonal therapy as a maintenance treatment of recurrent depression. *Archives of General Psychiatry, 48,* 1053–1059.

Frank, E., Swartz, H. A., Mallinger, A. G., Thase, M. E., Weaver, E. V., & Kupfer, D. J. (1999). Adjunctive psychotherapy for bipolar disorder: Effects of changing treatment modality. *Journal of Abnormal Psychology, 108*(4), 579–587.

Franklin, M. E., Abramowitz, J. S., Furr, J. M., Kalsy, S., & Riggs, D. S. (2003). A naturalistic examination of therapist experience and outcome of exposure and ritual prevention for OCD. *Psychotherapy Research, 13,* 153–167.

Franklin, M. E., Abramowitz, J. S., Kozak, M. J., Levitt, J. T., & Foa, E. B. (2000). Effectiveness of exposure and ritual prevention for obsessive–compulsive disorder: Randomized compared with nonrandomized samples. *Journal of Consulting and Clinical Psychology, 68*(4), 594–602.

Freedberg, E. J., & Johnson, W. E. (1978). *The effects of assertion training within the context of a multi-modal alcoholism treatment programme for employed alcoholics (Substudy 998).* Toronto, Ontario: Alcoholism and Drug Addiction Research Foundation.

Freeman, C. P. L., Barry, R., Dunkeld-Turnbull, J., & Henderson, A. (1988). Controlled trial of psychotherapy for bulimia nervosa. *British Medical Journal, 296,* 521–525.

Freeston, M. H., Ladouceur, R., Gagnon, F., Thibodeau, N., Rhéaume, J., Letarte, H., et al. (1997). Cognitive-behavioral treatment of obsessive thoughts: A controlled study. *Journal of Consulting and Clinical Psychology, 65,* 405–413.

Freiheit, S. R., & Overholser, J. C. (1997). Training issues in cognitive-behavioural psychotherapy. *Journal of Behavior Therapy and Experimental Psychiatry, 28,* 79–86.

Freud, S. (1964). An outline of psycho-analysis. In J. Strachey (Ed. and Trans.), *The standard edition of the complete psychological works of Sigmund Freud* (Vol. 23, pp. 139–207). London: Hogarth Press. (Original work published 1940)

Friedman, C. J., Shear, M. K., & Frances, A. J. (1987). DSM-III personality disorders in panic patients. *Journal of Personality Disorders, 1,* 132–135.

Friedman, L., Bliwise, D. L., Yesavage, J. A., & Salom, S. R. (1991). A preliminary study comparing sleep restriction and relaxation treatments for insomnia in older adults. *Journal of Gerontology, 46,* 1–8.

Friedman, M. J., Davidson, J. R. T., Mellman, T. A., & Southwick, S. M. (2000). Pharmacotherapy. In E. B. Foa, T. M. Keane, & M. J. Friedman (Eds.), *Effective treatments for PTSD: Practice guidelines from the International Society for Traumatic Stress Studies* (pp. 84–105). New York: Guilford Press.

Frost, R. O., & Hartl, T. L. (1996). A cognitive-behavioral model of compulsive hoarding. *Behaviour Research and Therapy, 34,* 341–350.

Frueh, B. C., Turner, S. M., & Beidel, D. C. (1995). Exposure therapy for combat-related PTSD: A critical review. *Clinical Psychology Review, 15,* 799–817.

Fuller, R., Branchey, L., Brightwell, D., Derman, R., Emrick, D., Iber, F., et al. (1986). Disulfiram treatment of alcoholism: A Veterans Administration cooperative study. *Journal of the American Medical Association, 256,* 1449–1455.

Fuller, R. K., & Roth, H. P. (1979). Disulfiram for the treatment of alcoholism: An evaluation in 128 men. *Annals of Internal Medicine, 90,* 901–904.

Funderburk, B. W., Eyberg, S. M., Newcomb, K., McNeil, C. B., Hembree Kigin, T., & Capage, L. (1998). Parent–child interaction therapy with behavior problem children: Maintenance of treatment effects in the school setting. *Child and Family Behavior Therapy, 20*(2), 17–38.

Gabbard, G. O., Coyne, L., Allen, J. G., Spohn, H., Colson, D. B., & Vary, M. (2000). Evaluation of intensive inpatient treatment of patients with severe personality disorders. *Psychiatric Services, 51*(7), 893–898.

Gabbard, G. O., Lazar, S. G., Hornberger, J., & Spiegel, D. (1997). The economic impact of psychotherapy: A review. *American Journal of Psychiatry, 154,* 147–155.

Gabbard, G. O., Takahashi, T., Davidson, J., Bauman-Bork, M., & Ensroth, K. (1991). A psychodynamic perspective on the clinical impact of insurance review. *American Journal of Psychiatry, 148,* 318–323.

Gaffan, E. A., Tsaousis, I., & Kemp-Wheeler, S. M. (1995). Researcher allegiance and meta-analysis: The case of cognitive therapy for depression. *Journal of Consulting and Clinical Psychology, 63,* 966–980.

Gallagher, D. E., & Thompson, L. W. (1983). Effectiveness of psychotherapy for both endogenous and non-endogenous depression in older adult outpatients. *Journal of Gerontology, 38,* 707–712.

Gallagher-Thompson, D., Hanley-Peterson, P., & Thompson, L. (1990). Maintenance of gains versus relapse following brief psychotherapy for depression. *Journal of Consulting and Clinical Psychology, 58,* 371–374.

Gallagher-Thompson, D., & Steffen, A. M. (1994). Comparative effects of cognitive-behavioral and brief psychodynamic psychotherapies for depressed family caregivers. *Journal of Consulting and Clinical Psychology, 62,* 543–549.

Gallant, D. M., Bishop, M. P., Camp, E., & Tisdale, C. (1968). A six-month controlled evaluation of metronidazole (Flagyl) in chronic alcoholic patients. *Current Therapeutic Research, 10,* 82–87.

Garb, H. N. (1989). Clinical judgment, clinical training, and professional experience. *Psychological Bulletin, 105,* 387–396.

Garcia-Palacios, A., Botella, C., Robert, C., Banos, R., Perpina, C., Quero, S., et al. (2002a). Clinical utility of cognitive-behavioural treatment for panic disorder: Results obtained in different settings: A research centre and a public mental health care unit. *Clinical Psychology and Psychotherapy, 9,* 373–383.

Garcia-Palacios, A., Hoffman, H., Carlin, A., Furness, T. A., III, & Botella, C. (2002b). Virtual reality in the treatment of spider phobia: A controlled study. *Behaviour Research and Therapy, 40*(9), 983–993.

Garety, P., Fowler, D., Kuipers, E., Freeman, D., Dunn, G., Bebbington, P., et al. (1997). London–East Anglia randomised controlled trial of cognitive-behavioural therapy for psychosis: II. Predictors of outcome. *British Journal of Psychiatry, 171,* 420–426.

Garety, P., & Freeman, D. (1999). Cognitive approaches to delusions: A critical review of theories and evidence. *British Journal of Clinical Psychology, 38,* 113–154.

Garety, P. A., Knipers, L., Fowler, D., Chamberlain, F., & Dunn, G. (1994). Cognitive behavioral therapy for drug-resistant psychosis. *British Journal of Psychiatry, 67,* 259–271.

Garfield, S. L. (1994). Research on client variables in psychotherapy. In A. E. Bergin & S. L. Garfield (Eds.), *Handbook of psychotherapy and behavior change* (4th ed., pp. 190–228). New York: Wiley.

Garfield, S. L. (1996). Some problems associated with "validated" forms of psychotherapy. *Clinical Psychology: Science and Practice, 3,* 218–229.

Garner, D. M., Olmsted, M. P., Davis, R., Rockert, W., Goldbloom, D., & Eagle, M. (1990). The association between bulimic symptoms and reported psychopathology. *International Journal of Eating Disorders, 9,* 1–15.

Garner, D. M., Rockert, W., Davis, R., & Garner, M. D. (1993). A comparison between CBT and supportive expressive therapy for bulimia nervosa. *American Journal of Psychiatry, 150,* 37–46.

Gaston, L. (1990). The concept of the alliance and its role in psychotherapy: Theoretical and empirical considerations. *Psychotherapy, 27,* 143–153.

Gaston, L., Marmar, C. R., Gallagher, D., & Thomson, L. W. (1991). Alliance prediction of outcome beyond in-treatment symptomatic change as psychotherapy progresses. *Psychotherapy Research, 1,* 104–112.

Gaston, L., Thompson, L., Gallagher, D., Cournoyer, L.-G., & Gagnon, R. (1998). Alliance, technique and their interactions in predicting outcome of behavioral, cognitive and brief dynamic therapy. *Psychotherapy Research, 8,* 190–209.

Geddes, J., Freemantle, N., Harrison, P., & Bebbington, P. (2000). Atypical antipsychotics in the treatment of schizophrenia: Systematic overview and meta-regression analysis. *British Medical Journal, 321*(7273), 1371–1376.

Geist, R., Heinmaa, M., Stephens, D., Davis, R., & Katzman, D. K. (2000). Comparison of family therapy and family group psychoeducation in adolescents with anorexia nervosa. *Canadian Journal of Psychiatry, 45*(2), 173–178.

Gelenberg, A. J., & Hopkins, H. S. (1993). Report on efficacy of treatments for bipolar disorder. *Psychopharmacology Bulletin, 29,* 447–456.

Gelernter, C. S., Uhde, T. W., & Cimbolic, P. (1991). Cognitive-behavioral and pharmacological treatments for social phobia: A controlled study. *Archives of General Psychiatry, 48,* 938–945.

Gerrein, J. R., Rosenberg, C. M., & Manohar, V. (1973). Disulfiram maintenance in outpatient treatment of alcoholism. *Archives of General Psychiatry, 28,* 633–635.

Ghaderi, A., & Andersson, G. (1999). Meta-analysis of CBT for bulimia nervosa: Investigating the effects using DSM-III-R and DSM-IV criteria. *Scandinavian Journal of Behaviour Therapy, 28,* 79–87.

Ghaderi, A., & Scott, B. (2003). Pure and guided self-help for full and sub-threshold bulimia nervosa and binge eating disorder. *British Journal of Clinical Psychology, 42*(3), 257–269.

Ghosh, R. A., & Marks, I. M. (1987). Self-treatment of agoraphobia by exposure. *Behavior Therapy, 18,* 2–16.

Gilbody, S., Whitty, P., Grimshaw, J., & Thomas, R. (2003). Educational and organizational interventions to improve the management of depression in primary care: A systematic review. *Journal of the American Medical Association, 289,* 3145–3151.

Gillespie, K., Duffy, M., Hackmann, A., & Clark, D. M. (2002). Community based cognitive therapy in the treatment of posttraumatic stress disorder following the Omagh bomb. *Behaviour Research and Therapy, 40*(4), 345–357.

Gittleson, M. (1962). The curative functions in psychotherapy. *International Journal of Psychoanalysis, 43,* 194–205.

Gledhill, A., Lobban, F., & Sellwood, W. (1998). Group CBT for people with schizophrenia: A preliminary evaluation. *Behavioural and Cognitive Psychotherapy, 26*(1), 63–75.

Glick, I. D., Clarkin, J. F., Haas, G. L., & Spencer, J. H. (1993). Clinical significance of inpatient family intervention: Conclusions from a clinical trial. *Hospital and Community Psychiatry, 44,* 869–873.

Gloaguen, V., Cottraux, J., Cucherat, M., & Blackburn, I. (1998). A meta-analysis of the effects of cognitive therapy in depressed patients. *Journal of Affective Disorders, 49*(1), 59–72.

Glynn, S. M., Marder, S. R., Liberman, R. P., Blair, K., Wirshing, W. C., Wirshing, D. A., et al. (2002). Supplementing clinic-based skills training with manual-based community support sessions: Effects on social adjustment of patients with schizophrenia. *American Journal of Psychiatry, 159*(5), 829–837.

Goddaer, J., & Abraham, I. L. (1994). Effects of relaxing music on agitation during meals among nursing home residents with severe cognitive impairment. *Archives of Psychiatric Nursing, 8*(3), 150–158.

Goenjian, A. K., Karayan, I., Pynoos, R. S., Minassian, D., Najarian, L. M., Steinberg, A. M., et al. (1997). Outcome of psychotherapy among early adolescents after trauma. *American Journal of Psychiatry, 154*(4), 536–542.

Goisman, R. M., Warshaw, M. G., & Keller, M. B. (1999). Psychosocial treatment prescriptions for generalized anxiety disorder, panic disorder, and social phobia, 1991–1996. *American Journal of Psychiatry, 156*(11), 1819–1821.

Gold, M. R., Siegal, J. E., Russell, L. B., & Weinstein, M. C. (1996). *Cost effectiveness in health and medicine.* New York: Oxford University Press.

Goldberg, D., & Huxley, P. (1980). *Mental illness in the community: The pathway to psychiatric care.* London: Tavistock.

Goldberg, S. C., Schulz, S. C., Schulz, P. M., Resnick, R. J., Hamer, R. M., & Friedel, R. O. (1986). Borderline and schizotypal personality disorders treated with low dose thiothoxine versus placebo. *Archives of General Psychiatry, 43,* 680–686.

Goldbloom, D. S., Olmsted, M., Davis, R., Clewes, J., Heinmaa, M., Rockert, W., et al. (1997). A randomized controlled trial of fluoxetine and cognitive behavioral therapy for bulimia nervosa: Short-term outcome. *Behaviour Research and Therapy, 35,* 803–811.

Goldfried, M. R. (1995). *From cognitive therapy to psychotherapy integration.* New York: Springer.

Goldner, E. M., Hsu, L., Waraich, P., & Somers, J. M. (2002). Prevalence and incidence studies of schizophrenic disorders: A systematic review of the literature. *Canadian Journal of Psychiatry, 47,* 833–843.

Goldstein, A. J., de Beurs, E., Chambless, D. L., & Wilson, K. A. (2000). EMDR for panic disorder with agoraphobia: Comparison with waiting list and credible attention–placebo control conditions. *Journal of Consulting and Clinical Psychology, 68*(6), 947–956.

Goldstein, M. J. (1991). Psychosocial (nonpharmacologic) treatments for schizophrenia. *Review of Psychiatry, 10,* 116–135.

Gonzales, L. R., Lewinsohn, P. M., & Clarke, G. N. (1985). Longitudinal follow-up of unipolar depressives: An investigation of predictors of relapse. *Journal of Consulting and Clinical Psychology, 53,* 461–469.

Goodwin, F. K. (2002). Rationale for long-term treatment of bipolar disorder and evidence for long-term lithium treatment. *Journal of Clinical Psychiatry, 63*(Suppl. 10), 5–12.

Goodwin, F. K., & Jamison, K. R. (1990). *Manic–depressive illness.* New York: Oxford University Press.

Gortner, E. T., Gollan, J. K., Dobson, K. S., & Jacobson, N. S. (1998). Cognitive-behavioral treatment for depression: Relapse prevention. *Journal of Consulting and Clinical Psychology, 66*(2), 377–384.

Gossop, M., Johns, A., & Green, L. (1986). Opiate withdrawal: Inpatient versus outpatient programmes and preferred versus random assignment to treatment. *British Medical Journal, 293*(6539), 103–104.

Gossop, M., Marsden, J., Stewart, D., & Kidd, T. (2003). The National Treatment Outcome Research Study (NTORS): 4–5 year follow-up results. *Addiction, 98*(3), 291–303.

Gossop, M., & Strang, J. (2000). Price, cost and value of opiate detoxification treatments: Reanalysis of data from two randomised trials. *British Journal of Psychiatry, 177,* 262–266.

Gottdiener, W., & Haslam, N. (2002). The benefits of individual psychotherapy for people diagnosed with schizophrenia: A meta-analytic review. *Ethical Human Sciences and Services, 4*(3), 163–187.

Gottesman, I. I., & Gould, T. D. (2003). The endophenotype concept in psychiatry: Etymology and strategic intentions. *American Journal of Psychiatry, 160*(4), 636–645.

Gottfredson, D. C., & Gottfredson, G. D. (1992). Theory-guided investigation: Three field experiments. In J. McCord & R. E. Tremblay (Eds.), *Preventing antisocial behavior: Interventions from birth through adolescence* (pp. 311–329). New York: Guilford Press.

Gottheil, E., Weinstein, S., Sterling, R., Lundy, A., & Serota, R. (1998). A randomized controlled study of the effectiveness of intensive outpatient treatment for cocaine dependence. *Psychiatric Services, 49*(6), 782–787.

— Gould, R., Buckminster, S., Pollack, M., Otto, M., & Yap, L. (1997). Cognitive-behavioral and pharmacological treatment for social phobia: A meta-analysis. *Psychology: Science and Practice, 4,* 291–306.

Gould, R. A., Clum, G. A., & Shapiro, D. (1993). The use of bibliotherapy in the treatment of panic: A preliminary investigation. *Behavior Therapy, 24,* 241–252.

Gould, R. A., Mueser, K. T., Bolton, E., Mays, V., & Goff, D. (2001). Cognitive therapy for psychosis in schizophrenia: An effect size analysis. *Schizophrenia Research, 48,* 335–342.

Gould, R. A., Otto, M. W., & Pollack, M. H. (1995). A meta-analysis of treatment outcome for panic disorder. *Clinical Psychology Review, 15,* 819–844.

Gowers, S., Norton, K., Halek, C., & Crisp, A. H. (1994). Outcome of outpatient psychotherapy in a random allocation treatment study of anorexia nervosa. *International Journal of Eating Disorders, 15,* 165–177.

Grayson, J. B., Foa, E. B., & Skeketee, G. S. (1986). Exposure *in-vivo* of obsessive–compulsives under distraction and attention focussing conditions: Replication and extension. *Behaviour Research and Therapy, 24,* 475–479.

Green, M. A., & Curtis, G. C. (1988). Personality disorders in panic patients: Response to termination of antipanic medication. *Journal of Personality Disorders, 2,* 303–314.

Green, M. F., Kern, R. S., Braff, D. L., & Mintz, J. (2000). Neurocognitive deficits and functional outcome in schizophrenia: Are we measuring the "right stuff"? *Schizophrenia Bulletin, 26*(1), 119–136.

Greenberg, R. P., Bornstein, R. F., Greenberg, M. D., & Fisher, S. (1992). A meta-analysis of antidepressant outcome under "blinder" conditions. *Journal of Consulting and Clinical Psychology, 60,* 664–669.

Greenwald, R. (1996). The information gap in the EMDR controversy. *Professional Psychology: Research and Practice, 27,* 67–72.

Gregoire, A. (1992). New treatments for erectile impotence. *British Journal of Psychiatry, 160,* 315–326.

Grey, N., Young, K., & Holmes, E. (2002). Cognitive restructuring within reliving: A treatment for peritraumatic emotional hotspots in PTSD. *Behavioural and Cognitive Psychotherapy, 30,* 63–82.

Griffith, J. D., Rowan-Szal, G. A., Roark, R. R., & Simpson, D. D. (2000). Contingency management in outpatient methadone treatment: A meta-analysis. *Drug and Alcohol Dependence, 58*(1–2), 55–66.

Grilo, C. M. (2002). Binge eating disorder. In C. G. Fairburn & K. D. Brownwell (Eds.), *Eating disorders and obesity: A comprehensive handbook* (2nd ed., pp. 178–182). New York: Guilford Press.

Grilo, C. M., Masheb, R. M., & Wilson, G. T. (2001). Subtyping binge eating disorder. *Journal of Consulting and Clinical Psychology, 69,* 1066–1072.

Grilo, C. M., Sanislow, C. A., Skodol, A. E., Gunderson, J. G., Stout, R. L., Shea, M. T., et al. (2003). Do eating disorders co-occur with personality disorders?: Comparison groups matter. *International Journal of Eating Disorders, 33*(2), 155–164.

Gruber, K., Chutuape, M. A., & Stitzer, M. L. (2000). Reinforcement-based intensive outpatient treatment for inner city opiate abusers: A short-term evaluation. *Drug and Alcohol Dependence, 57*(3), 211–223.

Grunhaus, L. (1988). Clinical and psychobiological characteristics of simultaneous panic disorder and major depression. *American Journal of Psychiatry, 145,* 1214–1221.

Guerra, N., & Slaby, R. G. (1990). Cognitive mediators of aggression in adolescent offenders: II. Intervention. *Developmental Psychology, 26,* 269–277.

Gumley, A., O'Grady, M., McNay, L., Reilly, J., Power, K., & Norrie, J. (2003). Early intervention for relapse in schizophrenia: Results of a 12-month randomized controlled trial of cognitive behavioural therapy. *Psychological Medicine, 33*(3), 419–431.

Gunderson, J. G., Frank, A. F., Katz, H. M., et al. (1984). Effects of psychotherapy in schizophrenia: II. Comparative outcome of two forms of treatment. *Schizophrenia Bulletin, 10,* 564–598.

Guthrie, E., Moorey, J., Margison, F., Barker, H., Palmer, S., McGrath, G., et al. (1999). Cost-effectiveness of brief psychodynamic–interpersonal therapy in high utilizers of psychiatric services. *Archives of General Psychiatry, 56,* 519–526.

Haaga, D. A. (2000). Introduction to special section on stepped care models in psychotherapy. *Journal of Consulting and Clinical Psychology, 68,* 547–548.

Hackman, A., & McLean, C. (1975). A comparison of flooding and thought stopping in the treatment of obsessional neurosis. *Behaviour Research and Therapy, 13,* 263–269.

Hadas-Lidor, N., Katz, N., Tyano, S., & Weizman, A. (2001). Effectiveness of dynamic cognitive intervention in rehabilitation of clients with schizophrenia. *Clinical Rehabilitation, 15*(4), 349–359.

Haddock, G., Slade, P. D., Bentall, R. P., Reid, D., & Faragher, E. B. (1998a). A comparison of the long-term effectiveness of distraction and focusing in the treatment of auditory hallucinations. *British Journal of Medical Psychology, 71*(Pt. 3), 339–349.

Haddock, G., Tarrier, N., Morrison, A., Hopkins, R., Drake, R., & Lewis, S. (1999). A pilot study evaluating the effectiveness of individual inpatient cognitive-behavioural therapy in early psychosis. *Social Psychiatry and Psychiatric Epidemiology, 34,* 254–258.

Haddock, G., Tarrier, N., Spaulding, W., Yusupoff, L., Kinney, C., & McCarthy, E. (1998b). Individual cognitive–behaviour therapy in the treatment of hallucinations and delusions: A review. *Clinical Psychology Review, 18,* 821–838.

Hadwin, J., Baron-Cohen, S., Howlin, P., & Hill, K. (1996). Can we teach children with autism to understand emotions, belief, or pretence? *Development and Psychopathology, 8*(2), 345–365.

Hadwin, J., Baron-Cohen, S., Howlin, P., & Hill, K. (1997). Does teaching theory of mind have an effect on the ability to develop conversation in children with autism? *Journal of Autism and Developmental Disorders, 27*(5), 519–537.

Hafner, J., & Marks, I. (1976). Exposure in vivo of agoraphobics: Contributions of diazepam, group exposure and anxiety evocation. *Psychological Medicine, 6,* 71–88.

Hahlweg, K., Fiegenbaum, W., Frank, M., Schroeder, B., & von Witzleben, I. (2001). Short- and long-term effectiveness of an empirically supported treatment for agoraphobia. *Journal of Consulting and Clinical Psychology, 69*(3), 375–382.

Halford, W. K., & Haynes, R. (1991). Psychosocial rehabilitation of chronic schizophrenic patients: Recent findings on social skills training and family psychoeducation. *Clinical Psychology Review, 11,* 23–44.

Halford, W. K., Steindl, S., Varhese, F. N., & Schweitzer, R. D. (1999). Observed family interaction and outcome in patients with first-admission psychoses. *Behavior Therapy, 30,* 555–580.

Hall, A., & Crisp, A. H. (1983). Brief psychotherapy in the treatment of anorexia nervosa. In A. J. Krawkowski & C. P. Kimball (Eds.), *Psychosomatic medicine* (pp. 703–717). New York: Plenum Press.

Hall, A., & Crisp, A. H. (1987). Brief psychotherapy in the treatment of anorexia nervosa. *British Journal of Psychiatry, 151,* 185–191.

Hall, W., & Heather, N. (1991). The issue of statistical power in comparison of minimal and intensive controlled drinking interventions. *Addictive Behaviors, 16,* 83–87.

Halmi, K. A., Agras, W. S., Mitchell, J., Wilson, G. T., Crow, S., Bryson, S. W., et al. (2002). Relapse predictors of patients with bulimia nervosa who achieved abstinence through cognitive behavioral therapy. *Archives of General Psychiatry, 59*(12), 1105–1109.

Hamilton, K. E., & Dobson, K. S. (2002). Cognitive therapy of depression: Pretreatment patient predictors of outcome. *Clinical Psychology Review, 22*(6), 875–893.

Hansen, N. B., & Lambert, M. J. (2003). An evaluation of the dose–response relationship in naturalistic treatment settings using survival analysis. *Mental Health Services Research, 5,* 1–12.

Hardy, G. E., Barkham, M., Shapiro, D. A., Reynolds, S., Rees, A., & Stiles, W. B. (1995a). Credibility and outcome of cognitive-behavioural and psychodynamic-interpersonal psychotherapy. *British Journal of Clinical Psychology, 34*(Pt. 4), 555–569.

Hardy, G. E., Barkham, M., Shapiro, D. A., Stiles, W. B., Rees, A., & Reynolds, S. (1995b). Impact of Cluster C personality disorders on outcomes of contrasting brief psychotherapies for depression. *Journal of Consulting and Clinical Psychology, 63*(6), 997–1004.

Hardy, G. E., Cahill, J., Shapiro, D. A., Barkham, M., Rees, A., & Macaskill, N. (2001). Client interpersonal and cognitive styles as predictors of response to time-limited cognitive therapy for depression. *Journal of Consulting and Clinical Psychology, 69*(5), 841–845.

Hare, R. D., Hart, S. D., & Harpur, T. J. (1991). Psychopathy and the DSM-IV criteria for antisocial personality disorder. *Journal of Abnormal Psychology, 100,* 391–398.

Harkavy-Friedman, J. M., Asnis, G. M., Boeck, M., & DiFiore, J. (1987). Prevalence of specific suicidal behaviors in a high school sample. *American Journal of Psychiatry, 144*(9), 1203–1206.

Harpin, R. E., Liberman, R. P., Marks, I., Stern, S., & Bohannon, W. E. (1982). Cognitive-behavior therapy for chronically depressed patients: A controlled pilot study. *Journal of Nervous and Mental Disease, 170,* 295–301.

Harrington, R., Bredenkamp, D., Groothues, C., Rutter, M., Fudge, H., & Pickles, A. (1994). Adult outcomes of childhood and adolescent depression: III. Links with suicidal behaviors. *Journal of Child Psychology and Psychiatry, 35,* 1309–1319.

Harrington, R., Fudge, H., Rutter, M., Pickles, A., & Hill, J. (1990). Adult outcomes of childhood and adolescent depression: I. Psychiatric status. *Archives of General Psychiatry, 47,* 465–473.

Harrington, R., Fudge, H., Rutter, M., Pickles, A., & Hill, J. (1991). Adult outcomes of childhood and adolescent depression: II. Links with antisocial disorders. *Journal of the American Academy of Child and Adolescent Psychiatry, 30,* 434–439.

Harrington, R., Kerfoot, M., Dyer, E., McNiven, F., Gill, J., Harrington, V., et al. (1998a). Randomized trial of a home-based family intervention for children who have deliberately poisoned themselves. *Journal of the American Academy of Child and Adolescent Psychiatry, 37*, 512–518.

Harrington, R., Whittaker, J., & Shoebridge, P. (1998b). Psychological treatment of depression in children and adolescents: A review of treatment research. *British Journal of Psychiatry, 173*, 291–298.

Harrington, R., Whittaker, J., Shoebridge, P., & Campbell, F. (1998c). Systematic review of efficacy of cognitive behaviour therapies in childhood and adolescent depressive disorder. *British Medical Journal, 316*, 1559–1563.

Harris, S. L., Handleman, J. S., Kristoff, B., Bass, L., & Gordon, R. (1990). Changes in language development among autistic and peer children in segregated and integrated preschool settings. *Journal of Autism and Developmental Disorders, 20*, 23–31.

Hartl, T. L., & Frost, R. (1999). Cognitive-behavioral treatment of compulsive hoarding: A multiple baseline experimental case study. *Behaviour Research and Therapy, 37*, 451–461.

Hartman, L. M., & Daly, E. M. (1983). Relationship factors in the treatment of sexual dysfunction. *Behaviour Research and Therapy, 21*, 153–160.

Hartman, R. R., Stage, S. A., & Webster-Stratton, C. (2003). A growth curve analysis of parent training outcomes: Examining the influence of child risk factors (inattention, impulsivity, and hyperactivity problems), parental and family risk factors. *Journal of Child Psychology and Psychiatry, 44*(3), 388–398.

Hartman, W. E., & Fithian, M. A. (1972). *Treatment of sexual dysfunctions: A biopsychosocial approach.* Long Beach, CA: Center for Marital and Sexual Studies.

Hartmann, A., Herzog, T., & Drinkman, A. (1992). Psychotherapy of bulimia nervosa: What is effective?: A meta-analysis. *Journal of Psychosomatic Research, 36*, 159–167.

Hartmann, U., & Langer, D. (1993). Combination of psychosexual therapy and intrapenile injections in the treatment of erectile dysfunctions: Rationale and predictors of outcome. *Journal of Sex Education and Therapy, 19*, 1–12.

Hattie, J. A., Sharpley, C. F., & Rogers, H. J. (1984). Comparative effectiveness of professional and paraprofessional helpers. *Psychological Bulletin, 95*, 534–541.

Haug, T. T., Blomhoff, S., Hellstrom, K., Holme, I., Humble, M., Madsbu, H. P., et al. (2003). Exposure therapy and sertraline in social phobia: 1-year follow-up of a randomised controlled trial. *British Journal of Psychiatry, 182*, 312–318.

Haug, T. T., Hellstrom, K., Blomhoff, S., Humble, M., Madsbu, H. P., & Wold, J. E. (2000). The treatment of social phobia in general practice: Is exposure therapy feasible? *Family Practice, 17*, 114–118.

Hawkins, E. J., Lambert, M. J., Vermeersch, D., Slade, K., & Tuttle, C. T. (2004). The therapeutic effects of providing patient progress information to therapists and patients. *Psychotherapy Research, 14*, 308–327.

Hawton, K. (1985). *Sex therapy: A practical guide.* Oxford, UK: Oxford University Press.

Hawton, K. (1995). Treatment of sexual dysfunctions by sex therapy and other approaches. *British Journal of Psychiatry, 167*, 307–314.

Hawton, K. (1996). Suicide and attempted suicide in young people. In A. MacFarlane (Ed.), *Adolescent medicine* (pp. 117–130). London: Royal College of Physicians.

Hawton, K., & Catalan, J. (1986). Prognostic factors in sex therapy. *Behaviour Research and Therapy, 24*, 377–385.

Hawton, K., & Catalan, J. (1990). Sex therapy for vaginismus: Characteristics of couples and treatment outcome. *Sexual and Marital Therapy, 5*, 39–48.

Hawton, K., Catalan, J., & Fagg, J. (1992). Sex therapy for erectile dysfunction: Characteristics of couples, treatment outcome, and prognostic factors. *Archives of Sexual Behavior, 21*, 61–175.

Hay, P. (1998). The epidemiology of eating disorder behaviors: An Australian community-based survey. *International Journal of Eating Disorders, 23*(4), 371–382.

Hay, P. J., & Bacaltchuk, J. (2001). Psychotherapy for bulimia nervosa and binging (Cochrane Review). In *The Cochrane Library*, Issue 4, 2002. Oxford, UK: Update Software.

Hayes, R. L., & McGrath, J. J. (2000). Cognitive rehabilitation for people with schizophrenia and related conditions (Cochrane Review). In *The Cochrane Library*, Issue 4, 2002. Oxford, UK: Update Software.

Haynes, B. R., Devereaux, P. J., & Guyatt, G. H. (2002). Physicians' and patients' choices in evidence-based practice: Evidence does not make decisions, people do. *British Medical Journal, 324,* 1350.

Hazell, P. L., & Stuart, J. E. (2003). A randomized controlled trial of clonidine added to psychostimulant medication for hyperactive and aggressive children. *Journal of the American Academy of Child and Adolescent Psychiatry, 42*(8), 886–894.

Head, D., Portnoy, S., & Woods, R. T. (1990). The impact of reminiscence groups in two different settings. *International Journal of Geriatric Psychiatry, 5,* 295–302.

Healey, A., & Knapp, M. (1994). *Economic evaluation and psychotherapy: A review for the Department of Health.* Unpublished manuscript.

Heather, N. (1995). Interpreting the evidence on brief interventions for excessive drinkers: The need for caution. *Alcohol and Alcoholism, 30,* 287–296.

Heather, N., Brodie, J., Wale, S., Wilkinson, G., Luce, A., Webb, E., et al. (2000). A randomized controlled trial of moderation-oriented cue exposure. *Journal of Studies on Alcohol, 61*(4), 561–570.

Heather, N., Campion, P. D., Neville, R. G., & MacCabe, D. (1987a). Evaluation of a controlled drinking minimal intervention for problem drinkers in general practice (the DRAMS scheme). *Journal of the Royal College of General Practitioners, 37,* 358–363.

Heather, N., & Robertson, I. (1989). *Problem drinking* (2nd ed.). London: Oxford University Press.

Heather, N., Robertson, I., MacPherson, B., Allsop, S., & Fulton, A. (1987b). The effectiveness of a controlled drinking self-help manual: One year follow-up results. *British Journal of Clinical Psychology, 26,* 279–287.

Hegel, M. T., Ravaris, C. L., & Ahles, T. A. (1994). Combined cognitive-behavioral and time-limited alprazolam treatment of panic disorder. *Behavior Therapy, 25,* 183–195.

Heiman, J. R. (2002). Psychologic treatments for female sexual dysfunction: Are they effective and do we need them? *Archives of Sexual Behavior, 31,* 445–450.

Heiman, J. R., & LoPiccolo, J. (1983). Clinical outcome of sex therapy: Effects of daily v weekly treatment. *Archives of General Psychiatry, 40,* 443–449.

Heimberg, R., Dodge, C., Hope, D., Kennedy, C., et al. (1990). Cognitive behavioral group treatment for social phobia: Comparison with a credible placebo control. *Cognitive Therapy and Research, 14*(1), 1–23.

Heimberg, R., Salzman, D., Holt, C., & Blendell, K. (1993). Cognitive-behavioral group treatment for social phobia: Effectiveness at five-year follow-up. *Cognitive Therapy and Research, 17*(4), 325–339.

Heimberg, R. G. (1996). Social phobia, avoidant personality disorder and the multiaxial conceptualizarion of interpersonal anxiety. In P. M. Salkovskis (Ed.), *Trends in cognitive and behavioural therapies* (pp. 43–61). Chichester, UK: Wiley.

Heimberg, R. G. (2001). Current status of psychotherapeutic interventions for social phobia. *Journal of Clinical Psychiatry, 62*(Suppl. 1), 36–42.

Heimberg, R. G. (2002). Cognitive-behavioral therapy for social anxiety disorder: Current status and future directions. *Biological Psychiatry, 51*(1), 101–108.

Heimberg, R. G., & Juster, H. R. (1994). Treatment of social phobia in cognitive-behavioral groups. *Journal of Clinical Psychiatry, 55*(Suppl. 6), 38–46.

Heimberg, R. G., Liebowitz, M. R., Hope, D. A., Schneier, F. R., Holt, C. S., Welkowitz, L. A., et al. (1998). Cognitive behavioral group therapy vs. phenelzine therapy for social phobia: 12-week outcome. *Archives of General Psychiatry, 55*(12), 1133–1141.

Heinssen, R. K., Liberman, R. P., & Kopelowicz, A. (2000). Psychosocial skills training for schizophrenia: Lessons from the laboratory. *Schizophrenia Bulletin, 26*(1), 21–46.

Hellerstein, D. J., Little, S. A., Samstag, L. W., Batchelder, S., Muran, J. C., Fedak, M., et al. (2001). Adding group psychotherapy to medication treatment in dysthymia: A randomized prospective pilot study. *Journal of Psychotherapy Practice and Research, 10*(2), 93–103.

Helzer, J. E., Canino, G. J., Yeh, E. K., Bland, R. C., Lee, C. K., Hwu, H. G., et al. (1991). Alcoholism—North America and Asia: A comparison of population surveys with the Diagnostic Interview Schedule. *Archives of General Psychiatry, 47,* 313–319.

Helzer, J. E., Robins, L., & McEvoy, L. (1987). Post-traumatic stress disorder in the general population: Findings of the epidemiological catchment area survey. *New England Journal of Medicine*, *317*, 1630–1634.

Hembree-Kigin, T. L., & McNeil, C. B. (1995). *Parent–child interaction therapy: A step-by-step guide for clinicans*. New York: Plenum Press.

Henggeler, S. W., Cunningham, P. B., Pickrel, S. G., Schoenwald, S. K., & Brondino, M. J. (1996a). Multisystemic therapy: An effective violence prevention approach for serious juvenile offenders. *Journal of Adolescence*, *19*, 47–61.

Henggeler, S. W., Melton, G. B., & Smith, L. A. (1992). Family preservation using multisystemic therapy: An effective alternative to incarcerating serious juvenile offenders. *Journal of Consulting and Clinical Psychology*, *60*, 953–961.

Henggeler, S. W., Melton, G. B., Smith, L. A., Schoenwald, S. K., & Hanley, J. H. (1993). Family preservation using multisystemic treatment: Long-term follow-up to a clinical trial with serious juvenile offenders. *Journal of Child and Family Studies*, *2*, 283–293.

Henggeler, S. W., Pickrel, S. G., Brondino, M. J., & Crouch, J. L. (1996b). Eliminating (almost) treatment dropout of substance abusing or dependent delinquents through home-based multisystemic therapy. *American Journal of Psychiatry*, *153*, 427–428.

Henggeler, S. W., Rodick, J., Borduin, C. M., Hanson, C., Watson, S., & Urey, J. (1986). Multisystemic treatment of juvenile offenders: Effects on adolescent behavior and family interaction. *Developmental Psychology*, *22*, 132–141.

Henry, W. P. (1998). Science, politics and the politics of science: The use and misuse of empirically validated treatment research. *Psychotherapy Research*, *8*, 126–140.

Henry, W. P., Schacht, T. E., & Strupp, H. H. (1986). Structural analysis of social behavior: Application to a study of interpersonal process of differential therapeutic outcome. *Journal of Consulting and Clinical Psychology*, *54*, 27–31.

Henry, W. P., Schacht, T. E., Strupp, H. H., Buffer, S. F., & Binder, J. L. (1993a). Effects of training in time-limited psychotherapy: Mediators of therapists responses to training. *Journal of Consulting and Clinical Psychology*, *61*, 441–447.

Henry, W. P., Strupp, H. H., Butler, S. F., Schacht, T. E., & Binder, J. L. (1993b). The effects of training in time-limited psychotherapy: Changes in therapists behavior. *Journal of Consulting and Clinical Psychology*, *61*, 434–440.

Herceg-Baron, R. L., Prussoff, B. A., Wismann, M. M., DiMascio, A., Ney, C., & Klerman, G. L. (1979). Pharmacotherapy and psychotherapy in acutely depressed patients: A study of attrition patterns in a clinical trial. *Comprehensive Psychiatry*, *20*, 315–325.

Hersen, M., Bellack, A. S., Himmelhoch, J. M., & Thase, M. E. (1984). Effects of social skills training, amitriptyline and psychotherapy in unipolar depressed women. *Behavior Therapy*, *15*, 21–40.

Herz, M. I., Lamberti, J. S., Mintz, J., Scott, R., O'Dell, S. P., McCartan, L., et al. (2000). A program for relapse prevention in schizophrenia: A controlled study. *Archives of General Psychiatry*, *57*, 277–283.

Herzog, D. B., Greenwood, D. N., Dorer, D. J., Flores, A. T., Ekeblad, E. R., Richards, A., et al. (2000). Mortality in eating disorders: A descriptive study. *International Journal of Eating Disorders*, *28*, 20–26.

Herzog, D. B., Keller, M. B., Lavori, P. W., & Sacks, N. R. (1991). The course and outcome of bulimia nervosa. *Journal of Clinical Psychiatry*, *52*(Suppl. 10), 4–8.

Hickman, M., Cox, S., Harvey, J., Howes, S., Farrell, M., Frischer, M., et al. (1999). Estimating the prevalence of problem drug use in inner London: A discussion of three capture-recapture studies. *Addiction*, *94*(11), 1653–1662.

Higgins, S., Badger, G., & Budney, A. (2000). Initial abstinence and success in achieving longer term cocaine abstinence. *Experimental and Clinical Psychopharmacology*, *8*, 377–386.

Higgins, S., & Petry, N. M. (1999). Contingency management: Incentives for sobriety. *Alcohol Research and Health*, *23*(2), 122–127.

Higgins, S., Wong, C., Badger, G., Ogden, D., & Dantona, R. (2000). Contingent reinforcement increases cocaine abstinence during outpatient treatment and 1 year of follow-up. *Journal of Consulting and Clinical Psychology*, *68*, 64–72.

Higgins, S. T., Budney, A. J., Bickel, W. K., Badger, G. J., Foerg, F. E., & Ogden, D. (1995). Outpatient behavioral treatment for cocaine dependence: One-year outcome. *Experimental and Clinical Psychopharmacology, 3*, 205–212.

Higgins, S. T., Budney, A. J., Bickel, W. K., Foerg, F. E., Donham, R., & Badger, G. J. (1994). Incentives improve outcome in outpatient behavioral treatment of cocaine dependence. *Archives of General Psychiatry, 51*, 568–576.

Higgins, S. T., Budney, A. J., Bickel, W. K., Hughes, J. R., Foerg, F., & Badger, G. (1993). Achieving cocaine abstinence with a behavioral approach. *American Journal of Psychiatry, 150*, 763–769.

Higgitt, A. (1992). Dependency on prescribed drugs. *Reviews in Clinical Gerontology, 2*, 151–155.

Higgitt, A., & Fonagy, P. (1993). Psychotherapy in borderline and narcissistic personality disorder. In P. Tyrer & G. Stein (Eds.), *Personality disorder reviewed* (pp. 225–261). London: Gaskell.

Higgitt, A., & Fonagy, P. (2002). Clinical effectiveness. *British Journal of Psychiatry, 181*(2), 170–174.

Hilsenroth, M. J., Ackerman, S. J., & Blagys, M. D. (2001). Evaluating the phase model of change during short-term psychodynamic psychotherapy. *Psychotherapy Research, 11*, 29–47.

Hilsenroth, M. J., Ackerman, S. J., Clemence, A. J., Strassle, C. G., & Handler, L. (2002). Effects of structured clinician training on patient and therapist perspectives of alliance early in psychotherapy. *Psychotherapy: Theory, Research, Practice, Training, 39*, 309–323.

Himle, J. A., Rassi, S., Haghighatgou, H., Krone, K. P., Nesse, R. M., & Abelson, J. (2001). Group behavioral therapy of obsessive–compulsive disorder: Seven vs. twelve-week outcomes. *Depression and Anxiety, 13*(4), 161–165.

Hinshaw, S. P., Owens, E. B., Wells, K. C., Kraemer, H. C., Abikoff, H. B., Arnold, L. E., et al. (2000). Family processes and treatment outcome in the MTA: Negative/ineffective parenting practices in relation to multimodal treatment. *Journal of Abnormal Child Psychology, 28*(6), 555–568.

Hiss, H., Foa, E. B., & Kozac, M. J. (1994). Relapse prevention program for treatment of obsessive–compulsive disorder. *Journal of Consulting and Clinical Psychology, 62*, 801–808.

Hlastala, S., Frank, E., Mallinger, A. G., Thase, M. E., Ritenour, A. M., & Kupfer, D. J. (1997). Bipolar depression: An underestimated treatment challenge. *Depression and Anxiety, 5*, 73–83.

Hoath, F., & Sanders, M. (2002). A feasibility study of Enhanced Group Triple P—Positive parenting program for parents of children with attention-deficit/hyperactivity disorder. *Behaviour Change, 19*, 191–206.

Hobbs, M., Mayou, R., Harrison, B., & Worlock, P. (1996). A randomised controlled trial of psychological debriefing for victims of road traffic accidents. *British Medical Journal, 313*(7070), 1438–1439.

Hodgson, R., Rachman, S., & Marks, I. M. (1972). The treatment of chronic obsessive–compulsive neurosis: Follow-up and further findings. *Behaviour Research and Therapy, 10*, 181–189.

Hoeffer, B., Rader, J., McKenzie, D., Lavelle, M., & Stewart, B. (1997). Reducing aggressive behaviour during bathing cognitively impaired nursing home residents. *Journal of Gerontological Nursing, 23*(5), 16–23.

Hoek, H. W. (2002). Distribution of eating disorders. In C. G. Fairburn & K. D. Brownwell (Eds.), *Eating disorders and obesity: A comprehensive handbook* (2nd ed., pp. 233–237). New York: Guilford Press.

Hoffart, A., & Martinsen, E. W. (1993). The effects of personality disorders and anxious depressive comorbidity on outcome in patients with unipolar depression and with panic disorder and agoraphobia. *Journal of Personality Disorders, 7*, 304–311.

Hofmann, S. G., Newman, M. G., Becker, E., Taylor, C. B., & Roth, W. T. (1995). Social phobia with and without avoidant personality disorder: Preliminary behavior therapy outcome findings. *Journal of Anxiety Disorders, 9*, 427–438.

Hogarty, G., Anderson, C., Reiss, D., Kornblith, S. J., Greenwald, D., Javna, C., et al. (1986). Family psychoeducation, social skills training, and maintenance chemotherapy in the aftercare treatment of schizophrenia: I. One-year effects of a controlled study on relapse and expressed emotion. *Archives of General Psychiatry, 43*, 633–642.

Hogarty, G., Anderson, C. M., & Reiss, D. J. (1987). Family psychoeducation, social skills training and medication in schizophrenia: The long and short of it. *Psychopharmacology Bulletin, 23*, 12–13.

Hogarty, G. E., Greenwald, D., Ulrich, R. F., Kornblith, S. J., DiBarry, A. L., Cooley, S., et al. (1997a). Three-year trials of personal therapy among schizophrenic patients living with or independent of family: II. Effects on adjustment of patients. *American Journal of Psychiatry, 154*(11), 1514–1524.

Hogarty, G. E., Kornblith, S. J., Greenwald, D., DiBarry, A. L., Cooley, S., Ulrich, R. F., et al. (1997b). Three-year trials of personal therapy among schizophrenic patients living with or independent of family: I. Description of study and effects on relapse rates. *American Journal of Psychiatry, 154*(11), 1504–1513.

Hoglend, P. (1993). Transference interpretations and long-term change after dynamic psychotherapy of brief to moderate length. *American Journal of Psychotherapy, 47*, 494–507.

Hohagen, F., Winkelmann, G., Rasche-Ruchle, H., Hand, I., Konig, A., Munchau, N., et al. (1998). Combination of behaviour therapy with fluvoxamine in comparison with behaviour therapy and placebo: Results of a multicentre study. *British Journal of Psychiatry, 173*(Suppl. 35), 71–78.

Holden, G. W., Lavigne, V. V., & Cameron, A. M. (1990). Probing the continuum of effectiveness in parent training: Characteristics of parents and preschoolers. *Journal of Clinical Child Psychology, 19*, 2–8.

Holden, J. M., Sagovsky, R., & Cox, J. L. (1989). Counselling in a general practice setting: Controlled study of health visitor intervention in treatment of postnatal depression. *British Medical Journal, 298*, 223–226.

Holden, N. L. (1990). Is anorexia nervosa an obsessive–compulsive disorder? *British Journal of Psychiatry, 157*, 1–5.

Holden, U. P., & Woods, R. T. (1995). *Positive approaches to dementia care* (3rd ed.). Edinburgh: Churchill Livingstone.

Holder, H., Longabaugh, R., Miller, W. R., & Rubois, A. V. (1991). The cost-effectiveness of treatment for alcoholism: A first approximation. *Journal of Studies on Alcohol, 52*, 517–520.

Holen, A. (1990). *A long term outcome study of survivors from a disaster: The Alexander L. Kielland disaster in perspective.* Monograph, University of Oslo, Norway.

Hollander, E., Allen, A., Lopez, R. P., Bienstock, C. A., Grossman, R., Siever, L. J., et al. (2001). A preliminary double-blind, placebo-controlled trial of divalproex sodium in borderline personality disorder. *Journal of Clinical Psychiatry, 62*, 199–203.

Hollon, S. D., & Beck, A. T. (1994). Cognitive and cognitive-behavioral therapies. In A. E. Bergin & S. L. Garfield (Eds.), *Handbook of psychotherapy and behavior change* (4th ed., pp. 428–466). New York: Wiley.

Hollon, S. D., & DeRubeis, R. J. (1981). Placebo–psychotherapy combinations: Inappropriate representations of psychotherapy in drug–psychotherapy comparative trials. *Psychological Bulletin, 90*(3), 467–477.

Hollon, S. D., DeRubeis, R. J., Evans, M. D., Weimer, M. J., Garvey, M. J., Grove, W. M., et al. (1992). Cognitive therapy and pharmacotherapy for depression: Singly or in combination. *Archives of General Psychiatry, 49*, 774–781.

Hollon, S. D., & Shelton, R. C. (2002, June 25). *Cognitive therapy and the prevention of relapse in severely depressed outpatients.* Paper presented at 33rd Annual Meeting of the Society for Psychotherapy Research, Santa Barbara, CA.

Holmes, J. (2002). All you need is cognitive behaviour therapy? *British Medical Journal, 324*(7332), 288–290; discussion 290–294.

Honig, A., Hofman, A., Hilwig, M., Noorthoorn, E., & Ponds, R. (1995). Psycho-education and expressed emotion in bipolar disorder: Preliminary findings. *Psychiatry Research, 56,* 299–301.

Honig, A., Hofman, A., Rozendaal, N., & Dingemans, P. (1997). Psychoeducation in bipolar disorder: Effect on expressed emotion. *Psychiatry Research, 72,* 17–22.

Hood, K. K., & Eyberg, S. M. (2003). Outcomes of parent–child interaction therapy: Mothers' reports of maintenance three to six years after treatment. *Journal of Clinical Child and Adolescent Psychology, 32*(3), 419–429.

Hoogduin, C. A. L., Duivenvoorden, H., Schaap, C., & de Haan, E. (1989). On the outpatient treatment of obsessive–compulsives: Outcome, prediction of outcome and follow-up. In P. Emmelkamp, W. T. Evaraerd, F. Kraaimaaat & M. van Son (Eds.), *Fresh perspectives on anxiety disorders* (pp. 173–185). Amsterdam: Swets.

Hoogduin, C. A. L., & Duivenvoorden, H. J. (1988). A decision model in the treatment of obsessive–compulsive neurosis. *British Journal of Psychiatry, 152,* 516–521.

Hope, D. A., Heimberg, R. G., & Bruch, M. A. (1990). *The importance of cognitive interventions in the treatment of social phobia.* Paper presented at the annual meeting of the Phobia Society of America, Washington, DC.

Hope, D. A., Heimberg, R. G., & Bruch, M. A. (1995a). Dismantling cognitive-behavioral group therapy for social phobia. *Behaviour Research and Therapy, 33,* 637–650.

Hope, D. A., Herbert, J. D., & White, C. (1995b). Diagnostic subtype, avoidant personality disorder and efficacy of cognitive-behavioral group therapy for social phobia. *Cognitive Therapy and Research, 19,* 399–417.

Hopman-Rock, M., Staats, P. G. M., Tak, E. C. P. M., & Droes, R. M. (1999). The effects of a psychomotor activation programme for use in groups of cognitively impaired people in homes for the elderly. *International Journal of Geriatric Psychiatry, 14,* 633–642.

Horn, W. F., Ialongo, N. S., Pascoe, J. M., Greenberg, G., Packard, T., Lopez, M., Wagner, et al. (1991). Additive effects of psychostimulants, parent training, and self-control therapy with ADHD children. *Journal of the American Academy of Child and Adolescent Psychiatry, 30*(2), 233–240.

Horowitz, K., Weine, S., & Jekel, J. (1995). PTSD symptoms in urban adolescent girls: Compounded community trauma. *Journal of the American Academy of Child and Adolescent Psychiatry, 34*(10), 1353–1361.

Horowitz, L. M., Rosenberg, S., Ureñio, G., Kalehzan, B., & O'Halloran, P. (1989). Psychodynamic formulation, consensual response method and interpersonal problems. *Journal of Consulting and Clinical Psychology, 57,* 599–606.

Horowitz, L. M., Rosenberg, S. E., Baer, B., Ureñio, G., & Villaseñor, G. (1988). Inventory of interpersonal problems: Psychometric properties and clinical applications. *Journal of Consulting and Clinical Psychology, 56,* 885–892.

Horowitz, L. M., Rosenberg, S. E., & Bartholomew, K. (1993). Interpersonal problems, attachment styles and outcome in brief dynamic therapy. *Journal of Consulting and Clinical Psychology, 61,* 549–560.

Horowitz, M. J. (1989). Relationship schema formulation: Role relationship models and intrapsychic conflicts. *Psychiatry, 52,* 260–274.

Horowitz, M. J., Marmar, C., Weiss, D. S., DeWitt, K. N., & Rosenbaum, R. (1984). Brief psychotherapy of bereavement reactions: The relationship of process to outcome. *Archives of General Psychiatry, 41,* 438–448.

Horvath, A. O., Gaston, L., & Luborsky, L. (1993). The therapeutic alliance and its measures. In N. Miller, L. Luborsky, J. P. Barber, & J. P. Docherty (Eds.), *Psychodynamic treatment research: A handbook for clinical practice* (pp. 247–273). New York: Basic Books.

Horvath, A. O., & Symonds, B. D. (1991). Relation between working alliance and outcome in psychotherapy: A meta-analysis. *Journal of Consulting and Clinical Psychology, 38,* 139–149.

Horvath, A. T. (1993). Enhancing motivation for treatment of addictive behavior: Guidelines for the psychotherapist. *Psychotherapy Research, 30,* 473–480.

Howard, B. L., & Kendall, P. C. (1996). Cognitive-behavioral family therapy for anxiety-disordered children: A multiple-baseline evaluation. *Cognitive Therapy and Research, 20,* 423–443.

Howard, K. I., Cornille, T. A., Lyons, J. S., Vessey, J. T., Lueger, R. J., & Saunders, S. M. (1996). Patterns of mental health service utilization. *Archives of General Psychiatry, 53,* 696–703.

Howard, K. I., Krause, M. S., & Orlinsky, D. E. (1986). The dose–effect relationship in psychotherapy. *American Psychologist, 41,* 159–164.

Howard, K. I., Lueger, R. J., Marling, M. S., & Martinovich, Z. (1993). A phase model of psychotherapy outcome: Causal mediation of change. *Journal of Consulting and Clinical Psychology, 61,* 678–685.

Howard, R. C. (1999). Treatment of anxiety disorders: Does specialty training help? *Professional Psychology: Research and Practice, 30,* 470–473.

Howlin, P., Baron-Cohen, S., & Hadwin, J. (1999). *Teaching children with autism to mind-read: A practical guide.* Chichester, UK: Wiley.

Howlin, P., & Rutter, M. (1987). *Treatment of autistic children.* New York: Wiley.

Hsu, L., Rand, W., Sullivan, S., Liu, D., Mulliken, B., McDonagh, B., et al. (2001). Cognitive therapy, nutritional therapy and their combination in the treatment of bulimia nervosa. *Psychological Medicine, 31*(5), 871–879.

Huey, W. C., & Rank, R. C. (1984). Effects of counselor and peer-led group assertiveness training on black adolescent aggression. *Journal of Counseling Psychology, 31,* 95–98.

Hughes, G., Hogue, T., Hollin, C., & Champion, H. (1997). First-stage evaluation of a treatment programme for personality disordered offenders. *Journal of Forensic Psychiatry, 8,* 515–527.

Hughes, I., Hailwood, R., Abbati-Yeoman, J., & Budd, R. (1996). Developing a family intervention service for serious mental illness: Clinical observations and experiences. *Journal of Mental Health, 5,* 145–159.

Humphreys, K., & Weisner, C. (2000). Use of exclusion criteria in selecting research subjects and its effect on the generalizability of alcohol treatment outcome studies. *American Journal of Psychiatry, 57,* 588–594.

Hunsley, J. (2003). Cost-effectiveness and medical cost-offset considerations in psychological service provision. *Canadian Psychology, 44,* 61–73.

Hunt, G. M., & Azrin, N. H. (1973). A community reinforcement approach to alcoholism. *Behaviour Research and Therapy, 11,* 91–104.

Huppert, J. D., Bufka, L. F., Barlow, D. H., Gorman, J. M., Shear, M. K., & Woods, S. W. (2001). Therapists, therapist variables, and cognitive-behavioral therapy outcome in a multicenter trial for panic disorder. *Journal of Consulting and Clinical Psychology, 69*(5), 747–755.

Hurlbert, D. F. (1993). A comparative study using orgasm consistency training in the treatment of women reporting hypoactive sexual desire. *Journal of Sex and Marital Therapy, 19,* 41–55.

Hurlbert, D. F., White, L. C., Powell, R. D., & Apt, C. (1993). Orgasm consistency training in the treatment of women reporting hypoactive sexual desire: An outcome comparison of women-only groups and couples-only groups. *Journal of Behavior Therapy and Experimental Psychiatry, 24,* 3–13.

Husband, H. J. (1999). The psychological consequences of learning a diagnosis of dementia: three case examples. *Aging and Mental Health, 3*(2), 179–183.

Huxley, N. A., Rendall, M., & Sederer, L. (2000). Psychosocial treatments in schizophrenia: A review of the past 20 years. *Journal of Nervous and Mental Disease, 188*(4), 187–201.

Hyer, L., Woods, M. G., Bruno, R., & Boudewyns, P. (1989). Treatment outcomes of Vietnam veterans with PTSD and the consistency of the MCMI. *Journal of Clinical Psychology, 45,* 547–552.

Ialongo, N. S., Edelsohn, G., Werthamer-Larsson, L., Crockett, L., & Kellam, S. (1994). The significance of self-reported anxious symptoms in first-grade children. *Journal of Abnormal Child Psychology, 22,* 441–455.

Ialongo, N. S., Edelsohn, G., Werthamer-Larsson, L., Crockett, L., & Kellam, S. (1995). The significance of self-reported anxious symptoms in first-grade children: Prediction to anxious symptoms and adaptive functioning in fifth grade. *Journal of Child Psychology and Psychiatry, 36*, 427–437.

Ialongo, N. S., Horn, W. F., Pascoe, J. M., Greenberg, G., Packard, T., Lopez, M., et al. (1993). The effects of a multimodal intervention with attention-deficit hyperactivity disorder children: A 9-month follow-up. *Journal of the American Academy of Child and Adolescent Psychiatry, 32*(1), 182–189.

Iguchi, M. Y., Belding, M. A., Morral, A. R., Lamb, R. J., & Husband, S. D. (1997). Reinforcing operants other than abstinence in drug abuse treatment: An effective alternative for reducing drug use. *Journal of Consulting and Clinical Psychology, 65*(3), 421–428.

Iliffe, S., Haines, A., Gallivan, S., Booroff, A., Goldenberg, E., & Morgan, P. (1991). Assessment of elderly people in general practice: I. Social circumstances and mental state. *British Journal of General Practice, 41*, 9–12.

Ingenmey, R., & Van Houten, R. (1991). Using time delay to promote spontaneous speech in an autistic child. *Journal of Applied Behaviour Analysis, 24*, 591–596.

Inouye, D. K. (1983). Mental health care: Access, stigma and effectiveness. *American Psychologist, 38*, 912–917.

Ironson, G., Freund, B., Strauss, J., & Williams, J. (2002). Comparison of two treatments for traumatic stress: A community-based study of EMDR and prolonged exposure. *Journal of Clinical Psychology, 58*, 113–128.

Irvin, J. E., Bowers, C. A., Dunn, M. E., & Wang, M. C. (1999). Efficacy of relapse prevention: A meta-analytic review. *Journal of Consulting and Clinical Psychology, 67*(4), 563–570.

Ito, L. M., de Araujo, L. A., Tess, V. L., de Barros-Neto, T. P., Asbahr, F. R., & Marks, I. (2001). Self-exposure therapy for panic disorder with agoraphobia: Randomised controlled study of external v. interoceptive self-exposure. *British Journal of Psychiatry, 178*, 331–336.

Ito, L. M., Noshirvani, H., Basoglu, M., & Marks, I. M. (1996). Does exposure to internal cues enhance exposure to external cues in agoraphobia with panic? *Psychotherapy and Psychosomatics, 65*, 24–28.

Jacobi, C., Dahme, B., & Dittmann, R. (2002). Cognitive-behavioural, fluoxetine and combined treatment for bulimia nervosa: Short- and long-term results. *European Eating Disorders Review, 10*, 179–198.

Jacobson, N. S., Dobson, K., Fruzzetti, A. E., Schmaling, D. B., & Salusky, S. (1991). Marital therapy as a treatment for depression. *Journal of Consulting and Clinical Psychology, 59*, 547–557.

Jacobson, N. S., Follette, W. C., & Revenstorf, D. (1984). Psychotherapy outcome research: Methods for reporting variability and evaluating clinical significance. *Behavior Therapy, 15*, 336–352.

Jacobson, N. S., & Hollon, S. D. (1996a). Cognitive-behavior therapy versus pharmacotherapy: Now that the jury's returned its verdict, it's time to present the rest of the evidence. *Journal of Consulting and Clinical Psychology, 64*(1), 74–80.

Jacobson, N. S., & Hollon, S. D. (1996b). Prospects for future comparisons between drugs and psychotherapy: Lessons from the CBT-versus-pharmacotherapy exchange. *Journal of Consulting and Clinical Psychology, 64*(1), 104–108.

Jacobson, N. S., & Revenstorf, D. (1988). Statistics for assessing the clinical significance of psychotherapy techniques: Issues, problems and new developments. *Behavioral Assessment, 10*, 133–145.

Jacobson, N. S., & Truax, P. (1991). Clinical significance: A statistical approach to defining meaningful clinical change in psychotherapy research. *Journal of Consulting and Clinical Psychology, 59*, 12–19.

Jacobson, N. S., Wilson, L., & Upper, C. (1988). The clinical significance of treatment gains resulting from exposure-based interventions for agoraphobia: A re-analysis of outcome data. *Behavior Therapy, 19*, 539–554.

Jaffe, A. J., Rounsaville, B., Chang, G., Schottenfeld, R. S., Meyer, R. E., & O'Malley, S. S. (1996). Naltrexone, relapse prevention, and supportive therapy with alcoholics: An analysis of patient treatment matching. *Journal of Consulting and Clinical Psychology, 64*(5), 1044–1053.

Jakes, S., Rhodes, J., & Turner, T. (1999). Effectiveness of cognitive therapy for delusions in routine clinical practice. *British Journal of Psychiatry, 175,* 331–335.

James, I., & Blackburn, I. (1995). Cognitive therapy with obsessive–compulsive disorder. *British Journal of Psychiatry, 166,* 444–450.

James, I. A., Blackburn, I. M., Milne, D. L., & Reichfelt, F. K. (2001). Moderators of trainee therapists' competence in cognitive therapy. *British Journal of Clinical Psychology, 40*(Pt. 2), 131–141.

Jamison, C., & Scogin, F. (1995). The outcome of cognitive bibliotherapy with depressed adults. *Journal of Consulting and Clinical Psychology, 63*(4), 644–650.

Jansen, A., Broekmate, J., & Heymans, M. (1992). Cue exposure vs. self-control in the treatment of binge eating: A pilot study. *Behaviour Research and Therapy, 30,* 235–241.

Jansen, A., van den Hout, M. A., de Loof, C., Zandenbergen, J., & Griez, E. (1989). A case of bulimia successfully treated by cue exposure. *Journal of Behavior Therapy and Experimental Psychiatry, 20,* 327–332.

Jansson, L., & Öst, L. G. (1982). Behavioral treatments for agoraphobia: An evaluative review. *Clinical Psychology Review, 2,* 311–336.

Jarrett, R. B., Basco, M. R., Risser, R., Ramanan, J., Marwill, M., Kraft, D., et al. (1998). Is there a role for continuation phase cognitive therapy for depressed outpatients? *Journal of Consulting and Clinical Psychology, 66,* 1036–1040.

Jarrett, R. B., Kraft, D., Doyle, J., Foster, B. M., Eaves, G., & Silver, P. (2001). Preventing recurrent depression using cognitive therapy with and without a continuation phase: A randomized clinical trial. *Archives of General Psychiatry, 58,* 381–388.

Jarrett, R. B., & Maguire, M. A. (1991). *Short-term psychotherapy for depression.* Unpublished technical report commissioned by the Agency for Health Care Policy and Research (AHCPR) Depression Panel, Rockville, MD.

Jarrett, R. B., & Rush, A. J. (1994). Short-term psychotherapy of depressive disorders: Current status and future directions. *Psychiatry: Interpersonal and Biological Processes, 57,* 115–132.

Jarrett, R. B., Schaffer, M., McIntire, D., Witt-Browder, A., Kraft, D., & Risser, R. C. (1999). Treatment of atypical depression with cognitive therapy or phenelzine: A double-blind, placebo-controlled trial. *Archives of General Psychiatry, 56*(5), 431–437.

Jaycox, L. H., Reivich, K. J., Gillham, J. E., & Seligman, M. E. P. (1994). Prevention of depressive symptoms in schoolchildren. *Behavioural Research and Therapy, 32,* 801–816.

Jenike, M. A., Baer, L., Minichiello, W. E., Schwartz, C. E., & Carey, R. J. (1986a). Concomitant obsessive–compulsive disorder and schizotypal personality disorders. *American Journal of Psychiatry, 143,* 530–532.

Jenike, M. A., Baer, L., Minichiello, W. E., Schwartz, C. E., & Carey, R. J., Jr. (1986b). Coexistent obsessive–compulsive disorder and schizotypal personality disorder: A poor prognostic indicator. *Archives of General Psychiatry, 43*(3), 296.

Jenner, J., van de Willige, G., & Wiersma, D. (1998). Effectiveness of cognitive therapy with coping training for persistent auditory hallucinations: A retrospective study of attenders of a psychiatric out-patient department. *Acta Psychiatrica Scandinavica, 98,* 384–389.

Jensen, J. A. (1994). An investigation of eye-movement desensitization and reprocessing (EMD/R) as a treatment for posttraumatic stress disorder (PTSD) symptoms of Vietnam combat veterans. *Behavior Therapy, 25,* 311–325.

Jensen, P. S., Hinshaw, S. P., Kraemer, H. C., Lenora, N., Newcorn, J. H., Abikoff, H. B., et al. (2001). ADHD comorbidity findings from the MTA study: Comparing comorbid subgroups. *Journal of the American Academy of Child and Adolescent Psychiatry, 40*(2), 147–158.

Johnson, J. A. W. (1976). The duration of maintenance therapy in chronic schizophrenia. *Acta Psychiatrica Scandinavica, 53,* 298–301.

Johnson, S. L., & Roberts, J. E. (1995). Life events and bipolar disorder: Implications from biological theories. *Journal of Consulting and Clinical Psychology, 117*, 434–449.

Jones, D. (1990/1991). Weaning elderly patients off psychotropic drugs in general practice: A randomized controlled trial. *Health Trends, 22*, 164–166.

Jones, E. E., Cumming, J. D., & Horowitz, M. J. (1988). Another look at the nonspecific hypothesis of therapeutic effectiveness. *Journal of Consulting and Clinical Psychology, 56*, 48–55.

Jones, M. K., & Mezies, R. G. (1997). Danger ideation reduction therapy (DIRT): Preliminary findings with three obsessive–compulsive washers. *Behaviour Research and Therapy, 35*, 955–960.

Jones, M. K., & Mezies, R. G. (1998). Danger ideation reduction therapy (DIRT) for treatment resistant compulsive washers: A controlled trial. *Behaviour Research and Therapy, 36*, 959–970.

Joyce, A. S., Ogrodniczuk, J., Piper, W. E., & McCallum, M. (2002). A test of the phase model of psychotherapy change. *Canadian Journal of Psychiatry, 47*(8), 759–766.

Joyce, A. S., & Piper, W. E. (1998). Expectancy, the therapeutic alliance, and treatment outcome in short-term individual psychotherapy. *Journal of Psychotherapy Practice and Research, 7*, 236–248.

Judd, L. L., Akiskal, H. S., Maser, J. D., Zeller, P. J., Endicott, J., Coryell, W., et al. (1998a). Major depressive disorder: A prospective study of residual subthreshold depressive symptoms as predictor of rapid relapse. *Journal of Affective Disorders, 50*(2–3), 97–108.

Judd, L. L., Akiskal, H. S., Maser, J. D., Zeller, P. J., Endicott, J., Coryell, W., et al. (1998b). A prospective 12-year study of subsyndromal and syndromal depressive symptoms in unipolar major depressive disorders. *Archives of General Psychiatry, 55*(8), 694–700.

Judd, L. L., Paulus, M. J., Schettler, P. J., Akiskal, H. S., Endicott, J., Leon, A. C., et al. (2000). Does incomplete recovery from first lifetime major depressive episode herald a chronic course of illness? *American Journal of Psychiatry, 157*, 1501–1504.

Kadden, R. M. (2001). Behavioral and cognitive-behavioral treatments for alcoholism: Research opportunities. *Addictive Behaviors, 26*(4), 489–507.

Kadden, R. M., Cooney, N. L., Getter, H., & Litt, M. D. (1989). Matching alcoholics to coping skills or interactional therapies: Posttreatment results. *Journal of Consulting and Clinical Psychology, 57*(6), 698–704.

Kadden, R. M., Litt, M., Cooney, N., & Busher, D. (1992). Relationship between role-play measures of coping skills and alcoholism treatment outcome. *Addictive Behaviors, 17*(5), 425–437.

Kadden, R. M., Litt, M. D., Cooney, N. L., Kabela, E., & Getter, H. (2001). Prospective matching of alcoholic clients to cognitive-behavioral or interactional group therapy. *Journal of Studies on Alcohol, 62*(3), 359–369.

Kadera, S. W., Lambert, M. J., & Andrews, A. A. (1996). How much therapy is really enough?: A session-by-session analysis of the psychotherapy dose–effect relationship. *Journal of Psychotherapy: Practice and Research, 5*, 1–20.

Kahan, M., Wilson, L., & Becker, L. (1995). Effectiveness of physician-based interventions with problem drinkers: A review. *Canadian Medical Association Journal, 152*(6), 851–859.

Kahle, A. L., & Kelley, M. L. (1994). Children's homework problems: A comparison of goal setting and parent training. *Behavior Therapy, 25*, 275–290.

Kahn, D. A., Carpenter, D., Docherty, J. P., & Frances, A. (1996). The expert consensus guideline series: Treatment of bipolar disorder. *Journal of Clinical Psychiatry, 57*, 1–76.

Kaltenthaler, E., Parry, G., & Catherine, B. (2004). Computerised cognitive behaviour therapy: A systematic review. *Behavioural and Cognitive Psychotherapy, 32*, 31–55.

Kamlet, M., & Kleinman, L. (1999). Assessing the cost–utility of psychotherapy. In N. E. Miller & K. M. Magruder (Eds.), *Cost effectiveness of psychotherapy* (pp. 109–121). New York: Oxford University Press.

Kamlet, M., Paul, N., Greenhouse, J. G., Kupfer, D., Frank, E., & Wade, M. (1995). Cost utility analysis of maintenance treatment for recurrent depression. *Controlled Clinical Trials, 16*, 17–40.

Kane, J. M. (1996). Treatment resistant schizophrenic patients. *Journal of Clinical Psychiatry, 57*(Suppl. 9), 35–40.

Kang, S. Y., Kleinman, P. H., Woody, G. E., Millman, R. B., Todd, T. C., Kemp, J., et al. (1991). Outcomes for cocaine abusers after once-a-week psychosocial therapy. *American Journal of Psychiatry, 148*(5), 630–635.

Kaplan, A. S. (2002). Psychological treatments for anorexia nervosa: A review of published studies and promising new directions. *Canadian Journal of Psychiatry, 47*(3), 235–242.

Kaplan, H. S. (1974). *The new sex therapy.* New York: Times Books.

Kaplan, R. M., & Groessl, E. J. (2002). Applications of cost-effectiveness methodologies in behavioral medicine. *Journal of Consulting and Clinical Psychology, 70,* 482–493.

Karel, M. J., & Hinrichsen, G. (2000). Treatment of depression in late life: Psychotherapeutic interventions. *Clinical Psychology Review, 20,* 707–729.

Karno, M., & Golding, J. M. (1991). Obsessive–compulsive disorder. In L. N. Robins & D. A. Reiger (Eds.), *Psychiatric disorders in America: The Epidemiologic Catchment Area study* (pp. 204–219). New York: Free Press.

Karno, M., Golding, J. M., Sorenson, S. B., & Burnham, M. A. (1988). The epidemiology of OCD in five US communities. *Archives of General Psychiatry, 45,* 1094–1099.

Karterud, S., Pedersen, G., Bjordal, E., Brabrand, J., Friis, S., Haaseth, O., et al. (2003). Day treatment of patients with personality disorders: Experiences from a Norwegian treatment research network. *Journal of Personality Disorders, 17*(3), 243–262.

Kashner, T. M., & Rush, A. J. (1999). Measuring medical offsets of psychotherapy. In N. E. Miller & K. M. Magruder (Eds.), *Cost effectiveness of psychotherapy* (pp. 109–121). New York: Oxford University Press.

Kasl-Godley, J., & Gatz, M. (2000). Psychosocial interventions for individuals with dementia: An integration of theory, therapy, and a clinical understanding of dementia. *Clinical Psychology Review, 20,* 755–782.

Kasvikis, Y., Bradley, B., Powell, J., Marks, I., & Gray, J. A. (1991). Postwithdrawal exposure treatment to prevent relapse in opiate addicts: A pilot study. *International Journal of Addiction, 26*(11), 1187–1195.

Kasvikis, Y., & Marks, I. M. (1988). Clomipramine, self-exposure and therapist accompanied exposure in obsessive–compulsive ritualizers: Two year follow-up. *Journal of Anxiety Disorders, 2,* 291–298.

Katon, W., Von Korff, M., Lin, E., Walker, E., Simon, G., & Bush, T. (1999). Collaborative management to achieve treatment guidelines: Impact on depression in primary care. *Journal of American Medical Association, 273,* 1026–1031.

Katon, W. J. (1991). Psychiatry and primary care. *General Hospital Psychiatry, 13,* 9–13.

Katz, E. C., Gruber, K., Chutuape, M. A., & Stitzer, M. L. (2001). Reinforcement-based outpatient treatment for opiate and cocaine abusers. *Journal of Substance Abuse Treatment, 20*(1), 93–98.

Kazdin, A. E. (1986). Comparative outcome studies of psychotherapy: Methodological issues and strategies. *Journal of Consulting and Clinical Psychology, 54,* 95–105.

Kazdin, A. E. (1991). Treatment research: The investigation and evaluation of psychotherapy. In M. Hersen, A. E. Kazdin & A. S. Bellack (Eds.), *The clinical psychology handbook* (2nd ed., pp. 293–312). New York: Wiley.

Kazdin, A. E. (1994a). Methodology, design and evaluation in psychotherapy research. In A. E. Bergin & S. L. Garfield (Eds.), *Handbook of psychotherapy and behavior change* (4th ed., pp. 19–71). New York: Wiley.

Kazdin, A. E. (1994b). Psychotherapy for children and adolescents. In A. E. Bergin & S. L. Garfield (Eds.), *Handbook of psychotherapy and behavior change* (4th ed., pp. 543–594). New York: Wiley.

Kazdin, A. E. (1995a). Child, parent, and family dysfunction as predictors of outcome in cognitive-behavioural treatment of antisocial children. *Behavioural Research and Therapy, 33,* 271–281.

Kazdin, A. E. (1995b). *Conduct disorder in childhood and adolescence* (2nd ed.). Thousand Oaks, CA: Sage.

Kazdin, A. E. (1996). Problem solving and parent management in treating aggressive and anti-social behaviour. In E. S. Hibbs & P. S. Jensen (Eds.), *Psychosocial treatments for child and adolescent disorders: Empirically based strategies for clinical practice* (pp. 377–408). Washington, DC: American Psychological Association.

Kazdin, A. E. (1997). A model for developing effective treatments: Progression and interplay of theory, research, and practice. *Journal of Clinical Child Psychology, 26*, 114–129.

Kazdin, A. E. (2004). Psychotherapy for children and adolescents. In M. Lambert (Ed.), *Bergin and Garfield's handbook of psychotherapy and behavior change* (5th ed., pp. 543–589). New York: Wiley.

Kazdin, A. E., Holland, L., & Crowley, M. (1997). Family experience of barriers to treatment and premature termination from child therapy. *Journal of Consulting and Clinical Psychology, 65*, 453–463.

Kazdin, A. E., & Kendall, P. C. (1998). Current progress and future plans for developing effective treatments: Comments and perspectives. *Journal of Clinical Child Psychology, 27*, 217–226.

Kazdin, A. E., Mazurick, J. L., & Siegel, T. C. (1994). Treatment outcome among children with externalizing disorder who terminate prematurely versus those who complete psychotherapy. *Journal of the American Academy of Child and Adolescent Psychiatry, 33*, 549–557.

Kazdin, A. E., & Nock, M. K. (2003). Delineating mechanisms of change in child and adolescent therapy: Methodological issues and research recommendations. *Journal of Child Psychology and Psychiatry, 44*(8), 1116–1129.

Kazdin, A. E., Siegel, T. C., & Bass, D. (1992). Cognitive problem-solving skills training and parent management training in the treatment of antisocial behavior in children. *Journal of Consulting and Clinical Psychology, 60*, 733–747.

Kazdin, A. E., & Wasser, G. (2000). Therapeutic changes in children, parents and families resulting from treatment of children with conduct problems. *Journal of the American Academy of Child and Adolescent Psychiatry, 39*(4), 414–420.

Keane, T. M., Fairbank, J. A., Caddell, J. M., & Zimering, R. T. (1989). Implosive therapy reduces symptoms of PTSD in Vietnam combat veterans. *Behavior Therapy, 20*, 245–260.

Keck, P. E., & McElroy, S. L. (2002). Carbamazepine and Valproate in the maintenance treatment of bipolar disorder. *Journal of Clinical Psychiatry, 63*(Suppl. 10), 13–17.

Keel, P. K., & Mitchell, J. E. (1997). Outcome in bulimia nervosa. *American Journal of Psychiatry, 154*(3), 313–321.

Keel, P. K., Mitchell, J. E., Miller, K. B., Davis, T. L., & Crow, S. J. (1999). Long-term outcome of bulimia nervosa. *Archives of General Psychiatry, 56*(1), 63–69.

Keisjers, G. P. J., Hoogduin, C. A. L., & Schaap, C. P. D. (1994). Predictors of treatment outcome in the behavioral treatment of obsessive–compulsive disorder. *British Journal of Psychiatry, 165*, 781–786.

Keller, M., McCullough, J., Klein, D., Arnow, B., Dunner, D., Gelenberg, A., et al. (2000). A comparison of nefazodone, the cognitive behavioral analysis system of psychotherapy, and their combination for the treatment of chronic depression. *New England Journal of Medicine, 342*(20), 1462–1470.

Keller, M. B., Lavori, P. W., Endicott, J., Coryell, W., & Klerman, G. L. (1983). Double depression: Two year follow-up. *American Journal of Psychiatry, 140*, 689–694.

Keller, M. B., Lavori, P. W., Friedman, B. L., Nielson, E., McDonald-Scott, P., Andreason, N. C., et al. (1987). The LIFE-II: A comprehensive method for assessing outcome in prospective longitudinal studies. *Archives of General Psychiatry, 44*, 540–549.

Keller, M. B., Lavori, P. W., Wunder, J., Beardslee, W. R., Schwartz, C. E., & Roth, J. (1992). Chronic course of anxiety disorders in children and adolescents. *Journal of the American Academy of Child and Adolescent Psychiatry, 31*(4), 595–599.

Keller, M. B., & Shapiro, R. W. (1982). Double depression: Superimposition of acute depressive episodes on chronic depressive disorders. *American Journal of Psychiatry, 139*, 438–442.

Kelly, T., Soloff, P. H., Cornelius, J., George, A., Lis, J. A., & Ulrich, R. (1992). Can we study (treat) borderline patients?: Attrition from research and open treatment. *Journal of Personality Disorders, 6*, 417–433.

Kemp, R., David, A., & Hayward, P. (1996). Compliance therapy: An intervention targeting insight and treatment adherence in psychotic patients. *Behavioural and Cognitive Psychotherapy, 24*, 331–350.

Kemp, R., Kirov, G., Everitt, B., Hayward, P., & David, A. (1998). Randomised controlled trial of compliance therapy: 18-month follow-up. *British Journal of Psychiatry, 172*, 413–419.

Kendall, P. C. (1993). Cognitive-behavioral therapies with youth: Guiding theory, current status and emerging developments. *Journal of Consulting and Clinical Psychology, 61*, 235–247.

Kendall, P. C. (1998). Empirically supported psychological therapies. *Journal of Consulting and Clinical Psychology, 66*, 3–6.

Kendall, P. C., Brady, E., & Verduin, T. (2001). Comorbidity in childhod anxiety disorders and treatment outcome. *Journal of the American Academy Child and Adolescent Psychiatry, 40*, 787–794.

Kendall, P. C., Flannery-Schroeder, E., Panichelli-Mindel, S. M., Southam-Gerow, M. A., Henin, A., & Warman, M. (1997). Therapy for youths with anxiety disorders: A second randomized clinical trial. *Journal of Consulting and Clinical Psychology, 65*, 366–380.

Kendall, R. E. (1993). Schizophrenia: Clinical features. In R. Michels (Ed.), *Psychiatry* (Vol. 1, Section 53). Philadelphia: Lippincott.

Kendall, T., Pilling, S., Barnes, T., Garety, P., et al. (2003). *Core interventions in the treatment and management of schizophrenia in primary and secondary care.* London: Gaskell.

Kendall-Tackett, K. A., Williams, L. M., & Finkelhor, D. (1993). Impact of sexual abuse on children: A review and synthesis of recent empirical studies. *Psychological Bulletin, 113*(1), 164–180.

Kessler, R. C. (2000). The epidemiology of pure and comorbid generalized anxiety disorder: A review and evaluation of recent research. *Acta Psychiatrica Scandinavica,* (Suppl. 406), 7–13.

Kessler, R. C., McGonagle, K. A., Zhao, S., Nelson, C. B., Hughes, M., Eshleman, S., et al. (1994). Lifetime and 12-month prevalence of DSM-III-R psychiatric disorders in the United States. *Archives of General Psychiatry, 51*, 8–19.

Kessler, R. C., Merikangas, K. R., Berglund, P., Eaton, W. W., Koretz, D. S., & Walters, E. E. (2003). Mild disorders should not be eliminated from the DSM-V. *Archives of General Psychiatry, 60*, 1117–1122.

Kessler, R. C., Nelson, C. B., McGonagle, K. A., Liu, J., Swartz, M., & Blazer, D. G. (1996). Comorbidity of DSM-III-R major depressive disorder in the general population: results from the US National Comorbidity Survey. *British Journal of Psychiatry, 168*(Suppl. 30), 17–30.

Kessler, R. C., Sonnega, A., Bromet, E., Hughes, M., & Nelson, C. B. (1995). Post-traumatic stress disorder in the National Comorbidity Survey. *Archives of General Psychiatry, 52*, 1048–1060.

Kessler, R. C., Stang, P., Wittchen, H. U., Stein, M., & Walters, E. E. (1999). Lifetime comorbidities between social phobia and mood disorders in the US National Comorbidity Survey. *Psychological Medicine, 29*(3), 555–567.

Kienhorst, C. W., De Wilde, E. J., Van den Bout, J., Diekstra, R. F., & Wolters, W. H. (1990). Characteristics of suicide attempters in a population-based sample of Dutch adolescents. *British Journal of Psychiatry, 156*, 243–248.

Kilmann, P. R., & Auerbach, R. (1979). Treatments of premature ejaculation and psychogenic impotence: A critical review of the literature. *Archives of Sexual Behavior, 8*, 81–100.

Kilmann, P. R., Milan, R. J., Boland, J. P., Nankin, H. R., Davidson, E., West, M. O., et al. (1987). Group treatment of secondary erectile dysfunction. *Journal of Sex and Marital Therapy, 13*, 168–182.

Kilmann, P. R., Mills, K. H., Caid, C., Davidson, E., Bella, B., Milan, R., et al. (1986). Treatment of secondary orgasmic dysfunction: An outcome study. *Archives of Sexual Behavior, 15*, 211–229.

Kilpatrick, D. G., & Resnick, H. S. (1993). PTSD associated with exposure to criminal victimization in clinical and community populations. In J. R. T. Davidson & E. B. Foa (Eds.), *PTSD in review: DSM-IV and beyond*. Washington, DC: American Psychiatric Press.

Kim-Cohen, J., Caspi, A., Moffitt, T. E., Harrington, H.-L., & Milne, B. J., & Poulton, R. (2003). Prior juvenile diagnoses in adults with mental disorder: Developmental followback of a prospective longitudinal cohort. *Archives of General Psychiatry, 60*, 709–717.

Kinder, B. N., & Curtiss, G. (1988). Specific components in the etiology, assessment and treatment of male sexual dysfunctions: Controlled outcome studies. *Journal of Sex and Marital Therapy, 14*, 40–48.

King, C. A., & Kirschenbaum, D. S. (1990). An experimental evaluation of a school-based program for children-at-risk: Wisconsin early intervention. *Journal of Community Psychology, 18*, 167–177.

King, M. B. (1989). Eating disorders in a general practice population: Prevalence, characteristics, and follow-up at 12 to 18 months. *Psychological Medicine, 22*, 951–959.

King, M. B. (1991). The natural history of eating pathology in attenders to primary care. *International Journal of Eating Disorders, 10*, 379–387.

King, N. J., Tonge, B. J., Heyne, D., Turner, S. M., Pritchard, M., Young, D., et al. (2001a). Cognitive-behavioural treatment of school-refusing children: Maintenance of improvement at 3- to 5-year follow-up. *Scandinavian Journal of Behaviour Therapy, 30*, 85–89.

King, N. J., Heyne, D., Gullone, E., & Molloy, G. N. (2001b). Usefulness of emotive imagery in the treatment of childhood phobias: Clinical guidelines, case examples and issues. *Counselling Psychology Quarterly, 14*, 95–101.

King, N. J., & Ollendick, T. H. (1997). Annotation: Treatment of childhood phobias. *Journal of Child Psychology and Psychiatry, 38*, 389–400.

King, N. J., Tonge, B. J., Heyne, D., Pritchard, M., Rollings, S., Young, D., et al. (1998). Cognitive-behavioral treatment of school-refusing children: A controlled evaluation. *Journal of the American Academy of Child and Adolescent Psychiatry, 37*, 395–403.

King, V. L., Kidorf, M. S., Stoller, K. B., Carter, J. A., & Brooner, R. K. (2001). Influence of antisocial personality subtypes on drug abuse treatment response. *Journal of Nervous and Mental Disease, 189*(9), 593–601.

Kirby, K. C., Marlowe, D. B., Festinger, D. S., Garvey, K. A., & La Monaca, V. (1999). Community reinforcement training for family and significant others of drug abusers: A unilateral intervention to increase treatment entry of drug users. *Drug and Alcohol Dependence, 56*(1), 85–96.

Kirby, K. C., Marlowe, D. B., Festinger, D. S., Lamb, R. J., & Platt, J. J. (1998). Schedule of voucher delivery influences initiation of cocaine abstinence. *Journal of Consulting and Clinical Psychology, 66*(5), 761–767.

Kirk, J. W. (1983). Behavioral treatment of obsessive–compulsive patients in routine clinical practice. *Behaviour Research and Therapy, 21*, 57–62.

Kirley, B. G., Schneider, J. A., Agras, W. S., & Bachman, J. A. (1985). Comparison of two group treatments for bulimia. *Journal of Consulting and Clinical Psychology, 53*, 43–48.

Kissin, B., & Gross, M. M. (1968). Drug therapy in alcoholism. *American Journal of Psychiatry, 125*, 31–41.

Kissin, B., Platz, A., & Su, W. H. (1970). Social and psychological factors in the treatment of chronic alcoholism. *Journal of Psychiatric Research, 8*, 13–27.

Kitwood, T. (1993). Towards a theory of dementia care: the interpersonal process. *Ageing and Society, 13*, 51–67.

Klein, D. F. (1990). NIMH Collaborative Research on Treatment of Depression [Letter]. *Archives of General Psychiatry, 47*, 683–685.

Klein, D. F. (1996). Preventing hung juries about therapy studies. *Journal of Consulting and Clinical Psychology, 64*(1), 81–87.

Klein, D. N., & Hayden, E. P. (2000). Dysthymic disorder: Current status and future directions. *Current Opinion in Psychiatry*, *13*, 171–177.

Klein, D. N., Lewinsohn, P. M., & Seeley, J. R. (1997). Psychosocial characteristics of adolescents with a past history of dysthymic disorder: Comparison with adolescents with past histories of major depressive and non-affective disorders, and never mentally ill controls. *Journal of Affective Disorder*, *42*, 127–135.

Klein, D. N., Schwartz, J. E., Rose, S., & Leader, J. B. (2000). Five-year course and outcome of dysthymic disorder: A prospective, naturalistic follow-up study. *American Journal of Psychiatry*, *157*(6), 931–939.

Klein, D. N., Schwartz, J. E., Santiago, N. J., Vivian, D., Vocisano, C., Castonguay, L. G., et al. (2003). Therapeutic alliance in depression treatment: Controlling for prior change and patient characteristics. *Journal of Consulting and Clinical Psychology*, *71*(6), 997–1006.

Klerman, G. L. (1983). The efficacy of psychotherapy as the basis for public policy. *American Psychologist*, *38*, 929–934.

Klerman, G. L., & Weissman, M. M. (1989). Increasing rates of depression. *Journal of the American Medical Association*, *261*, 2229–2235.

Klerman, G. L., Weissman, M. M., Markowitz, J., Glick, I., Wilner, P., Mason, B., et al. (1994). Medication and psychotherapy. In A. E. Bergin & S. L. Garfield (Eds.), *Handbook of psychotherapy and behavior change* (4th ed., pp. 734–782). New York: Wiley.

Klerman, G. L., Weissman, M. M., Rounsaville, B. J., & Chevron, E. S. (1984). *Interpersonal therapy of depression*. New York: Basic Books.

Kliewer, W., Lepore, S. J., Oskin, D., & Johnson, P. D. (1998). The role of social and cognitive processes in children's adjustment to community violence. *Journal of Consulting and Clinical Psychology*, *66*(1), 199–209.

Klosko, J. S., Barlow, D. H., Tassinari, R., & Cerny, J. A. (1990). A comparison of alprazolam and behavior therapy in treatment of panic disorder. *Journal of Consulting and Clinical Psychology*, *58*, 77–84.

Kluznik, J. C., Speed, N., Van Valkenburg, C., & Magraw, R. (1986). 40 year follow-up of United States prisoners of war. *American Journal of Psychiatry*, *143*, 1443–1446.

Knapp, M., & Healey, A. (1999). Psychotherapy: Individual differences in costs and outcomes. In N. E. Miller & K. M. Magruder (Eds.), *Cost effectiveness of psychotherapy* (pp. 122–133). New York: Oxford University Press.

Knight, B. G. (1988). Factors influencing therapist-rated change in older adults. *Journal of Gerontology*, *43*, 111–112.

Kobak, K. A., Greist, J. H., Jefferson, J. W., Katzelnick, D. J., & Henk, H. J. (1998). Behavioral versus pharmacological treatments of obsessive compulsive disorder: A meta-analysis. *Psychopharmacology (Berlin)*, *136*(3), 205–216.

Kocakulah, M. C., & Valadares, K. J. (2003). Cost offset effect strategies for the provision of mental health care services. *Journal of Health Care Finance*, *30*, 31–40.

Koder, D. A., Brodaty, H., & Anstey, K. J. (1996). Cognitive therapy for depression in the elderly. *International Journal of Geriatric Psychiatry*, *11*(2), 97–107.

Kohler, F. W., Strain, P. S., Hoyson, M., Davis, L., Donina, W. M., & Rapp, N. (1995). Using a group-oriented contingency to increase social interactions between children with autism and their peers. *Behaviour Modification*, *19*, 10–32.

Kohut, H. (1977). *The restoration of the self*. New York: International Universities Press.

Kok, A. J., Kong, T. Y., & Bernard-Opitz, V. (2002). A comparison of the effects of structured play and facilitated play approaches on preschoolers with autism: A case study. *Autism*, *6*(2), 181–196.

Kokotovic, A. M., & Tracey, T. J. (1990). Working alliance in the early phase of counselling. *Journal of Counselling Psychology*, *37*, 16–21.

Kolada, J. L., Bland, R. C., & Newman, S. C. (1994). Obsessive–compulsive disorder. *Acta Pyschiatrica Scandinavica* (Suppl. 376), 24–35.

Koons, C. R., Robins, C. J., Tweed, J. L., Lynch, T. R., Gonzalez, A. M., Morse, J. Q., et al.

(2001). Efficacy of dialectical behavior therapy in women veterans with borderline personality disorder. *Behavior Therapy, 32*, 371–390.

Kopta, S. M., Howard, K. I., Lowry, J. L., & Beutler, L. E. (1994). Patterns of symptomatic recovery in psychotherapy. *Journal of Consulting and Clinical Psychology, 62*(5), 1009–1016.

Kornblith, S. J., Rehm, L. P., O'Hara, M. W., & Lamparski, D. M. (1983). The contribution of self-reinforcement training and behavioral assignments to the efficacy of self-control therapy for depression. *Cognitive Therapy and Research, 7*, 499–528.

Kottgen, C., Sonnichsen, I., Mollenhauser, K., & Jurth, R. (1984). Group therapy with families of schizophrenia patients: Results of the Hamburg Camberwell family interview study III. *International Journal of Family Psychiatry, 5*, 84–94.

Kovacs, M., & Devlin, B. (1998). Internalizing disorders in childhood. *Journal of Child Psychology and Psychiatry, 39*, 47–63.

Kovacs, M., Obrosky, S., Gatsonis, C., & Richards, C. (1997). First episode of major depressive and dysthymic disorder in childhood: Clinical and socio-demographic factors in recovery. *Journal of the American Academy of Child and Adolescent Psychiatry, 36*, 777–784.

Kovacs, M., Rush, A. J., Beck, A. T., & Hollon, S. D. (1981). Depressed outpatients treated with cognitive therapy and pharmacotherapy: A one year follow-up. *Archives of General Psychiatry, 38*, 33–39.

Kozac, M. J., Lieboowitz, M. R., & Foa, E. B. (2000). Cognitive behavior therapy and pharmacotherapy for OCD: The NIMH-ponsored colloaborative study. In W. Goodman, M. Rudorfer & J. Maser (Eds.), *Obsessive–compulsive disorder: Contemporary issues in treatment* (pp. 501–530). Mahwah, NJ: Erlbaum.

Kraft, M. K., Rothbard, A. B., Hadley, T. R., McLellan, A. T., & Asch, D. A. (1997). Are supplementary services provided during methadone maintenance really cost-effective? *American Journal of Psychiatry, 154*(9), 1214–1219.

Kranzler, H. R., & Van Kirk, J. (2001). Efficacy of naltrexone and acamprosate for alcoholism treatment: A meta-analysis. *Alcoholism: Clinical and Experimental Research, 25*(9), 1335–1341.

Kraus, L., Augustin, R., Frischer, M., Kummler, P., Uhl, A., & Wiessing, L. (2003). Estimating prevalence of problem drug use at national level in countries of the European Union and Norway. *Addiction, 98*(4), 471–485.

Krauskopf, C., Baumgardner, A., & Mandraccia, S. (1981). Return rate following intake revisited. *Journal of Counselling Psychology, 28*, 519–521.

Kripke, D., & Robinson, D. (1985). Ten years with a lithium group. *McLean Hospital Journal, 10*, 1–11.

Kristenson, H., Ohlin, H., Hulten-Nosslin, M. B., Trell, E., & Hood, B. (1983). Identification and intervention of heavy drinking in middle-aged men: Results and follow-up of 24–60 months of long-term study with randomized controls. *Alcoholism: Clinical and Experimental Research, 7*, 203–209.

Krochmalik, A., Jones, M. K., & Mezies, R. G. (2001). Danger ideation reduction therapy (DIRT) for treatment resistant compulsive washing. *Behaviour Research and Therapy, 39*, 897–912.

Kroll, L., Harrington, R., Jayson, D., Fraser, J., & Gowers, S. (1996). Pilot study of continuation cognitive-behavioral therapy for major depression in adolescent psychiatric patients. *Journal of the American Academy of Child and Adolescent Psychiatry, 35*, 1156–1161.

Krupnick, J. L., Sotsky, S. M., Simmens, S., Moyer, J., Elkin, I., Watkins, J., et al. (1996). The role of the therapeutic alliance in psychotherapy and pharmacotherapy outcome: Findings in the National Institute of Mental Health Treatment of Depression Collaborative Research Program. *Journal of Consulting and Clinical Psychology, 64*(3), 532–539.

Krystal, J. H., Cramer, J. A., Krol, W. F., Kirk, G. F., & Rosenheck, R. A. (2001). Naltrexone in the treatment of alcohol dependence. *New England Journal of Medicine, 345*(24), 1734–1739.

Kuipers, E., & Bebbington, P. (1988). Expressed emotion research in schizophrenia: Theoretical and clinical implications. *Psychological Medicine, 18*, 893–909.

Kuipers, E., Fowler, D., Garety, P., Chisholm, D., Freeman, D., Dunn, G., et al. (1998). London–East Anglia randomised controlled trial of cognitive-behavioural therapy for psychosis: III. Follow-up and economic evaluation at 18 months. *British Journal of Psychiatry, 173,* 61–68.

Kuipers, E., Garety, P., Fowler, D., Dunn, G., Bebbington, P., Freeman, D., et al. (1997). London–East Anglia randomised controlled trial of cognitive-behavioural therapy for psychosis: I. Effects of the treatment phase. *British Journal of Psychiatry, 171,* 319–327.

Kukla, A. (1989). Nonempirical issues in psychology. *American Psychologist, 44,* 785–794.

Kupfer, D. J., Frank, E., Perel, J. M., Cornes, Mallinger, A. G., Thase, M. E., et al. (1992). Five year outcome for maintenance therapies in recurrent depression. *Archives of General Psychiatry, 49,* 769–773.

Kuruvilla, K. (1984). Treatment of single impotent males. *Indiana Journal of Psychology, 26,* 160–163.

Kusumakar, V. (2002). Antidepressants and antipsychotics in the long-term treatment of bipolar disorder. *Journal of Clinical Psychiatry, 63*(Suppl. 10), 23–28.

Kuyken, W., Kurzer, N., DeRubeis, R. J., Beck, A. T., & Brown, G. K. (2001). Response to cognitive therapy in depression: The role of maladaptive beliefs and personality disorders. *Journal of Consulting and Clinical Psychology, 69*(3), 560–566.

Lacey, J. H. (1983). Bulimia nervosa, binge eating and psychogenic vomiting: A controlled treatment study and long-term outcome. *British Medical Journal, 286,* 1609–1613.

LaCrosse, M. B. (1980). Perceived counsellor social influence and counselling outcomes: Validity of the counsellor rating form. *Journal of Consulting and Clinical Psychology, 27,* 320–327.

Ladouceur, R., Dugas, M. J., Freeston, M. H., Leger, E., Gagnon, F., & Thibodeau, N. (2000). Efficacy of a cognitive-behavioral treatment for generalized anxiety disorder: Evaluation in a controlled clinical trial. *Journal of Consulting and Clinical Psychology, 68*(6), 957–964.

Laessle, R. G., Kittl, S., & Fichter, M. (1987a). Major affective disorders in anorexia nervosa and bulimia: A descriptive diagnostic study. *Psychiatry, 151,* 785–789.

Laessle, R. G., Zoettl, C., & Pirke, K.-M. (1987b). Meta-analysis of treatment studies for bulimia. *International Journal of Eating Disorders, 5,* 647–653.

Lafferty, P., Beutler, L. E., & Crago, M. (1989). Differences between more and less effective psychotherapists: A study of select therapist variables. *Journal of Consulting and Clinical Psychology, 57*(1), 76–80.

Lahey, B. B., & Carlson, C. (1992). Validity of the diagnostic category of attention deficit disorder without hyperactivity: A review of the literature. In S. E. Shaywitz & B. A. Shaywitz (Eds.), *Attention deficit disorder comes of age: Toward the twenty-first century* (pp. 119–144). Austin, TX: Pro-Ed.

Lam, D., Bright, J., Jones, S., Hayward, P., Schuck, N., Chisholm, D., et al. (2000). Cognitive therapy for bipolar illness—a pilot study of relapse prevention. *Cognitive Therapy and Research, 24*(5), 503–520.

Lam, D., Wong, G., & Sham, P. (2001). Prodromes, coping strategies and course of illness in bipolar affective disorder—a naturalistic study. *Psychological Medicine, 31*(8), 1397–1402.

Lam, D., Wright, K., & Smith, N. (2004). Dysfunctional assumptions in bipolar disorder. *Journal of Affective Disorders, 79,* 193–199.

Lam, D. H. (1991). Psychosocial family intervention in schizophrenia: A review of empirical studies. *Psychological Medicine, 21,* 423–441.

Lam, D. H., Jones, S., Bright, J., & Hayward, P. (1999). *Cognitive therapy for bipolar disorder: A therapist's guide to concepts, methods and practice.* New York: Wiley.

Lam, D. H., Watkins, E. R., Hayward, P., Bright, J., Wright, K., Kerr, N., et al. (2003). A randomized controlled study of cognitive therapy for relapse prevention for bipolar affective disorder: Outcome of the first year. *Archives of General Psychiatry, 60*(2), 145–152.

Lam, D. H., & Wong, G. (1997). Prodromes, coping strategies, insight and social functioning in bipolar affective disorders. *Psychological Medicine, 27,* 1091–1100.

Lam, D. H., & Woods, R. T. (1986). Ward orientation training in dementia: A single-case study. *International Journal of Geriatric Psychiatry, 1,* 145–147.

Lambert, M. J. (2001). Psychotherapy outcome and quality improvement: Introduction to the special section on client-focused research. *Journal of Consulting and Clinical Psychology, 69,* 147–149.

Lambert, M. J., Burlinghame, G. M., Umphress, V. J., Hansen, N. B., Vermeersch, D., Clouse, G., et al. (1996). The reliability and validity of the Outcome Questionnaire. *Clinical Psychology and Psychotherapy, 3,* 106–116.

Lambert, M. J., Hansen, N. B., & Finch, A. E. (2001a). Patient-focused research: Using patient outcome data to enhance treatment effects. *Journal of Consulting and Clinical Psychology, 69*(2), 159–172.

Lambert, M. J., Whipple, J. L., Hawkins, E. J., Vermeersch, D. A., Nielsen, S. L., & Smart, D. W. (2003). Is it time for clinicians to routinely track patient outcome?: A meta-analysis. *Clinical Psychology: Science and Practice, 10,* 288–301.

Lambert, M. J., Whipple, J. L., Smart, D. W., Vermeersch, D. A., Nielsen, S. L., & Hawkins, E. J. (2001b). The effects of providing therapists with feedback on patient progress during psychotherapy: Are outcomes enhanced? *Psychotherapy Research, 11,* 49–68.

Larsson, B. S., Melin, L., Breitholtz, E., & Andersson, G. (1991). Short-term stability of depressive symptoms and suicide attempts in Swedish adolescents. *Acta Psychiatrica Scandinavica, 83*(5), 385–390.

Last, C. G., Hansen, C., & Franco, N. (1998). Cognitive-behavioral treatment of school phobia. *Journal of the American Academy of Child and Adolescent Psychiatry, 37,* 404–411.

Last, C. G., Hersen, M., Kazdin, A. E., Finkelstein, R., & Strauss, C. C. (1987). Comparison of DSM-III separation anxiety and overanxious disorders: Demographic characteristics and patterns of co-morbidity. *Journal of the American Academy of Child and Adolescent Psychiatry, 26*(4), 527–531.

Laverty, S. G. (1966). Aversion therapies in the treatment of alcoholism. *Psychosomatic Medicine, 28,* 651–666.

Lay, B., Jennen-Steinmetz, C., Reinhard, I., & Schmidt, M. H. (2002). Characteristics of inpatient weight gain in adolescent anorexia nervosa: Relation to speed of relapse and readmission. *European Eating Disorders Review, 10,* 22–40.

Layne, A. E., Bernstein, G. A., Egan, E. A., & Kushner, M. G. (2003). Predictors of treatment response in anxious-depressed adolescents with school refusal. *Journal of the American Academy Child and Adolescent Psychiatry, 42,* 319–326.

Layne, C. M., Pynoos, R. S., & Cardenas, J. (2001a). Wounded adolescence: School-based group psychotherapy for adolescents who sustained or witnessed violent injury. In M. Shafii & S. L. Shafii (Eds.), *School violence: Assessment, management, prevention* (pp. 163–186). Washington, DC: American Psychiatric Association.

Layne, C. M., Pynoos, R. S., Saltzman, W. R., Arslanagic, B., Black, M., Savjak, N., et al. (2001b). Trauma/grief-focused group psychotherapy: School-based postwar intervention with traumatized Bosnian adolescents. *Group Dynamics, 5*(4), 277–290.

Leckman, J. F., & Cohen, D. J. (1994). Tic disorders. In M. Rutter, E. Taylor & L. Hersov (Eds.), *Child and adolescent psychiatry: Modern approaches* (pp. 455–466). Oxford, UK: Blackwell.

Lecompte, D., & Pelc, I. (1996). A cognitive-behavioural program to improve compliance with medication in patients with schizophrenia. *International Journal of Mental Health, 25,* 51–56.

Lee, C., Gavriel, H., Drummond, P., Richards, J., & Greenwald, R. (2002). Treatment of PTSD: Stress inoculation training with prolonged exposure compared to EMDR. *Journal of Clinical Psychology, 58*(9), 1071–1089.

Lee, D. A., Scragg, P., & Turner, S. (2001). The role of shame and guilt in traumatic events: A clinical model of shame-based and guilt-based PTSD. *British Journal of Medical Psychology, 74,* 451–466.

Lee, N. F., & Rush, A. J. (1986). Cognitive-behavioral group therapy for bulimia. *International Journal of Eating Disorders, 5*(4), 599–615.

Leff, J., & Everitt, B. (2001). "Is couple therapy better than antidepressant drugs?": Commentary reply. *British Journal of Psychiatry, 178*, 181–182.

Leff, J., Sharpley, M., Chisholm, D., Bell, R., & Gamble, C. (2001). Training community psychiatric nurses in schizophrenia family work: A study of clinical and economic outcomes for patients and relatives. *Journal of Mental Health, 10*, 189–197.

Leff, J., Vearnals, S., Brewin, C. R., Wolff, G., Alexander, B., Asen, E., et al. (2000). The London Depression Intervention Trial: Randomised controlled trial of antidepressants v. couple therapy in the treatment and maintenance of people with depression living with a partner: Clinical outcome and costs. *British Journal of Psychiatry, 177*, 95–100.

Leff, J. P., Berkowitz, R., Shavit, N., Strachan, A., Glass, I., & Vaughn, C. (1988). A trial of family therapy vs. a relatives group for schizophrenia. *British Journal of Psychiatry, 153*, 58–66.

Leff, J. P., Berkowitz, R., Shavit, N., Strachan, A., Glass, I., & Vaughn, C. (1990). A trial of family therapy vs. a relatives group for schizophrenia: Two year follow-up. *British Journal of Psychiatry, 157*, 571–577.

Leff, J. P., Kuipers, L., Berkowitz, R., & Sturgeon, D. (1982). A controlled trial of social intervention in schizophrenia families. *British Journal of Psychiatry, 141*, 121–134.

Leff, J. P., Kuipers, L., Berkowitz, R., & Sturgeon, D. (1985). A controlled trial of social intervention in the families of schizophrenia patients: Two year follow-up. *British Journal of Psychiatry, 146*, 594–600.

Leff, J. P., & Vaughn, C. (1985). *Expressed emotion in families*. New York: Guilford Press.

Leff, J. P., & Wing, J. K. (1971). Trial of maintenance therapy in schizophrenia. *British Medical Journal, 3*, 599–604.

LeGrange, D., Eisler, I., Dare, C., & Russell, G. F. (1992). Evaluation of family treatments in adolescent anorexia nervosa: A pilot study. *International Journal of Eating Disorders, 12*, 347–357.

Leibenluft, E., & Goldberg, R. L. (1987). Guidelines for short-term inpatient psychotherapy. *Hospital and Community Psychiatry, 38*, 38–43.

Leiblum, S. R., Rosen, R. C., & Pierce, D. (1976). Group treatment format: Mixed sexual dysfunction. *Archives of Sexual Behavior, 5*, 313–322.

Leichsenring, F. (2001). Comparative effects of short-term psychodynamic psychotherapy and cognitive-behavioral therapy in depression: A meta-analytic approach. *Clinical Psychology Review, 21*(3), 401–419.

Leichsenring, F., & Leibing, E. (2003). The effectiveness of psychodynamic therapy and cognitive behavior therapy in the treatment of personality disorders: A meta-analysis. *American Journal of Psychiatry, 160*(7), 1223–1232.

Leigh, G., Osborne, A. C., & Cleland, P. (1984). Factors associated with patient drop-out from an out-patient alcoholism treatment service. *Journal of Studies on Alcohol, 45*, 359–362.

Leitenberg, H., Rosen, J., Gross, J., Nudelman, S., & Vara, L. S. (1988). Exposure plus response prevention treatment of bulimia nervosa. *Journal of Consulting and Clinical Psychology, 56*, 535–541.

Leitenberg, H., Rosen, J. C., Wolf, J., Vara, L. S., Detzer, M. J., & Srebnik, D. (1994). Comparison of cognitive-behavior therapy and desipramine in the treatment of bulimia nervosa. *Behaviour Research and Therapy, 32*, 37–45.

Lelliot, P. T., Noshirvani, H. F., Basoglu, M., Marks, I. M., & Monteiro, W. O. (1988). Obsessive–compulsive beliefs and treatment outcome. *Psychological Medicine, 18*, 697–702.

Lenior, M. E., Dingemans, P. M. A. J., Linszen, D. H., de Haan, L., & Schene, A. H. (2001). Social functioning and the course of early-onset schizophrenia: Five-year follow-up of a psychosocial intervention. *British Journal of Psychiatry, 179*, 53–58.

Lenze, E. J., Dew, M. A., Mazumdar, S., Begley, A. E., Cornes, C., Miller, M. D., et al.

(2002). Combined pharmacotherapy and psychotherapy as maintenance treatment for late-life depression: Effects on social adjustment. *American Journal of Psychiatry, 159*(3), 466–468.

Leon, S. C., Kopta, S. M., Howard, K. I., & Lutz, W. (1999). Predicting patients' responses to psychotherapy: Are some more predictable than others? *Journal of Consulting and Clinical Psychology, 67*(5), 698–704.

Leone, N. F. (1982). Response of borderline patents to loxapine and chlorpromazine. *Journal of Clinical Psychiatry, 43*, 148–150.

Lesser, I. M., Rubin, R. T., & Pecknold, J. C. (1988). Secondary depression in panic disorder and agoraphobia. *Archives of General Psychiatry, 45*, 437–443.

Leung, N., Waller, G., & Thomas, G. (1999). Group cognitive-behavioural therapy for anorexia nervosa: A case for treatment? *European Eating Disorders Review, 7*, 351–361.

Leung, S. N. M., & Orrell, M. W. (1993). A brief cognitive behavioural therapy group for the elderly: Who benefits? *International Journal of Geriatric Psychiatry, 8*, 593–598.

Levene, J. E., Newman, F., & Jefferies, J. J. (1989). Focal family therapy outcome study: I. Patient and family functioning. *Canadian Journal of Psychiatry, 34*(7), 641–647.

Levin, E., Sinclair, I., & Gorbach, P. (1989). *Families, services and confusion in old age.* Aldershot, UK: Gower Press.

Levine, J., Barak, Y., & Granek, I. (1998). Cognitive group therapy for paranoid schizophrenics: Applying cognitive dissonance. *Journal of Cognitive Psychotherapy: An International Quarterly, 12*, 3–12.

Levinson, T., & Sereny, G. (1969). An experimental evaluation of insight therapy for the chronic alcoholic. *Canadian Psychiatric Association Journal, 14*, 143–146.

Levitz, L. S., & Stunkard, A. J. (1974). A therapeutic coalition for obesity: Behavior modification and patient self-help. *American Journal of Psychiatry, 131*, 423–427.

Lewandowski, L. M., Gebing, T. A., Anthony, J. L., & O'Brien, W. H. (1997). Meta-analysis of cognitive-behavioral treatment studies for bulimia. *Clinical Psychology Review, 17*(7), 703–718.

Lewinsohn, P. M., & Clarke, G. N. (1999). Psychosocial treatments for adolescent depression. *Clinical Psychology Review, 19*, 329–342.

Lewinsohn, P. M., Clarke, G. N., Hops, H., & Andrews, J. (1990). Cognitive-behavioural treatment for depressed adolescents. *Behaviour Therapy, 21*, 385–401.

Lewinsohn, P. M., Clarke, G. N., & Rohde, P. (1994). Psychological approaches to the treatment of depression in adolescents. In W. M. Reynolds & H. F. Johnston (Eds.), *Handbook of depression in children and adolescents* (pp. 309–344). New York: Plenum Press.

Lewinsohn, P. M., Clarke, G. N., Rohde, P., Hops, H., & Seeley, J. R. (1996). A course in coping: A cognitive-behavioral approach to the treatment of adolescent depression. In E. D. Hibbs & P. S. Jensen (Eds.), *Psychosocial treatments for child and adolescent disorders: Empirically based strategies for clinical practice* (pp. 109–135). Washington, DC: American Psychological Association.

Lewis, S., Tarrier, N., Haddock, G., Bentall, R., Kinderman, P., Kingdon, D., et al. (2002). Randomised controlled trial of cognitive-behavioural therapy in early schizophrenia: Acute-phase outcomes. *British Journal of Psychiatry*, (Suppl. 43), S91–S97.

Liberman, R. P. (1994). Psychosocial treatments for schizophrenia. *Psychiatry, 57*, 104–114.

Liberman, R. P., & Eckman, T. (1981). Behavior therapy vs. insight oriented therapy for repeated suicide attempters. *Archives of General Psychiatry, 38*, 1126–1130.

Libman, E., Fichten, C. S., Brender, W., Burstein, R., Cohen, J., & Binik, Y. M. (1984). A comparison of three therapeutic formats in the treatment of secondary orgasmic dysfunction. *Journal of Sex and Marital Therapy, 10*, 147–159.

Lichtein, K. L., Riedel, B. W., Wilson, N. M., Lester, K. W., & Aguillard, R. N. (2001). Relaxation and sleep compression for late-life insomnia: A placebo-controlled trial. *Journal of Consulting and Clinical Psychology, 69*, 227–239.

Liddell, A., di Fazio, L., Blackwood, J., & Ackerman, C. (1994). Long-term follow-up of treated dental phobics. *Behaviour Research and Therapy, 32*, 605–610.

Liddle, B., & Spence, S. H. (1990). Cognitive-behavioral therapy with depressed primary school children: A cautionary note. *Behavioural Psychotherapy, 18*, 85–102.

Lidren, D. M., Watkins, P. L., Gould, R. A., Clum, G. A., Asterino, M., & Tulloch, H. L. (1994). A comparison of bibliotherapy and group therapy in the treatment of panic disorder. *Journal of Consulting and Clinical Psychology, 62*(4), 865–869.

Liebowitz, M. R., Heimberg, R. G., Schneier, F. R., Hope, D. A., Davies, S., Holt, C. S., et al. (1999). Cognitive-behavioral group therapy versus phenelzine in social phobia: Long-term outcome. *Depression Anxiety, 10*(3), 89–98.

Likierman, H., & Rachman, S. (1982). Obsessions: An experimental investigation of thought stopping and habituation training. *Behavioral Psychotherapy, 10*, 324–338.

Lincoln, T. M., Rief, W., Hahlweg, K., Frank, M., von Witzleben, I., Schroeder, B., et al. (2003). Effectiveness of an empirically supported treatment for social phobia in the field. *Behaviour Research and Therapy, 41*(11), 1251–1269.

Lindesay, J., Briggs, K., & Murphy, E. (1989). The Guys/Age Concern survey: Prevalence rates of cognitive impairment, depression and anxiety in an urban elderly community. *British Journal of Psychiatry, 155*, 317–329.

Lindsay, M., Crino, R., & Andrews, G. (1997). Controlled trial of exposure and response prevention in obsessive–compulsive disorder. *British Journal of Psychiatry, 171*, 135–139.

Lindsay, W. R., Gamsu, C. V., McLaughlin, E., Hood, E. M., & Espie, C. A. (1987). A controlled trial of treatments for generalized anxiety. *British Journal of Clinical Psychology, 26*, 3–15.

Lindy, J. D., Green, B. L., Grace, M., & Tichener, J. (1983). Survivors of the Beverly Hills supper-club fire. *American Journal of Psychotherapy, 4*, 593–610.

Linehan, M. M. (1993). *Skills training manual for treating borderline personality disorder.* New York: Guilford Press.

Linehan, M. M., Armstrong, H. E., Suarez, A., Allmon, D., & Heard, H. (1991). Cognitive-behavioral treatment of chronically parasuicidal borderline patients. *Archives of General Psychiatry, 48*, 1060–1064.

Linehan, M. M., Dimeff, L. A., Reynolds, S. K., Comtois, K. A., Welch, S. S., Heagerty, P., et al. (2002). Dialectical behavior therapy versus comprehensive validation therapy plus 12-step for the treatment of opioid dependent women meeting criteria for borderline personality disorder. *Drug and Alcohol Dependence, 67*(1), 13–26.

Linehan, M. M., Heard, H., & Armstrong, H. E. (1993). Naturalistic follow-up of a behavioral treatment for chronically parasuicidal borderline patients. *Archives of General Psychiatry, 50*, 971–974.

Linehan, M. M., Schmidt, H., Dimeff, L. A., Craft, J. C., Kanter, J., & Comtois, K. A. (1999). Dialectical behavior therapy for patients with borderline personality disorder and drug dependence. *American Journal on Addictions, 8*, 279–292.

Links, P. S., Steiner, M., Boigo, I., & Irwin, D. (1990). Lithium therapy for borderline patients: Preliminary findings. *Journal of Personality Disorders, 4*, 173–181.

Linszen, D. H., Dingemans, P., Van der Does, J. W., Nugter, A., Scholte, P., Lenior, R., et al. (1996). Treatment, expressed emotion and relapse in recent onset schizophrenic disorders. *Psychological Medicine, 26*(2), 333–342.

Linszen, D. H., Dingemans, M. A. J., Scholte, W., Lenior, M., & Goldstein, M. J. (1998). Early recognition, intensive intervention and other protective and risk factors for psychotic episodes in schizophrenia. *International Clinical Psychopharmacology, 13*(Suppl. 3), S7–S12.

Lipman, R. S., Covi, I., & Shapiro, A. K. (1979). The Hopkins Symptom Check List: Factors derived from the HSCL-90. *Journal of Affective Disorders, 1*, 9–24.

Lipsey, M. W., & Wilson, D. B. (1993). The efficacy of psychological, educational, and behavioral treatment: Confirmation from meta-analysis. *American Psychologist, 48*, 1181–1209.

Lipsitz, J. D., Markowitz, J. C., Cherry, S., & Fyer, A. J. (1999). Open trial of interpersonal psychotherapy for the treatment of social phobia. *American Journal of Psychiatry, 156*(11), 1814–1816.

Lipsius, S. H. (1991). Combined individual and group psychotherapy: Guidelines at the interface. *International Journal of Group Psychotherapy, 41,* 313–327.

Litt, M. D., Kadden, R. M., Cooney, N. L., & Kabela, E. (2003). Coping skills and treatment outcomes in cognitive-behavioral and interactional group therapy for alcoholism. *Journal of Consulting and Clinical Psychology, 71*(1), 118–128.

Little, R. J. A., & Rubin, D. B. (1987). *Statistical analysis with missing data.* New York: Wiley.

Livingston, G., & Hinchliffe, A. C. (1993). The epidemiology of psychiatric disorders in the elderly. *International Review of Psychiatry, 5,* 317–326.

Lochman, J. E., Coie, J. D., Underwood, M. K., & Terry, R. (1993). Effectiveness of a social relations intervention program for aggressive and nonaggressive, rejected children. *Journal of Consulting and Clinical Psychology, 61,* 1053–1058.

Loeb, K. L., Wilson, G. T., Gilbert, J. S., & Labouvie, E. (2000). Guided and unguided self-help for binge eating. *Behaviour Research and Therapy, 38*(3), 259–272.

Loerch, B., Graf-Morgenstern, M., Hautzinger, M., Schlegel, S., Hain, C., Sandmann, J., et al. (1999). Randomised placebo-controlled trial of moclobemide, cognitive-behavioural therapy and their combination in panic disorder with agoraphobia. *British Journal of Psychiatry, 174,* 205–212.

Lohr, J. M., Tolin, D. F., & Lilienfeld, S. O. (1998). Efficacy of eye movement desensitization and reprocessing: Implications for behaviour therapy. *Behavior Therapy, 29,* 123–156.

Long, P., Forehand, R., Wierson, M., & Morgan, A. (1994). Moving into adulthood: Does parent training with young noncompliant children have long-term effects? *Behaviour Research and Therapy, 32,* 101–107.

Longabaugh, R., & Morgenstern, J. (1999). Cognitive-behavioral coping-skills therapy for alcohol dependence: Current status and future directions. *Alcohol Research and Health, 23,* 78–85.

Longabaugh, R., Wirtz, P. W., Zweben, A., & Stout, R. L. (1998). Network support for drinking, Alcoholics Anonymous and long-term matching effects. *Addiction, 93*(9), 1313–1333.

LoPiccolo, J., Heiman, J. R., Hogan, D. R., & Roberts, C. W. (1985). Effectiveness of single therapists versus cotherapy teams in sex therapy. *Journal of Consulting and Clinical Psychology, 53,* 287–294.

LoPiccolo, J., & Stock, W. E. (1986). Treatment of sexual dysfunctions. *Journal of Consulting and Clinical Psychology, 54,* 158–167.

Lord, C., & Rutter, M. (1994). Autism and pervasive developmental disorders. In M. Rutter, E. Taylor & L. Hersov (Eds.), *Child and adolescent psychiatry: Modern approaches* (3rd ed., pp. 569–593). Oxford, UK: Blackwell Scientific.

Lovaas, O. I. (1987). Behavioral treatment and normal educational/intellectual functioning in young autistic children. *Journal of Consulting and Clinical Psychology, 55,* 3–9.

Lovell, K., Marks, I. M., Noshirvani, H., & O'Sullivan, G. (1994). Should treatment distinguish anxiogenic from anxiolytic obsessive–compulsive ruminations?: Results of a pilot controlled study and of a clinical audit. *Psychotherapy and Psychosomatics, 61*(3–4), 150–155.

Low, G., Jones, D., Duggan, C., Power, M., & MacLeod, A. (2001). The treatment of deliberate self-harm in borderline personality disorder using dialectical behaviour therapy: A pilot study in a high security hospital. *Behavioural and Cognitive Psychotherapy, 29*(1), 85–92.

Lowe, B., Zipfel, S., Buchholz, C., Dupont, Y., Reas, D. L., & Herzog, W. (2001). Long-term outcome of anorexia nervosa in a prospective 21-year follow-up study. *Psychological Medicine, 31*(5), 881–890.

Luborsky, L. (1984). *Principles of psychoanalytic psychotherapy: A manual for supportive–expressive treatment.* New York: Basic Books.

Luborsky, L., & Crits-Christoph, P. (1990). *Understanding transference: The CCRT method (the core conflictual relationship theme).* New York: Basic Books.

Luborsky, L., Crits-Christoph, P., McLellan, T., Woody, G., Piper, W., Liberman, B., et al.

(1986). Do therapists vary much in their success?: Findings from four outcome studies. *American Journal of Orthopsychiatry, 51*, 501–512.

Luborsky, L., Diguer, L., Seligman, D. A., Rosenthal, R., Krause, E. D., Johnson, S., et al. (1999). The researcher's own therapy allegiances: A "wild card" in comparisons of treatment efficacy. *Clinical Psychology: Science and Practice, 6*, 95–106.

Luborsky, L., McLellan, A. T., Diguer, L., Woody, G., & Seligman, D. (1997). The psychotherapist matters: Comparison of outcome across twenty-two therapists and seven patient samples. *Clinical Psychology: Science and Practice, 4*, 53–65.

Luborsky, L., McLellan, A. T., Woody, G. E., O'Brien, C. P., & Auerbach, A. (1985). Therapists success and its determinants. *Archives of General Psychiatry, 42*, 602–611.

Luborsky, L., Popp, C., & Barber, J. P. (1994). Common and special factors in different transference-related measures. *Psychotherapy Research, 4*, 277–286.

Lueger, R. J., Howard, K. I., Martinovich, Z., Lutz, W., Anderson, E. E., & Grissom, G. (2001). Assessing treatment progress of individual patients using expected treatment response models. *Journal of Consulting and Clinical Psychology, 69*(2), 150–158.

Lutz, W., Martinovich, Z., & Howard, K. I. (1999). Patient profiling: An application of random coefficient regression models to depicting the response of a patient to outpatient psychotherapy. *Journal of Consulting and Clinical Psychology, 67*(4), 571–577.

Lutzker, J. R. (1996). Timeout from emotion, time for science: A response to Kemp. *Child and Family Behavior Therapy, 18*, 29–34.

Lynskey, M. T. (1998). The comorbidity of alcohol dependence and affective disorders: Treatment implications. *Drug and Alcohol Dependence, 52*(3), 201–209.

Lyons, L. C., & Woods, P. J. (1991). The efficacy of rational–emotive therapy: A quantitative review of the outcome research. *Clinical Psychology Review, 11*, 357–369.

MacDonald, A. (1986). Do general practitioners miss depression in elderly patients? *British Medical Journal, 292*, 1365–1367.

Macklin, M. L., Metzger, L. J., Lasko, N. B., Berry, N. J., Orr, S. P., & Pitman, R. K. (2000). Five-year follow-up study of eye movement desensitization and reprocessing therapy for combat-related posttraumatic stress disorder. *Comprehensive Psychiatry, 41*(1), 24–27.

Malan, D. (1976). *The frontiers of brief psychotherapy.* New York: Plenum Press.

Malinckrodt, B., Gantt, D., & Coble, H. M. (1995). Attachment patterns in the psychotherapy relationship: Development of a client attachment to therapy scale. *Journal of Counselling Psychology, 42*, 307–317.

Malkoff-Schwartz, S., E., F., & Andersen, B. (1998). Stressful life events and social rhythm disruption in the onset of manic and depressive bipolar episodes. *Archives of General Psychiatry, 55*, 702–707.

Malmberg, L., & Fenton, M. (2001). Individual psychodynamic psychotherapy and psychoanalysis for schizophrenia and severe mental illness (Cochrane Review). In *The Cochrane Library*, Issue 4, 2002 (p. CD001360). Oxford, UK: Update Software.

Manassis, K., Mendlowitz, S. L., Scapillato, D., Avery, D., Fiksenbaum, L., Freire, M., et al. (2002). Group and individual cognitive-behavioral therapy for childhood anxiety disorders: A randomized trial. *Journal of the American Academy of Child and Adolescent Psychiatry, 41*, 1423–1430.

Mann, J. (1973). *Time-limited psychotherapy.* Cambridge, MA: Harvard University Press.

Manning, D. W., Markowitz, J. C., & Frances, A. J. (1992). A review of combined psychotherapy and pharmacotherapy in the treatment of depression. *Journal of Psychotherapy Practice and Research, 1*, 103–116.

March, J. S. (1995). Cognitive-behavioral psychotherapy for children and adolescents with OCD: A review and recommendations for treatment. *Journal of the American Academy of Child and Adolescent Psychiatry, 34*, 7–18.

March, J. S., Amaya-Jackson, L., Murray, M. C., & Schulte, A. (1998). Cognitive-behavioral psychotherapy for children and adolescents with posttraumatic stress disorder after a single-incident stressor. *Journal of the American Academy of Child and Adolescent Psychiatry, 37*(6), 585–593.

March, J. S., Franklin, M., Nelson, A., & Foa, E. (2001). Cognitive-behavioral psychotherapy for pediatric obsessive–compulsive disorder. *Journal of Clinical Child Psychology*, *30*(1), 8–18.

March, J. S., & Leonard, H. L. (1996). Obsessive–compulsive disorder in children and adolescents: A review of the past 10 years. *Journal of the American Academy of Child and Adolescent Psychiatry*, *35*, 1265–1273.

March, J. S., & Mulle, K. (1995). Behavioral psychotherapy for obsessive–compulsive disorder: A preliminary single-case study. *Journal of Anxiety Disorders*, *9*, 175–184.

March, J. S., Mulle, K., & Herbel, B. (1994). Behavioral psychotherapy for children and adolescents with obsessive–compulsive disorder: An open trial of a new protocol-driven treatment package. *Journal of the American Academy of Child and Adolescent Psychiatry*, *33*, 333–341.

March, J. S., Swanson, J. M., Arnold, L. E., Hoza, B., Conners, C. K., Hinshaw, S. P., et al. (2000). Anxiety as a predictor and outcome variable in the multimodal treatment study of children with ADHD (MTA). *Journal of Abnormal Child Psychology*, *28*(6), 527–541.

Marchand, A., Goyer, L. R., Dupuis, G., & Mainguy, N. (1998). Personality disorders and the outcome of cognitive-behavioural treatment of panic disorder with agoraphobia. *Canadian Journal of Behavioral Science*, *30*, 14–23.

Marchione, K. E., Michelson, L., Greenwald, M., & Dancu, C. (1987). Cognitive behavioral treatment of agoraphobia. *Behaviour Research and Therapy*, *25*(5), 319–328.

Marcotte, D., & Baron, P. (1993). L'efficacité d'une strategie d'intervention emotio–rationelle auprès d'adolescents dépressifs du milieu scolaire [The efficacy of a school-based rational–emotive intervention strategy with depressive adolescents]. *Canadian Journal of Counselling*, *27*, 77–92.

Marcus, S. V., Marquis, P., & Sakai, C. (1997). Controlled study of treatment of PTSD using EMDR in an HMO setting. *Psychotherapy*, *34*, 307–315.

Margraf, J., Ehlers, A., Roth, W. T., Clark, D. B., Sheikh, J., Agras, W. S., et al. (1991). How "blind" are double-blind studies? *Journal of Consulting and Clinical Psychology*, *59*, 184–187.

Mari, J. J., & Streiner, D. L. (1994). An overview of family interventions and relapse on schizophrenia: Meta-analysis of research findings. *Psychological Medicine*, *24*(3), 565–578.

Markowitz, J. (1996). Psychotherapy for dysthymic disorder. *Psychiatric Clinics of North America*, *19*, 133–149.

Markowitz, J. C. (1994). Psychotherapy of dysthymia: Is it effective? *American Journal of Psychiatry*, *151*, 1114–1121.

Marks, I. (1999). Computer aids to mental health care. *Canadian Journal of Psychiatry*, *44*(6), 548–555.

Marks, I., Lovell, K., Noshirvani, H., Livanou, M., & Thrasher, S. (1998). Treatment of post traumatic stress disorder by exposure and/or cognitive restructuring. *Archives of General Psychiatry*, *55*, 317–325.

Marks, I. M. (1987). *Fears, phobias and rituals*. Oxford, UK: Oxford University Press.

Marks, I. M., Gray, S., & Cohen, D. (1983). Imipramine and brief therapist-aided exposure in agoraphobics having self-exposure homework. *Archives of General Psychiatry*, *40*, 153–162.

Marks, I. M., Hodgson, R., & Rachman, S. (1975). Treatment of chronic obsessive–compulsive neurosis by *in-vivo* exposure. *British Journal of Psychiatry*, *127*, 349–364.

Marks, I. M., & Mathews, A. M. (1979). Brief standard self-rating for phobic patients. *Behaviour Research and Therapy*, *17*, 263–267.

Marks, I. M., & O'Sullivan, G. (1988). Drugs and psychological treatments for agoraphobia/panic and obsessive–compulsive disorders: A review. *British Journal of Psychiatry*, *153*, 650–658.

Marks, I. M., Stern, R. S., Mawson, D., Cobb, J., & McDonald, D. (1980). Clomipramine and exposure for obsessive–compulsive rituals. *British Journal of Psychiatry*, *152*, 522–534.

Marks, I. M., Swinson, R. P., Basoglu, M., Kuch, K., Noshirvani, H., Kuch, K., et al.

(1993a). Reply to comment on the London/Toronto study. *British Journal of Psychiatry*, *162*, 790–793.

Marks, I. M., Swinson, R. P., Basoglu, M., Kuch, K., Noshirvani, H., O'Sullivan, G., et al. (1993b). Alprazolam and exposure alone and combined in panic disorder with agoraphobia. *Journal of Psychiatry*, *162*, 776–787.

Marmar, C. R., Gaston, L., Gallagher, D., & Thompson, L. W. (1989). Alliance and outcome in late-life depression. *Journal of Nervous and Mental Disease*, *177*, 464–472.

Marmar, C. R., Horowitz, M. J., Weiss, D. S., Wilner, N. R., & Kaltreider, N. B. (1988). A controlled trial of brief psychotherapy and mutual-help group treatment of conjugal bereavement. *American Journal of Psychiatry*, *145*, 203–209.

Marriott, A., Donaldson, C., Tarrier, N., & Burns, A. (2000). Effectiveness of cognitive-behavioural family intervention in reducing the burden of care in carers of patients with Alzheimer's disease. *British Journal of Psychiatry*, *176*, 557–562.

Marshall, W. L. (1985). Variable exposure in flooding. *Behavior Therapy*, *16*, 119–135.

Marshall, W. L. (1988). Behavioural indices of habituation and sensitisation during exposure to phobic stimuli. *Behaviour Research and Therapy*, *26*, 67–77.

Martin, C., & Tarrier, N. (1992). The importance of cultural factors in exposure to obsessive ruminations: A case example. *Behavior Psychotherapy*, *20*, 181–184.

Martin, D. J., Garske, J. P., & Davis, M. K. (2000). Relation of the therapeutic alliance with outcome and other variables: A meta-analytic review. *Journal of Consulting and Clinical Psychology*, *68*(3), 438–450.

Martinsen, E. W., Olsen, T., Tonset, E., Nyland, K. E., & Aarre, T. F. (1998). Cognitive-behavioral group therapy for panic disorder in the general clinical setting: A naturalistic study with 1-year follow-up. *Journal of Clinical Psychiatry*, *59*(8), 437–442; quiz, 443.

Marzillier, J. S., Lambert, C., & Kellett, J. (1976). A controlled evaluation of systematic desensitization and social skills training for socially inadequate psychiatric patients. *Behaviour Research and Therapy*, *14*, 225–238.

Mason, B. J., Markowitz, J. C., & Klerman, G. L. (1993). IPT for dysthymic disorder. In G. L. Klerman & M. M. Weissman (Eds.), *New applications of interpersonal therapy* (pp. 225–364). Washington, DC: American Psychiatric Press.

Massion, A. O., Dyck, I. R., Shea, M. T., Phillips, K. A., Warshaw, M. G., & Keller, M. B. (2002). Personality disorders and time to remission in generalized anxiety disorder, social phobia, and panic disorder. *Archives of General Psychiatry*, *59*(5), 434–440.

Masters, W. H., & Johnson, V. E. (1966). *Human sexual response*. Boston: Little, Brown.

Masters, W. H., & Johnson, V. E. (1970). *Human sexual inadequacy*. Boston: Little, Brown.

Mathews, A., Bancroft, J., Whitehead, A., Hackmann, A., Julier, D., Bancroft, J., et al. (1976). The behavioral treatment of sexual inadequacy: A comparative study. *Behaviour Research and Therapy*, *14*, 427–436.

Matson, J. L. (1989). *Treating depression in children and adolescents*. New York: Pergamon Press.

Matson, J. L., Sevin, J. A., Box, M. L., & Francis, K. L. (1993). An evaluation of two methods for increasing self-initiated verbalisations in autistic children. *Journal of Applied Behaviour Analysis*, *26*, 389–398.

Matson, J. L., Sevin, J. A., Fridley, D., & Love, S. R. (1990). Increasing spontaneous language in three autistic children. *Journal of Applied Behavioural Analysis*, *23*, 227–234.

Matson, J. L., & Swiezy, N. (1994). Social skills training with autistic children. In J. L. Matson (Ed.), *Autism in children and adults: Etiology assessment and intervention* (pp. 241–260). Pacific Grove, CA: Brooks/Cole.

Mattick, R., & Jarvis, T. (1993). *An outline for the management of alcohol problems: Quality Assurance Project*. Sydney: National Drug and Alcohol Research Centre.

Mattick, R. P., Andrews, G., Hadzi-Pavlovic, D., & Christensen, H. (1990). Treatment of panic and agoraphobia: An integrative review. *Journal of Nervous and Mental Disease*, *178*, 567–576.

Mattick, R. P., & Newman, C. R. (1991). Social phobia and avoidant personality disorder. *International Journal of Psychiatry*, *3*, 163–173.

Mattick, R. P., & Peters, L. (1988). Treatment of severe social phobia: Effects of guided exposure with and without cognitive restructuring. *Journal of Consulting and Clinical Psychology*, *56*, 251–260.

Mattick, R. P., Peters, L., & Clarke, J. C. (1989). Exposure and cognitive restructuring for social phobia: A controlled study. *Behavior Therapy*, *20*, 3–23.

Maude-Griffin, P. M., Hohenstein, J. M., Humfleet, G. L., Reilly, P. M., Tusel, D. J., & Hall, S. M. (1998). Superior efficacy of cognitive-behavioral therapy for urban crack cocaine abusers: Main and matching effects. *Journal of Consulting and Clinical Psychology*, *66*(5), 832–837.

Mavissakalian, M. (1993). Combined behavioral and pharmacological treatment of anxiety disorders. In J. M. Oldham, M. B. Riba, & A. Tasman (Eds.), *Review of psychiatry* (Vol. 12, pp. 541–564). Washington, DC: American Psychiatric Press.

Mavissakalian, M., & Hamann, M. S. (1988). Correlates of DSM-III personality disorder in panic disorder and agoraphobia. *Comprehensive Psychiatry*, *29*, 535–544.

Mavissakalian, M., & Michelson, L. (1986). Two year follow-up of exposure and imipramine treatment of agoraphobia. *American Journal of Psychiatry*, *143*, 1106–1112.

Mavissakalian, M., Michelson, L., & Dealy, R. S. (1983). Pharmacological treatment of agoraphobia: Imipramine versus imipramine with programmed practice. *British Journal of Psychiatry*, *1983*, 348–355.

Mawson, D., Marks, I. M., & Ramm, L. (1982). Clomipramine and exposure for chronic obsessive–compulsive rituals: III. Two year follow-up and further findings. *British Journal of Psychiatry*, *140*, 11–18.

Maxfield, L., & Hyer, L. (2002). The relationship between efficacy and methodology in studies investigating EMDR treatment of PTSD. *Journal of Clinical Psychology*, *58*(1), 23–41.

May, P. R., Tuma, A. H., & Dixon, W. J. (1976). Schizophrenia: A follow-up study of results of treatment: I. Design and other problems. *Archives of General Psychiatry*, *33*, 474–478.

Mayerovitch, J. I., du Fort, G. G., Kakuma, R., Bland, R. C., Newman, S. C., & Pinard, G. (2003). Treatment seeking for obsessive–compulsive disorder: Role of obsessive–compulsive disorder symptoms and comorbid psychiatric diagnoses. *Comprehensive Psychiatry*, *44*(2), 162–168.

Mayou, R. A., Ehlers, A., & Hobbs, M. (2000). Psychological debriefing for road traffic accident victims: Three-year follow-up of a randomised controlled trial. *British Journal of Psychiatry*, *176*, 589–593.

McCallum, M., & Piper, W. E. (1997). The psychological mindedness assessment procedure. In M. McCallum & W. E. Piper (Eds.), *Psychological mindedness: A contemporary understanding* (pp. 27–58). Mahwah, NJ: Erlbaum.

McCrady, B. S., Epstein, E. E., & Hirsch, L. S. (1999). Maintaining change after conjoint behavioral alcohol treatment for men: Outcomes at 6 months. *Addiction*, *94*(9), 1381–1396.

McCrady, B. S., Longabaugh, R., Fink, E., & Stout, R. (1986). Cost-effectiveness of alcoholism treatment in partial hospital versus in-patient settings after brief in-patient treatment: 12 month outcomes. *Journal of Consulting and Clinical Psychology*, *54*, 708–713.

McCrady, B. S., Moreau, J., Paolino, T. J., & Longabaugh, R. (1982). Joint hospitalization and couples therapy for alcoholism: A four year follow-up. *Journal of Studies on Alcohol*, *43*, 1244–1250.

McCrady, B. S., Paolino, T. J., Longaborough, R., & Rossi, J. (1979). Effects of joint hospital admission and couples treatment for hospitalized alcoholics: A pilot study. *Addictive Behaviors*, *4*, 1244–1250.

McCullough, J. P. (1991). Psychotherapy for dysthymia: A naturalistic study of ten patients. *Journal of Nervous and Mental Disease*, *179*, 734–740.

McCullough, J. P., Klein, D. N., Shea, M. T., & Miller, I. (1992). *Review of DSM-IV mood disorder data in the field trials*. Paper presented at the 100th Meeting of the American Psychological Association, Washington, DC.

McDermut, W., Miller, I. W., & Brown, R. A. (2001). The efficacy of group psychotherapy for depression: A meta-analysis and review of the empirical research. *Clinical Psychology: Science and Practice, 8,* 98–116.

McEachin, J. J., Smith, T., & Lovaas, O. I. (1993). Long-term outcome for children with autism who received early intensive behavioral treatment. *American Journal of Mental Retardation, 97,* 359–372.

McFarlane, W. R., Link, B., Dushay, R., Marchal, J., & Crilly, J. (1995a). Psychoeducational multiple family groups: Four-year relapse outcome in schizophrenia. *Family Process, 34*(2), 127–144.

McFarlane, W. R., Lukens, E., Link, B., Dushay, R., Deakins, S. A., Newmark, M., et al. (1995b). Multiple-family groups and psychoeducation in the treatment of schizophrenia. *Archives of General Psychiatry, 52*(8), 679–687.

McFarlane, W. R., McNary, S., Dixon, L., Hornby, H., & Cimett, E. (2001). Predictors of dissemination of family psychoeducation in community mental health centers in Maine and Illinois. *Psychiatric Services, 52*(7), 935–942.

McGill, C. W., Falloon, I. R. H., Boyd, J. L., & Wood-Siverio, C. (1983). Family educational intervention in the treatment of schizophrenia. *Hospital and Community Psychiatry, 34,* 934–938.

McGilton, K. S., Rivera, T. M., & Dawson, P. (2003). Can we help persons with dementia find their way in a new environment? *Aging and Mental Health, 7*(5), 363–371.

McGlashan, T. (1986). The Chestnut Lodge follow-up study: III. Long-term outcome of borderline personalities. *Archives of General Psychiatry, 43,* 2–30.

McGorry, P. D., Yung, A. R., Phillips, L. J., Yuen, H. P., Francey, S., Cosgrave, E. M., et al. (2002). Randomized controlled trial of interventions designed to reduce the risk of progression to first-episode psychosis in a clinical sample with subthreshold symptoms. *Archives of General Psychiatry, 59*(10), 921–928.

McGuire, H., & Hawton, K. (2003). Interventions for vaginismus (Cochrane Review). In *The Cochrane Library,* Issue 2. Oxford, UK: Update Software.

McKay, J. R., Alterman, A. I., Cacciola, J. S., Rutherford, M. J., O'Brien, C. P., & Koppenhaver, J. (1997). Group counseling versus individualized relapse prevention aftercare following intensive outpatient treatment for cocaine dependence: Initial results. *Journal of Consulting and Clinical Psychology, 65*(5), 778–788.

McLean, P. D., & Hakstian, A. R. (1979). Clinical depression: Comparative efficacy of outpatient treatments. *Journal of Consulting and Clinical Psychology, 47,* 818–836.

McLean, P. D., & Hakstian, A. R. (1990). Relative endurance of unipolar depression treatment effects: Longitudinal follow-up. *Journal of Consulting and Clinical Psychology, 58,* 482–488.

McLean, P. D., Whittal, M. L., Thordarson, D. S., Taylor, S., Sochting, I., Koch, W. J., et al. (2001). Cognitive versus behavior therapy in the group treatment of obsessive–compulsive disorder. *Journal of Consulting and Clinical Psychology, 69*(2), 205–214.

McLellan, A. T., Arndt, I. O., Metzger, D. S., Woody, G. E., & O'Brien, C. P. (1993). The effects of psychosocial services in substance abuse treatment. *Journal of the American Medical Association, 269*(15), 1953–1959.

McLellan, A. T., Childress, A. R., O'Brien, C. P., & Ehrman, R. N. (1986). Extinguishing conditioned responses during treatment for opiate dependence: Turning laboratory findings into clinical procedures. *Journal of Substance Abuse and Treatment, 3,* 33–40.

McLellan, A. T., Grissom, G. R., Zanis, D., Randall, M., Brill, P., & O'Brien, C. P. (1997). Problem-service "matching" in addiction treatment: A prospective study in 4 programs. *Archives of General Psychiatry, 54*(8), 730–735.

McMahon, C. G., & Samali, R. (1999). Pharmacological treatment of premature ejaculation. *Current Opinion in Urology, 9,* 553–561.

McMahon, R. J., Forehand, R., Griest, D. L., & Wells, K. C. (1981). Who drops out of treatment during parent behavioural training? *Behavioural Counselling Quarterly, 1,* 79–95.

McNamee, G., O'Sullivan, G., Lelliot, P., & Marks, I. M. (1989). Telephone-guided treatment for housebound agoraphobics with panic disorder: Exposure vs. relaxation. *Behavior Therapy, 20,* 491–497.

McNeil, C. B., Capage, L. C., Bahl, A., & Blanc, H. (1999). Importance of early intervention for disruptive behavior problems: Comparison of treatment and wait-list control groups. *Early Education and Development, 10,* 445–454.

McNeil, C. B., Eyberg, S., Eisenstadt, T. H., Newcomb, K., & Funderburk, B. (1991). Parent–child interaction therapy with behaviour problem children: Generalisation of treatment effects to the school setting. *Journal of Clinical Child Psychology, 20,* 140–151.

McQuay, H. J., & Moore, R. A. (1997). Using numerical results from systematic reviews in clinical practice. *Annals of Internal Medicine, 126,* 712–720.

McShane, R., Keene, J., Gedling, K., Fairburn, C., Jacoby, R., & Hope, T. (1997). Do neuroleptic drugs hasten cognitive decline in dementia?: Prospective study with necropsy follow-up. *British Medical Journal, 314,* 266–270.

Meads, C., Gold, L., & Burls, A. (2001). How effective is outpatient care compared to inpatient care for the treatment of anorexia nervosa?: A systematic review. *European Eating Disorders Review, 9,* 229–241.

Meares, R., Stevenson, J., & Comerford, A. (1999). Psychotherapy with borderline patients: I. A comparison between treated and untreated cohorts. *Australian and New Zealand Journal of Psychiatry, 33*(4), 467–472.

Medical Research Council. (2000). *A framework for development and evaluation of RCTs for complex interventions to improve health.* London: Author.

Mellman, T. A., Leverich, G. S., Hasuer, P., Kramlinger, K., Post, R. M., & Uhde, T. W. (1992). Axis II pathology in panic and affective disorders: Relationship to diagnosis, course of illness, and treatment response. *Journal of Personality Disorders, 6,* 53–63.

Melman, A., Tiefler, L., & Pederson, R. (1988). Evaluation of first 406 patients in urology department based center for male sexual dysfunction. *Urology, 32,* 6–10.

Mendlowitz, S. L., Manassis, K., Bradley, S., Scalpillato, D., Miezitis, S., & Shaw, B. F. (1999). Cognitive-behavioral group treatments in childhood anxiety disorders: The role of parental involvement. *Journal of the American Academy of Child and Adolescent Psychiatry, 38*(10), 1223–1229.

Mennin, D. S., & Heimberg, R. G. (2000). The impact of comorbid mood and personality disorders in the cognitive-behavioral treatment of panic disorder. *Clinical Psychology Review, 20*(3), 339–357.

Mercier, M. A., Stewart, J. W., & Quitkin, F. M. (1992). A pilot sequential study of cognitive therapy and pharmacotherapy of atypical depression. *Journal of Clinical Psychiatry, 53,* 166–170.

Merckelbach, H., van den Hout, M. A., Hoekstra, R., & van Oppen, P. (1988). Are prepared fears less severe but more resistant to treatment? *Behaviour Research and Therapy, 26,* 527–530.

Merikangas, K. R., Mehta, R. L., Molnar, B. E., Walters, E. E., Swendsen, J. D., Aguilar-Gaziola, S., et al. (1998). Comorbidity of substance use disorders with mood and anxiety disorders: Results of the International Consortium in Psychiatric Epidemiology. *Addictive Behaviors, 23*(6), 893–907.

Merinder, L. B. (2000). Patient education in schizophrenia: A review. *Acta Psychiatrica Scandinavica, 102*(2), 98–106.

Merry, J., & Whitehead, A. (1968). Metronidazole and alcoholism. *British Journal of Psychiatry, 114,* 859–861.

Mersch, P. P. A. (1995). The treatment of social phobia: The differential effectiveness of exposure *in vivo* and an integration of exposure *in vivo*, rational emotive therapy and social skills training. *Behaviour Research and Therapy, 33,* 259–269.

Mersch, P. P. A., Emmelkamp, P. M., Bogels, S. M., & van der Sleen, J. (1989). Social phobia: Individual response patterns and the effects of behavioral and cognitive interventions. *Behaviour Research and Therapy, 27*(4), 421–434.

Mersch, P. P. A., Emmelkamp, P. M., & Lips, C. (1991). Social phobia: Individual response patterns and the long-term effects of behavioral and cognitive interventions: A follow-up study. *Behaviour Research and Therapy, 29*(4), 357–362.

Mesibov, G. B. (1986). A cognitive program for teaching social behaviours in verbal autistic adolescents and adults. In E. Schopler & G. B. Mesibov (Eds.), *Social behavior in autism.* New York: Plenum Press.

Messer, S. B. (2001). Empirically supported treatments: What's a nonbehaviorist to do? In B. D. Slife, D. Brent, R. N. Williams & S. H. Barlow (Eds.), *Critical issues in psychotherapy: Translating new ideas into practice* (pp. 3–19). Thousand Oaks, CA: Sage.

Meterissian, G. B., & Bradwejn, J. (1989). Comparative studies on the efficacy of psychotherapy, pharmacotherapy, and their combination in depression: Was adequate pharmacotherapy provided? *Journal of Clinical Psychopharmacology, 9,* 334–339.

Meyer, B., Pilkonis, P. A., Krupnick, J. L., Egan, M. K., Simmens, S. J., & Sotsky, S. M. (2002). Treatment expectancies, patient alliance, and outcome: Further analyses from the National Institute of Mental Health Treatment of Depression Collaborative Research Program. *Journal of Consulting and Clinical Psychology, 70*(4), 1051–1055.

Meyer, J. K., Schmidt, C. W., & Wise, T. N. (1983). *Clinical management of sexual disorders.* Baltimore: Williams & Wilkins.

Meyer, R. E. (1989). Prospects for a rational pharmacotherapy of alcoholism. *Journal of Clinical Psychiatry, 50,* 403–412.

Meyer, T. D., & Hautzinger, M. (2000). Psychotherapie bei bipolaren affektiven storungen—ein uberblick uber den stand der forschung [Psychotherapy of bipolar affective disorder—A review of the research evidence]. *Verhaltenstherapie, 10,* 177–186.

Meyers, R. J., Miller, W. R., Hill, D. E., & Tonigan, R. S. (1999). Community reinforcement and family training (CRAFT): Engaging unmotivated drug users in treatment. *Journal of Substance Abuse, 10*(3), 1–18.

Meyers, R. J., Miller, W. R., Smith, J. E., & Tonigan, J. S. (2002). A randomized trial of two methods for engaging treatment-refusing drug users through concerned significant others. *Journal of Consulting and Clinical Psychology, 70*(5), 1182–1185.

Michelson, L., Marchione, K., Greenwald, M., Testa, S., & Marchione, N. J. (1996). A comparative outcome and follow-up investigation of panic disorder with agoraphobia: The relative and combined efficacy of cognitive therapy, relaxation training and therapist-assisted exposure. *Journal of Anxiety Disorders, 10,* 297–330.

Miklowitz, D., & Goldstein, M. (1990). Behavioral family treatment for patients with bipolar affective disorder. *Behavior Modification, 14,* 457–489.

Miklowitz, D., Goldstein, M., Nuechterlein, K., Snyder, K., & Mintz, J. (1988). Family factors and the course of bipolar affective disorder. *Archives of General Psychiatry, 45,* 225–231.

Miklowitz, D. J., & Craighead, W. E. (2001). Bipolar affective disorder: Does psychosocial treatment add to the efficacy of drug therapy? *Trends in Evidence-Based Neuropsychiatry, 3,* 58–64.

Miklowitz, D. J., George, E. L., Richards, J. A., Simoneau, T. L., & Suddath, R. L. (2003). A randomized study of family-focused psychoeducation and pharmacotherapy in the outpatient management of bipolar disorder. *Archives of General Psychiatry, 60*(9), 904–912.

Miklowitz, D. J., Simoneau, T. L., George, E. L., Richards, J. A., Kalbag, A., Sachs-Ericsson, N., et al. (2000). Family-focused treatment of bipolar disorder: 1-year effects of a psychoeducational program in conjunction with pharmacotherapy. *Biological Psychiatry, 48*(6), 582–592.

Milan, R. J., Kilmann, P. R., & Boland, J. P. (1988). Treatment outcome of secondary orgasmic dysfunction: A two to six year follow-up. *Archives of Sexual Behavior, 17,* 463–480.

Milby, J. B., Schumacher, J. E., McNamara, C., Wallace, D., Usdan, S., McGill, T., et al. (2000). Initiating abstinence in cocaine abusing dually diagnosed homeless persons. *Drug and Alcohol Dependence, 60*(1), 55–67.

Milby, J. B., Schumacher, J. E., Raczynski, J. M., Caldwell, E., Engle, M., Michael, M., et al. (1996). Sufficient conditions for effective treatment of substance abusing homeless persons. *Drug and Alcohol Dependence, 43*(1–2), 39–47.

Milby, J. B., Schumacher, J. E., Wallace, D., Frison, S., McNamara, C., Usdan, S., et al. (2003). Day treatment with contingency management for cocaine abuse in homeless persons: 12-month follow-up. *Journal of Consulting and Clinical Psychology, 71*(3), 619–621.

Millar, H. R. (1998). New eating disorder service. *Psychiatric Bulletin, 22*, 751–754.

Miller, A. L., & Glinski, J. (2000). Youth suicidal behavior: Assessment and intervention. *Journal of Clinical Psychology, 56*(9), 1131–1152.

Miller, G. E., & Prinz, R. J. (1990). The enhancement of social learning family interventions for childhood conduct disorders. *Psychological Bulletin, 108*, 291–307.

Miller, I. W., Norman, W. H., Keitner, G. I., Bishop, S., & Dow, M. G. (1989). Cognitive-behavioral treatment of depressed in-patients. *Behavior Therapy, 20*, 25–47.

Miller, N. E., & Magruder, K. M. (Eds.). (1996). *The cost-effectiveness of psychotherapy: A guide for practitioners, researchers, and policy-makers.* New York: Wiley.

Miller, W. R., & Hester, R. K. (1986). The effectiveness of alcoholism treatment: What research reveals. In W. R. Miller & N. Heather (Eds.), *Treating addictive behaviors: The process of change* (pp. 121–174). New York: Plenum Press.

Miller, W. R., Meyers, R. J., & Tonigan, J. S. (1999). Engaging the unmotivated in treatment for alcohol problems: A comparison of three strategies for intervention through family members. *Journal of Consulting and Clinical Psychology, 67*(5), 688–697.

Miller, W. R., & Sanchez, V. C. (1993). Motivating young adults for treatment and lifestyle change. In G. Howard (Ed.), *Issues in alcohol use and abuse in young adults* (pp. 55–79). Notre Dame, IN: University of Notre Dame Press.

Miller, W. R., Walters, S. T., & Bennett, M. E. (2001). How effective is alcoholism treatment? *Journal of Studies on Alcohol, 62*, 211–220.

Miller, W. R., & Wilbourne, P. L. (2002). Mesa Grande: A methodological analysis of clinical trials of treatments for alcohol use disorders. *Addiction, 97*, 265–277.

Miller, W. R., Wilbourne, P. L., & Hettema, J. E. (2003). What works?: A summary of alcohol treatment outcome research. In R. K. Hester & W. R. Miller (Eds.), *Handbook of alcoholism treatment approaches: Effective alternatives* (3rd ed., pp. 13–63). Boston, MA: Allyn & Bacon.

Milne, D. L., Baker, C., Blackburn, I. M., James, I., & Reichelt, K. (1999). Effectiveness of cognitive therapy training. *Journal of Behavior Therapy and Experimental Psychiatry, 30*(2), 81–92.

Milrod, B., & Busch, F. (1996). Long-term outcome of panic disorder treatment: A review of the literature. *Journal of Nervous and Mental Disease, 184*(12), 723–730.

Milrod, B., Busch, F., Leon, A. C., Aronson, A., Roiphe, J., Rudden, M., et al. (2001). A pilot open trial of brief psychodynamic psychotherapy for panic disorder. *Journal of Psychotherapy Practice and Research, 10*, 239–245.

Milrod, B., & Shear, M. K. (1991). Dynamic treatment of panic disorder: A review. *Journal of Nervous and Mental Disease, 179*, 741–743.

Minichiello, W., Baer, L., & Jenike, M. A. (1987). Schizotypal personality disorder: A poor prognostic indicator for behavior therapy in the treatment of obsessive–compulsive disorder. *Journal of Anxiety Disorders, 1*, 273–276.

Mitchell, J. E. (1991). A review of the controlled trials of psychotherapy for bulimia nervosa. *Journal of Psychosomatic Research, 35*, 23–31.

Mitchell, J. E., Fletcher, L., Hanson, K., Mussell, M. P., Seim, H., Crosby, R., et al. (2001). The relative efficacy of fluoxetine and manual-based self-help in the treatment of outpatients with bulimia nervosa. *Journal of Clinical Psychopharmachology, 21*(3), 298–304.

Mitchell, J. E., Halmi, K., Wilson, G. T., Agras, W. S., Kraemer, H., & Crow, S. (2002). A randomized secondary treatment study of women with bulimia nervosa who fail to respond to CBT. *International Journal of Eating Disorders, 32*(3), 271–281.

Mitchell, J. E., Pyle, R. L., Eckert, E. D., Hatsukami, D., et al. (1990). A comparison study of antidepressants and structured intensive group psychotherapy in the treatment of bulimia nervosa. *Archives of General Psychiatry, 47*, 149–157.

Mitchell, J. E., Specker, S. M., & de Zwaan, M. (1991). Comorbidity and medical complications of bulimia nervosa. *Journal of Clinical Psychiatry, 52*(Suppl. 10), 13–20.

Mitchell, J. T., & Everly, G. S. (1994). *Critical Incident Stress Debriefing: CISD—an operations manual for the prevention of traumatic stress among emergency service and disaster workers.* Baltimore: Chevron.

Mittelman, M. S., Ferris, S. H., Shulman, E., Steinberg, G., Ambinder, A., Mackell, J. A., et al. (1995). A comprehensive support program: Effect on depression in spouse–caregivers of AD patients. *Gerontologist, 35*, 792–802.

Moffitt, T. E., Caspi, A., Dickson, N., Silva, P., & Stanton, W. (1996). Childhood-onset versus adolescent-onset antisocial problems in males: Natural history from ages 3 to 18 years. *Developmental Psychopathology, 9*, 399–424.

Mohlman, J., Gorenstein, E. E., Kleber, M., DeJesus, M., Gorman, J. M., & Papp, L. (2003). Standard and enhanced cognitive-behavior therapy for late-life generalized anxiety disorder: Two pilot investigations. *American Journal of Geriatric Psychiatry, 11*, 24–32.

Mohr, D. C., & Beutler, L. E. (1990). Erectile dysfunction: A review of diagnostic and treatment procedures. *Clinical Psychology Review, 10*, 123–150.

Mojtabai, R., Nicholson, R. A., & Carpenter, B. N. (1998). Role of psychosocial treatments in management of schizophrenia: A meta-analytic review of controlled outcome studies. *Schizophrenia Bulletin, 24*(4), 569–587.

Monahan, S. C., & Finney, J. W. (1996). Explaining abstinence rates following treatment for alcohol abuse: A quantitative synthesis of patient, research design and treatment effects. *Addiction, 91*(6), 787–805.

Moncrieff, J. (1995). Lithium revisited: A re-examination of the placebo-controlled trials of lithium prophylaxis in manic–depressive disorder. *British Journal of Psychiatry, 167*, 569–573.

Moncrieff, J., Wessley, S., & Hardy, R. (1998). Meta-analysis of trials comparing antidepressants with active placebos. *British Journal of Psychiatry, 172*, 227–231.

Moniz-Cook, E., Agar, S., Silver, M., Woods, R., Wang, M., Elston, C., et al. (1998). Can staff training reduce behavioural problems in residential care for the elderly mentally ill? *International Journal of Geriatric Psychiatry, 13*, 149–158.

Moniz-Cook, E., Stokes, G., & Agar, S. (2003). Difficult behaviour and dementia in nursing homes: Five cases of psychosocial intervention. *Clinical Psychology and Psychotherapy, 10*(3), 197–208.

Moniz-Cook, E., Woods, R. T., & Richards, K. (2001). Functional analysis of challenging behaviour in dementia: The role of superstition. *International Journal of Geriatric Psychiatry, 16*(1), 45–56.

Monsen, J. T., Odland, T., Faugli, A., Daae, E., & Eilertsen, D. E. (1995). Personality disorders: Changes and stability after intensive psychotherapy focusing on affect consciousness. *Psychotherapy Research, 5*, 33–48.

Montgomery, P. (2003). Media-based behavioural treatmnets for behavioural disorders in children (Cochrane Review). In *The Cochrane Library*, Issue 4. Chichester, UK: Wiley.

Montgomery, P., & Dennis, J. (2003). Cognitive behavioural interventions for sleep problems in adults aged 60+ (Cochrane Review). *The Cochrane Library*, Issue 3. Chichester, UK: Wiley.

Montgomery, R. W., & Allyon, T. (1994). Eye movement desensitization across subjects: Subjective and physiological measures of treatment efficacy. *Journal of Behavior Therapy and Experimental Psychiatry, 25*, 217–230.

Monti, P. M., Rohsenow, D. J., Hutchinson, K. E., Swift, R. M., Mueller, T. I., Colby, S. M., et al. (1999). Naltrexone's effect on cue-elicited craving among alcoholics in treatment. *Alcoholism: Clinical and Experimental Research, 23*, 1386–1394.

Monti, P. M., Rohsenow, D. J., Michalec, E., Martin, R. A., & Abrams, D. B. (1997). Brief coping skills treatment for cocaine abuse: Substance use outcomes at three months. *Addiction, 92*(12), 1717–1728.

Monti, P. M., Rohsenow, D. J., Rubonis, A. V., Niaura, R. S., Sirota, A. D., Colby, S. M., et al. (1993). Cue exposure with coping skills treatment for male alcoholics: A preliminary investigation. *Journal of Consulting and Clinical Psychology, 61*(6), 1011–1019.

Moore, R. G., & Blackburn, I.-M. (1997). Cognitive therapy in the treatment of non-responders to antidepressant medication: A controlled pilot study. *Behavioural and Cognitive Psychotherapy, 25*, 251–259.

Moras, K., & Strupp, H. H. (1982). Pretherapy interpersonal relations, patient's alliance and the outcome in brief psychotherapy. *Archives of General Psychiatry, 39*, 397–402.

Moreau, D., Mufson, L., Weissman, M. M., & Klerman, G. L. (1991). Interpersonal psychotherapy for adolescent depression: Description of modification and preliminary application. *Journal of the American Academy of Child and Adolescent Psychiatry, 30*, 642–651.

Moreno, J. L. (1953). *Who shall survive?* New York: Beacon House.

Morgan, H., & Raffle, C. (1999). Does reducing safety behaviours improve treatment response in patients with social phobia? *Australian and New Zealand Journal of Psychiatry, 33*(4), 503–510.

Morgan, K. (1987). *Sleep and ageing.* London: Croom Helm.

Morgan, K. (1992). Sleep, insomnia, and mental health. *Reviews in Clinical Gerontology, 2*, 246–253.

Morgan, L., Scourfield, J., Williams, D., Jasper, A., & Lewis, G. (2003). The Aberfan disaster: 33-year follow-up of survivors. *British Journal of Psychiatry, 182*, 532–536.

Morgenstern, J., Blanchard, K. A., Morgan, T. J., Labouvie, E., & Hayaki, J. (2001). Testing the effectiveness of cognitive-behavioral treatment for substance abuse in a community setting: Within treatment and posttreatment findings. *Journal of Consulting and Clinical Psychology, 69*(6), 1007–1017.

Morgenstern, J., & Longabaugh, R. (2000). Cognitive-behavioral treatment for alcohol dependence: A review of evidence for its hypothesized mechanisms of action. *Addiction, 95*(10), 1475–1490.

Moritz, S., Fricke, S., Jacobsen, D., Kloss, M., Wein, C., Rufer, M., et al. (2004). Positive schizotypal symptoms predict treatment outcome in obsessive–compulsive disorder. *Behaviour Research and Therapy, 42*, 217–227.

Morley, S. (1987). Single case methodology in behavior therapy. In S. J. Lindsay & G. E. Powell (Eds.), *A handbook of clinical adult psychology.* London: Gower Press.

Morley, S. (1989). Single case research. In G. Parry & F. N. Watts (Eds.), *Behavioral and mental health research: A handbook of skills and methods* (pp. 233–264). Hillsdale, NJ: Erlbaum.

Morokoff, P. J., & LoPiccolo, J. (1986). A comparative evaluation of minimal therapist contact and 15-session treatment for female orgasmic dysfunction. *Journal of Consulting and Clinical Psychology, 54*, 294–300.

Morris, R. G., Morris, L. W., & Britton, P. G. (1988). Factors affecting the emotional well-being of the caregivers of dementia sufferers. *British Journal of Psychiatry, 153*, 147–156.

Morrison, A., Bentall, R., French, P., Walford, L., Kilcommons, A., Knight, A., et al. (2002). Randomised controlled trial of early detection and cognitive therapy for preventing transition to psychosis in high-risk individuals: Study design and interim analysis of transition rate and psychological risk factors. *British Journal of Psychiatry, 181*(Suppl. 43), S78–S84.

Morrow-Bradley, C., & Elliot, R. (1986). Utilization of psychotherapy research by practicing psychotherapists. *American Psychologist, 41*, 188–197.

Moyer, A., Finney, J. W., Swearingen, C. E., & Vergun, P. (2002). Brief interventions for alcohol problems: A meta-analytic review of controlled investigations in treatment-seeking and non-treatment-seeking populations. *Addiction, 97*(3), 279–292.

MTA Cooperative Group, The. (1999). A 14-month randomized clinical trial of treatment strategies for attention-deficit/hyperactivity disorder: The MTA Cooperative Group multimodal treatment study of children with ADHD. *Archives of General Psychiatry, 56*(12), 1073–1086.

Mueller, T. I., Leon, A. C., Keller, M. B., Solomon, D. A., Endicott, J., Coryell, W., et al. (1999). Recurrence after recovery from major depressive disorder during 15 years of observational follow-up. *American Journal of Psychiatry, 156*(7), 1000–1006.

Mueser, K. T., & Berenbaum, H. (1990). Psychodynamic treatment of schizophrenia: Is there a future? *Psychological Medicine, 20*, 253–262.

Mufson, L., Morean, D., Weissman, M. M., & Wickramaratne, P. (1994). Modification of interpersonal psychotherapy with depressed adolescents. *Journal of the American Academy of Child and Adolescent Psychiatry, 33*, 695–705.

Mufson, L., Weissman, M. M., Moreau, D., & Garfinkel, R. (1999). Efficacy of interpersonal psychotherapy for depressed adolescents. *Archives of General Psychiatry, 56,* 573–579.

Mulder, R. T. (2002). Personality pathology and treatment outcome in major depression: A review. *American Journal of Psychiatry, 159*(3), 359–371.

Müller-Oerlinghausen, B., Ahrens, B., Grof, E., Grof, P., Lenz, G., Schou, M., et al. (1992). The effect of long-term lithium treatment on the mortality of patients with manic–depressive and schizoaffective illness. *Acta Psychiatrica Scandinavica, 86,* 218–222.

Munjack, D. J., Schlaks, A., Sanchez, V. C., Usigli, R., Zulueta, A., & Leonard, M. (1984). Rational emotive therapy in the treatment of erectile dysfunction: An initial study. *Journal of Sex and Marital Therapy, 10,* 170–175.

Muratori, F., Picchi, L., Bruni, G., Patarnello, M., & Romagnoli, G. (2003). A two-year follow-up of psychodynamic psychotherapy for internalizing disorders in children. *Journal of the American Academy of Child and Adolescent Psychiatry, 42*(3), 331–339.

Muris, P., Meesters, C., Merckelbach, H., Sermon, A., & Zwakhalen, S. (1998). Worry in normal children. *Journal of the American Academy of Child and Adolescent Psychiatry, 37,* 703–710.

Murphy, G. E., Simons, A. D., Wetzel, R. D., & Lustman, P. J. (1984). Cognitive therapy and pharmacotherapy: Singly and together in the treatment of depression. *Archives of General Psychiatry, 41,* 33–41.

Mussell, M. P., Mitchell, J. E., Crosby, R. D., Fulkerson, J. A., Hoberman, H. M., & Romano, J. L. (2000). Commitment to treatment goals in prediction of group cognitive-behavioral therapy treatment outcome for women with bulimia nervosa. *Journal of Consulting and Clinical Psychology, 68*(3), 432–437.

Myers, J. K., Weissman, M. M., Tischler, G. L., et al. (1984). Six month prevalence of psychiatric disorders in three communities. *Archives of General Psychiatry, 41,* 959–967.

Mynors-Wallis, L. M., Gath, D. H., Day, A., & Baker, F. (2000). Randomised controlled trial of problem solving treatment, antidepressant medication, and combined treatment for major depression in primary care. *British Medical Journal, 320*(7226), 26–30.

Mynors-Wallis, L. M., Gath, D. H., Lloyd-Thomas, A. R., & Tomlinson, D. (1995). Randomised controlled trial comparing problem solving treatment with amitriptyline and placebo for major depression in primary care. *British Medical Journal, 310*(6977), 441–445.

Nagy, L. M., Krystal, J. H., Charney, D. S., Merikangas, K. R., & Woods, S. W. (1993). Long-term outcome of panic disorder after short-term imipramine and behavioral group treatment: 2.9 year naturalistic follow-up study. *Journal of Clinical Psychopharmacology, 13,* 16–24.

Nagy, L. M., Krystal, J. H., Woods, S. W., & Charney, D. S. (1989). Clinical and medication outcome after short term alprazolam and behavioral group treatment in panic disorder. *Archives of General Psychiatry, 46,* 993–999.

Najavits, L. M., & Weiss, R. D. (1994). Variations in therapist effectiveness in the treatment of patients with substance use disorders: An empirical review. *Addiction, 89,* 679–688.

Najavits, L. M., Weiss, R. G., Shaw, S. R., & Dierberger, A. E. (2000). Psychotherapists' views of treatment manuals. *Professional Psychology: Research and Practice, 31,* 404–408.

Narrow, W. E., Rae, D. S., Robins, L. N., & Regier, D. A. (2002). Revised prevalence estimates of mental disorders in the United States: Using a clinical significance criterion to reconcile 2 surveys' estimates. *Archives of General Psychiatry, 59*(2), 115–123.

National Institute for Clinical Excellence. (2004). Depression: The management of depression in primary and secondary care. Available online at *www.nice.org.uk.*

Neal, M., & Briggs, M. (1999). Validation therapy for dementia (Cochrane review). In *The Cochrane Library,* Issue 3. Chichester, UK: Wiley.

Neitzel, M. T., Russell, R. L., Hemmings, K. A., & Gretter, M. L. (1987). Clinical significance of psychotherapy for unipolar depression: A meta-analytic approach to social comparison. *Journal of Consulting and Clinical Psychology, 55,* 156–161.

Nemeroff, C. B. (1996). The corticotropin-releasing factor (CRF) hypothesis of depression: New findings and new directions. *Molecular Psychiatry, 1,* 326–342.

Newman, C., & Beck, A. T. (1993). *Cognitive therapy of rapid cycling bipolar affective disorder—treatment manual*. Philadelphia: Center for Cognitive Therapy, University of Pennsylvania.

Newman, D. L., Moffitt, T. E., Caspi, A., & Silva, P. A. (1998). Comorbid mental disorders: Implications for treatment and sample selection. *Journal of Abnormal Psychology, 107*(2), 305–311.

Newman, M. G., Kenardy, J., Herman, S., & Taylor, C. B. (1997). Comparison of palmtop-computer-assisted brief cognitive-behavioral treatment to cognitive-behavioral treatment for panic disorder. *Journal of Consulting and Clinical Psychology, 65*(1), 178–183.

Newton, N. A., & Lazarus, L. W. (1992). Behavioral and psychotherapeutic interventions. In J. E. Birren, R. B. Sloane, & G. D. Cohen (Eds.), *Handbook of mental health and ageing* (2nd ed., pp. 699–719). San Diego: Academic Press.

Neziroglu, F. (1979). A combined behavioural pharmacotherapy approach to obsessive compulsive disorders. In J. Oriols, C. Ballus, M. Gonzales, & J. Prijol (Eds.), *Biological psychiatry today*. Amsterdam: Elsevier/North Holland.

Neziroglu, F., Yaryura-Tobias, J. A., Walz, J., & McKay, D. (2000). The effect of fluvoxamine and behavior therapy on children and adolescents with obsessive–compulsive disorder. *Journal of Child and Adolescent Psychopharmacology, 10*(4), 295–306.

Nixon, R. D., Sweeney, L., Erickson, D. B., & Touyz, S. W. (2003). Parent–child interaction therapy: A comparison of standard and abbreviated treatments for oppositional defiant preschoolers. *Journal of Consulting and Clinical Psychology, 71*(2), 251–260.

Nofzinger, E. A., Thase, M. E., Reynolds, C. F., Frank, E., Jennings, J. R., Garamoni, G. L., et al. (1993). Sexual functioning in depressed men: Assessment using self-report, behavioral and nocturnal penile tumescence measures before and after treatment with cognitive behavioral therapy. *Archives of General Psychiatry, 50*, 24–30.

Norcross, J. C. (2001). Empirically supported therapy relationships: Summary report of the Division 29 Task Force. *Psychotherapy Research, 38*, 345–497.

Norcross, J. C. (2002). *Psychotherapy relationships that work: Therapist contributions and responsiveness to patients' needs*. New York: Oxford University Press.

Nordentoft, M., Jeppsen, P., Abel, M., Kassow, P., Petersen, L., Thorup, A., et al. (2002). Opus study: Suicidal behaviour, suicidal ideation and hopelessness among patients with first-episode psychosis: One-year follow-up of a randomised controlled trial. *British Journal of Psychiatry, 181*(Suppl. 43), S98–S106.

Nordhus, I. H., & Pallesen, S. (2003). Psychological treatment of late-life anxiety: An empirical review. *Journal of Consulting and Clinical Psychology, 71*(4), 643–651.

Noyes, R., Reich, J., Christiansen, J., Suelzer, M., Pfohl, B., & Coryell, W. A. (1990). Outcome of panic disorder: Relationship to diagnostic subtypes and comorbidity. *Archives of General Psychiatry, 47*, 809–818.

Nugent, W. R., Carpenter, D., & Parks, J. (1993). A statewide evaluation of family preservation and family reunification services. *Research on Social Work Practice, 3*, 40–65.

Nye, C. L., Zucker, R. A., & Fitzgerald, H. E. (1995). Early intervention in the path to alcohol problems through conduct problems: Treatment involvement and child behaviour change. *Journal of Consulting and Clinical Psychology, 63*, 831–840.

Oakley-Brown, M. (1991). The epidemiology of anxiety disorders. *International Journal of Psychiatry, 3*, 243–252.

Oates, R. K., O'Toole, B. I., Lynch, D. L., Stern, A., & Cooney, G. (1994). Stability and change in outcomes for sexually abused children. *Journal of the American Academy of Child and Adolescent Psychiatry, 33*(7), 945–953.

O'Brien, C. P., Hamm, K. B., Ray, B. A., & Pierce, J. F. (1972). Group versus individual psychotherapy with schizophrenics. *Archives of General Psychiatry, 27*, 474–478.

O'Brien, C. P., & Lynch, K. G. (2003). Can we design and replicate clinical trials with a multiple drug focus. *Drug and Alcohol Dependence, 70*(2), 135–137.

O'Brien, K. M., & Vincent, N. K. (2003). Psychiatric comorbidity in anorexia and bulimia nervosa: Nature, prevalence, and causal relationships. *Clinical Psychology Review, 23*(1), 57–74.

Ockene, J. K., Adams, A., Hurley, T. G., Wheeler, E. V., & Hebert, J. R. (1999). Brief physician- and nurse practitioner-delivered counseling for high-risk drinkers: Does it work? *Archives of Internal Medicine, 159*(18), 2198–2205.

O'Connor, D. W., Pollitt, P. A., Hyde, J. B., Brook, C. P. B., Reiss, B. B., & Roth, M. (1988). Do general practitioners miss dementia in elderly patients? *British Medical Journal, 297,* 1107–1110.

O'Connor, K., Todorov, C., Robillard, S., Borgeat, F., & Brault, M. (1999). Cognitive-behaviour therapy and medication in the treatment of obsessive–compulsive disorder: A controlled study. *Canadian Journal of Psychiatry, 44*(1), 64–71.

O'Donohue, W., Dopke, C. A., & Swingen, D. N. (1997). Psychotherapy for female sexual dysfunction: A review. *Clinical Psychology Review, 17*(5), 537–566.

O'Donohue, W. T., Swingen, D. N., Dopke, C. A., & Regev, L. G. (1999). Psychotherapy for male sexual dysfunction: A review. *Clinical Psychology Review, 19*(5), 591–630.

Oei, T. P. S., & Jackson, P. R. (1980). Long-term effects of group and individual social skills training with alcoholics. *Addictive Behaviors, 5,* 129–136.

Oei, T. P. S., & Jackson, P. R. (1982). Social skills and cognitive behavioral approaches to the treatment of problem drinking. *Journal of Studies on Alcohol, 43,* 532–547.

Oei, T. P. S., Llamas, M., & Devilly, G. J. (1999). The efficacy and cognitive processes of cognitive behaviour therapy in the treatment of panic disorder with agoraphobia. *Behavioural and Cognitive Psychotherapy, 27,* 63–88.

O'Farrell, T. J., Choquette, K. A., & Cutter, H. S. (1998). Couples relapse prevention sessions after behavioral marital therapy for male alcoholics: Outcomes during the three years after starting treatment. *Journal of Studies on Alcohol, 59*(4), 357–370.

O'Farrell, T. J., Choquette, K. A., Cutter, H. S., Brown, E. D., & McCourt, W. F. (1993). Behavioral marital therapy with and without additional couples relapse prevention sessions for alcoholics and their wives. *Journal of Studies on Alcohol, 54*(6), 652–666.

O'Farrell, T. J., Cutter, H. S., Choquette, K. A., Floyd, F. J., & Bayog, R. D. (1992). Behavioral marital therapy for male alcoholics: Marital and drinking adjustment during the two years after treatment. *Behavior Therapy, 23*(4), 529–549.

O'Farrell, T. J., Cutter, H. S., & Floyd, F. J. (1985). Evaluating behavior therapy for male alcoholics: Effects on marital adjustment and communication from before to after treatment. *Behavior Therapy, 16,* 147–167.

Office of National Statistics. (2000). *Psychiatric morbidity among adults living in private households.* London: Author.

Ogles, B. M., Lambert, M. J., & Sawyer, J. D. (1995). Clinical significance of the National Institute of Mental Health Treatment of Depression Collaborative Research Program data. *Journal of Consulting and Clinical Psychology, 63,* 321–326.

Ogrodniczuk, J. S., Piper, W. E., McCallum, M., Joyce, A. S., & Rosie, J. S. (2002). Interpersonal predictors of group therapy outcome for complicated grief. *International Journal of Group Psychotherapy, 52,* 511–535.

Oliver, P. C., Piachaud, J., Done, D. J., Regan, A., Cooray, S. E., & Tyrer, P. J. (2003). Difficulties developing evidence-based approaches in learning disabilities. *Evidence-Based Mental Health, 6,* 37–38.

Oliver, P. C., Piachaud, J., Done, J., Regan, A., Cooray, S., & Tyrer, P. (2002). Difficulties in conducting a randomized controlled trial of health service interventions in intellectual disability: Implications for evidence-based practice. *Journal of Intellectual Disability Research, 46*(Pt. 4), 340–345.

Ollendick, T. H., & King, N. J. (1998). Empirically supported treatments for children with phobic and anxiety disorders. *Journal of Clinical Child Psychology, 27,* 156–167.

O'Malley, S. S., Foley, S. H., Rounsaville, B. J., Watkins, J. T., Imber, S. D., Sotsky, S. M., et al. (1988). Therapist competence and patient outcome in interpersonal psychotherapy of depression. *Journal of Consulting and Clinical Psychology, 56,* 496–501.

O'Malley, S. S., Jaffe, A. J., Chang, G., Rode, S., Schottenfeld, R., Meyer, R. E., et al. (1996). Six-month follow-up of naltrexone and psychotherapy for alcohol dependence. *Archives of General Psychiatry, 53*(3), 217–224.

O'Malley, S. S., Jaffe, A. J., Chang, G., Schottenfeld, R. S., Meyer, R., & Rounsaville, B. (1992). Naltrexone and coping skills therapy for alcohol dependence. *Archives of General Psychiatry, 49,* 881–887.

Ong, Y., Martineau, F., Lloyd, C., & Robbins, I. (1987). A support group for the depressed elderly. *International Journal of Geriatric Psychiatry, 2,* 119–123.

Oosterbaan, D. B., van Balkom, A. J., Spinhoven, P., de Meij, T. G., & van Dyck, R. (2002). The influence on treatment gain of comorbid avoidant personality disorder in patients with social phobia. *Journal of Nervous and Mental Disease, 190*(1), 41–43.

Oosterbaan, D. B., van Balkom, A. J., Spinhoven, P., Van Oppen, P., & Van Dyck, R. (2001). Cognitive therapy versus moclobemide in social phobia: A controlled study. *Clinical Psychology and Psychotherapy, 8,* 263–273.

Orford, J., Oppenheimer, E., & Edwards, G. (1976). Abstinence or control: The outcome for excessive drinkers two years after consultation. *Behaviour Research and Therapy, 14,* 409–418.

Orlinsky, D. E., Grawe, K., & Parks, B. K. (1994). Process and outcome in psychotherapy. In A. E. Bergin & S. L. Garfield (Eds.), *Handbook of psychotherapy and behavior change* (4th ed., pp. 270–376). New York: Wiley.

Öst, L. G. (1987). Applied relaxation: Description of a coping technique and a review of controlled studies. *Behaviour Research and Therapy, 25,* 397–409.

Öst, L. G. (1988). Applied relaxation vs. progressive relaxation in the treatment of panic disorder. *Behaviour Research and Therapy, 26,* 13–22.

Öst, L. G. (1989). One session treatment for specific phobias. *Behaviour Research and Therapy, 27,* 1–7.

Öst, L. G., Alm, T., Brandberg, M., & Breitholtz, E. (2001a). One vs. five sessions of exposure and five sessions of cognitive therapy in the treatment of claustrophobia. *Behaviour Research and Therapy, 39*(2), 167–183.

Öst, L. G., Brandberg, M., & Alm, T. (1997a). One versus five sessions of exposure in the treatment of flying phobia. *Behaviour Research and Therapy, 35,* 987–996.

Öst, L. G., & Breitholtz, E. (2000). Applied relaxation vs. cognitive therapy in the treatment of generalized anxiety disorder. *Behaviour Research and Therapy, 38*(8), 777–790.

Öst, L. G., Fellenius, J., & Sterner, U. (1991a). Applied tension, exposure in vivo, and tension-only in the treatment of blood phobia. *Behaviour Research and Therapy, 29,* 561–574.

Öst, L. G., Ferebee, I., & Furmark, T. (1997b). One-session group therapy of spider phobia: Direct versus indirect treatments. *Behaviour Research and Therapy, 35*(8), 721–732.

Öst, L. G., Jerramalm, A., & Johansson, J. (1981). Individual response patterns and the effects of different behavioral methods in the treatment of social phobia. *Behaviour Research and Therapy, 19,* 1–16.

Öst, L. G., Lindahl, I. L., Sterner, U., & Jerremalm, A. (1984). Exposure *in-vivo* vs. applied relaxation in the treatment of blood phobia. *Behaviour Research and Therapy, 22,* 205–216.

Öst, L. G., Salkovskis, P., & Hellstrom, K. (1991b). One session therapist directed exposure vs. self-exposure in the treatment of spider phobia. *Behavior Therapy, 22,* 407–422.

Öst, L. G., Sterner, U., & Fellenius, J. (1989). Applied tension, applied relaxation in the treatment of blood phobia. *Behaviour Research and Therapy, 27,* 109–121.

Öst, L. G., Svensson, L., Hellstrom, K., & Lindwall, R. (2001b). One-session treatment of specific phobias in youths: A randomized clinical trial. *Journal of Consulting and Clinical Psychology, 69,* 814–824.

Öst, L. G., & Westling, B. E. (1995). Applied relaxation vs. cognitive behavior therapy in the treatment of panic disorder. *Behaviour Research and Therapy, 33,* 145–158.

Öst, L. G., Westling, B. E., & Hellstrom, K. (1993). Applied relaxation, exposure *in-vivo* and cognitive methods in the treatment of panic disorder with agoraphobia. *Behaviour Research and Therapy, 31,* 383–394.

O'Sullivan, G., & Marks, I. M. (1990). Long-term outcome of phobic and obsessive–compulsive disorders after treatment. In R. Noyes, M. Roth, & G. D. Burrows (Eds.), *Handbook of anxiety: Vol. 4. The treatment of anxiety* (pp. 87–108). Amsterdam: Elsevier Science.

Otto, M. W., Gould, R. A., & McLean, R. Y. S. (1996). The effectiveness of cognitive-behavior therapy for panic disorder without concurrent medication treatment: A reply to Power and Sharp [letter]. *Journal of Psychopharmacology, 10,* 254–256.

Otto, M. W., Pollack, M. H., Gould, R. A., Worthington, J. J., III, McArdle, E. T., & Rosenbaum, J. F. (2000). A comparison of the efficacy of clonazepam and cognitive-behavioral group therapy for the treatment of social phobia. *Journal of Anxiety Disorders, 14*(4), 345–358.

Otto, M. W., Pollack, M. H., Sachs, G. S., Reiter, S. R., Meltzer-Brody, S., & Rosenbaum, J. F. (1993). Discontinuation of benzodiazepine treatment: Efficacy of cognitive-behavioural therapy for patients with panic disorder. *American Journal of Psychiatry, 150,* 1485–1490.

Ouimette, P. C., Finney, J. W., & Moos, R. H. (1997). Twelve-step and cognitive-behavioral treatment for substance abuse: A comparison of treatment effectiveness. *Journal of Consulting and Clinical Psychology, 65*(2), 230–240.

Owens, E. B., Hinshaw, S. P., Kraemer, H. C., Arnold, L. E., Abikoff, H. B., Cantwell, D. P., et al. (2003). Which treatment for whom for ADHD?: Moderators of treatment response in the MTA. *Journal of Consulting and Clinical Psychology, 71*(3), 540–552.

Oxman, T. E., Barrett, J. E., Sengupta, A., Katon, W., Williams, J. W., Jr., Frank, E., et al. (2001). Status of minor depression or dysthymia in primary care following a randomized controlled treatment. *General Hospital Psychiatry, 23*(6), 301–310.

Ozonoff, S., & Miller, J. N. (1995). Teaching theory of mind: A new approach to social skills training for individuals with autism. *Journal of Autism and Developmental Disorders, 25,* 415–433.

Paley, G., & Shapiro, D. A. (2002). Lessons from psychotherapy research for psychological interventions for people with schizophrenia. *Psychology and Psychotherapy: Theory, Research and Practice, 75,* 5–17.

Pallesen, S., Nordhus, I. H., Kvale, G., Nielsen, G. H., Havik, O. E., Johnsen, B. H., et al. (2003). Behavioral treatment of insomnia in older adults: An open clinical trial comparing two interventions. *Behaviour Research and Therapy, 41,* 31–48.

Palmer, A. G., Williams, H., & Adams, M. (1995). CBT in a group format for bipolar affective disorder. *Behavioral and Cognitive Psychotherapy, 23,* 153–168.

Palmer, C., & Fenner, J. (1999). *Getting the message across: Review of research and theory about disseminating information within the NHS.* London: Gaskell.

Palmer, R. L., Birchall, H., McGrain, L., & Sullivan, V. (2002). Self-help for bulimic disorders: A randomised controlled trial comparing minimal guidance with face-to-face or telephone guidance. *British Journal of Psychiatry, 181,* 230–235.

Paris, J., Brown, R., & Nowlis, D. (1987). Long term follow-up of borderline patients in a general hospital. *Comprehensive Psychiatry, 28,* 530–535.

Park, J. M., Mataix-Cols, D., Marks, I. M., Ngamthipwatthana, T., Marks, M., Araya, R., et al. (2001). Two-year follow-up after a randomised controlled trial of self- and clinician-accompanied exposure for phobia/panic disorders. *British Journal of Psychiatry, 178,* 543–548.

Parmelee, P. A., & Lawton, M. P. (1990). The design of special environments for the aged. In J. E. Birren & K. W. Schaie (Eds.), *Handbook of the psychology of ageing* (3rd ed., pp. 465–489). San Diego: Academic Press.

Parry, G. (1986). The case of the anxious executive: A study from the research clinic. *British Journal of Medical Psychology, 59,* 221–233.

Parry, G. (1992). Improving psychotherapy services: Applications of research, audit and evaluation. *British Journal of Clinical Psychology, 31,* 3–19.

Parry, G. (1996). Psychotherapy services in the English National Health Service. In N. E. Miller & K. M. Magruder (Eds.), *The cost-effectiveness of psychotherapy: A guide for practitioners, researchers and policy-makers* (pp. 317–326). New York: Wiley.

Parry, G. (2000). Evidence based psychotherapy: Special case or special pleading. *Evidence-Based Mental Health, 3,* 35–37.

Parry, G., Cape, J., & Pilling, S. (2003). Clinical practice guidelines in clinical psychology and psychotherapy. *Clinical Psychology and Psychotherapy, 10,* 337–351.

Parsons, B., Quitkin, F. M., McGrath, P. J., Stewart, J. W., Tricarno, E., Ocepek-Welikson, et al. (1989). Phenelzine, imipramine and placebo in borderline patients meeting criteria for atypical depression. *Psychopharmacology Bulletin, 25*, 524–534.

Patelis-Siotis, I. (2001). Cognitive-behavioral therapy: Applications for the management of bipolar disorder. *Bipolar Disorders, 3*, 1–10.

Patelis-Siotis, I., Young, L. T., Robb, J. C., Marriott, M., Bieling, P. J., Cox, L. C., et al. (2001). Group cognitive behavioral therapy for bipolar disorder: A feasibility and effectiveness study. *Journal of Affective Disorders, 65*(2), 145–153.

Pato, M. T., Zoka-Kadouch, R., Zohar, J., & Murphy, D. L. (1988). Return of symptoms after desensitization of clomipramine in patients with obsessive–compulsive disorder. *American Journal of Psychiatry, 145*, 1521–1525.

Patterson, G. R. (1976). *Living with children: New methods for parents and teachers* (rev. ed.). Champaign, IL: Research Press.

Patterson, G. R. (1982). *Coercive family processes.* Aegean, OR: Castalia.

Patterson, G. R., & Chamberlain, P. (1988). Treatment process: A problem at three levels. In L. C. Wynne (Ed.), *The state of the art in family therapy research: Controversies and recommendations* (pp. 189–223). New York: Family Process Press.

Patterson, G. R., & Forgatch, M. S. (1987). *Parents and adolescents living together: Part 1. The basics.* Eugene, OR: Castalia.

Patterson, G. R., Reid, J. B., Jones, R. R., & Conger, R. E. (1975). *A social learning approach to family intervention: Vol. 1. Families with aggressive children.* Eugene, OR: Castalia.

Pattison, E. M., Brissenden, A., & Wohl, T. (1967). Assessing specific aspects of in-patient group psychotherapy. *International Journal of Group Psychotherapy, 17*, 283–297.

Paunovic, N., & Ost, L. G. (2001). Cognitive-behavior therapy vs. exposure therapy in the treatment of PTSD in refugees. *Behaviour Research and Therapy, 39*(10), 1183–1197.

Paykel, E. S., Brayne, C., Huppert, F. A., Gill, C., Barkley, C., Gehlbaar, E., et al. (1994). Incidence of dementia in a population older than 75 years in the United Kingdom. *Archives of General Psychiatry, 51*, 325–332.

Paykel, E. S., Ramana, R., Cooper, Z., Hayhurst, H., Kerr, J., & Barocka, A. (1995). Residual symptoms after partial remission: An important outcome in depression. *Psychological Medicine, 25*, 1171–1180.

Paykel, E. S., Scott, J., Teasdale, J. D., Johnson, A. L., Garland, A., Moore, R., et al. (1999). Prevention of relapse in residual depression by cognitive therapy: A controlled trial. *Archives of General Psychiatry, 56*(9), 829–835.

Peachey, J. E., Annis, H. M., Bornstein, E. R., Sykora, K., Maglana, S. M., & Shamai, S. (1989). Calcium carbimide in alcoholism treatment: Part 1. A placebo controlled double-blind clinical trial of short-term efficacy. *British Journal of Addiction, 84*, 877–887.

Peet, M. (1994). Induction of mania with selective serotonin re-uptake inhibitors and tricyclic antidepressants. *British Journal of Psychiatry, 164*, 549–550.

Pekkala, E., & Merinder, L. (2002). Psychoeducation for schizophrenia (Cochrane Review). In *The Cochrane Library*, Issue 4, 2002. Oxford, UK: Update Software.

Pendleton, V. R., Goodrick, G. K., Poston, W. S. C., Reeves, R. S., & Foreyt, J. P. (2002). Exercise augments the effects of cognitive-behavioral therapy in the treatment of binge eating. *International Journal of Eating Disorders, 31*, 172–184.

Peniston, E. G. (1986). EMG biofeedback assisted desensitization treatment for Vietnam combat veterans PTSD. *Clinical Biofeedback and Health, 9*, 35–41.

Perkonigg, A., Kessler, R. C., Storz, S., & Wittchen, H. U. (2000). Traumatic events and post-traumatic stress disorder in the community: Prevalence, risk factors and comorbidity. *Acta Psychiatrica Scandinavica, 101*(1), 46–59.

Perl, M., Westlin, A. B., & Peterson, L. G. (1985). The female rape survivor: Time limited therapy with female/male co-therapists. *Journal of Psychosomatic Obstetrics and Gynaecology, 4*, 197–205.

Perlick, D., Clarkin, J. F., Sirey, J., Raue, P., Greenfield, S., Struening, E., et al. (1999). Burden experienced by care-givers of persons with bipolar affective disorder. *British Journal of Psychiatry, 175*, 56–62.

Perlick, D. A., Rosenheck, R. A., Clarkin, J. F., Sirey, J. A., Salahi, J., Struening, E. L., et al. (2001). Stigma as a barrier to recovery: Adverse effects of perceived stigma on social adaptation of persons diagnosed with bipolar affective disorder. *Psychiatric Services, 52*(12), 1627–1632.

Perry, A., Tarrier, N., Morriss, R., McCarthy, E., & Limb, K. (1999). Randomised controlled trial of efficacy of teaching patients with bipolar disorder to identify early symptoms of relapse and obtain treatment. *British Medical Journal, 318*(7177), 149–153.

Perry, J. C. (1985). Depression in borderline personality disorders: Lifetime prevalence at interview and longitudinal course of symptoms. *American Journal of Psychiatry, 142*, 15–21.

Perry, J. C., Augusto, F., & Cooper, S. H. (1989). Assessing psychodynamic conflicts: 1. Reliability of the idiographic conflict formulation method. *Psychiatry, 52*, 289–301.

Perry, J. C., Banon, E., & Ianni, F. (1999). Effectiveness of psychotherapy for personality disorders. *American Journal of Psychiatry, 156*(9), 1312–1321.

Perry, S. (1990). Combining anti-depressants and psychotherapy: Rationale and strategies. *Journal of Clinical Psychiatry, 51*(Suppl.), 16–20.

Perse, T. (1988). Obsessive–compulsive disorder: A treatment review. *Journal of Clinical Psychiatry, 49*, 48–55.

Persons, J. (1989). *Cognitive therapy in practice: The case formulation approach.* New York: Norton.

Persons, J. B. (1991). Psychotherapy outcome studies do not accurately represent current models of psychotherapy: A proposed remedy. *American Psychologist, 46*, 99–106.

Peterson, C. B., Mitchell, J. E., Engbloom, S., Nugent, S., Mussell, M. P., & Miller, J. P. (1998). Group cognitive-behavioral treatment of binge eating disorder: A comparison of therapist-led versus self-help formats. *International Journal of Eating Disorders, 24*(2), 125–136.

Peterson, C. B., Mitchell, J. E., Engbloom, S., Nugent, S., Pederson Mussell, M., Crow, S. J., et al. (2001). Self-help versus therapist-led group cognitive-behavioral treatment of binge eating disorder at follow-up. *International Journal of Eating Disorders, 30*(4), 363–374.

Petry, N. M., & Martin, B. (2002). Low-cost contingency management for treating cocaine- and opioid-abusing methadone patients. *Journal of Consulting and Clinical Psychology, 70*(2), 398–405.

Petry, N. M., Martin, B., Cooney, J. L., & Kranzler, H. R. (2000). Give them prizes, and they will come: Contingency management for treatment of alcohol dependence. *Journal of Consulting and Clinical Psychology, 68*(2), 250–257.

Pharoah, F. M., Rathbone, J., Mari, J.J., & Streiner, D. (2002). Family intervention for schizophrenia (Cochrane Review). In *The Cochrane Library*, Issue 4. Chichester, UK: Wiley.

Piccinelli, M., Pini, S., Bellantuono, C., & Wilkinson, G. (1995). Efficacy of drug treatment in obsessive–compulsive disorder: A meta-analytic review. *British Journal of Psychiatry, 166*, 424–443.

Piccinelli, M., & Wilkinson, G. (1994). Outcome of depression in psychiatric settings. *British Journal of Psychiatry, 164*, 297–304.

Pierce, K., & Schreibman, L. (1995). Increasing complex social behaviors in children with autism: Effects of peer-implemented pivotal response training. *Journal of Applied Behavior Analysis, 28*(3), 285–295.

Pike, K. (1998). Long-term course of anorexia nervosa: Response, relapse, remission, and recovery. *Clinical Psychology Review, 18*(4), 447–475.

Pike, K. M., Walsh, B. T., Vitousek, K., Wilson, G. T., & Bauer, J. (2003). Cognitive behavior therapy in the posthospitalization treatment of anorexia nervosa. *American Journal of Psychiatry, 160*(11), 2046–2049.

Pilling, S., Bebbington, P., Kuipers, E., Garety, P., Geddes, J., Martindale, B., et al. (2002a). Psychological treatments in schizophrenia: II. Meta-analyses of randomized controlled trials of social skills training and cognitive remediation. *Psychological Medicine, 32*(5), 783–791.

Pilling, S., Bebbington, P., Kuipers, E., Garety, P., Geddes, J., Orbach, G., et al. (2002b). Psychological treatments in schizophrenia: I. Meta-analysis of family intervention and cognitive behaviour therapy. *Psychological Medicine, 32,* 763–782.

Piorkowsky, G. K., & Mann, E. T. (1975). Issues in treatment efficacy research with alcoholics. *Perceptual and Motor Skills, 41,* 695–700.

Piper, W. E., Azim, H. F., Joyce, A. S., & McCallum, M. (1991a). Transference interpretations, therapeutic alliance, and outcome in short-term individual psychotherapy. *Archives of General Psychiatry, 48*(10), 946–953.

Piper, W. E., Azim, H. F., McCallum, M., & Joyce, A. S. (1990). Patient suitability and outcome in short-term individual psychotherapy. *Journal of Consulting and Clinical Psychology, 58*(4), 475–481.

Piper, W. E., Azim, H. F. A., Joyce, A. S., McCallum, M., Nixon, G. W. H., & Segal, P. S. (1991b). Quality of object relations vs. interpersonal functioning as a predictor of the therapeutic alliance and psychotherapy outcome. *Journal of Nervous and Mental Disease, 179,* 432–438.

Piper, W. E., Joyce, A. S., Azim, H. F. A., & Rosie, J. S. (1994). Patient characteristics and success in day treatment. *Journal of Nervous and Mental Disease, 182,* 381–386.

Piper, W. E., Joyce, A. S., McCallum, M., & Azim, H. F. (1998). Interpretive and supportive forms of psychotherapy and patient personality variables. *Journal of Consulting and Clinical Psychology, 66*(3), 558–567.

Piper, W. E., Joyce, A. S., McCallum, M., & Azim, H. F. A. (1993). Concentration and correspondence of transference interpretations in short term therapy. *Journal of Consulting and Clinical Psychology, 61,* 586–595.

Piper, W. E., McCallum, M., Joyce, A. S., Azim, H. F., & Ogrodniczuk, J. S. (1999). Follow-up findings for interpretive and supportive forms of psychotherapy and patient personality variables. *Journal of Consulting and Clinical Psychology, 67*(2), 267–273.

Piper, W. E., McCallum, M., Joyce, A. S., Rosie, J. S., & Ogrodniczuk, J. (2001). Patient personality and time-limited group psychotherapy for complicated grief. *International Journal of Group Psychotherapy, 51,* 525–552.

Pisterman, S., Firestone, P., McGrath, P., Goodman, J. T., Webster, I., Mallory, R., et al. (1992). The role of parent training in treatment of preschoolers with ADDH. *American Journal of Orthopsychiatry, 62,* 397–408.

Pisterman, S., McGrath, P., Firestone, P., Goodman, J. T., Webster, I., & Mallory, R. (1989). Outcome of parent-mediated treatment of preschoolers with attention deficit disorder with hyperactivity. *Journal of Consulting and Clinical Psychology, 57,* 628–635.

Pitman, R. K., Orr, S. P., Altman, B., Longpre, R. E., & Macklin, M. L. (1996). Emotional processing during eye movement desensitization and reprocessing (EMDR) therapy of Vietnam veterans with posttraumatic stress disorder. *Comprehensive Psychiatry, 37,* 419–429.

Pitschel-Walz, G., Leucht, S., Bauml, J., Kissling, W., & Engel, R. R. (2001). The effect of family interventions on relapse and rehospitalization in schizophrenia—a meta-analysis. *Schizophrenia Bulletin, 27*(1), 73–92.

Pittman, D. J., & Tate, R. L. (1972). A comparison of two treatment programs for alcoholics. *International Journal of Social Psychiatry, 18,* 183–193.

Plomin, R., & McGuffin, P. (2003). Psychopathology in the postgenomic era. *Annual Review of Psychology, 54,* 205–228.

Poikolainen, K. (1999). Effectiveness of brief interventions to reduce alcohol intake in primary health care populations: A meta-analysis. *Preventive Medicine, 28*(5), 503–509.

Pollack, M. H., Otto, M. W., Sabatino, S., Majcher, D., Worthington, J. J., McArdle, E. T., et al. (1996). Relationship of childhood anxiety to adult panic disorder: Correlates and influence on course. *American Journal of Psychiatry, 153,* 376–381.

Pomerleau, O., Pertshuk, M., Adkins, D., & d'Aquili, E. (1978). Treatment for middle-income problem drinkers. In P. E. Nathan, G. A. Marlatt, & T. Loberg (Eds.), *Alcoholism: New directions in behavioral research and treatment* (pp. 143–160). New York: Plenum Press.

Pope, H. G., Jonas, M. J., & Hudson, J. I. (1983). The validity of DSM-III borderline personality disorders. *Archives of General Psychiatry, 40*, 23–30.

Powell, J., Gray, J., & Bradley, B. (1993). Subjective craving for opiates: evaluation of a cue exposure protocol for use with detoxified opiate addicts. *British Journal of Clinical Psychology, 32*(Pt. 1), 39–53.

Power, K., McGoldrick, T., Brown, K., Buchanan, R., Sharp, D., Swanson, V., & Karatzias, A. (2002). Controlled comparison of eye movement desensitization and reprocessing versus exposure plus cognitive restructuring versus waiting list in the treatment of posttraumatic stress disorder. *Clinical Psychology and Psychotherapy, 9*, 299–318.

Power, K. G., Jerrom, D. W., Simpson, R. J., Mitchell, M. J., & Swanson, V. (1989). A controlled comparison of cognitive-behaviour therapy, diazepam and placebo in the management of generalized anxiety. *Behavioural Psychotherapy, 17*, 1–14.

Power, K. G., & Sharp, D. M. (1995). Keep taking the tablets?: Inadequate controls for concurrent psychotropic medication in studies of psychological treatments for panic disorder [letter]. *Journal of Psychopharmacology, 9*, 71–72.

Power, K. G., Simpson, R. J., Swanson, V., & Wallace, L. A. (1990). A controlled comparison of cognitive-behavior therapy, diazepam, and placebo, alone and in combination, for the treatment of generalized anxiety disorder. *Journal of Anxiety Disorders, 4*, 267–292.

Prendergast, M. L., Podus, D., Chang, E., & Urada, D. (2002). The effectiveness of drug abuse treatment: A meta-analysis of comparison group studies. *Drug and Alcohol Dependence, 67*(1), 53–72.

Preston, K. L., Silverman, K., Umbricht, A., DeJesus, A., Montoya, I. D., & Schuster, C. R. (1999). Improvement in naltrexone treatment compliance with contingency management. *Drug and Alcohol Dependence, 54*(2), 127–135.

Preston, K. L., Umbricht, A., Wong, C. J., & Epstein, D. H. (2001). Shaping cocaine abstinence by successive approximation. *Journal of Consulting and Clinical Psychology, 69*(4), 643–654.

Price, S. C., Reynolds, B. S., Cohen, B. D., & Anderson, A. J. (1981). Group treatment of erectile dysfunction for men without partners: A controlled evaluation. *Archives of Sexual Behavior, 8*, 127–138.

Prien, R. F., Carpenter, L. L., & Kupfer, D. J. (1991). The definition and operational criteria for treatment outcome of major depressive disorder. *Archives of General Psychiatry, 48*, 796–800.

Prien, R. F., Kupfer, D. J., Mansky, P. A., Small, J. G., Tuason, V. B., Voss, C. B., et al. (1984). Drug therapy in the prevention of recurrences in unipolar and bipolar affective disorders. *Archives of General Psychiatry, 41*, 1096–1104.

Prien, R. F., & Potter, W. Z. (1990). NIMH workshop report on treatment of bipolar disorder. *Psychopharmacology Bulletin, 26*, 409–427.

Proctor, R., Burns, A., Stratton-Powell, H., Tarrier, N., Faragher, B., Richardson, G., et al. (1999). Behavioural management in nursing and residential homes: A randomised controlled trial. *Lancet, 354*, 26–29.

Project MATCH Research Group. (1997a). Matching alcoholism treatments to client heterogeneity: Project MATCH posttreatment drinking outcomes. *Journal of Studies on Alcohol, 58*, 7–29.

Project MATCH Research Group. (1997b). Project MATCH secondary a priori hypotheses. *Addiction, 92*(12), 1671–1698.

Project MATCH Research Group. (1998a). Matching patients with alcohol disorders to treatments: Clinical implications from Project MATCH. *Journal of Mental Health, 7*(6), 589–602.

Project MATCH Research Group. (1998b). Therapist effects in three treatments for alcohol problems. *Psychotherapy Research, 8*(4), 455–474.

Pronovost, J., Cote, L., & Ross, C. (1990). Epidemiological study of suicidal behaviour among secondary-school students. *Canada's Mental Health, 38*(1), 9–14.

Proudfoot, J., Goldberg, D., Mann, A., Everitt, B., Marks, I., & Gray, J. A. (2003). Computerized, interactive, multimedia cognitive-behavioural program for anxiety and depression in general practice. *Psychological Medicine, 33*(2), 217–227.

Prout, H. R., & Nowak-Drabik, K. M. (2003). Psychotherapy with persons who have mental retardation: An evaluation of effectiveness. *American Journal on Mental Retardation, 108,* 82–93.

Pusey, H., & Richards, D. (2001). A systematic review of the effectiveness of psychosocial interventions for carers of people with dementia. *Aging and Mental Health, 5*(2), 107–119.

Pyle, R. L., Mitchell, J. E., Eckert, E. D., Hatsukami, D., et al. (1990). Maintenance treatment and six month outcome for bulimic patients who respond to initial treatment. *American Journal of Psychiatry, 147,* 871–875.

Quality Assurance Project. (1983). A treatment outline for depressive disorders. *Australian and New Zealand Journal of Psychiatry, 17,* 129–146.

Quay, H. C., & LaGreca, A. M. (1986). Disorders of anxiety, withdrawal, and dysphoria. In H. C. Quay & J. S. Werry (Eds.), *Psychopathological disorders of childhood* (3rd ed., pp. 111–155). New York: Wiley.

Quayhagen, M. P., Quayhagen, M., Corbeil, R. R., Roth, P. A., & Rodgers, J. A. (1995). A dyadic remediation program for care recipients with dementia. *Nursing Research, 44,* 153–159.

Quayle, M., & Moore, E. (1998). Evaluating the impact of structured groupwork with men in a high security hospital. *Criminal Behaviour and Mental Health, 8,* 77–92.

Quinn, M. M., Kavale, K. A., Mathur, S. R., Rutherford, R. B., & Forness, S. R. (1999). A meta-analysis of social skill interventions for students with emotional or behavioral disorders. *Journal of Emotional and Behavioral Disorders, 7,* 54–64.

Rabavilas, A. D., Boulougouris, J. C., & Stefanis, C. (1979). Duration of flooding sessions in the treatment of obsessive–compulsive patients. *Behaviour Research and Therapy, 14,* 349–355.

Rachman, S. (1983). Obstacles to the successful treatment of obsessions. In E. Foa & P. Emmelkamp (Eds.), *Failures in behavior therapy.* New York: Wiley.

Rachman, S., Cobb, J., Grey, B., McDonald, D., Mawson, D., Sartory, G., et al. (1979). The behavioral treatment of obsessive disorders with and without clomipramine. *Behaviour Research and Therapy, 17,* 467–478.

Rachman, S., Hodgson, R., & Marks, I. M. (1971). The treatment of chronic obsessive–compulsive neurosis. *Behaviour Research and Therapy, 9,* 237–247.

Rachman, S., Marks, I. M., & Hodgson, R. (1973). The treatment of obsessive–compulsive neurotics by modeling and flooding *in-vivo. Behaviour Research and Therapy, 11,* 463–471.

Ramsay, R. (1990). Post-traumatic stress disorder: A new clinical entity? *Journal of Psychosomatic Research, 34,* 355–365.

Randolph, E. T., Eth, S., Glynn, S. M., Paz, G. G., Leong, G. B., Shaner, A. L., et al. (1994). Behavioral family management in schizophrenia: Outcome of a clinic-based intervention. *British Journal of Psychiatry, 164,* 501–506.

Rankin, H., Hodgson, R., & Stockwell, T. (1983). Cue exposure and response prevention with alcoholics: A controlled trial. *Behaviour Research and Therapy, 21,* 435–446.

Rapee, R. M., & Heimberg, R. G. (1997). A cognitive-behavioral model of anxiety in social phobia. *Behaviour Research and Therapy, 35*(8), 741–756.

Rapee, R. M., & Lim, L. (1992). Discrepancy between self- and observer ratings of performance in social phobics. *Journal of Abnormal Psychology, 101,* 728–731.

Raphael, B. (1979). Preventative intervention with the recently bereaved. *Archives of General Psychiatry, 34,* 1450–1454.

Raphael, B., Meldrum, L., & McFarlane, A. C. (1995). Does debriefing after psychological trauma work? *British Medical Journal, 3310,* 1479–1480.

Rastam, M., & Gillberg, C. (1992). Background factors in anorexia nervosa: A controlled study of 51 teenage cases including a population sample. *European Child and Adolescent Psychiatry, 1,* 54–65.

Rathus, J. H., Sanderson, W. C., Miller, A. L., & Wetzler, S. (1995). Impact of personality functioning on cognitive behavioral treatment of panic disorder: A preliminary report. *Journal of Personality Disorders, 9,* 160–168.

Raue, P., Castonguay, L., & Goldfried, M. R. (1993). The working alliance: A comparison of two therapies. *Psychotherapy Research, 3,* 197–207.

Raue, P. J., Goldfried, M. R., & Barkham, M. (1997). The therapeutic alliance in psychodynamic-interpersonal and cognitive-behavioral therapy. *Journal of Consulting and Clinical Psychology, 65*(4), 582–587.

Ravindran, A. V., Anisman, H., Merali, Z., Charbonneau, Y., Telner, J., Bialik, R. J., et al. (1999). Treatment of primary dysthymia with group cognitive therapy and pharmacotherapy: Clinical symptoms and functional impairments. *American Journal of Psychiatry, 156*(10), 1608–1617.

Raw, S. D. (1993, March). Does psychotherapy research teach us anything about psychotherapy? *Behavior Therapist,* pp. 75–76.

Rawson, R., Huber, A., McCann, M., Shoptaw, S., Farabee, D., Reiber, C., et al. (2002). A comparison of contingency management and cognitive-behavioral approaches during methadone maintenance treatment for cocaine dependence. *Archives of General Psychiatry, 59*(9), 817–824.

Rea, M. M., Tompson, M. C., Miklowitz, D. J., Goldstein, M. J., Hwang, S., & Mintz, J. (2003). Family-focused treatment versus individual treatment for bipolar disorder: Results of a randomized clinical trial. *Journal of Consulting and Clinical Psychology, 71*(3), 482–492.

Rector, N. A., & Beck, A. T. (2001). Cognitive behavioral therapy for schizophrenia: An empirical review. *Journal of Nervous and Mental Disease, 189,* 278–287.

Rector, N. A., Seeman, M. V., & Segal, Z. V. (2003). Cognitive therapy for schizophrenia: A preliminary randomized controlled trial. *Schizophrenia Research, 63,* 1–11.

Reed, G. F. (1983). Obsessive compulsive disorder: A cognitive/structural approach. *Canadian Psychology, 24,* 169–180.

Rees, D. W., & Farmer, R. (1985). Health beliefs and attendance for specialist alcoholism treatment. *British Journal of Psychiatry, 147,* 317–319.

Reeve, W., & Ivison, D. (1985). Use of environmental manipulation and classroom and modified informal reality orientation with institutionalized, confused elderly patients. *Age and Ageing, 14,* 119–121.

Regier, D. A., Farmer, M. E., & Goodwin, F. K. (1992). Comorbidity of mental and substance abuse disorders. In R. Michaels (Ed.), *Psychiatry* (Vol. 3, Section 17.1). Philadelphia: Lippincott.

Regier, D. A., Farmer, M. E., Rae, D. S., Locke, B. Z., Keith, S. J., Judd, L. L., et al. (1990). Comorbidity of mental disorders with alcohol and other drug abuse: Results from the Epidemiologic Catchment Area (ECA) Study. *Journal of the American Medical Association, 264*(19), 2511–2518.

Reich, J., Noyes, R., & Troughton, E. (1987). Dependent personality disorder associated with phobic avoidance in patients with panic disorder. *American Journal of Psychiatry, 144,* 323–326.

Reich, J. H. (1986). The epidemiology of anxiety. *Journal of Nervous and Mental Disease, 174,* 129–136.

Reinecke, M. A., Ryan, N. E., & DuBois, D. L. (1998). Cognitive-behavioral therapy of depression and depressive symptoms during adolescence: A review and meta-analysis. *Journal of the American Academy of Child and Adolescent Psychiatry, 37,* 26–34.

Reinert, R. E. (1958). A comparison of reserpine and disulfiram in the treatment of alcoholism. *Quarterly Journal of Studies on Alcohol, 19,* 617–622.

Reiss, D., Grubin, D., & Meux, C. (1996). Young psychopaths in special hospital: Treatment and outcome. *British Journal of Psychiatry, 168,* 99–104.

Renfrey, G., & Spates, C. R. (1994). Eye movement desensitization: A partial dismantling study. *Journal of Behavior Therapy and Experimental Psychiatry, 25,* 231–239.

Renneberg, B., Goldstein, A. M., Phillips, D., & Chambless, D. L. (1990). Intensive behavioral group treatment of avoidant personality disorder. *Behavior Therapy, 21,* 363–377.

Resick, P. A., Jordan, C. G., Girelli, S. A., Hutter, C. K., & Marhoefer-Dvorak, S. (1988). A comparative outcome study of behavioral group therapy for sexual assault victims. *Behavior Therapy, 19*, 385–401.

Resick, P. A., Nishith, P., Weaver, T. L., Astin, M. C., & Feuer, C. A. (2002). A comparison of cognitive-processing therapy with prolonged exposure and a waiting condition for the treatment of chronic posttraumatic stress disorder in female rape victims. *Journal of Consulting and Clinical Psychology, 70*(4), 867–879.

Resick, P. A., & Schnicke, M. K. (1992). Cognitive processing therapy for sexual assault victims. *Journal of Consulting and Clinical Psychology, 60*, 784–756.

Rettew, D. C. (2000). Avoidant personality disorder, generalized social phobia, and shyness: Putting the personality back into personality disorders. *Harvard Review of Psychiatry, 8*, 283–297.

Reynolds, B. S. (1982). Biofeedback and facilitation of erection in men with erectile dysfunction. *Archives of Sexual Behavior, 9*, 101–113.

Reynolds, B. S. (1991). Psychological treatment of erectile dysfunction in men without partners: Outcome results and a new direction. *Journal of Sex and Marital Therapy, 17*, 136–146.

Reynolds, B. S., Cohen, B. D., Shochet, B. V., Price, S. C., & Anderson, A. J. (1981). Dating skills training in the group treatment of erectile dysfunction for men without partners. *Journal of Sex and Marital Therapy, 7*, 184–194.

Reynolds, C. F., III, Frank, E., Perel, J. M., Imber, S. D., Cornes, C., Miller, M. D., et al. (1999a). Nortriptyline and interpersonal psychotherapy as maintenance therapies for recurrent major depression: A randomized controlled trial in patients older than 59 years. *Journal of the American Medical Association, 281*(1), 39–45.

Reynolds, C. F., III, Miller, M. D., Pasternak, R. E., Frank, E., Perel, J. M., Cornes, C., et al. (1999b). Treatment of bereavement-related major depressive episodes in later life: A controlled study of acute and continuation treatment with nortriptyline and interpersonal psychotherapy. *American Journal of Psychiatry, 156*(2), 202–208.

Richards, D. (1999). The eye movement desensitization and reprocessing debate: Commentary on Rosen et al. and Poole et al. *Behavioural and Cognitive Psychotherapy, 27*, 13–17.

Richards, D. A., Lovell, K., & Marks, I. M. (1994). Post-traumatic stress disorder: Evaluation of a treatment program. *Journal of Traumatic Stress, 7*, 319–325.

Richters, J. E., Arnold, L. E., Jensen, P. S., Abikoff, H., Conners, K., Greenhill, L. L., et al. (1995). NIMH collaborative multisite multimodal treatment study of children with ADHD: I. Background and rationale. *Journal of the American Academy of Child and Adolescent Psychiatry, 34*, 987–1000.

Rieppi, R., Greenhill, L. L., Ford, R. E., Chuang, S., Wu, M., Davies, M., et al. (2002). Socioeconomic status as a moderator of ADHD treatment outcomes. *Journal of the American Academy of Child and Adolescent Psychiatry, 41*(3), 269–277.

Ritsher, J. B., Moos, R. H., & Finney, J. W. (2002). Relationship of treatment orientation and continuing care to remission among substance abuse patients. *Psychiatric Services, 53*(5), 595–601.

Ritterband, L. M., Gonder-Frederick, L. A., Cox, D. J., Clifton, A. D., West, R. W., & Borowitz, S. M. (2003). Internet interventions: In review, in use and into the future. *Professional Psychology: Research and Practice, 34*, 527–534.

Robin, A. L., Siegel, P. T., Koepke, T., Moye, A., & Tice, S. (1994). Family therapy versus individual therapy for adolescent females with anorexia nervosa. *Journal of Developmental and Behavioral Pediatrics, 15*, 111–116.

Robin, A. L., Siegel, P. T., & Moye, A. (1995). Family versus individual therapy for anorexia: Impact on family conflict. *International Journal of Eating Disorders, 17*, 313–322.

Robin, A. L., Siegel, P. T., Moye, A. W., Gilroy, M., Baker-Dennis, A., & Sikard, A. (1999). A controlled comparison of family versus individual therapy for adolescents with anorexia nervosa. *Journal of the American Academy of Child and Adolescent Psychiatry, 38*, 1482–1489.

Robins, L. N., & Regier, D. A. (Eds.). (1991). *Psychiatric disorders in America: The Epidemiologic Catchment Area Study*. New York: Free Press.

Robinson, L. A., Berman, J. S., & Neimeyer, R. A. (1990). Psychotherapy for the treatment of depression: A comprehensive review of controlled outcome research. *Psychological Bulletin, 108*, 30–49.

Robinson, S., Birchwood, M., & Eastman, C. (unpublished report). *A trial of group cognitive therapy for panic disorder with agoraphobia in a dedicated service setting*.

Robson, R. A. H., Paulus, I., & Clarke, G. G. (1965). An evaluation of the effects of a clinic program on the rehabilitation of chronic alcoholic patients. *Quarterly Journal of Studies on Alcohol, 26*, 264–278.

Rogers, C. R. (1951). *Client-centered therapy*. Cambridge, MA: Riverside Press.

Rogers, S., Silver, S. M., Goss, J., Obenchain, J., Willis, A., & Whitney, R. L. (1999). A single session, group study of exposure and eye movement desensitization and reprocessing in treating posttraumatic stress disorder among Vietnam war veterans: Preliminary data. *Journal of Anxiety Disorders, 13*, 119–130.

Rohde, P., Clarke, G. N., Lewinsohn, P. M., Seeley, J. R., & Kaufman, N. K. (2001). Impact of comorbidity on a cognitive-behavioral group treatment for adolescent depression. *Journal of the American Academy Child and Adolescent Psychiatry, 40*, 795–802.

Rohsenow, D. J., Monti, P. M., Binkoff, J. A., Liepman, M. R., Nirenberg, T. D., & Abrams, D. B. (1991). Patient-treatment matching for alcoholic men in communication skills versus cognitive-behavioral mood management training. *Addictive Behaviors, 16*(1–2), 63–69.

Rohsenow, D. J., Monti, P. M., Martin, R. A., Michalec, E., & Abrams, D. B. (2000). Brief coping skills treatment for cocaine abuse: 12-month substance use outcomes. *Journal of Consulting and Clinical Psychology, 68*(3), 515–520.

Rohsenow, D. J., Monti, P. M., Rubonis, A. V., Gulliver, S. B., Colby, S. M., Binkoff, J. A., et al. (2001). Cue exposure with coping skills training and communication skills training for alcohol dependence: 6- and 12-month outcomes. *Addiction, 96*(8), 1161–1174.

Rollnick, S., & Miller, W. R. (1995). What is motivational interviewing? *Behavioural and Cognitive Psychotherapy, 29*, 457–471.

Roozen, H. G., Kerkhof, A. J., & van den Brink, W. (2003). Experiences with an outpatient relapse program (community reinforcement approach) combined with naltrexone in the treatment of opioid-dependence: Effect on addictive behaviors and the predictive value of psychiatric comorbidity. *European Addiction Research, 9*(2), 53–58.

Roper, G., Rachman, S., & Marks, I. M. (1975). Passive and participant modelling in exposure treatment of obsessive–compulsive neurotics. *Behaviour Research and Therapy, 13*, 271–279.

Rose, S., Bisson, J., & Wessely, S. (2003). Psychological debriefing for preventing post traumatic stress disorder (PTSD) (Cochrane Review). In *The Cochrane Library*, Issue 2. Oxford, UK: Update Software.

Rose, S., Brewin, C. R., Andrews, B., & Kirk, M. (1999). A randomized controlled trial of individual psychological debriefing for victims of violent crime. *Psychological Medicine, 29*(4), 793–799.

Rosen, R. C. (1999). The process of care model for evaluation and treatment of erectile dysfunction. *International Journal of Impotence Research, 11*, 59–70.

Rosen, R. C. (2000). Medical and psychological interventions for erectile dysfunction: Towards a combined treatment approach. In S. R. Leiblum & R. C. Rosen (Eds.), *Principles and practice of sex therapy* (pp. 276–304). New York: Guilford Press.

Rosenberg, S. D. (1974). Drug maintenance in the outpatient treatment of chronic alcoholics. *Archives of General Psychiatry, 30*, 373–377.

Rosenvinge, J. H., Martinussen, M., & Ostensen, E. (2000). The comorbidity of eating disorders and personality disorders: A meta-analytic review of studies published between 1983 and 1998. *Eating and Weight Disorders, 5*, 52–61.

Ross, H. E. (1995). DSM-IIIR alcohol abuse and dependence and psychiatric comorbidity in Ontario: Results from the mental health supplement to the Ontario Health Survey. *Drug and Alcohol Dependence, 39*, 111–128.

Ross, M., & Scott, M. (1985). An evaluation of the effectiveness of individual and group cognitive therapy in the treatment of depressed patients in an inner city health centre. *Journal of the Royal College of General Practitioners, 35*, 239–242.

Rosselló, J., & Bernal, G. (1999). The efficacy of cognitive-behavioral and interpersonal treatments for depression in Puerto Rican adolescents. *Journal of Consulting and Clinical Psychology, 67*, 734–745.

Rosser, R. M., Birch, S., Bond, H., Denford, J., & Schachter, J. (1987). Five year follow-up of patients treated with psychotherapy at the Cassel Hospital for nervous diseases. *Journal of the Royal Society of Medicine, 80*, 549–555.

Rossiter, E. M., Agras, W. S., Losch, M., & Telch, C. F. (1988). Dietary restraint of bulimic subjects following cognitive behavioral or pharmacological treatment. *Behaviour Research and Therapy, 26*, 495–432.

Rossiter, E. M., & Wilson, G. T. (1985). Cognitive restructuring and response prevention in the treatment of bulimia nervosa. *Behaviour Research and Therapy, 23*, 349–359.

Roth, A. D., & Church, J. A. (1994). The use of revised habituation in the treatment of obsessive–compulsive disorders. *British Journal of Clinical Psychology, 33*, 201–204.

Roth, A. D., & Fonagy, P. (1996). *What works for whom?: A critical review of psychotherapy research.* New York: Guilford Press.

Roth, A. D., & Parry, G. (1997). The implications of psychotherapy research for clinical practice and service development: Lessons and limitations. *Journal of Mental Health, 6*, 367–380.

Roth, S., Dye, E., & Lebowitz, L. (1988). Group therapy for sexual-assault victims. *Psychotherapy, 25*, 82–93.

Rothbaum, B. O. (1997). A controlled study of eye movement desensitization and reprocessing in the treatment of posttraumatic stress disordered sexual assault victims. *Bulletin of the Menninger Clinic, 61*, 317–334.

Rothbaum, B. O., & Astin, M. C. (2000). Integration of pharmacotherapy and psychotherapy for bipolar disorder. *Journal of Clinical Psychiatry, 61*(Suppl. 9), 68–75.

Rothbaum, B. O., Foa, E. B., Riggs, D. S., Murdock, T., & Walsh, W. (1992). A prospective examination of PTSD in rape victims. *Journal of Traumatic Stress, 5*, 455–475.

Rothbaum, B. O., Hodges, L., Smith, S., Lee, J. H., & Price, L. (2000). A controlled study of virtual reality exposure therapy for the fear of flying. *Journal of Consulting and Clinical Psychology, 68*(6), 1020–1026.

Rothenberg, J. L., Sullivan, M. A., Church, S. H., Seracini, A., Collins, E., Kleber, H. D., et al. (2002). Behavioral naltrexone therapy: An integrated treatment for opiate dependence. *Journal of Substance Abuse Treatment, 23*(4), 351–360.

Rotheram-Borus, M., Piacentini, J., Van Rossem, R., Graae, F., Cantwell, C., Castro-Blanco, D., et al. (1999). Treatment adherence among Latina female adolescent suicide attempters. *Suicide and Life-Threatening Behavior, 29*(4), 319–331.

Rotheram-Borus, M. J., Piacentini, J., Van Rossem, R., Graae, F., Cantwell, C., Castro-Blanco, D., et al. (1996). Enhancing treatment adherence with a specialized emergency room program for adolescent suicide attempters. *Journal of the American Academy of Child and Adolescent Psychiatry, 35*, 654–663.

Rounsaville, B. J., Glazer, W., Wilber, C. H., Weissman, M. M., & Kleber, H. D. (1983). Short-term interpersonal psychotherapy in methadone-maintained opiate addicts. *Archives of General Psychiatry, 40*(6), 629–636.

Rounsaville, B. J., O'Malley, S., Foley, S., & Weissman, M. M. (1988). Role of manual guided training in the conduct and efficacy of interpersonal therapy for depression. *Journal of Consulting and Clinical Psychology, 56*, 681–688.

Rounsaville, B. J., Petry, N. M., & Carroll, K. M. (2003). Single versus multiple drug focus in substance abuse clinical trials research. *Drug and Alcohol Dependence, 70*(2), 117–125.

Rounsaville, B. J., Weissman, M. M., & Prusoff, B. A. (1981). Psychotherapy with depressed outpatients: Patient and process variables as predictors of outcome. *British Journal of Psychiatry, 13*, 67–74.

Routh, C. P., Hill, J. W., Steele, H., Elliott, C. E., & Dewey, M. E. (1995). Maternal attachment status, psychosocial stressor and problem behaviour: Follow-up after parent training course for conduct disorder. *Journal of Child Psychology and Psychiatry, 36*, 1179–1198.

Roy, S., & Tyrer, P. (2001). Treatment of personality disorders. *Current Opinion in Psychiatry, 14*, 555–558.

Rubin, A., Bischofshausen, S., Conroy Moore, K., Dennis, B., Hastie, M., Melnick, L., et al. (2001). The effectiveness of EMDR in a child guidance center. *Research on Social Work Practice, 11*(4), 435–457.

Rubino, G., Barker, C., Roth, A. D., & Fearon, P. (2000). Therapist empathy and depth of interpretation in response to potential alliance ruptures: The role of therapist and patient attachment styles. *Psychotherapy Research, 10*, 408–420.

Ruma, P. R., Burke, R. V., & Thompson, R. W. (1996). Group parent training: Is it effective for children of all ages? *Behavior Therapy, 27*, 159–169.

Rush, A. J., Beck, A. T., Kovacs, M., & Hollon, S. D. (1977). Comparative efficacy of cognitive therapy and imipramine in the treatment of depressed patients. *Cognitive Therapy and Research 1*, 17–37.

Russell, C. J., & Keel, P. K. (2002). Homosexuality as a specific risk factor for eating disorders in men. *International Journal of Eating Disorders, 31*(3), 300–306.

Russell, G. F. M., Szmukler, G. I., Dare, C., & Eisler, I. (1987). An evaluation of family therapy in anorexia nervosa and bulimia nervosa. *Archives of General Psychiatry, 44*, 1047–1056.

Ryan, E. R., & Cicchetti, D. V. (1985). Predicting quality of alliance in the initial psychotherapy interview. *Journal of Nervous and Mental Disease, 173*, 717–725.

Rychtarik, R. G., Connors, G. J., Whitney, R. B., McGillicuddy, N. B., Fitterling, J. M., & Wirtz, P. W. (2000). Treatment settings for persons with alcoholism: Evidence for matching clients to inpatient versus outpatient care. *Journal of Consulting and Clinical Psychology, 68*(2), 277–289.

Ryle, A. (1990). *Cognitive analytic therapy: Active participation in change.* Chichester, UK: Wiley.

Ryle, A. (Ed.). (1995). *Cognitive analytic therapy: Developments in theory and practice.* Chichester, UK: Wiley.

Ryle, A., & Golynkina, K. (2000). Effectiveness of time-limited cognitive analytic therapy of borderline personality disorder: Factors associated with outcome. *British Journal of Medical Psychology, 73*(Pt. 2), 197–210.

Ryle, A., & Kerr, I. B. (2002). *Introducing cognitive analytic therapy.* Chichester, UK: Wiley.

Sachs, G. S., Thase, M. E., Otto, M. W., Bauer, M., Miklowitz, D., Wisniewski, S. R., et al. (2003). Rationale, design, and methods of the systematic treatment enhancement program for bipolar disorder (STEP-BD). *Biological Psychiatry, 53*(11), 1028–1042.

Sackett, D., Richardson, W. S., Rosenberg, W., & Haynes, B. (1996). *Evidence Based Medicine.* London: Churchill Livingstone.

Safer, D. L., Telch, C. F., & Agras, W. S. (2001). Dialectical behavior therapy for bulimia nervosa. *American Journal of Psychiatry, 158*(4), 632–634.

Safran, J. D., Crocker, P., McMain, S., & Murray, P. (1990). The therapeutic alliance rupture as a therapy event for empirical investigation. *Psychotherapy, 27*, 154–165.

Safran, J. D., & Muran, J. C. (1996). The resolution of ruptures in the therapeutic alliance. *Journal of Consulting and Clinical Psychology, 55*, 379–384.

Safran, J. D., & Muran, J. C. (2000). *Negotiating the therapeutic alliance: A relational treatment guide.* New York: Guilford Press.

Safran, J. D., & Segal, Z. V. (1990). *Interpersonal process in cognitive therapy.* New York: Basic Books.

Safren, S. A., Heimberg, R. G., & Juster, H. R. (1997). Clients' expectancies and their relationship to pretreatment symptomatology and outcome of cognitive-behavioral group treatment for social phobia. *Journal of Consulting and Clinical Psychology, 65*(4), 694–698.

Salkovskis, P. M. (1985). Obsessional–compulsive problems: A cognitive behavioural analysis. *Behaviour Research and Therapy, 23*, 571–583.

Salkovskis, P. M. (1995). Demonstrating specific effects in cognitive and behavioral therapy. In

M. Aveline & D. Shapiro (Eds.), *Research foundations for psychotherapy practice* (pp. 191–228). Chichester, UK: Wiley.

Salkovskis, P. M., & Clark, D. (1991). Cognitive therapy for panic attacks. *Journal of Cognitive Psychotherapy, 5*, 215–226.

Salkovskis, P. M., Jones, D. R., & Clark, D. M. (1986). Respiratory control in the treatment of panic attacks: Replication and extension with concurrent measurement of behaviour and pCO_2. *British Journal of Psychiatry, 148*, 526–532.

Salkovskis, P. M., & Warwick, H. M. (1985). Cognitive therapy of obsessive–compulsive disorder: Treating treatment failures. *Behavioural Psychotherapy, 13*, 243–255.

Salkovskis, P. M., & Westbrook, D. (1989). Behavior therapy and obsessional ruminations: Can failure be turned into success? *Behaviour Research and Therapy, 27*, 149–160.

Salkovskis, P. M., Wroe, A. L., Morrison, N., Forrester, E., Richards, C., Reynolds, M., et al. (2000). Responsibility attitudes and interpretations are characteristic of obsessive compulsive disorder. *Behaviour Research and Therapy, 38*, 347–372.

Salloum, A., Avery, L., & McClain, R. P. (2001). Group psychotherapy for adolescent survivors of homicide victims: A pilot study. *Journal of the American Academy of Child and Adolescent Psychiatry, 40*(11), 1261–1267.

Saltzman, W. R., Pynoos, R. S., Layne, C. M., Steinberg, A. M., & Aisenberg, E. (2001). Trauma- and grief-focused intervention for adolescents exposed to community violence: Results of a school-based screening and group treatment protocol. *Group Dynamics, 5*(4), 291–303.

Salzman, C., Wolfson, A. N., Schatzberg, A., Looper, J., Henke, R., Albanese, M., et al. (1995). Effect of fluoxetine on anger in symptomatic volunteers with borderline personality disorder. *Journal of Clinical Psychopharmacology, 15*, 23–29.

Samuels, J., Eaton, W. W., Bienvenu, O. J., III, Brown, C. H., Costa, P. T., Jr., & Nestadt, G. (2002). Prevalence and correlates of personality disorders in a community sample. *British Journal of Psychiatry, 180*, 536–542.

Sanchez, L. M., & Turner, S. M. (2003). Practicing psychology in the era of managed care: Implications for practice and training. *American Psychologist, 58*, 116–129.

Sandahl, C., Herlittz, K., Ahlin, G., & Rönnberg, S. (1998). Time-limited group therapy for moderately alcohol dependent patients: A randomised controlled trial. *Psychotherapy Research, 8*, 361–378.

Sanderson, W. C., Beck, A. T., & McGinn, L. K. (1994). Cognitive therapy for generalized anxiety disorder: Significance of comorbid personality disorders. *Journal of Cognitive Psychotherapy, 8*, 13–18.

Sanislow, C. A., & McGlashan, T. H. (1998). Treatment outcome of personality disorders. *Canadian Journal of Psychiatry, 43*, 237–250.

Santiseban, D. A., Perez-Vidal, A., Coatsworth, J. D., Kurtines, W. M., Schwartz, S., LaPierre, A., et al. (2003). The efficacy of brief strategic family therapy in modifying Hispanic adolescent behavior problems and substance use. *Journal of Family Psychology, 17*, 121–133.

Santor, D. A., & Kusumakar, V. (2001). Open trial of interpersonal therapy in adolescents with moderate to severe major depression: Effectiveness of novice IPT therapists. *Journal of the American Academy Child and Adolescent Psychiatry, 40*, 236–240.

Satterfield, J. H., Satterfield, B. T., & Cantwell, D. P. (1981). Three-year multimodality treatment study of 100 hyperactive boys. *Journal of Pediatrics, 98*, 650–655.

Satterfield, J. H., Satterfield, B. T., & Schell, A. M. (1987). Therapeutic interventions to prevent delinquency in hyperactive boys. *Journal of the American Academy of Child and Adolescent Psychiatry, 26*, 56–64.

Satterfield, W. A., & Lyddon, W. J. (1998). Client attachment and the working alliance. *Counselling Psychology Quarterly, 11*, 407–415.

Saunders, D. G. (1996). Feminist cognitive-behavioral and process-psychodynamic treatments for men who batter: Interaction of abuser traits and treatment models. *Violence and Victims, 11*, 393–414.

Saxena, S., Maidment, K. M., Vapnik, T., Golden, G., Rishawain, T., Rosen, R. M., et al. (2002). Obsessive–compulsive hoarding: Symptom severity and response to multimodal treatment. *Journal of Clinical Psychiatry, 63,* 21–27.

Schachar, R., Jadad, A. R., Gauld, M., Boyle, M., Booker, L., Snider, A., et al. (2002). Attention-deficit hyperactivity disorder: Critical appraisal of extended treatment studies. *Canadian Journal of Psychiatry, 47*(4), 337–348.

Schaffer, N. D. (1982). Multi-dimensional measures of therapist behavior as a predictor of outcome. *Psychological Bulletin, 92,* 670–681.

Scheck, M. M., Schaeffer, J. A., & Gillette, C. (1998). Brief psychological intervention with traumatized young women: The efficacy of eye movement desensitization and reprocessing. *Journal of Traumatic Stress, 11*(1), 25–44.

Scheidlinger, S. (1994). On overview of nine decades of group psychotherapy. *Hospital and Community Psychiatry, 45,* 217–225.

Schenk, J., Pfang, H., & Rausche, A. (1983). Personality traits versus the quality of the marital relationship as the determinant of marital sexuality. *Archives of Sexual Behavior, 12,* 31–42.

Schleien, S. J., Mustonen, T., & Rynders, J. E. (1995). Participation of children with autism and nondisabled peers in a cooperatively structured community art program. *Journal of Autism and Developmental Disorders, 25,* 397–413.

Schmidt, N. B., Woolaway-Bickel, K., Trakowski, J., Santiago, H., Storey, J., Koselka, M., et al. (2000). Dismantling cognitive-behavioral treatment for panic disorder: Questioning the utility of breathing retraining. *Journal of Consulting and Clinical Psychology, 68*(3), 417–424.

Schmidt, U., Hodes, M., & Treasure, J. (1992). Early onset bulimia nervosa—who is at risk? *Psychological Medicine, 22,* 623–628.

Schmidt, U., & Marks, I. M. (1988). Cue exposure to food plus response prevention of binges for bulimia: A pilot study. *International Journal of Eating Disorders, 7,* 663–672.

Schmidt, U., & Marks, I. M. (1989). Exposure plus prevention of binging vs. exposure plus prevention of vomiting in bulimia nervosa. *Journal of Nervous and Mental Disease, 177,* 259–266.

Schnelle, J. F., Newman, D., White, M., Abbey, J., Wallston, K. A., Fogarty, T., et al. (1993). Maintaining continence in nursing home residents through the application of industrial quality control. *Gerontologist, 33,* 114–121.

Schnelle, J. F., Traughber, B., Sowell, V. A., Newman, D. R., Petrilli, C. O., & Ory, M. (1989). Prompted voiding treatment of urinary incontinence in nursing home patients: A behavior management approach for nursing home staff. *Journal of the American Geriatrics Society, 37,* 1051–1057.

Schnyder, U., Schnyder-Luthi, C., Ballinari, P., & Blaser, A. (1998). Therapy for vaginismus: *In vivo* versus *in vitro* desensitization. *Canadian Journal of Psychiatry, 43*(9), 941–944.

Scholey, K. A., & Woods, B. T. (2003). A series of brief cognitive therapy interventions with people experiencing both dementia and depression: A description of techniques and common themes. *Clinical Psychology and Psychotherapy, 10,* 175–185.

Scholing, A., & Emmelkamp, P. M. G. (1993). Exposure with and without cognitive therapy for generalized social phobia: Effects of individual and group treatment. *Behaviour Research and Therapy, 31,* 667–681.

Scholing, A., & Emmelkamp, P. M. G. (1999). Prediction of treatment outcome in social phobia: A cross-validation. *Behaviour Research and Therapy, 37*(7), 659–670.

Schooler, N. R., Keith, S. J., Severe, J. B., Matthews, S. M., Bellack, A. S., Glick, I. D., et al. (1997). Relapse and rehospitalization during maintenance treatment of schizophrenia: The effects of dose reduction and family treatment. *Archives of General Psychiatry, 54*(5), 453–463.

Schover, L. R., & Leiblum, S. R. (1994). Commentary: The stagnation of sex therapy. *Journal of Psychology and Human Sexuality, 6,* 5–30.

Schover, L. R., & LoPiccolo, J. (1982). Treatment effectiveness for dysfunctions of sexual desire. *Journal of Sex and Marital Therapy, 8,* 179–197.

Schuhmann, E. M., Foote, R. C., Eyberg, S. M., Boggs, S. R., & Algina, J. (1998). Efficacy of parent–child interaction therapy: Interim report of a randomized trial with short-term maintenance. *Journal of Clinical Child Psychology, 27,* 34–45.

Schulberg, H. C., Block, M. R., Madonia, M. J., Scott, C. P., Rodriguez, E., Imber, S. D., et al. (1996). Treating major depression in primary care practice: Eight-month clinical outcomes. *Archives of General Psychiatry, 53*(10), 913–919.

Schulberg, H. C., Katon, W., Simon, G. E., & Rush, A. J. (1998). Treating major depression in primary care practice: An update of the Agency for Health Care Policy and Research Practice Guidelines. *Archives of General Psychiatry, 55*(12), 1121–1127.

Schulte, D., Rainer, K., Pepping, G., & Schute-Bahrenberg, T. (1992). Tailor-made versus standardized therapy of phobic patients. *Advances in Behaviour Research and Therapy, 14,* 67–92.

Schulz, R., & Beach, S. R. (1999). Caregiving as a risk factor for mortality: The caregiver health effects study. *Journal of American Medical Association, 282*(23), 2215–2219.

Schwartz, D., & Lellouch, J. (1967). Explanatory and pragmatic attitudes in therapeutic trials. *Journal of Chronic Disease, 20,* 637–648.

Schwartz, D. M., & Thompson, M. G. (1981). Do anorectics get well?: Current research and future needs. *American Journal of Psychiatry, 138,* 319–323.

Schwartz, R. C., Barrett, M. J., & Saba, G. (1985). Family therapy for bulimia. In D. M. Garner & P. E. Garfinkel (Eds.), *Handbook of psychotherapy for anorexia nervosa and bulimia.* New York: Guilford Press.

Scogin, F., Jamison, C., & Davis, N. (1990). Two-year follow-up of bibliotherapy for depression in older adults. *Journal of Consulting and Clinical Psychology, 58,* 665–667.

Scogin, F., Jamison, C., & Gochneaur, K. (1989). Comparative efficacy of cognitive and behavioral bibliotherapy for mildly and moderately depressed older adults. *Journal of Consulting and Clinical Psychology, 57,* 403–407.

Scogin, F., & McElreath, L. (1994). Efficacy of psychosocial treatments for geriatric depression: A quantitative review. *Journal of Consulting and Clinical Psychology, 62,* 69–74.

Scott, A. I. F., & Freeman, C. P. L. (1992). Edinburgh primary care depression study: Treatment outcome, patient satisfaction and costs after 16 weeks. *British Medical Journal, 304,* 883–887.

Scott, C., Tacchi, M. J., Jones, R., & Scott, J. (1997). Acute and one-year outcome of a randomised controlled trial of brief cognitive therapy for major depressive disorder in primary care. *British Journal of Psychiatry, 171,* 131–134.

Scott, J. (1992). Chronic depression: Can cognitive therapy succeed when other treatments fail? *Behavioural Psychotherapy, 20,* 25–36.

Scott, J. (2001). Cognitive therapy as an adjunct to medication in bipolar disorder. *British Journal of Psychiatry, 178*(Suppl. 41), S164–S168.

Scott, J., Garland, A., & Moorhead, S. (2001). A pilot study of cognitive therapy in bipolar disorders. *Psychological Medicine, 31*(3), 459–467.

Scott, J., Palmer, S., Paykel, E., Teasdale, J., & Hayhurst, H. (2003). Use of cognitive therapy for relapse prevention in chronic depression: Cost-effectiveness study. *British Journal of Psychiatry, 182,* 221–227.

Scott, J., & Pope, M. (2003). Cognitive styles in individuals with bipolar disorders. *Psychological Medicine, 33,* 1081–1088.

Scott, M. J., & Stradling, S. G. (1997). Client compliance with exposure treatments for posttraumatic stress disorder. *Journal of Traumatic Stress, 10*(3), 523–526.

Scott, S., Spender, Q., Doolan, M., Jacobs, B., & Aspland, H. (2001). Multicentre controlled trial of parenting groups for childhood antisocial behaviour in clinical practice. *British Medical Journal, 323*(7306), 194–198.

Segal, Z. V., Williams, J. M. G., & Teasdale, J. D. (2002). *Mindfulness-based cognitive therapy for depression: A new approach to preventing relapse.* New York: Guilford Press.

Segraves, K. A., Segraves, R. T., & Schoenberg, H. W. (1987). Use of sexual history to differentiate organic from psychogenic impotence. *Archives of Sexual Behavior, 9,* 457–575.

Segraves, R. T., Knopf, J., & Cammic, P. (1982). Spontaneous remission in erectile dysfunction. *Behaviour Research and Therapy, 20*, 89–91.

Sellman, J. D., Sullivan, P. F., Dore, G. M., Adamson, S. J., & MacEwan, I. (2001). A randomized controlled trial of motivational enhancement therapy (MET) for mild to moderate alcohol dependence. *Journal of Studies on Alcohol, 62*(3), 389–396.

Sellwood, W., Barrowclough, C., Tarrier, N., Quinn, J., Mainwaring, J., & Lewis, S. (2001). Needs-based cognitive-behavioural family intervention for carers of patients suffering from schizophrenia: 12-month follow-up. *Acta Psychiatrica Scandinavica, 104*(5), 346–355.

Selmi, P. M., Klein, M. H., Greist, J. H., Sorrell, S. P., & Erdman, H. P. (1990). Computer-administered cognitive-behavioral therapy for depression. *American Journal of Psychiatry, 147*(1), 51–56.

Sensky, T., & Scott, J. (2002). All you need is cognitive behaviour therapy?: Critical appraisal of evidence base must be understood and respected. *British Medical Journal, 324*(7352), 1522.

Sensky, T., Turkington, D., Kingdon, D., Scott, J. L., Scott, J., Siddle, R., et al. (2000). A randomized controlled trial of cognitive-behavioral therapy for persistent symptoms in schizophrenia resistant to medication. *Archives of General Psychiatry, 57*(2), 165–172.

Serfaty, M. A., Turkington, D., Heap, M., Ledsham, L., & Jolley, E. (1999). Cognitive therapy versus dietary counselling in the outpatient treatment of anorexia nervosa: Effects of the treatment phase. *European Eating Disorders Review, 7*, 334–350.

Shadish, W. R., Matt, G. E., Navarro, A. M., & Phillips, G. (2000). The effects of psychological therapies under clinically representative conditions: A meta-analysis. *Psychological Bulletin, 126*(4), 512–529.

Shaffer, D., Fisher, P., Duclan, M., Davies, M., Piacentini, J., Schwab-Stone, M., et al. (1996). The NIMH Diagnostic Interview Schedule for Children Version 2.3 (DISC 2.3): Description, acceptability, prevalence rates, and performances in the MECA study. *Journal of American Academy of Child and Adolescent Psychiatry, 35*, 865–877.

Shakeshaft, A. P., Bowman, J. A., Burrows, S., Doran, C. M., & Sanson-Fisher, R. W. (2002). Community-based alcohol counselling: A randomized clinical trial. *Addiction, 97*(11), 1449–1463.

Shakir, S., Volkmar, F., Bacon, S., & Pfefferbaum, A. (1979). Group psychotherapy as an adjunct to lithium maintenance. *American Journal of Psychiatry, 136*, 455–456.

Shalev, A. Y., Bonne, O., & Eth, S. (1996). Treatment of post-traumatic stress disorder: A review. *Psychosomatic Medicine, 58*, 165–182.

Shapiro, B. (1943). Premature ejaculation: A review of 1130 cases. *Journal of Urology, 50*, 374–379.

Shapiro, D. A., & Shapiro, D. (1982a). Meta-analysis of comparative outcome studies: A replication and refinement. *Psychological Bulletin, 92*, 581–604.

Shapiro, D. A. (1996). "Validated" treatments and evidence-based psychological services. *Clinical Psychology: Science and Practice, 3*, 256–259.

Shapiro, D. A., Barkham, M., Rees, A., Hardy, G. E., Reynolds, S., & Startup, M. (1994). Effects of treatment duration and severity of depression on the effectiveness of cognitive-behavioral and psychodynamic-interpersonal psychotherapy. *Journal of Consulting and Clinical Psychology, 62*(3), 522–534.

Shapiro, D. A., Rees, A., Barkham, M., Hardy, G., Reynolds, S., & Startup, M. (1995). Effects of treatment duration and severity of depression on the maintenance of gains following cognitive behavioral and psychodynamic interpersonal psychotherapy. *Journal of Consulting and Clinical Psychology, 63*, 378–387.

Shapiro, D. A., & Shapiro, D. (1982b). Meta-analysis of comparative outcome studies: A replication and refinement. *Psychological Bulletin, 92*, 581–604.

Shapiro, F. (1989a). Efficacy of the eye movement desensitization procedure in the treatment of traumatic memories. *Journal of Traumatic Stress, 2*, 199–223.

Shapiro, F. (1989b). Eye movement desensitization: A new treatment for post-traumatic stress disorder. *Journal of Behavior Therapy and Experimental Psychiatry, 20*, 211–217.

Sharp, D. M., Power, K. G., Simpson, R. J., Swanson, V., Moodie, E., Anstee, J. A., et al. (1996). Fluvoxamine, placebo and cognitive behavior therapy used alone and in combination in the treatment of panic disorder and agoraphobia. *Journal of Anxiety Disorders, 10*, 219–242.

Sharp, D. M., Power, K. G., & Swanson, V. (2000). Reducing therapist contact in cognitive behaviour therapy for panic disorder and agoraphobia in primary care: Global measures of outcome in a randomised controlled trial. *British Journal of General Practice, 12*, 963–968.

Shaw, B. F., Elkin, I., Yamaguchi, J., Olmsted, M., Vallis, T. M., Dobson, K. S., et al. (1999). Therapist competence ratings in relation to clinical outcome in cognitive therapy of depression. *Journal of Consulting and Clinical Psychology, 67*(6), 837–846.

Shea, M. T. (1993). Psychosocial treatment of personality disorder. *Journal of Personality Disorders, 7*(Suppl.), 167–180.

Shea, M. T., Elkin, I., Imber, S. D., Sotsky, S. M., Watkins, J. T., Collins, J. F., et al. (1992a). Course of depressive symptoms over follow-up: Findings from the NIMH Treatment of Depression Collaborative Research Program. *Archives of General Psychiatry, 49*, 782–787.

Shea, M. T., Pilkonis, P. A., Beckham, E., Collins, J. F., Elkin, I., Sotsky, S. M., et al. (1992b). Personality disorders and treatment outcome in the NIMH Treatment of Depression Collaborative Research Program. *American Journal of Psychiatry, 147*, 711–718.

Shear, M. K., Houck, P., Greeno, C., & Masters, S. (2001). Emotion-focused psychotherapy for patients with panic disorder. *American Journal of Psychiatry, 158*(12), 1993–1998.

Shear, M. K., Pilkonis, P. A., Cloitre, M., & Leon, A. C. (1994). Cognitive behavioral treatment compared with non-prescriptive treatment of panic disorder. *Archives of General Psychiatry, 51*, 395–401.

Sheldon, T. A., Song, F., & Davey-Smith, G. (1993). Critical appraisal of the medical literature: How to assess whether health care interventions do more good than harm. In M. F. Drummond & A. Maynard (Eds.), *Purchasing and providing cost effective health care* (pp. 31–48). London: Churchill Livingstone.

Shepherd, J., Stein, K., & Milne, R. (2000). Eye movement desensitization and reprocessing in the treatment of post-traumatic stress disorder: A review of an emerging therapy. *Psychological Medicine, 30*, 863–871.

Shepherd, M., Watt, D., Falloon, I., & Smeeton, N. (1989). The natural history of schizophrenia: A five year follow-up of outcome and prediction in a representative sample of schizophrenics. In *Psychological Medicine Monograph 16*. Cambridge, UK: Cambridge University Press.

Sherbourne, C. D., Wells, K. B., Duan, N., Miranda, J., Unutzer, J., Jaycox, L., et al. (2001). Long-term effectiveness of disseminating quality improvement for depression in primary care. *Archives of General Psychiatry, 58*(7), 696–703.

Sherman, J. J. (1998). Effects of psychotherapeutic treatments for PTSD: A meta-analysis of controlled clinical trials. *Journal of Traumatic Stress, 11*(3), 413–435.

Shirk, S. (1998, November). *Adult versus child psychodynamic outcomes: Why the disparity?* Paper presented at the meeting of the Research Committee on Psychodynamic Treatment Techniques, Athens, Greece.

Shirk, S. R., & Russell, R. L. (1992). A reevaluation of estimates of child therapy effectiveness. *Journal of the American Academy of Child and Adolescent Psychiatry, 31*, 703–709.

Shore, J. H., Vollmer, W. M., & Tatum, E. L. (1986). Community patterns of post-traumatic stress disorders. *Journal of Nervous and Mental Disease, 177*, 681–685.

Siever, L. J., Klar, J., & Coccaro, E. (1985). Psychobiologic substrates of personality. In L. S. Siever & H. Klar (Eds.), *Biologic response styles: Clinical implications*. Washington, DC: American Psychiatric Press.

Sifneos, P. E. (1972). *Short-term psychotherapy and emotional crisis*. Cambridge, MA: Harvard University Press.

Sifneos, P. E. (1987). *Short-term dynamic psychotherapy: Evaluation and technique* (2nd ed.). New York: Plenum Press.

Silver, M., & Oakes, P. (2001). Evaluation of a new computer intervention to teach people with autism or Asperger syndrome to recognize and predict emotions in others. *Autism, 5*(3), 299–316.

Silver, S. M., Brooks, A., & Obenchain, J. (1995). Treatment of Vietnam war veterans with PTSD: A comparison of eye movement desensitization and reprocessing and reprocessing, biofeedback, and relaxation training. *Journal of Traumatic Stress, 8,* 337–342.

Silverman, K., Chutuape, M. A., Bigelow, G. E., & Stitzer, M. L. (1999). Voucher-based reinforcement of cocaine abstinence in treatment-resistant methadone patients: Effects of reinforcement magnitude. *Psychopharmacology, 146*(2), 128–138.

Silverman, W. K., Kurtines, W. M., Ginsburg, G. S., Weems, C. F., Rabian, B., & Serafini, L. T. (1999). Contingency management, self-control, and education support in the treatment of childhood phobic disorders: A randomized clinical trial. *Journal of Consulting and Clinical Psychology, 67*(5), 675–687.

Simons, A. D., Murphy, G. E., Levine, J. E., & Wetzel, R. D. (1986). Cognitive therapy and pharmacotherapy for depression: Sustained improvement over one year. *Archives of General Psychiatry, 43,* 43–48.

Simons, A. D., & Thase, M. E. (1992). Biological markers, treatment outcome and one year follow-up of endogenous depression: Electroencephalographic studies sleep studies and response to cognitive therapy. *Journal of Consulting and Clinical Psychology, 60,* 392–401.

Simons, J. S., & Carey, M. P. (2001). Prevalence of sexual dysfunctions: Results from a decade of research. *Archives of Sexual Behavior, 30,* 177–219.

Simpson, D. D., Joe, G. W., & Broome, K. M. (2002). A national 5-year follow-up of treatment outcomes for cocaine dependence. *Archives of General Psychiatry, 59*(6), 538–544.

Simpson, D. D., Joe, G. W., Fletcher, B. W., Hubbard, R. L., & Anglin, M. D. (1999). A national evaluation of treatment outcomes for cocaine dependence. *Archives of General Psychiatry, 56*(6), 507–514.

Simpson, S., Corney, R., Fitzgerald, P., & Beecham, J. (2000). A randomised controlled trial to evaluate the effectiveness and cost-effectiveness of counselling patients with chronic depression. *Health Technology Assessment, 4*(36).

Simpson, S., Corney, R., Fitzgerald, P., & Beecham, J. (2003). A randomized controlled trial to evaluate the effectiveness and cost-effectiveness of psychodynamic counselling for general practice patients with chronic depression. *Psychological Medicine, 33*(2), 229–239.

Siqueland, L., Crits-Christoph, P., Frank, A., Daley, D., Weiss, R., Chittams, J., Blaine, J., et al. (1998). Predictors of dropout from psychosocial treatment of cocaine dependence. *Drug and Alcohol Dependence, 52*(1), 1–13.

Sitharthan, T., Sitharthan, G., Hough, M. J., & Kavanagh, D. J. (1997). Cue exposure in moderation drinking: A comparison with cognitive-behavior therapy. *Journal of Consulting and Clinical Psychology, 65*(5), 878–882.

Skea, D., & Lindesay, J. (1996). An evaluation of two models of long-term residential care for elderly people with dementia. *International Journal of Geriatric Psychiatry, 11,* 233–241.

Skoog, G., & Skoog, I. (1999). A 40-year follow-up of patients with obsessive–compulsive disorder. *Archives of General Psychiatry, 56,* 121–127.

Slavson, S. R. (1964). *A textbook in analytic group psychotherapy.* New York: International Universities Press.

Slife, B. D. (2004). Theoretical challenges to therapy practice and research: The constraint of naturalism. In M. J. Lambert (Ed.), *Bergin and Garfield's handbook of psychotherapy and behavior change* (5th ed., pp. 44–83). New York: Wiley.

Slipp, S., & Kressel, K. (1978). Difficulties in family therapy evaluation: I. A comparison of insight vs. problem solving: II. Design, critique, and recommendations. *Family Process, 17,* 409–422.

Sloane, P. D., Lindeman, D. A., Phillips, C., Moritz, D. J., & Koch, G. (1995). Evaluating Alzheimer's special care units: Reviewing the evidence and identifying potential sources of bias. *Gerontologist, 35,* 103–111.

Smart, R. G., & Gray, G. (1978). Minimal, moderate and long-term treatment for alcoholism. *British Journal of Addiction, 73,* 35–38.

Smith, J., & Birchwood, M. J. (1987). Specific and non-specific effects of educational interventions with families living with schizophrenic relatives. *British Journal of Psychiatry, 150,* 645–652.

Smith, J. E., Meyers, R. J., & Delaney, H. D. (1998). The community reinforcement approach with homeless alcohol-dependent individuals. *Journal of Consulting and Clinical Psychology, 66*(3), 541–548.

Smith, J. W., & Fawley, P. J. (1990). Long-term abstinence from alcohol in patients receiving aversion therapy as part of a multimodal in-patient program. *Journal of Substance Abuse Treatment, 7,* 77–82.

Smith, J. W., Frawley, P. J., & Polissar, N. L. (1997). Six- and twelve-month abstinence rates in inpatient alcoholics treated with either faradic aversion or chemical aversion compared with matched inpatients from a treatment registry. *Journal of Addictive Disorders, 16*(1), 5–24.

Smith, K., & Crawford, S. (1986). Suicidal behavior among "normal" high school students. *Suicide and Life-Threatening Behavior, 16*(3), 313–325.

Smith, M. L., & Glass, G. V. (1977). Meta-analysis of psychotherapy outcome studies. *American Psychologist, 32,* 752–760.

Smith, M. L., Glass, G. V., & Miller, T. I. (1980). *The benefits of psychotherapy.* Baltimore: Johns Hopkins University Press.

Smith, N. M., Floyd, M. R., Scogin, F., & Jamison, C. S. (1997). Three-year follow-up of bibliotherapy for depression. *Journal of Consulting and Clinical Psychology, 65*(2), 324–327.

Smith, T., Bellack, A. S., & Liberman, R. P. (1996). Social skills training for schizophrenia: Review and future directions. *Clinical Psychology Review, 16,* 599–617.

Smith, T. A., Kroeger, R. F., Lyon, H. E., & Mullins, M. R. (1990). Evaluating a behavioral method to manage dental fears: A two year study of dental practices. *Journal of the American Dental Association, 121,* 525–530.

Smyer, M. A., Zarit, S. H., & Qualls, S. H. (1990). Psychological intervention with the ageing individual. In J. E. Birren & K. W. Schaie (Eds.), *Handbook of the psychology of ageing* (3rd ed., pp. 375–403). San Diego: Academic Press.

Sobell, M. B., & Sobell, L. C. (2000). Stepped care as a heuristic approach to the treatment of alcohol problems. *Journal of Consulting and Clinical Psychology, 68,* 573–579.

Soberman, G. B., Greenwald, R., & Rule, D. L. (2002). A controlled study of eye movement desensitization and reprocessing (EMDR) for boys with conduct problems. *Journal of Aggression, Maltreatment and Trauma, 6*(1), 217–236.

Sohn, D. (1996). Publication bias and the evaluation of psychotherapy efficacy in reviews of the research literature. *Clinical Psychology Review, 16,* 147–156.

Soloff, P. H. (1994). Is there any drug treatment of choice for the borderline patient? *Acta Psychiatrica Scandinavica, 89*(Suppl. 379), 50–55.

Soloff, P. H., George, A., Nathan, R. S., Schulz, P. M., Cornelius, J. R., Herring, J., et al. (1989). Amitripyline versus haloperidol in borderlines: Final outcomes and predictors of response. *Journal of Clinical Pharmacology, 9,* 238–246.

Soloff, P. H., George, A., Nathan, R. S., Schulz, P. M., Ulrich, R. F., & Perel, J. M. (1986). Progress in the pharmacotherapy of borderline disorders: A double blind study of amitriptyline, haloperidol, and placebo. *Archives of General Psychiatry, 43,* 691–697.

Solomon, D. A., Keitner, G. I., Shea, M. T., & Keller, M. B. (1995). Course of illness and maintenance treatments for patients with bipolar disorder. *Journal of Clinical Psychiatry, 56,* 5–13.

Solomon, S. D., Gerrity, E. T., & Muff, A. M. (1992). Efficacy of treatments for post-traumatic stress disorder. *Journal of the American Medical Association, 268,* 633–638.

Sonuga-Barke, E. J., Daley, D., & Thompson, M. (2002). Does maternal ADHD reduce the effectiveness of parent training for preschool children's ADHD? *Journal of the American Academy of Child and Adolescent Psychiatry, 41*(6), 696–702.

Sonuga-Barke, E. J., Daley, D., Thompson, M., Laver-Bradbury, C., & Weeks, A. (2001). Parent-based therapies for preschool attention-deficit/hyperactivity disorder: A randomized, controlled trial with a community sample. *Journal of the American Academy of Child and Adolescent Psychiatry, 40*(4), 402–408.

Sotsky, S. M., Glass, D. R., Shea, M. T., Pilkonis, P. A., Collins, J. F., Elkin, I., et al. (1991). Patient predictors of response to psychotherapy and pharmacotherapy: Findings in the NIMH Treatment of Depression Collaborative Research Program. *American Journal of Psychiatry, 148*(8), 997–1008.

Southam-Gerow, M., Kendall, P. C., & Weersing, V. R. (2001). Examining outcome variability: Correlates of treatment response in a child and adolescent anxiety clinic. *Journal of Consulting and Clinical Psychology, 30*, 422–436.

Spector, A., Davies, S., Woods, B., & Orrell, M. (2000). Reality orientation for dementia: A systematic review of the evidence for its effectiveness. *Gerontologist, 40*(2), 206–212.

Spector, A., Orrell, M., Davies, S., & Woods, R. T. (1998). Reminiscence therapy for dementia: A review of the evidence of effectiveness (Cochrane review). *The Cochrane Library*, Issue 3. Chichester, UK: Wiley.

Spector, A., Thorgrimsen, L., Woods, B., Royan, L., Davies, S., Butterworth, M., et al. (2003). Efficacy of an evidence-based cognitive stimulation therapy programme for people with dementia: Randomised controlled trial. *British Journal of Psychiatry, 183*, 248–254.

Spector, I. P., & Carey, M. P. (1990). Incidence and prevalence of the sexual dysfunctions: A critical review of the empirical literature. *Archives of Sexual Behavior, 19*, 389–408.

Spector, J. (2001). EMDR: Current developments and review update. *Psicoterapia Cognitiva e Comportamentale, 7*, 25–34.

Spector, J., & Read, J. (1999). The current status of eye movement desensitization and reprocessing (EMDR). *Clinical Psychology and Psychotheapy, 6*, 165–174.

Spiegel, D. A., & Bruce, T. J. (1997). Benzodiazepines and exposure-based cognitive behavior therapies for panic disorder: Conclusions from combined treatment trials. *American Journal of Psychiatry, 154*(6), 773–781.

Spiegel, D. A., Roth, M., Weissman, M., et al. (1993). Comment on the London/Toronto study of alprazolam and exposure in panic disorder with agoraphobia. *British Journal of Psychiatry, 162*, 788–789.

Spielberger, C. D., Gorsuch, R. L., & Lushene, R. (1983). *Manual for the State–Trait Anxiety Inventory*. Palo Alto, CA: Consulting Psychologists Press.

Spirito, A., Boergers, J., Donaldson, D., Bishop, D., & Lewander, W. (2002). An intervention trial to improve adherence to community treatment by adolescents after a suicide attempt. *Journal of the American Academy of Child and Adolescent Psychiatry, 41*(4), 435–442.

Spirito, A., Plummer, B., Gispert, M., Levy, S., Kurkjian, J., Lewander, W., et al. (1992). Adolescent suicide attempts: Outcomes at follow-up. *American Journal of Orthopsychiatry, 62*(3), 464–468.

Spitzer, R. L., Endicott, J., & Ronin, E. (1978). Research diagnostic criteria. *Archives of General Psychiatry, 35*, 773–782.

Srisurapanont, M., & Jarusuraisin, N. (2002). Opioid antagonists for alcohol dependence. *Cochrane Database of Systematic Reviews, 2*. Chichester, UK: Wiley

St. Lawrence, J. S., & Madakasira, S. (1992). Evaluation and treatment of premature ejaculation: A critical review. *International Journal of Psychiatry in Medicine, 22*, 77–97.

Stallard, P., & Law, F. (1993). Screening and psychological debriefing of adolescent survivors of life-threatening events. *British Journal of Psychiatry, 163*, 660–665.

Stangier, U., Heidenreich, T., Peitz, M., Lauterbach, W., & Clark, D. M. (2003). Cognitive therapy for social phobia: Individual versus group treatment. *Behaviour Research and Therapy, 41*(9), 991–1007.

Stanley, M. A., & Beck, J. G. (2000). Anxiety disorders. *Clinical Psychology Review, 20*(6), 731–754.

Stanley, M. A., Beck, J. G., & Glassco, J. D. (1996). Treatment of generalized anxiety in older adults: A preliminary comparison of behavioral and supportive approaches. *Behavior Therapy, 27,* 565–581.

Stanley, M. A., Beck, J. G., Novy, D. M., Averill, P. M., Swann, A. C., Diefenbach, G. J., et al. (2003). Cognitive-behavioral treatment of late-life generalized anxiety disorder. *Journal of Consulting and Clinical Psychology, 71*(2), 309–319.

Stanley, M. A., & Novy, D. M. (2000). Cognitive-behavior therapy for generalized anxiety in late life: An evaluative overview. *Journal of Anxiety Disorders, 14*(2), 191–207.

Stanton, M. D., & Shadish, W. R. (1997). Outcome, attrition, and family-couples treatment for drug abuse: A meta-analysis and review of the controlled, comparative studies. *Psychological Bulletin, 122*(2), 170–191.

Stark, M. J. (1992). Dropping out of substance abuse treatment: A clinically oriented review. *Clinical Psychology Review, 12,* 93–116.

Stein, D. J., Simeon, D., Frenkel, M., Islam, M. N., & Hollander, E. (1995). An open trial of valproate in borderline personality disorder. *Journal of Clinical Psychiatry, 56,* 506–510.

Stein, D. M., & Lambert, M. J. (1984). On the relationship between therapist experience and psychotherapy outcome. *Clinical Psychology Review, 4,* 127–142.

Stein, D. M., & Lambert, M. J. (1995). Graduate training in psychotherapy: Are therapy outcomes enhanced? *Journal of Consulting and Clinical Psychology, 63,* 182–196.

Steinbruek, S. M., Maxwell, S. E., & Howard, G. S. (1983). A meta-analysis of psychotherapy and drug therapy in the treatment of unipolar depression with adults. *Journal of Consulting and Clinical Psychology, 51,* 856–863.

Steinhausen, H. C. (1995). Treatment and outcome of adolescent anorexia nervosa. *Hormone Research, 43*(4), 168–170.

Steinhausen, H. C. (1997). Annotation: Outcome of anorexia nervosa in the younger patient. *Journal of Child Psychology and Psychiatry, 38,* 271–276.

Steinhausen, H. C., & Glanville, K. (1983). A long-term follow-up of adolescent anorexia nervosa. *Acta Psychiatrica Scandinavica, 68,* 1–10.

Steinhausen, H. C., Seidel, R., & Winkler Metzke, C. (2000). Evaluation of treatment and intermediate and long-term outcome of adolescent eating disorders. *Psychological Medicine, 30*(5), 1089–1098.

Steketee, G. (1990). Personality traits and disorder in obsessive–compulsives. *Journal of Anxiety Disorders, 4,* 351–364.

Steketee, G., & Cleere, L. (1990). Obsessional–compulsive disorders. In A. S. Bellack, M. Hersen & A. E. Kazdin (Eds.), *International handbook of behavior modification and therapy* (2nd ed., pp. 307–332). New York: Plenum Press.

Steketee, G., Frost, R. O., Wincze, J., Greene, K. A. I., & Douglass, H. (2000). Group and individual treatment of compulsive hoarding: A pilot study. *Behavioural and Cognitive Psychotherapy, 28,* 259–268.

Steketee, G., & Shapiro, L. J. (1995). Predicting behavioral treatment outcome for agoraphobia and obsessive–compulsive disorder. *Clinical Psychology Review, 15,* 317–346.

Stern, R., Lipsedge, M., & Marks, I. M. (1973). Obsessive ruminations: A controlled trial of thought stopping techniques. *Behaviour Research and Therapy, 11,* 659–662.

Steuer, J., Mintz, J., Hammen, C., Hill, M. A., Jarvik, L. F., McCarley, T., et al. (1984). Cognitive-behavioral and psychodynamic group psychotherapy in treatment of geriatric depression. *Journal of Consulting and Clinical Psychology, 52,* 180–192.

Stevenson, J., & Meares, R. (1992). An outcome study of psychotherapy for patients with borderline personality disorder. *American Journal of Psychiatry, 149,* 358–362.

Stevenson, J., & Meares, R. (1999). Psychotherapy with borderline patients: II. A preliminary cost benefit study. *Australian and New Zealand Journal of Psychiatry, 33*(4), 473–477.

Stice, E., Agras, W. S., Telch, C. F., Halmi., K. A., Mitchell, J. E., & Wilson, G. T. (2001). Subtyping binge eating disordered women along dieting and negative affect dimensions. *International Journal of Eating Disorders, 30,* 11–27.

Stiles, W. B., Agnew-Davies, R., Hardy, G. E., Barkham, M., & Shapiro, D. A. (1998). Relations of the alliance with psychotherapy outcome: Findings in the Second Sheffield Psychotherapy Project. *Journal of Consulting and Clinical Psychology*, *66*(5), 791–802.

Stiles, W. B., Leach, C., Barkham, M., Lucock, M., Iveson, S., Shapiro, D. A., et al. (2003). Early sudden gains in psychotherapy under routine clinic conditions: Practice-based evidence. *Journal of Consulting and Clinical Psychology*, *71*(1), 14–21.

Stiles, W. B., & Shapiro, D. A. (1989). The abuse of the drug metaphor in psychotherpy process–outcome research. *Clinical Psychology Review*, *9*, 521–543.

Stiles, W. B., & Shapiro, D. A. (1994). Disabuse of the drug metaphor—psychotherapy process outcome correlations. *Journal of Consulting and Clinical Psychology*, *62*, 942–948.

Stitzer, M. L., Iguchi, M. Y., & Felch, L. J. (1992). Contingent take-home incentive: Effects on drug use of methadone maintenance patients. *Journal of Consulting and Clinical Psychology*, *60*(6), 927–934.

Stone, M. H. (1993). Long-term outcome in personality disorders. In P. Tyrer & G. Stein (Eds.), *Personality disorder reviewed* (pp. 321–345). London: Gaskell.

Strachan, A. M. (1986). Family intervention for the rehabilitation of schizophrenia: Towards protection and coping. *Schizophrenia Bulletin*, *12*, 678–698.

Strang, J., Marks, I., Dawe, S., Powell, J., Gossop, M., Richards, D., et al. (1997). Type of hospital setting and treatment outcome with heroin addicts: Results from a randomised trial. *British Journal of Psychiatry*, *171*, 335–339.

Strauss, C. C., & Last, C. G. (1993). Social and simple phobias in children. *Journal of Anxiety Disorders*, *7*, 141–152.

Stravynski, A. (1986). Indirect behavioral treatment of erectile failure and premature ejaculation in a man without a partner. *Archives of Sexual Behavior*, *15*, 355–361.

Stravynski, A., Belisle, M., Marcouiller, M., Lavallée, Y. J., & Elie, R. (1994). The treatment of avoidant personality disorder by social skills training in the clinic or in real-life settings. *Canadian Journal of Psychiatry*, *39*, 377–383.

Stravynski, A., Gaudette, G., Lesage, A., Arbel, N., Petit, P., Clerc, D., et al. (1997). The treatment of sexually dysfunctional men without partners: A controlled study of three behavioural group approaches. *British Journal of Psychiatry*, *170*, 338–344.

Stravynski, A., & Greenberg, D. (1990). The treatment of sexual dysfunction in single men. *Sexual and Marital Therapy*, *5*, 115–122.

Stravynski, A., & Greenberg, D. (1998). The treatment of social phobia: A critical assessment. *Acta Psychiatrica Scandinavica*, *98*(3), 171–181.

Stravynski, A., Marks, I., & Yule, W. (1982). Social skills problems in neurotic outpatients: Social skills training with and without cognitive modification. *Archives of General Psychiatry*, *39*, 1378–1385.

Stravynski, A., Sahar, A., & Verreault, R. (1991). A pilot study of the cognitive treatment of dsythymic disorder. *Behavioural Psychotherapy*, *4*, 369–372.

Streeton, C., & Whelan, G. (2001). Naltrexone, a relapse prevention maintenance treatment of alcohol dependence: A meta-analysis of randomized controlled trials. *Alcohol*, *36*(6), 544–552.

Strong, S. R. (1968). Counselling: An interpersonal influence process. *Journal of Consulting and Clinical Psychology*, *15*, 215–224.

Stroudemire, A., Frank, R., Hedemark, N., Kamlet, M., & Blazer, D. (1986). The economic burden of depression. *General Hospital Psychiatry*, *8*, 387–394.

Strupp, H. H. (1978). Psychotherapy research and practice—an overview. In A. E. Bergin & S. L. Garfield (Eds.), *Handbook of psychotherapy and behavior change* (2nd ed., pp. 3–22). New York: Wiley.

Strupp, H. H., & Binder, J. (1984). *Psychotherapy in a new key: A guide to time limited dynamic psychotherapy*. New York: Basic Books.

Strupp, H. H., Butler, S. F., & Rosser, C. L. (1988). Training in psychodynamic psychotherapy. *Journal of Consulting and Clinical Psychology*, *56*, 689–695.

Stuart, G. L., Treat, T. A., & Wade, W. A. (2000). Effectiveness of an empirically based treatment for panic disorder delivered in a service clinic setting: 1-year follow-up. *Journal of Consulting and Clinical Psychology, 68*(3), 506–512.

Stuart, S., Simons, A. D., Thase, M. E., & Pilkonis, P. (1992). Are personality assessments valid in acute major depression? *Journal of Affective Disorders, 24*(4), 281–289.

Sue, S., McKinney, H., & Allan, D. (1976). Predictors of duration of therapy for clients in the community mental health system. *Community Mental Health Journal, 12*, 365–375.

Suhr, J., Anderson, S., & Tranel, D. (1999). Progressive muscle relaxation in the management of behavioural disturbance in Alzheimer's disease. *Neuropsychological Rehabilitation, 9*, 31–44.

Suinn, R. M. (1993, February). Psychotherapy: Can the practitioner learn from the researcher? *Behavior Therapist*, pp. 47–49.

Sullivan, C. F., Copeland, J. R. M., Dewey, M. E., Davidson, I. A., McWilliam, C., Saunders, P., et al. (1988). Benzodiazepine usage amongst the elderly: Findings of the Liverpool Community Survey. *International Journal of Geriatric Psychiatry, 3*, 289–292.

Sullivan, H. S. (1953). *The interpersonal theory of psychiatry*. New York: Norton.

Sullivan, P. F. (1995). Mortality in anorexia nervosa. *American Journal of Psychiatry, 152*(7), 1073–1074.

Sutton, A. J., Duval, S. J., Tweedie, R. I., Abrams, K. R., & Jones, D. R. (2000). Empirical assessment of effect of publication bias on meta-analyses. *British Medical Journal, 320*, 1574–1577.

Suzuki, M., Morita, H., & Kamoshita, S. (1990). Epidemiological survey of psychiatric disorders in Japanese school children: Part III. Prevalence of psychiatric disorders in junior high school children. *Nippon Koshu Eisei Zasshi, 37*, 991–1000.

Svartberg, M., & Stiles, T. C. (1991). Comparative effects of short-term psychodynamic psychotherapy: A meta-analysis. *Journal of Consulting and Clinical Psychology, 59*, 704–714.

Svartberg, M., & Stiles, T. C. (1994). Therapeutic alliance, therapist competence and client change in short-term anxiety-provoking psychotherapy. *Psychotherapy Research, 4*, 20–33.

Swartz, H. A., & Frank, E. (2001). Psychotherapy for bipolar depression: A phase-specific treatment strategy? *Bipolar Disorders, 3*(1), 11–22.

Swartz, M., Blazer, D., & Winfield, I. (1990). Estimating the prevalence of borderline personality disorder in the community. *Journal of Personality Disorders, 4*, 257–272.

Swinson, R. P., Fergus, K. D., Cox, B. J., & Wickwire, K. (1995). Efficacy of telephone-administered behavioral therapy for panic disorder with agoraphobia. *Behaviour Research and Therapy, 33*(4), 465–469.

Szapocznik, J., Rio, A., Murray, E., Cohen, R., Scopetta, M., Rivas-Valquez, A., et al. (1989). Structural family versus psychodynamic child therapy for problematic Hispanic boys. *Journal of Consulting and Clinical Psychology, 57*, 571–578.

Szmukler, G. I. (1983). Weight and food preoccupation in a population of English schoolgirls. In G. J. Bargman (Ed.), *Understanding anorexia nervosa and bulimia* (pp. 21–27). Columbus: Ross Laboratories.

Takefman, J., & Brender, W. (1984). An analysis of the effectiveness of two components in the treatment of erectile dysfunction. *Archives of Sexual Behavior, 13*, 321–340.

Tang, T. Z., & DeRubeis, R. J. (1999). Sudden gains and critical sessions in cognitive-behavioral therapy for depression. *Journal of Consulting and Clinical Psychology, 67*(6), 894–904.

Tang, T. Z., Luborsky, L., & Andrusyna, T. (2002). Sudden gains in recovering from depression: Are they also found in psychotherapies other than cognitive-behavioral therapy? *Journal of Consulting and Clinical Psychology, 70*(2), 444–447.

Target, M., & Fonagy, P. (1994a). The efficacy of psychoanalysis for children with emotional disorders. *Journal of the American Academy of Child and Adolescent Psychiatry, 33*, 361–371.

Target, M., & Fonagy, P. (1994b). The efficacy of psychoanalysis for children: Prediction of outcome in a developmental context. *Journal of the American Academy of Child and Adolescent Psychiatry, 33*, 1134–1144.

Tarrier, N. (1991a). Some aspects of family intervention programmes in schizophrenia: I. Adherence to intervention programmes. *British Journal of Psychiatry, 159*, 475–480.

Tarrier, N. (1991b). Some aspects of family intervention programmes in schizophrenia: II. Financial considerations. *British Journal of Psychiatry, 159,* 481–484.

Tarrier, N. (2001). What can be learned from clinical trials? Reply to Devilly and Foa. *Journal of Consulting and Clinical Psychology, 69,* 117–118.

Tarrier, N., Barrowclough, C., Vaughn, C., Bamrah, J. S., Porceddu, K., Watts, S., et al. (1988). The community management of schizophrenia: A controlled trial of a behavioral intervention with families to reduce relapse. *British Journal of Psychiatry, 153,* 532–542.

Tarrier, N., Barrowclough, C., Vaughn, C., Bamrah, J. S., Porceddu, K., Watts, S., et al. (1989). The community management of schizophrenia: A two year follow-up of a behavioral intervention with families. *British Journal of Psychiatry, 154,* 625–628.

Tarrier, N., Beckett, R., Harwood, S., Baker, A., Yusupoff, L., & Ugarterburu, I. (1993a). A trial of two cognitive-behavioral methods of treating drug-resistant residual psychotic symptoms in schizophrenic patients: I. Outcome. *British Journal of Psychiatry, 162,* 524–532.

Tarrier, N., Haddock, G., Barrowclough, C., & Wykes, T. (2002). Are all psychological treatments for psychosis equal?: The need for CBT in the treatment of psychosis and not for psychodynamic psychotherapy (invited commentary on Paley and Shapiro). *Psychology and Psychotherapy: Theory, Research and Practice, 75,* 365–374.

Tarrier, N., Kinney, C., McCarthy, E., Humphreys, L., Wittkowski, A., & Morris, J. (2000). Two-year follow-up of cognitive-behavioral therapy and supportive counseling in the treatment of persistent symptoms in chronic schizophrenia. *Journal of Consulting and Clinical Psychology, 68*(5), 917–922.

Tarrier, N., Lewis, S., Haddock, G., Bentall, R., Drake, R., Kinderman, P., et al. (2004). Cognitive-behavioural therapy in first-episode and early schizophrenia: 18 month follow-up of a randomised, controlled trial. *British Journal of Psychiatry, 184,* 231–239.

Tarrier, N., Pilgrim, H., Sommerfield, C., Faragher, B., Reynolds, M., Graham, E., et al. (1999a). A randomized trial of cognitive therapy and imaginal exposure in the treatment of chronic posttraumatic stress disorder. *Journal of Consulting and Clinical Psychology, 67*(1), 13–18.

Tarrier, N., Sharpe, L., & Beckett, R. (1993b). A trial of two cognitive-behavioral methods of treating drug-resistant residual psychotic symptoms in schizophrenic patients: II. Treatment specific changes in coping and problem solving skills. *Social Psychiatry and Psychiatric Epidemiology, 28,* 5–10.

Tarrier, N., Sommerfield, C., Pilgrim, H., & Humphreys, L. (1999b). Cognitive therapy or imaginal exposure in the treatment of post-traumatic stress disorder: Twelve-month follow-up. *British Journal of Psychiatry, 175,* 571–575.

Tarrier, N., Wittkowski, A., Kinney, C., McCarthy, E., Morris, J., & Humphreys, L. (1999c). Durability of the effects of cogitive-behavioural therapy in the treatment of chronic schizophrenia: 12 month follow-up. *British Journal of Psychiatry, 174,* 500–504.

Tarrier, N., Yusupoff, L., Kinney, C., McCarthy, E., Gledhill, A., Haddock, G., et al. (1998). Randomised controlled trial of intensive cogitive-behavioural therapy for patients with chronic schizophrenia. *British Medical Journal, 317,* 303–307.

Taube, C. A., & Barrett, S. A. (Eds.). (1985). *Mental health, United States 1985* (National Institute of Mental Health, DHHS Publication No. ADM 85-1378). Washington, DC: Superintendent of Documents, U.S. Government Printing Office.

Taylor, C. B., & Luce, K. H. (2003). Computer- and Internet-based psychotherapy interventions. *Current Directions in Psychological Science, 12,* 18–22.

Taylor, R. (2000). *A seven year reconviction study of HMP Grendon Therapeutic Community.* London: Home Office Research, Development, and Statistics Directorate.

Taylor, S. (1996). Meta-analysis of cognitive-behavioral treatments for social phobia. *Journal of Behavior Therapy and Experimental Psychiatry, 27,* 1–9.

Taylor, S., Thordarson, D. S., Maxfield, L., Fedoroff, I. C., Lovell, K., & Ogrodniczuk, J. (2003). Comparative efficacy, speed, and adverse effects of three PTSD treatments: Exposure therapy, EMDR, and relaxation training. *Journal of Consulting and Clinical Psychology, 71*(2), 330–338.

Taylor, T. K., Schmidt, F., Pepler, D., & Hodgins, C. (1998). A comparison of eclectic treatment with Webster-Stratton's Parents and Children Series in a children's mental health center: A randomized controlled trial. *Behavior Therapy, 29*, 221–240.

Teasdale, J. D. (1999). Emotional processing: Three modes of mind and the prevention of relapse in depression. *Behaviour Research and Therapy, 37*(Suppl. 1), S53–S78.

Teasdale, J. D., Fennell, M. J., Hibbert, G. A., & Amies, P. L. (1984). Cognitive therapy for major depressive disorder in primary care. *British Journal of Psychiatry, 144*, 400–406.

Teasdale, J. D., Segal, Z. V., Williams, J. M. G., Ridgeway, V. A., Soulsby, J. M., & Lau, M. A. (2000). Prevention of relapse/recurrence in major depression by mindfulness-based cognitive therapy. *Journal of Consulting and Clinical Psychology, 68*, 615–623.

Tebbutt, J., Swanston, H., Oates, R. K., & O'Toole, B. I. (1997). Five years after child sexual abuse: Persisting dysfunction and problems of prediction. *Journal of the American Academy of Child and Adolescent Psychiatry, 36*(3), 330–339.

Telch, C. F., Agras, W. S., & Linehan, M. M. (2001). Dialectical behavior therapy for binge eating disorder. *Journal of Consulting and Clinical Psychology, 69*(6), 1061–1065.

Telch, C. F., Agras, W. S., Rossiter, E. M., Wilfley, D., & Kenardy, J. (1990). Group cognitive-behavioral treatment for the nonpurging bulimic: An initial evaluation. *Journal of Consulting and Clinical Psychology, 58*, 629–635.

Telch, M. J., Agras, W. S., & Taylor, C. B. (1985). Combined pharmacological and behavioral treatment for agoraphobia. *Behaviour Research and Therapy, 23*, 325–335.

Telch, M. J., Luca, J. A., Schmidt, N. B., Hanna, H. H., Jaimez, T. L., & Lucas, R. A. (1993). Group cognitive-behavioral treatment of panic disorder. *Behaviour Research and Therapy, 31*, 279–287.

Teri, L., & Gallagher-Thompson, D. (1991). Cognitive-behavioural interventions for treatment of depression in Alzheimer's disease. *Gerontologist, 31*, 413–416.

Teri, L., Logsdon, R. G., Peskind, E., Raskind, M., Weiner, M. F., Tractenberg, R. E., et al. (2000). Treatment of agitation in AD: A randomized, placebo-controlled clinical trial. *Neurology, 55*, 1271–1278.

Teri, L., Logsdon, R. G., Uomoto, J., & McCurry, S. M. (1997). Behavioral treatment of depression in dementia patients: A controlled clinical trial. *Journal of Gerontology, 52*(B), 159–166.

Teusch, L., Bohme, H., & Gastpar, M. (1997). The benefit of an insight-oriented and experiential approach on panic and agoraphobia symptoms: Results of a controlled comparison of client-centered therapy alone and in combination with behavioral exposure. *Psychotherapy and Psychosomatics, 66*(6), 293–301.

Thase, M., Bowler, K., & Harden, T. (1991). Cognitive behavior therapy of endogenous depression. Part 2: Preliminary findings in 16 unmedicated in-patients. *Behavior Therapy, 22*, 469–477.

Thase, M. E., & Friedman, E. S. (1999). Is psychotherapy an effective treatment for melancholia and other severe depressive states? *Journal of Affective Disorders, 54*(1–2), 1–19.

Thase, M. E., Greenhouse, J. B., Frank, E., Reynolds, C. F., Pilkonis, P. A., Hurley, K., et al. (1997). Treatment of major depression with psychotherapy or psychotherapy–pharmacotherapy combinations. *Archives of General Psychiatry, 54*, 1009–1015.

Thase, M. E., Simons, A. D., McGeary, J., Cahalane, J. F., Hughes, C., Harden, T., et al. (1992). Relapse after cognitive behavior therapy of depression: Potential implications for longer courses of treatment. *American Journal of Psychiatry, 149*, 1046–1052.

Thase, M. E., Simons, A. D., & Reynolds, C. F. (1993). Psychobiological correlates of poor response to cognitive behavior therapy: Potential indications for antidepressant pharmacotherapy. *Psychopharmacology Bulletin, 29*, 293–301.

Thiels, C., Schmidt, U., Treasure, J., Garthe, R., & Troop, N. (1998). Guided self-change for bulimia nervosa incorporating use of a self-care manual. *American Journal of Psychiatry, 155*(7), 947–953.

Thom, A., Sartory, G., & Johren, P. (2000). Comparison between one-session psychological treatment and benzodiazepine in dental phobia. *Journal of Consulting and Clinical Psychology, 68*(3), 378–387.

Thom, B., Browne, C., Drummond, D. C., Edwards, G., & Mullan, M. (1992). Engaging patients with alcohol problems in treatment: The first consultation. *British Journal of Addiction, 87*, 601–611.

Thom, B., Foster, R., Keaney, F., & Salazar, C. (1994, February). *Alcohol treatment since 1983: A review of the research literature.* Report to the Alcohol Education and Research Council, London.

Thompson, E., Eggert, L., & Herting, J. (2000). Mediating effects of an indicated prevention program for reducing youth depression and suicide risk behaviors. *Suicide and Life-Threatening Behavior, 30*(3), 252–271.

Thompson, J. A., Charlton, P. F. C., Kerry, R., Lee, D., & Turner, S. W. (1995). An open trial of exposure therapy based on deconditioning for post-traumatic stress disorder. *British Journal of Clinical Psychology, 34*, 407–416.

Thompson, L. W., Coon, D. W., Gallagher-Thompson, D., Sommer, B. R., & Koin, D. (2001). Comparison of desipramine and cognitive/behavioral therapy in the treatment of elderly outpatients with mild-to-moderate depression. *American Journal of Geriatric Psychiatry, 9*, 225–240.

Thompson, L. W., Gallagher, D., & Breckenridge, J. S. (1987). Comparative effectiveness of psychotherapies for depressed elders. *Journal of Consulting and Clinical Psychology, 55*, 385–390.

Thompson, L. W., Gallagher, D., & Czirr, R. (1988). Personality disorder and outcome in the treatment of late-life depression. *Journal of Geriatric Psychiatry, 21*, 133–146.

Thompson, L. W., Wagner, B., Zeiss, A., & Gallagher, D. (1990). Cognitive behavioral therapy with early stage Alzheimer's patients: An exploratory view of the utility of this approach. In E. Light & B. D. Lebowitz (Eds.), *Alzheimers disease: Treatment and family stress.* New York: Hemisphere.

Thompson-Brenner, H., Glass, S., & Westen, D. (2003). A multidimensional meta-analysis of psychotherapy for bulimia nervosa. *Clinical Psychology: Science and Practice, 10*, 269–287.

Thornton, D., Mann, R., Bowers, L., et al. (1996). Sex offenders in a therapeutic community. In J. Shine (Ed.), *Grendon: A compilation of Grendon research.* Unpublished manuscript.

Thyer, B. A. (1985). Audiotaped exposure therapy in a case of obsessional neurosis. *Journal of Behavior Therapy and Experimental Psychiatry, 16*, 271–273.

Tolin, D. F., Abramowitz, J. S., Kozak, M. J., & Foa, E. B. (2001). Fixity of belief, perceptual aberration, and magical ideation in obsessive–compulsive disorder. *Journal of Anxiety Disorders, 15*(6), 501–510.

Tomsovic, M. (1970). A follow-up study of discharged alcoholics. *Hospital and Community Psychiatry, 21*, 94–97.

Toren, P., Wolmer, L., Rosental, B., Eldar, S., Koren, S., Lask, M., et al. (2000). Case series: Brief parent–child group therapy for childhood anxiety disorders using a manual-based cognitive-behavioral technique. *Journal of the American Academy of Child and Adolescent Psychiatry, 39*(10), 1309–1312.

Torgersen, S., Kringlen, E., & Cramer, V. (2001). The prevalence of personality disorders in a community sample. *Archives of General Psychiatry, 58*(6), 590–596.

Torrance, G. W. (1986). Measurement of health state utilities for economic appraisal: A review. *Journal of Health Economics, 5*, 1–30.

Toseland, R. W., Diehl, M., Freeman, K., Manzanares, T., & McCallion, P. (1997). The impact of validation group therapy on nursing home residents with dementia. *Journal of Applied Gerontology, 16*(1), 31–50.

Towell, D. B., Woodford, S., Reid, S., Rooney, B., & Towell, A. (2001). Compliance and outcome in treatment-resistant anorexia and bulimia: A retrospective study. *British Journal of Clinical Psychology, 40*(Pt. 2), 189–195.

Tracey, S. A., Patterson, M., Mattis, S. G., Chorpita, B. F., Albano, A. M., Heimberg, R. G., et al. (1999). *Cognitive behavioral group treatment of social phobia in adolescents: Preliminary examination of the contribution of parental involvement.* Paper presented at the annual meeting of the Anxiety Disorders Association of America, San Diego, CA.

Treasure, J., & Kordy, H. (1998). Evidence based care of eating disorders: Beware the glitter of the randomised controlled trial [Invited article]. *European Eating Disorders Review, 6,* 85–95.

Treasure, J., Schmidt, U., Troop, N., Tiller, J., Todd, G., & Turnbull, S. (1996). Sequential treatment for bulimia nervosa incorporating a self-care manual. *British Journal of Psychiatry, 168*(1), 94–98.

Treasure, J., Schmidt, U., Troop, N., Tiller, J. M., Todd, G., Keilen, M., et al. (1994). First step in managing bulimia nervosa: Controlled trial of therapeutic manual. *British Medical Journal, 308,* 686–689.

Treasure, J., Todd, G., Brolly, M., Tiller, J., Nehmed, A., & Denman, F. (1995). A pilot study of a randomised trial of cognitive analytical therapy versus educational behavioral therapy for adult anorexia nervosa. *Behaviour Research and Therapy, 33,* 363–367.

Troop, N. A., Schmidt, U. H., Tiller, J. M., Todd, G., Keilen, M., & Treasure, J. L. (1996). Compliance with self-directed treatment manual for bulimia nervosa: Predictors and outcome. *British Journal of Clinical Psychology, 35,* 435–438.

Trowell, J., Kolvin, I., Weeramanthri, T., Sadowski, H., Berelowitz, M., Glaser, D., et al. (2002). Psychotherapy for sexually abused girls: Psychopathological outcome findings and patterns of change. *British Journal of Psychiatry, 180,* 234–247.

Trowell, J., Ugarte, B., Kolvin, I., Berelowitz, M., Sadowski, H., & Le Couteur, A. (1999). Behavioural psychopathology of child sexual abuse in schoolgirls referred to a tertiary centre: A North London study. *European Journal of Child and Adolescent Psychiatry, 8*(2), 107–116.

Trull, T. J., Nietzel, M. T., & Main, A. (1988). The use of meta-analysis to assess the clinical significance of behavior therapy for agoraphobia. *Behavior Therapy, 19,* 527–538.

Tsang, H. W. (2001). Applying social skills training in the context of vocational rehabilitation for people with schizophrenia. *Journal of Nervous and Mental Disease, 189*(2), 90–98.

Tucker, L., Bauer, S. F., Wagner, S., Harlam, D., & Sher, I. (1987). Long-term hospital treatment of borderline patients: A descriptive outcome study. *American Journal of Psychiatry, 144,* 1443–1448.

Tunis, S. R., Stryer, D. B., & Clancy, C. M. (2003). Practical clinical trials: Increasing the value of clinical research for decision making in clinical and health policy. *Journal of the American Medical Association, 290,* 1624–1632.

Turkat, I. D., & Maisto, S. A. (1985). Personality disorders: Application of the experimental method to the formulation of personality disorders. In D. H. Barlow (Ed.), *Clinical handbook of psychological disorders.* New York: Guilford Press.

Turkington, D., Kingdon, D., & Turner, T. (2002). Effectiveness of a brief cognitive-behavioural therapy intervention in the treatment of schizophrenia. *British Journal of Psychiatry, 180,* 523–527.

Turner, S. M., Beidel, D. C., Cooley, M. R., Woody, S. R., & Messer, S. C. (1994a). A multi-component behavioral treatment for social phobia: Social effectiveness therapy. *Behaviour Research and Therapy, 32,* 381–390.

Turner, S. M., Beidel, D. C., & Cooley-Quille, M. R. (1995). Two-year follow-up of social phobics treated with social effectiveness therapy. *Behaviour Research and Therapy, 33,* 553–555.

Turner, S. M., Beidel, D. C., & Jacob, R. G. (1994b). Social phobia: A comparison of behavior therapy and atenolol. *Journal of Consulting and Clinical Psychology, 62,* 350–358.

Turner, S. M., Beidel, D. C., Wolff, P. L., Spaulding, S., & Jacob, R. G. (1996). Clinical features affecting treatment outcome in social phobia. *Behaviour Research and Therapy, 34*(10), 795–804.

Turner, S. W., McFarlane, A. C., & van der Kolk, B. A. (1996). The therapeutic environment and new explorations in the treatment of posttraumatic stress disorder. In B. A. van der Kolk, A. C. McFarlane, & L. Weisaeth (Eds.), *Traumatic stress: The effects of overwhelming experience on mind, body, and society* (pp. 537–558). New York: Guilford Press.

Tuschen-Caffier, B., Pook, M., & Frank, M. (2001). Evaluation of manual-based cognitive-behavioral therapy for bulimia nervosa in a service setting. *Behaviour Research and Therapy*, *39*(3), 299–308.

Tutty, S., Gephart, H., & Wurzbacher, K. (2003). Enhancing behavioral and social skill functioning in children newly diagnosed with attention-deficit hyperactivity disorder in a pediatric setting. *Journal of Developmental and Behavioral Pediatrics*, *24*(1), 51–57.

Tyrell, C. L., Dozier, M., Teague, G. B., & Fallott, R. B. (1999). Effective treatment relationships for persons with severe psychiatric disorders: The importance of attachment states of mind. *Journal of Consulting and Clinical Psychology*, *67*, 725–733.

Tyrer, P., Merson, S., Onyett, S., & Johnson, T. (1994). The effect of personality disorder on clinical outcome, social networks and adjustment: A controlled clinical trial of psychiatric emergencies. *Psychological Medicine*, *24*, 731–740.

Tyrer, P., Seivewright, N., Ferguson, B., Murphy, S., & Johnson, A. L. (1993). The Nottingham study of neurotic disorder: Effect of personality status on response to drug treatment, cognitive therapy and self-help over two years. *British Journal of Psychiatry*, *162*, 219–226.

Tyrer, P., Thompson, S., Schmidt, U., Jones, V., Knapp, M., Davidson, K., et al. (2003). Randomized controlled trial of brief cognitive behaviour therapy versus treatment as usual in recurrent deliberate self-harm: The POPMACT study. *Psychological Medicine*, *33*(6), 969–976.

Uhlenhuth, E. H., Balter, M. B., Mellinger, G. D., et al. (1983). Symptom checklist syndromes in the general population: Correlations with psychotherapeutic drug use. *Archives of General Psychiatry*, *40*, 1167–1172.

UKATT Research Team. (2001). United Kingdom Alcohol Treatment Trial (UKATT): Hypotheses, design and methods. *Alcoholism and Alcohol*, *36*, 11–21.

Vallis, T. M., Shaw, B. F., & Dobson, K. S. (1986). The cognitive therapy scale: Psychometric properties. *The Cognitive Therapy Scale: Psychometric Properties*, *54*, 381–385.

van Balkom, A. J., Bakker, A., Spinhoven, P., Blaauw, B. M., Smeenk, S., & Ruesink, B. (1997). A meta-analysis of the treatment of panic disorder with or without agoraphobia: A comparison of psychopharmacological, cognitive-behavioral, and combination treatments. *Journal of Nervous and Mental Disease*, *185*(8), 510–516.

van Balkom, A. J. L., de Haan, E., van Oppen, P., Spinhoven, I., Hoogduin, K. A. L., & van Dyke, R. (1998). Cognitive and behavioural therapies alone versus in combination with and without clomipramine. *Behaviour Research and Therapy*, *17*, 467–478.

van Balkom, A. J. L. M., Nauta, M. C. E., & Bakker, A. (1995). Meta-analysis on the treatment of panic disorder with agoraphobia: Review and examination. *Clinical Psychology and Psychotherapy*, *2*, 1–14.

van Balkom, A. J. L. M., van Oppen, P., Wermeulen, A. W. A., van Dyck, R., Nauta, M. C. E., & Vorst, H. C. M. (1994). Meta-analysis on the treatment of obsessive–compulsive disorder: A comparison of antidepressants, behavior, and cognitive therapy. *Clinical Psychology Review*, *14*, 359–381.

van Dam Baggen, R., & Kraaimaat, F. (2000). Group social skills training or cognitive group therapy as the clinical treatment of choice for generalized social phobia? *Journal of Anxiety Disorders*, *14*(5), 437–451.

van den Hout, M., Arntz, A., & Hoekstra, R. (1994). Exposure reduced agoraphobia but not panic and cognitive therapy reduced panic but not agoraphobia. *Behaviour Research and Therapy*, *32*, 447–451.

van den Hout, M. A., Emmelkamp, P. M. J., Kraaykamp, J., & Griez, E. (1988). Behavioral treatment of obsessive–compulsives: In-patient vs. out-patient. *Behaviour Research and Therapy*, *26*, 331–332.

van der Ham, T., van Strien, D. C., & van Engeland, H. (1994). A four-year prospective follow-up study of 49 eating-disordered adolescents: Differences in course of illness. *Acta Psychiatrica Scandinavica*, *90*, 229–235.

van Emmerik, A. A., Kamphuis, J. H., Hulsbosch, A. M., & Emmelkamp, P. M. (2002). Single session debriefing after psychological trauma: A meta-analysis. *Lancet*, *360*(9335), 766–771.

Van Etten, M. L., & Taylor, S. (1998). Comparative efficacy of treatments for PTSD: A meta-analysis. *Clinical Psychology and Psychotherapy, 5*(3), 126–145.

Van Gent, E. M., & Zwart, F. M. (1994). A long follow-up after group therapy in conjunction with lithium prophylaxis. *Nordic Journal of Psychiatry, 48*, 9–12.

van Lankveld, J. J. (1998). Bibliotherapy in the treatment of sexual dysfunctions: A meta-analysis. *Journal of Consulting and Clinical Psychology, 66*(4), 702–708.

Van Londen, L., Molenaar, R. P., Goekoop, J. G., Zwinderman, A. H., & Rooijmans, H. G. (1988). Three- to 5-year prospective follow-up of outcome in major depression. *Psychological Medicine, 28*, 731–735.

Van Noppen, B., Steketee, G., McCokle, B. H., & Pato, M. (1997). Group and multifamily behavioral treatment for obsessive–compulsive disorder: A pilot study. *Journal of Anxiety Disorders, 11*, 431–446.

van Oppen, P., de Haan, E., van Balkom, A. J., Spinhoven, P., Hoogduin, K., & van Dyck, R. (1995). Cognitive therapy and exposure *in vivo* in the treatment of obsessive compulsive disorder. *Behaviour Research and Therapy, 33*(4), 379–390.

van Velzen, C. J., Emmelkamp, P. M., & Scholing, A. (1997). The impact of personality disorders on behavioral treatment outcome for social phobia. *Behaviour Research and Therapy, 35*(10), 889–900.

Vanderhoof, J. C., & Campbell, P. (1967). Evaluation of an aversive technique as a treatment for alcoholism. *Quarterly Journal of Studies on Alcoholism, 28*, 476–485.

Vaughan, M., & Beech, H. R. (1985). Which obsessionals fail to change? In D. T. Mays & C. M. Franks (Eds.), *Negative outcome in psychotherapy and what to do about it* (pp. 195–198). New York: Springer.

Vaughn, C. E., & Leff, J. P. (1976). The influence of family and social factors on the course of psychiatric illness. *British Journal of Psychiatry, 129*, 125–137.

Vaughn, K., Armstrong, M. S., Gold, R., O'Connor, N., Jenneke, W., & Tarrier, N. (1994). A trial of eye movement desensitization compared to image habituation training and applied muscle relaxation training in PTSD. *Journal of Behavior Therapy and Experimental Psychiatry, 25*, 283–291.

Vaughn, K., & Tarrier, N. (1992). The use of image habituation training with PTSD. *British Journal of Psychiatry, 161*, 658–664.

Verheul, R., van den Bosch, L., Koeter, M., de Ridder, M., Stijnen, T., & van den Brink, W. (2003). Dialectical behaviour therapy for women with borderline personality disorder: 12-month, randomised clinical trial in The Netherlands. *British Journal of Psychiatry, 182*(2), 135–140.

Viney, L. L. (1998). Should we use personal construct therapy?: A paradigm for outcomes evaluation. *Psychotherapy, 35*, 366–338.

Visser, S., Hoekstra, R. J., & Emmelkamp, P. M. G. (1992). Long-term follow-up of obsessive–compulsive patients after exposure treatment. In A. Ehlers (Ed.), *Perspectives and promises of clinical psychology* (pp. 157–170). New York: Plenum Press.

Vitiello, B., Severe, J. B., Greenhill, L. L., Arnold, L. E., Abikoff, H. B., Bukstein, O. G., et al. (2001). Methylphenidate dosage for children with ADHD over time under controlled conditions: Lessons from the MTA. *Journal of the American Academy of Child and Adolescent Psychiatry, 40*(2), 188–196.

Volkmar, F., Shakir, S., Bacon, S., & Pfefferbaum, A. (1981). Group psychotherapy in the management of manic–depressive illness. *American Journal of Psychotherapy, 35*, 226–234.

Volpicelli, J. R., Alterman, A. I., Hayashida, M., & O'Brien, C. P. (1992). Naltrexone in the treatment of alcohol dependence. *Archives of General Psychiatry, 49*, 876–880.

Wade, W. A., Treat, T. A., & Stuart, G. L. (1998). Transporting an empirically supported treatment for panic disorder to a service clinic setting: A benchmarking strategy. *Journal of Consulting and Clinical Psychology, 66*(2), 231–239.

Wakefield, J. C., & Spitzer, R. L. (2002). Lowered estimates—but of what? *Archives of General Psychiatry, 59*, 129–130.

Waldinger, R. J., & Frank, A. F. (1989). Clinicians' experiences in combining medication and psychotherapy in the treatment of borderline patients. *Hospital and Community Psychiatry, 40*, 712–718.

Waldinger, R. J., & Gunderson, J. G. (1984). Completed therapies with borderline patients. *American Journal of Psychotherapy, 38*, 190–202.

Walker, H. M., Hops, H., & Greenwood, C. R. (1984). The CORBEH research and development model: Programmatic issues and strategies. In S. C. Paine, G. T. Bellamy, & B. Wilcox (Eds.), *Human services that work: From innovation to clinical practice* (pp. 57–77). Baltimore: Brookes.

Wallace, C. J., Nelson, C. J., Liberman, R. P., Aitchison, R. A., Lukoff, D., Elder, J. P., et al. (1980). A review and critique of social skills training with schizophrenics. *Schizophrenia Bulletin, 6*, 42–63.

Wallace, P., Cutler, S., & Haines, A. (1988). Randomized controlled trial of general practitioner intervention in patients with excessive alcohol consumption. *British Medical Journal, 297*, 663–668.

Wallerstein, R. S. (1989). The psychotherapy research project of the Menninger Foundation: An overview. *Journal of Consulting and Clinical Psychology, 57*, 195–205.

Wallerstein, R. S., Chotlos, J. W., Friend, M. B., Hammersley, D. W., Perlswig, E. A., & Winship, G. M. (1957). *Hospital treatment of alcoholism: A comparative experimental study.* New York: Basic Books.

Walsh, B. T., Wilson, G. T., Loeb, K. L., Devlin, M. J., Pike, K. M., Roose, S. P., et al. (1997). Medication and psychotherapy in the treatment of bulimia nervosa. *American Journal of Psychiatry, 154*(4), 523–531.

Wampold, B. E. (1997). Methodological problems in identifying efficacious psychotherapies. *Psychotherapy Research, 7*, 21–44.

Wampold, B. E. , Minami, T., Baskin, T., & Callen-Tierney, S. (2002). A meta-(re)analysis of the effects of cognitive therapy versus "other therapies" for depression. *Journal of Affective Disorders, 68*(2–3), 159–165.

Wampold, B. E., Mondin, G. W., Moody, M., Stich, F., Benson, K., & Ahn, H. (1997). A meta-analysis of outcome studies comparing bona fide psychotherapies: Empiricially, "all must have prizes." *Psychological Bulletin, 122*, 203–215.

Ward, E., King, M., Lloyd, M., Bower, P., Sibbald, B., Farrelly, S., et al. (2000). Randomised controlled trial of non-directive counselling, cognitive-behaviour therapy, and usual general practitioner care for patients with depression: I. Clinical effectiveness. *British Medical Journal, 321*(7273), 1383–1388.

Wardle, J. (1990). Behavior therapy and benzodiazepines: Allies or antagonists? *British Journal of Psychiatry, 156*, 163–168.

Wardle, J., Hayward, P., Higgitt, A., Stabl, M., Blizard, R., & Gray, J. (1994). Effects of concurrent diazepam treatment on the outcome of exposure therapy in agoraphobia. *Behaviour Research and Therapy, 32*, 203–215.

Warheit, G. J., & Auth, J. B. (1993). Epidemiology of alcohol abuse in adulthood. In R. Michaels (Ed.), *Psychiatry* (Vol. 3, Section 18). Philadelphia: Lippincott.

Warner, P., Bancroft, J., & Members of the Edinburgh Human Sexuality Group. (1987). A regional clinical service for psychosexual problems: A three year study. *Sex and Marital Therapy, 2*, 115–126.

Warren, F., Preedy-Fayers, K., McGauley, G., Pickering, A., Norton, K., Geddes, J. R., et al. (2003). *Review of treatments for severe personality disorder.* Home Office Online Report 30/03 (*http://www.homeoffice.gov.uk/rds/pdfs2/rdsolr3003.pdf*).

Warren, R., & Thomas, J. C. (2001). Cognitive-behavior therapy of obsessive–compulsive disorder in private practice: An effectiveness study. *Journal of Anxiety Disorders, 15*(4), 277–285.

Watson, J. P., & Brockman, B. (1982). A follow-up of couples attending a psychosexual problems clinic. *British Journal of Clinical Psychology, 21*, 143–144.

Webster-Stratton, C. (1981). Modification of mothers' behaviours and attitudes through a videotape modelling group discussion programme. *Behaviour Therapy, 12*, 634–642.

Webster-Stratton, C. (1982). Teaching mothers through videotape modelling to change their children's behaviour. *Journal of Pediatric Psychology, 7*, 279–294.

Webster-Stratton, C. (1984). Randomized trial of two parent-training programmes for families with conduct-disordered children. *Journal of Consulting and Clinical Psychology, 52*, 666–678.

Webster-Stratton, C. (1990). Enhancing the effectiveness of self-administered videotape parent training for families with conduct-problem children. *Journal of Abnormal Child Psychology, 18*, 479–492.

Webster-Stratton, C. (1994). Advancing videotape parent training: A comparison study. *Journal of Consulting and Clinical Psychology, 62*, 583–593.

Webster-Stratton, C. (1996a). Early intervention with videotape modelling: Programmes for families of children with oppositional defiant disorder or conduct disorder. In E. S. Hibbs & P. S. Jensen (Eds.), *Psychosocial treatments for child and adolescent disorders: Empirically based strategies for clinical practice* (pp. 435–474). Washington, DC: American Psychological Association.

Webster-Stratton, C. (1996b). Early-onset conduct problems: Does gender make a difference? *Journal of Consulting and Clinical Psychology, 64*, 540–551.

Webster-Stratton, C. (1998). Preventing conduct problems in Head Start children: Strengthening parenting competencies. *Journal of Consulting and Clinical Psychology, 66*, 715–730.

Webster-Stratton, C., & Hammond, M. (1997). Treating children with early-onset conduct problems: A comparison of child and parent training interventions. *Journal of Consulting and Clinical Psychology, 65*, 93–109.

Webster-Stratton, C., Hollinsworth, T., & Kolpacoff, M. (1989). The long-term cost effectiveness and clinical significance of three cost-effective training programs for families with conduct-problem children. *Journal of Consulting and Clinical Psychology, 57*, 550–553.

Webster-Stratton, C., Kolpacoff, M., & Hollinsworth, T. (1988). Self-administered videotape therapy for families with conduct-problem children: Comparison with two cost-effective treatments and a control group. *Journal of Consulting and Clinical Psychology, 56*, 558–566.

Webster-Stratton, C., & Reid, M. J. (2003). The Incredible Years Parents, Teachers and Children Training Series. In A. E. Kazdin & J. R. Weisz (Eds.), *Evidence-based psychotherapies for children and adolescents* (pp. 224–240). New York: Guilford Press.

Weersing, V. R., & Weisz, J. R. (2002). Community clinic treatment of depressed youth: Benchmarking usual care against CBT clinical trials. *Journal of Consulting and Clinical Psychology, 70*, 299–310.

Weiden, P., & Havens, L. (1994). Psychotherapeutic management techniques in the treatment of outpatients with schizophrenia. *Hospital and Community Psychiatry, 45*, 549–555.

Weisaeth, L. (1989). Importance of high response rates in traumatic stress research. *Acta Psychiatrica Scandinavica, 355*(Suppl.), 131–137.

Weiss, L. J., & Lazarus, L. W. (1993). Psychosocial treatment of the geropsychiatric patient. *International Journal of Geriatric Psychiatry, 8*, 95–100.

Weiss, R. D., Griffin, M. L., Greenfield, S. F., Najavits, L. M., Wyner, D., Soto, J. A., et al. (2000). Group therapy for patients with bipolar disorder and substance dependence: Results of a pilot study. *Journal of Clinical Psychiatry, 61*(5), 361–367.

Weissman, M. M. (1993). The epidemiology of personality disorders. In R. Michels (Ed.), *Psychiatry* (Vol. I, Section 15.2). Philadelphia: Lippincott.

Weissman, M. M., Leaf, P. J., & Blaser, D. G. (1986). Panic disorder: Clinical characteristics, epidemiology and treatment. *Psychopharmacology Bulletin, 22*, 787–791.

Weissman, M. M., Leaf, P. J., Holzer, C. E., & Merikangas, K. R. (1985). Epidemiology of anxiety disorders. *Psychopharmacology Bulletin, 26*, 543–545.

Weissman, M. M., Leaf, P. J., Tishler, G. L., et al. (1988). Affective disorders in five communities. *Psychological Medicine, 18*, 141–153.

Weissman, M. M., & Markowitz, J. (1994). Interpersonal psychotherapy—current status. *Archives of General Psychiatry, 51*, 599–606.

Weissman, M. M., Prusoff, B. A., & DiMascio, A. (1979). The efficacy of drugs and psychotherapy in the treatment of acute depressive episodes. *American Journal of Psychiatry, 136,* 555–558.

Weissman, M. M., Warner, V., Wickramaratne, P., Moreau, D., & Olfson, M. (1997). Offspring of depressed parents: 10 years later. *Archives of General Psychiatry, 54,* 932–940.

Weisz, J. R., Donenberg, G. R., Han, S. S., & Weiss, B. (1995a). Bridging the gap between laboratory and clinic in child and adolescent psychotherapy. *Journal of Consulting and Clinical Psychology, 63,* 688–701.

Weisz, J. R., & Weiss, B. (1989). Assessing the effects of clinic-based psychotherapy with children and adolescents. *Journal of Consulting and Clinical Psychology, 57,* 741–746.

Weisz, J. R., Weiss, B., Han, S. S., Granger, D. A., & Morton, T. (1995b). Effects of psychotherapy with children and adolescents revisited: A meta-analysis of treatment outcome studies. *Psychological Bulletin, 117,* 450–468.

Wells, A. (1995). Meta-cognition and worry: A cognitive model of generalized anxiety disorder. *Behavioural and Cognitive Psychotherapy, 23,* 301–320.

Wells, A., & Papageorgiou, C. (2001). Brief cognitive therapy for social phobia: A case series. *Behaviour Research and Therapy, 39*(6), 713–720.

Wells, E. A., Peterson, P. L., Gainey, R. R., Hawkins, J. D., & Catalano, R. F. (1994). Outpatient treatment for cocaine abuse: A controlled comparison of relapse prevention and twelve-step approaches. *American Journal of Drug and Alcohol Abuse, 20*(1), 1–17.

Wells, J. E., Bushnell, J. A., Hornblow, A. R., Joyce, P. R., & Oakley-Browne, M. A. (1989). Christchurch psychiatric epidemiology study: Methodology and lifetime prevalence for specific psychiatric disorders. *Australian and New Zealand Journal of Psychiatry, 23,* 315–326.

Wells, K. B. (1985). *Depression as a tracer condition for the National Study of Medical Care Outcomes: Background review* [R-3293 RWJ/HJK]. Santa Monica, CA: RAND Corporation.

Wells, K. B., Burnam, M. A., Rogers, W., et al. (1992). The course of depression in adult outpatients: Results from the medical outcomes study. *Archives of General Psychiatry, 49,* 788–794.

Wells, K. C., Epstein, J. N., Hinshaw, S. P., Conners, C. K., Klaric, J., Abikoff, H. B., et al. (2000). Parenting and family stress treatment outcomes in attention deficit hyperactivity disorder (ADHD): An empirical analysis in the MTA study. *Journal of Abnormal Child Psychology, 28*(6), 543–553.

Werble, B. (1970). Second follow-up of borderline patients. *Archives of General Psychiatry, 23,* 3–7.

Westen, D. (2002). Manualizing manual development. *Clinical Psychology: Science and Practice, 9,* 416–418.

Westen, D., & Morrison, K. (2001). A multidimensional meta-analysis of treatments for depression, panic, and generalized anxiety disorder: An empirical examination of the status of empirically supported therapies. *Journal of Consulting and Clinical Psychology, 69*(6), 875–899.

Westerberg, V. S., Miller, W. R., & Tonigan, J. S. (2000). Comparison of outcomes for clients in randomized versus open trials of treatment for alcohol use disorders. *Journal of Studies on Alcohol, 61*(5), 720–727.

Wetherell, J. L., Gatz, M., & Craske, M. G. (2003). Treatment of generalized anxiety disorder in older adults. *Journal of Consulting and Clinical Psychology, 71*(1), 31–40.

Wetzel, C., Bents, H., & Florin, I. (1999). High-density exposure therapy for obsessive–compulsive inpatients: A 1-year follow-up. *Psychotherapy and Psychosomatics, 68,* 186–192.

Wexler, B. E., & Cicchetti, D. (1992). The outpatient treatment of depression: Implications of outcome research for clinical practice. *Journal of Nervous and Mental Disease, 180,* 277–286.

Whalen, C., & Schreibman, L. (2003). Joint attention training for children with autism using behavior modification procedures. *Journal of Child Psychology and Psychiatry, 44*(3), 456–468.

Whipple, J. L., Lambert, M. J., Vermeersch, D. A., Smart, D. W., Nielsen, S. L., & Hawkins, E. J. (2003). Improving the effects of psychotherapy: The use of early identification of treatment failure and problem-solving strategies in routine practice. *Journal of Counselling Psychology, 50*, 59–68.

White, J. (1998). "Stress control" large group therapy for generalized anxiety disorder: Two year follow-up. *Behavioural and Cognitive Psychotherapy, 26*, 237–245.

White, J., Keenan, M., & Brooks, N. (1992). Stress control: A controlled comparative investigation of large group therapy for generalized anxiety disorder. *Behavioural Psychotherapy, 20*, 97–114.

Whitehead, A., Mathews, A., & Ramage, M. (1987). The treatment of sexually unresponsive women: A comparative evaluation. *Behaviour Research and Therapy, 25*, 195–205.

Whittal, M., Agras, W., & Gould, R. (1999). Bulimia nervosa: A meta-analysis of psychosocial and pharmacological treatments. *Behavior Therapy, 30*(1), 117–135.

Whittle, P. (2000). Experimental psychology and psychoanalysis: What we can learn from a century of misunderstanding. *Neuro-Psychoanalysis, 1*, 233–245.

Wiborg, I. M., & Dahl, A. A. (1996). Does brief dynamic psychotherapy reduce the relapse rate of panic disorder? *Archives of General Psychiatry, 53*(8), 689–694.

Wiedemann, G., Hahlweg, K., Hank, G., Feinstein, E., Muller, U., & Dose, M. (1994). Deliverability of psychoeducational family management. *Schizophrenia Bulletin, 20*(3), 547–556.

Wiersma, D., Jenner, J., van de Willige, G., Spakman, M., & Nienhuis, F. (2001). Cognitive behaviour therapy with coping training for persistent auditory hallucinations in schizophrenia: A naturalistic follow-up study of the durability of effects. *Acta Psychiatrica Scandinavica, 103*, 393–399.

Wierzbicki, M., & Pekarik, G. (1993). A meta-analysis of psychotherapy dropout. *Professional Psychology: Research and Practice, 24*, 190–195.

Wilberg, T., Friis, S., Karterud, S., Mehlum, L., Urnes, O., & Vaglum, P. (1998). Outpatient group psychotherapy: A valuable continuation treatment for patients with borderline personality disorder treated in a day hospital?: A three year follow-up study. *Nordic Journal of Psychiatry, 52*, 213–221.

Wildgoose, A., Clarke, S., & Waller, G. (2001). Treating personality fragmentation and dissociation in borderline personality disorder: A pilot study of the impact of cognitive analytic therapy. *British Journal of Medical Psychology, 74*(Pt. 1), 47–55.

Wilfley, D. E., Agras, W. S., Telch, C. F., Rossiter, E. M., Schneider, J. A., Golomb, A. G., et al. (1993). Group cognitive behavioral therapy and group interpersonal psychotherapy for the non-purging bulimic individual: A controlled comparison. *Journal of Consulting and Clinical Psychology, 61*, 296–303.

Wilfley, D. E., Friedman, M. A., Dounchis, J. Z., Stein, R. I., Welch, R. R., & Ball, S. A. (2000). Comorbid psychopathology in binge eating disorder: Relation to eating disorder severity at baseline and following treatment. *Journal of Consulting and Clinical Psychology, 68*(4), 641–649.

Wilfley, D. E., Welch, R. R., Stein, R. I., Spurrell, E. B., Cohen, L. R., Saelens, B. E., et al. (2002). A randomized comparison of group cognitive-behavioral therapy and group interpersonal psychotherapy for the treatment of overweight individuals with binge-eating disorder. *Archives of General Psychiatry, 59*(8), 713–721.

Wilhelm, F. H., & Roth, W. T. (1997). Acute and delayed effects of alprazolam on flight phobics during exposure. *Behaviour Research and Therapy, 35*(9), 831–841.

Wilk, A. I., Jensen, N. M., & Havighurst, T. C. (1997). Meta-analysis of randomized control trials addressing brief interventions in heavy alcohol drinkers. *Journal of General Internal Medicine, 12*(5), 274–283.

Willems, E. P. (1973). Go ye into all the world and modify behavior: An ecologist's view. *Representative Research in Social Psychology, 4*, 93–105.

Williams, C., & Whitfield, G. (2001). Written and computer-based self-help treatments for depression. *British Medical Bulletin, 57*, 133–144.

Williams, J. M. (1992). *Psychological treatment of depression.* London: Routledge.

Williams, J. W., Jr., Barrett, J., Oxman, T., Frank, E., Katon, W., Sullivan, M., et al. (2000). Treatment of dysthymia and minor depression in primary care: A randomized controlled trial in older adults. *Journal of the American Medical Association, 284*(12), 1519–1526.

Williams, R., Reeve, W., Ivison, D., & Kavanagh, D. (1987). Use of environmental manipulation and modified informal reality orientation with institutionalized confused elderly subjects: A replication. *Age and Ageing, 16,* 315–318.

Williams, S. L., & Falbo, J. (1996). Cognitive and performance-based treatments for panic attacks in people with varying degrees of agoraphobic disability. *Behaviour Research and Therapy, 34*(3), 253–264.

Williamson, I., & Hartley, P. (1998). British research into the increased vulnerability of young gay men to eating disturbance and body dissatisfaction. *European Eating Disorders Review, 7,* 1–4.

Wilson, A., White, J., & Lange, D. E. (1978). Outcome evaluation of a hospital-based alcoholism treatment programme. *British Journal of Addiction, 73,* 39–45.

Wilson, G. T. (1998). Manual-based treatment and clinical practice. *Clinical Psychology: Science and Practice, 5,* 363–375.

Wilson, G. T., Eldredge, K. L., Smith, D., & Niles, B. (1991). Cognitive-behavioral treatment with and without response prevention for bulimia. *Behaviour Research and Therapy, 29*(6), 575–583.

Wilson, G. T., & Fairburn, C. G. (1993). Cognitive treatments for eating disorders. *Journal of Consulting and Clinical Psychology, 61,* 261–269.

Wilson, G. T., Loeb, K. L., Walsh, B. T., Labouvie, E., Petkova, E., Liu, X., et al. (1999). Psychological versus pharmacological treatments of bulimia nervosa: Predictors and processes of change. *Journal of Consulting and Clinical Psychology, 67*(4), 451–459.

Wilson, G. T., Rossiter, E. M., Kleinfield, E. l., & Lindholm, L. (1986). Cognitive-behavioral treatment of bulimia nervosa: A controlled evaluation. *Behaviour Research and Therapy, 24,* 277–288.

Wilson, G. T., Vitousek, K. M., & Loeb, K. L. (2000). Stepped care treatment for eating disorders. *Journal of Consulting and Clinical Psychology, 68*(4), 564–572.

Wilson, S. A., Becker, L. A., & Tinker, R. H. (1995). Eye movement desensitization and reprocessing (EMDR) treatment for psychologically traumatized individuals. *Journal of Consulting and Clinical Psychology, 63*(6), 928–937.

Wilson, S. A., Becker, L. A., & Tinker, R. H. (1997). Fifteen-month follow-up of eye movement desensitization and reprocessing (EMDR) treatment for posttraumatic stress disorder and psychological trauma. *Journal of Consulting and Clinical Psychology, 65*(6), 1047–1056.

Wing, J. K., Cooper, J. E., & Sartorius, N. (1974). *Measurement and classification of psychiatric symptoms.* Cambridge, UK: Cambridge University Press.

Winston, A., Flegheimer, W., Pollack, J., Laikin, M., Kestenbaum, R., & McCullough, L. (1987). A brief psychotherapy fidelity scale-reliability, validity and relation to outcome. *Abstracts from the Society for Psychotherapy Research 18th Annual Meeting,* Ulm, West Germany.

Winston, A., Laikin, M., Pollack, J., Samstag, L. W., McCullough, L., & Muran, J. C. (1994). Short-term psychotherapy of personality disorders. *American Journal of Psychiatry, 151,* 190–194.

Winston, A., Pollack, J., McCullough, L., Flegenheimer, W., Kestenbaum, R., & Trujillo, M. (1991). Brief psychotherapy of personality disorders. *Journal of Nervous and Mental Disease, 179,* 188–193.

Winter, D. A. (2003). Personal construct psychotherapy: The evidence base. In F. Fransella (Ed.), *Personal construct psychology handbook* (pp. 265–272). Chichester, UK: Wiley.

Winters, J., Fals-Stewart, W., O'Farrell, T. J., Birchler, G. R., & Kelley, M. L. (2002). Behavioral couples therapy for female substance-abusing patients: Effects on substance use and relationship adjustment. *Journal of Consulting and Clinical Psychology, 70*(2), 344–355.

Wittchen, H. U. (1988). Natural course and spontaneous remission of untreated anxiety disorders: Results of the Munich follow-up study. In I. Hand & H. U. Wittchen (Eds.), *Panic and phobias* (2nd ed., pp. 3–17). Heidelberg: Springer.

Wittchen, H. U., Essau, C. A., & Krieg, C. (1991). Comorbidity: Similarities and differences in treated and untreated groups. *British Journal of Psychiatry, 159*(Suppl. 12), 23–33.

Wittchen, H. U., Zhao, S., Kessler, R. C., & Eaton, W. W. (1994). DSM-III-R generalized anxiety disorder in the National Comorbidity Survey. *Archives of General Psychiatry, 51*, 355–364.

Wlazlo, Z., Schroeder-Hartwig, K., Hand, I., Kaiser, G., & Munchau, N. (1990). Exposure in vivo vs. social skills training for social phobia: Long-term outcome and differential effects. *Behaviour Research and Therapy, 28*(3), 181–193.

Wolchik, S. A., Weiss, L., & Katzman, M. A. (1986). An empirically validated, short term psychoeducational group treatment program for bulimia. *International Journal of Eating Disorders, 5*, 21–34.

Wolfberg, P. J., & Schuler, A. L. (1993). Integrated play groups: A model for promoting the social and cognitive dimensions of play in children with autism. *Journal of Autism and Developmental Disorders, 23*, 467–489.

Wolfberg, P. J., & Schuler, A. L. (1999). Fostering peer interaction, imaginative play and spontaneous language in children with autism. *Child Language Teaching and Therapy, 15*(1), 41–52.

Wood, A., Trainor, G., Rothwell, J., Moore, A., & Harrington, R. (2001). Randomized trial of group therapy for repeated deliberate self-harm in adolescents. *Journal of the American Academy of Child and Adolescent Psychiatry, 40*(11), 1246–1253.

Wood, A. J., Harrington, R. C., & Moore, A. (1996). Controlled trial of a brief cognitive-behavioural intervention in adolescent patients with depressive disorders. *Journal of Child Psychology and Psychiatry, 37*, 737–746.

Woods, B. (2003). Evidence-based practice in psychosocial intervention in early dementia: How can it be achieved? *Aging and Mental Health, 7*, 5–6.

Woods, R. T. (1999a). Institutional care. In R. T. Woods (Ed.), *Psychological problems of ageing* (pp. 195–217). Chichester, UK: Wiley.

Woods, R. T. (1999b). Promoting well-being and independence for people with dementia. *International Journal of Geriatric Psychiatry, 14*, 97–109.

Woods, R. T. (1999c). Psychological "therapies" in dementia. In R. T. Woods (Ed.), *Psychological problems of ageing* (pp. 311–344). Chichester, UK: Wiley.

Woods, R. T. (2002). Non-pharmacological techniques. In N. Qizilbash (Ed.), *Evidence-based dementia practice* (pp. 428–446). Oxford, UK: Blackwell.

Woods, R. T., & Bird, M. (1999). Non-pharmacological approaches to treatment. In G. Wilcock, K. Rockwood, & R. Bucks (Eds.), *Diagnosis and management of dementia: A manual for memory disorders teams* (pp. 311–331). Oxford, UK: Oxford University Press.

Woods, R. T., & McKiernan, F. (1995). Evaluating the impact of reminiscence on older people with dementia. In B. K. Haight & J. Webster (Eds.), *The art and science of reminiscing: theory, research, methods and applications* (pp. 233–242). Washington, DC: Taylor & Francis.

Woods, R. T., Wills, W., Higginson, I., Hobbins, J., & Whitby, M. (2003). Support in the community for people with dementia and their carers: A comparative outcome study of specialist mental health service interventions. *International Journal of Geriatric Psychiatry, 18*, 298–307.

Woodside, D. B., Garfinkel, P. E., Lin, E., Goering, P., Kaplan, A. S., Goldbloom, D. S., et al. (2001). Comparisons of men with full or partial eating disorders, men without eating disorders, and women with eating disorders in the community. *American Journal of Psychiatry, 158*(4), 570–574.

Woody, G. E., Luborsky, L., McLellan, A. T., O'Brien, C. P., Beck, A. T., Blaine, J., et al. (1983). Psychotherapy for opiate addicts: Does it help? *Archives of General Psychiatry, 40*(6), 639–645.

Woody, G. E., McLellan, T., Luborsky, L., & O'Brien, C. P. (1985). Sociopathy and psycho-therapy outcome. *Archives of General Psychiatry, 179,* 188–193.

Woody, G., McLellan, A., Luborsky, L., & O'Brien, C. (1987). Twelve-month follow-up of psychotherapy for opiate dependence. *American Journal of Psychiatry, 144*(5), 590–596.

Woody, G. E., McLellan, A. T., Luborsky, L., & O'Brien, C. P. (1995). Psychotherapy in community methadone programs: A validation study. *American Journal of Psychiatry, 152*(9), 1302–1308.

Woody, G. E., McLellan, A. T., Luborsky, L., O'Brien, C. P., Blaine, J., Fox, S., et al. (1984). Psychiatric severity as a predictor of benefits from psychotherapy. *American Journal of Psychiatry, 141,* 1172–1177.

Woolfenden, S. R., Williams, K., & Peat, J. K. (2002). Family and parenting interventions for conduct disorder and delinquency: A meta-analysis of randomised controlled trials. *Archives of Disease in Childhood, 86*(4), 251–256.

Woolfenden, S. R., Williams, K., & Peat, J. (2003). Family and parenting interventions in children and adolescents with conduct disorder and delinquency aged 10–17 (Cochrane Review). In *The Cochrane Library,* Issue 4. Chichester, UK: Wiley.

World Health Organization. (1992). *International statistical classification of diseases and related health problems* (10th ed.). Geneva: Author.

World Health Organization Brief Intervention Study Group. (1996). A cross-national trial of brief interventions with heavy drinkers. *American Journal of Public Health, 86,* 948–955.

Wright, J., Clum, G. A., Roodman, A., & Febbraro, G. A. (2000). A bibliotherapy approach to relapse prevention in individuals with panic attacks. *Journal of Anxiety Disorders, 14*(5), 483–499.

Wulpsin, L., Bachop, M., & Hoffman, D. (1988). Group therapy in manic–depressive illness. *American Journal of Psychotherapy, 42,* 263–271.

Wutzke, S. E., Conigrave, K. M., Saunders, J. B., & Hall, W. D. (2001). The long-term effectiveness of brief interventions for unsafe alcohol consumption: A 10-year follow-up. *Addiction, 97,* 665–675.

Wykes, T., Parr, A.-M., & Landau, S. (1999a). Group treatment of auditory hallucinations: Exploratory study of effectiveness. *British Journal of Psychiatry, 175,* 180–185.

Wykes, T., Reeder, C., Corner, J., Williams, C., & Everitt, B. (1999b). The effects of neurocognitive remediation on executive processing in patients with schizophrenia. *Schizophrenia Bulletin, 25*(2), 291–307.

Wykes, T., Reeder, C., Williams, C., Corner, J., Rice, C., & Everitt, B. (2003). Are the effects of cognitive remediation therapy (CRT) durable?: Results from an exploratory trial in schizophrenia. *Schizophrenia Research, 61,* 163–174.

Wykes, T., & van der Gaag, M. (2001). Is it time to develop a new cognitive therapy for psychosis—cognitive remediation therapy (CRT)? *Clinical Psychology Review, 21*(8), 1227–1256.

Yalom, I. (1975). *The theory and practice of group psychotherapy.* New York: Basic Books.

Yarnall, K. S. H., Pollak, K. I., Østbye, T., Krause, K. M., & Michener, J. L. (2003). Primary care: Is there enough time for prevention? *American Journal of Public Health, 93,* 635–641.

Yonkers, K. A., Dyck, I. R., Warshaw, M., & Keller, M. B. (2000). Factors predicting the clinical course of generalised anxiety disorder. *British Journal of Psychiatry, 176,* 544–549.

Yost, E. B., Beutler, L. E., Corbishley, M. A., & Allender, J. R. (1986). *Group cognitive therapy: A treatment approach for depressed older adults.* Oxford, UK: Pergamon Press.

Young, J. E. (1999). *Cognitive therapy for personality disorders: A schema-focused approach* (3rd ed.). Sarasota, FL: Professional Resource Press/Professional Resource Exchange, Inc.

Young, J. E., Klosko, J., & Weishaar, M. (2003). *Schema therapy: A practitioner's guide.* New York: Guilford Press.

Young, J. E., & Lindemann, M. D. (1992). An integrative schema-focused model for personality disorders. *Journal of Cognitive Psychotherapy, 6,* 11–23.

Yulis, S. (1976). Generalization of therapeutic gain in the treatment of premature ejaculation. *Behavior Therapy, 7,* 355–358.

Zanarini, M. C., Frankenburg, F. R., Hennen, J., & Silk, K. R. (2003). The longitudinal course of borderline psychopathology: 6-year prospective follow-up of the phenomenology of borderline personality disorder. *American Journal of Psychiatry, 160*(2), 274–283.

Zaretsky, A. E., Segal, Z. V., & Gemar, M. (1999). Cognitive therapy for bipolar depression: A pilot study. *Canadian Journal of Psychiatry, 44*(5), 491–494.

Zeiss, R. A. (1978). Self-directed treatment for premature ejaculation. *Journal of Consulting and Clinical Psychology, 46,* 1234–1241.

Zetzel, E. R. (1956). Current concepts of transference. *International Journal of Psychoanalysis, 37,* 369–376.

Zimberg, S. (1974). Evaluation of alcoholism treatment in Harlem. *Quarterly Journal of Studies on Alcohol, 35,* 550–557.

Zimmer, D. (1987). Does marital therapy enhance the effectiveness of treatment for sexual dysfunction? *Journal of Sex and Marital Therapy, 13,* 193–209.

Zimmerman, J. K., Asnis, G. M., & Schwartz, B. J. (1995). Enhancing outpatient treatment compliance. In J. K. Zimmerman & G. M. Asnis (Eds.), *Treatment approaches with suicidal adolescents* (pp. 106–134). New York: Wiley.

Zimmerman, M., & Coryell, W. H. (1990). Diagnosing personality disorders within the community: A comparison of self-report and interview measures. *Archives of General Psychiatry, 47,* 527–531.

Zitrin, C. M., Klein, D. F., & Woerner, M. G. (1980). Treatment of agoraphobia with group exposure *in vivo* and imipramine. *Archives of General Psychiatry, 37,* 63–72.

Zitrin, C. M., Klein, D. F., Woerner, M. G., & Ross, D. C. (1983). Treatment of phobias. *Archives of General Psychiatry, 40,* 125–138.

Zuroff, D. C., Blatt, S. J., Sotsky, S. M., Krupnick, J. L., Martin, D. J., Sanislow, C. A., III, et al. (2000). Relation of therapeutic alliance and perfectionism to outcome in brief outpatient treatment of depression. *Journal of Consulting and Clinical Psychology, 68*(1), 114–124.

Zweben, A., Pearlan, S., & Li, S. (1988). A comparison of brief advice and conjoint therapy in the treatment of alcohol abuse: The results of the marital systems study. *British Journal of Addiction, 83,* 899–916.

AUTHOR INDEX

SUBJECT INDEX

"n" following a page number indicates a note.

Benzodiazepines
  generalized anxiety disorder, 171, 172
  interference with exposure, 191, 192
  and opiate abuse, 355
  panic disorder, 186–189
    versus exposure, 191, 192
  posttraumatic stress disorder, 223
  sleep disorders, elderly, 427, 436
  social phobia, 161, 162
Bereavement
  counseling, 121
  interpersonal psychotherapy and nortriptyline,
    104
Bibliotherapy
  depression, 108, 109
  panic disorder, 182, 183
  sexual dysfunctions, 381
Binge-eating disorder, 236, 239, 483
Bipolar disorder, 135–149
  anticonvulsant medications, 137, 138
  bipolar I disorders, 136
  bipolar II disorders, 136
  characteristics of, 135, 136
  cognitive therapy, 142–144
  comorbidity, 137, 147
  couple therapy, 145
  DSM-IV definition, 135, 136
  and expressed emotion, families, 138, 147
  family therapy, 145–147
  group therapy, 139–141
  interpersonal and social rhythm therapy, 144,
    145
  lithium treatment, 137, 138
  manic phase interventions, 147, 148
  medication compliance, 138, 141–143
  natural course of, 137
  psychoeducation, 141, 142
  psychosocial interventions, 138, 139
  psychotherapy, 139, 148, 149
  recurrence of, 138, 139, 148, 149
  relapse indicators, 138, 139
  and substance abuse, 147
  treatment, 137–149, 481, 482
"Blindness," in medication trials, 98
Blood-injury phobias, 155, 156, 482
Binge-eating disorder, 258–260, 263, 264
  cognitive-behavioral therapy, 259, 260
  dialectical behavior therapy, 260
  guided self-help, 260
  interpersonal psychotherapy, 259, 260
  treatment, 258–260
Borderline personality disorder
  characteristics, 298
  cognitive analytic therapy, 313
  cognitive-behavioral therapy, 309, 310
  comorbidity, 301, 303
  and depression, 303

dialectical behavior therapy, 310–312, 484
inpatient programs, 312
medication, 303, 304
natural course of, 301
nonspecific factors, 318, 319
partial hospitalization, 309
prevalence of, 300
psychodynamic therapy, 472, 473
and suicide, 298, 309–311
therapeutic community, 308, 312
treatment of, 305–313
Breathing retraining, panic disorder, 181, 182
Brief strategic family therapy, childhood anxiety
  disorders, 411
Brief therapy
  alcohol abuse, 323, 325, 326, 343–345, 359
    versus extended treatment, 326
  depression, 92, 93, 106, 107, 111
  elderly depressed, 433, 434
  panic disorder, 181, 185
  posttraumatic stress disorder, 223, 224
  problem drinkers, 344, 345
Bright-light treatment, 439
Bulimia nervosa, 246–258, 261–263, 483
  behavior therapy, 248, 249
  children/adolescents, 412–416
  characteristics of, 237, 412, 413
  cognitive-behavioral therapy, 250–255
    versus antidepressants, 250–252
  combination therapies, 248
  comorbidity, 239
  dialectical behavior therapy, 255
  exposure and response prevention, 248, 249
  interpersonal psychotherapy, 253, 254
  medication, 250–252
  meta-analysis of treatment approaches, 246–
    248
  natural course of, 239–241
  prediction of response to treatment, 258
  prevalence of, 238, 239, 413, 414
  psychotherapy, 254, 255, 414, 415
  recovery and relapse, 255
  self-help, 255–258
  stepped care, 255–258
  subtypes of, 237
  supportive expressive therapy, 252, 262
Buprenorphine, 354
Buspirone, 171, 172

Carbamazepine, bipolar disorder, 137, 138
Care environment interventions, dementia, 437,
  438
Caregiver burden
  bipolar disorder relapse, 138
  dementia intervention, 443, 444
  elderly, 427
Case reports, psychodynamic psychotherapy, 41

Hierarchy of evidence, 18, 59
Histrionic personality disorder, 299, 300
Hoarding, 214
Homogeneity assumption
　in DSM-based diagnosis, 37
　in meta-analysis, 23, 24
"Hotline" services, adolescent suicidality, 401, 403
"Hour-glass" model, 57, 58
Hyperactivity (see Attention-deficit/hyperactivity disorder)
Hypnosis, posttraumatic stress disorder, 223, 224
Hypoactive sexual desire disorder, 363, 379
Hypomania, 136

Imaginal exposure, posttraumatic stress disorder, 225, 226, 228
Imipramine
　bulimia nervosa, 250, 251
　depression, 71–77, 81–83, 94, 95
　panic disorder, 186, 187, 190–193
Impulsivity, 318
In vivo exposure
　manualized therapy adherence, 457
　obsessive–compulsive disorder, 200–207
　panic disorder with agoraphobia, 175–177
　　effectiveness trials, 180, 181
　　versus pharmacotherapy, 185–193
　social phobia, 158
　specific phobias, 155, 156
Inclusion criteria, and external validity, 92
Incredible Years Training Series, 392
"Incubation effect"
　cognitive-behavioral therapy, 285, 294
　interpersonal psychotherapy, 262
Informant inconsistency, children, 420
Inhibited female organism, 375–377
Inpatient treatment
　alcohol dependency, 342, 343
　borderline personality disorder, 312
　depression, 116–118
Insight-oriented therapy, 472, 473
Insomnia, 435, 436
"Integrity promoting care," 437, 438
Intention-to-treat sample, attrition, 31
Internal validity, 16–18, 26, 27
Internet
　information dissemination, 497, 498
　treatment delivery, 48, 49
Interoceptive exposure, panic disorder, 182
Interpersonal psychotherapy
　adolescent depression, 405
　basic elements, 9, 10
　bereavement therapy, 104
　binge-eating disorder, 259, 260
　bulimia nervosa, 253, 254
　　"incubation effect," 262

　depression, 71–76, 78–84, 89–95, 103, 104, 107, 120–123, 131
　dysthymia, 125, 126
　elderly, 432, 433
　manual adherence and outcome, 457, 458
　medication combination, depression, 103, 104
　opiate abuse, 356
　in primary care, depression, 120–123
　quality of life, 82
　social phobia, 163
　therapeutic alliance and outcome, 463
　therapist competence and outcome, 458, 459
　Ugandan study, 107
"Interpersonal and social rhythm therapy," 144, 145
Interpretative therapy, matching patients to, 471, 472

"Joint attention," autism, 390, 391
Juvenile delinquency, 395–397

Lamotrigine, 137
Length of treatment, 473–475
　alcohol dependence, 342, 343
　depression, 78–81
　randomized controlled trials limitation, 21
　in "stepped-care" approach, 48, 49
　and tracking system feedback, 473–475
Lithium, bipolar disorder, 137, 138
Long-term follow-up data, 489, 490
Lorazepam, generalized anxiety disorder, 171

Maintenance therapy/treatment, 494, 495
　depression, 81–84, 132, 134
　　relapse prevention, 112–116
　role of, 494, 495
Major depression, 66–69 (see also Depression)
Male erectile dysfunction
　Masters and Johnson's data, 369
　medication, 370, 371
　organic pathology underestimation, 382
　rational–emotive therapy, 372, 373
　relapse, 374, 375
　sensate focus techniques, 372
　somatic methods, 371
　systematic desensitization, 372
　treatment of men without partners, 373, 374
Managed care
　effect on psychotherapy innovation, 54
　evidence-based practice use, 49, 50
　influence of, 44
Mania, 147, 148
Manualized treatment, 456–458, 495, 496
　adherence, 456–458
　and case formulation neglect, 52
　in clinical practice guidelines, 60
　limitations and strengths, 21